D1766500

WITHDRAWN
BRITISH MEDICAL ASSOCIATION
FROM LIBRARY
0810199

Non-motor Symptoms of Parkinson's Disease

SECOND EDITION

Editor in chief:

K. Ray Chaudhuri

Co-Editors:

Eduardo Tolosa

Anthony H. V. Schapira

Werner Poewe

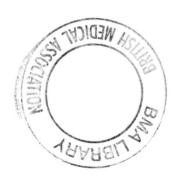

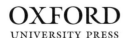

OXFORD

UNIVERSITY PRESS

Great Clarendon Street, Oxford, OX2 6DP,
United Kingdom

Oxford University Press is a department of the University of Oxford.
It furthers the University's objective of excellence in research, scholarship,
and education by publishing worldwide. Oxford is a registered trade mark of
Oxford University Press in the UK and in certain other countries

© Oxford University Press 2014

The moral rights of the authors have been asserted

First Edition published in 2009
Second Edition published in 2014

Impression: 1

All rights reserved. No part of this publication may be reproduced, stored in
a retrieval system, or transmitted, in any form or by any means, without the
prior permission in writing of Oxford University Press, or as expressly permitted
by law, by licence or under terms agreed with the appropriate reprographics
rights organization. Enquiries concerning reproduction outside the scope of the
above should be sent to the Rights Department, Oxford University Press, at the
address above

You must not circulate this work in any other form
and you must impose this same condition on any acquirer

Published in the United States of America by Oxford University Press
198 Madison Avenue, New York, NY 10016, United States of America

British Library Cataloguing in Publication Data

Data available

Library of Congress Control Number: 2014937429

ISBN 978–0–19–968424–3

Printed and bound by
CPI Group (UK) Ltd, Croydon, CR0 4YY

Oxford University Press makes no representation, express or implied, that the
drug dosages in this book are correct. Readers must therefore always check
the product information and clinical procedures with the most up-to-date
published product information and data sheets provided by the manufacturers
and the most recent codes of conduct and safety regulations. The authors and
the publishers do not accept responsibility or legal liability for any errors in the
text or for the misuse or misapplication of material in this work. Except where
otherwise stated, drug dosages and recommendations are for the non-pregnant
adult who is not breast-feeding

Links to third party websites are provided by Oxford in good faith and
for information only. Oxford disclaims any responsibility for the materials
contained in any third party website referenced in this work.

Preface to the Second Edition

Non-motor symptoms were recognized by James Parkinson and many other notable neurologists such as Gowers, Charcot and Wilson. However, they had remained the 'poor cousin' of the oft discussed, widely researched and extensively recognized motor features of Parkinson's disease (PD). In the 21st century, the focus has shifted, and in many senses the burden of non-motor symptoms in PD has emerged as one of the key determinants of translational research, novel treatment targets as well as the delivery of 'holistic' care. People with PD and their carers often rate the challenges of dealing with the non-motor aspects of the disease as more significant than the motor issues.

The first edition of this comprehensive textbook was a great success and received a commendation for a prestigious BMA book prize. We now are delighted to bring out the second edition of this book. New chapters have been added addressing continuous drug delivery and non-motor symptoms and thermoregulatory issues and there are updates on genetics, imaging, phenomenology, subtypes and treatment. The book brings together an impressive list of international leaders in the field and we hope this will be of benefit to all healthcare professionals as well as to all our patients with PD.

Professor K. Ray Chaudhuri

Preface to the First Edition

James Parkinson, the remarkable physician who described what we now call Parkinson's disease (PD), recognized the classical motor symptoms of PD but also referred to a host of non-motor problems such as sleep disturbance, constipation, dysarthria, dysphonia, dysphagia, sialorrhoea, urinary incontinence and delirium. For years, physicians, scientists and translational researchers have concentrated on improving the lives of people with PD, focusing on clinical research based on motor problems of PD, the bradykinesia, the dyskinesias, wearing off, gait problems and so on. For years therefore, the non-motor symptoms of PD, which range from cognitive to gastrointestinal, from sleep disorders to visual dysfunction, have remained under-researched, misunderstood, misrepresented and under-reported. This is in spite of clear evidence that some non-motor symptoms (NMS) of PD may pre-date the motor syndrome of PD and thus may in future allow detection of people at risk of PD. This may become a key issue that will underpin the efforts to discover effective neuroprotective therapy for PD. Furthermore, studies have now indicated that NMS have a robust correlation with the health-related quality of life of people with PD, in addition to being the chief cause of morbidity, hospitalization and mortality.

While some symptoms such as depression, dementia, dysautonomia and sleep problems are well known, others such as dysphagia, dribbling of saliva, weight changes, sexual problems and diplopia are less well recognized. Some NMS can also be precipitated by dopaminergic treatment of PD itself—and these include the dopamine dysregulation syndromes, drug-induced hallucinations or psychosis and postural hypotension. Others may occur during reduced level of central dopaminergic stimulation as would occur when the patient is wearing off, or 'off'. The non-recognition and poor awareness of NMS of PD was reported in a study in 2002 where the authors reported that depression, anxiety and fatigue are not identified by neurologists in over 50% of consultations, and existing sleep disturbance in over 40%. In 2006, a group of neuroscientists developed and internationally validated the first non-motor questionnaire for PD (NMSQuest) which empowered patients to report the often non-declared and under-treated NMS to healthcare professionals. Further studies using NMSQuest have underlined the global burden of NMS in PD irrespective of cultural origin, language and clinics. New tools have emerged thereafter, the Non-Motor Symptoms Scale for PD (NMSS), the revised version of the Unified Parkinson's Disease Rating Scale, the MDS-UPDRS which incorporates a new non-motor section, the wearing off questionnaire, and individual scales as included in the SCOPA programme, to assess the NMS of PD in a holistic manner.

In this book, which we believe is the first to be truly comprehensive in dealing with the range of NMS seen in PD, we have brought together the cumulative experience and expertise of key international experts and opinion leaders in writing 29 chapters on various

NMS of PD. The topics range from pre-motor NMS such as olfactory problems, depression and sleep disorders to those posing considerable therapeutic challenge such as dementia, pain and bladder or bowel disorders, and lesser researched NMS such as visual dysfunction and dribbling of saliva. Additional chapters include those concentrating on assessment of NMS, NMS as applied to genetic patterns of PD and the effect of surgery on NMS, among others.

Non-motor symptoms of PD dominate the lives of our patients and their carers, and for many, effective understanding of the symptoms and treatment options remains a key unmet need. We hope this book will go some way towards improving these deficiencies in our knowledge and culminate in better treatment delivery and a better quality of life for our patients and their carers.

Professor K. Ray Chaudhuri

Acknowledgement

The editors and in particular Prof. K. Ray Chaudhuri would like to thank Miss Sandeep Bassi for her work towards the compilation of the chapters for the book and also acting as a central liaison person for the project. We also thank all our colleagues at Kings College, London including allied health therapists for constructive feedback towards the book. We are indebted to the authors who have contributed to this new edition. They have freely given their time and effort and their help is greatly appreciated.

Contents

Contributors

Angelo Antonini
Department for Parkinson's disease,
IRCCS San Camillo, Venice, Italy

T. Baba
Department of Behavioral Neurology
Tohoku University Graduate School of
Medicine
Sendai, Japan

Italo Biaggioni
Department of Medicine
Division of Clinical Pharmacology
and the Autonomic Dysfunction Center
Vanderbilt University School of Medicine
Nashville, Tennessee, USA

Christine Brefel-Courbon
Department of Clinical Pharmacology
and Department of Neurosciences,
INSERM U825
University Hospital
Toulouse, France

David J. Brooks
MRC Clinical Sciences Centre
Faculty of Medicine, Imperial College
Hammersmith Hospital
London, UK

Gila Bronner
Sex Therapy Service
Sexual Medicine Center
Department of Urology, Sheba Medical
Center
Tel Hashomer, Israel

Richard G. Brown
Department of Psychology
King's College Hospital

Institute of Psychiatry
London, UK

David J. Burn
Institute for Ageing and Health
Newcastle University
Newcastle upon Tyne, UK

Francisco J. Carod-Artal
Neurology Department
Raigmore Hospital
Inverness
Scotland, UK

K. Ray Chaudhuri
King's College and Institute of
Psychiatry and University Hospital
Lewisham
National Parkinson Foundation Centre of
Excellence
King's College Hospital
London, UK

Miguel Coelho
Centro de Estudos Egas Moniz
Faculdade de Medicina de Lisboa
Lisbon, Portugal

Yaroslau Compta
Neurology Service
Hospital Clinic and Institut d'Investigacio
Biomediques August Pi I Sunyer (IDIBAPS)
Barcelona, Spain

Jesus de Pedro Cuesta
Applied Epidemiology Area
National Center for Epidemiology and
CIBERNED
Carlos III Institute of Health
Madrid, Spain

Estelle Dellapina
Department of Clinical Pharmacology and
Department of Neurosciences
INSERM U825
University Hospital
Toulouse, France

Nico J. Diederich
Department of Neurosciences
Centre Hospitalier de Luxembourg
Luxembourg

I. Estrada-Bellmann
Parkinson and Abnormal Movements
Outpatient Clinic
Department of Neurology
University Hospital UANL
Monterrey, Mexico

Andrew Evans
Movement Disorders Service
Department of Neurology
Royal Melbourne Hospital
Parkville, Victoria, Australia

Marian L. Evatt
Emory University School
of Medicine
Atlanta, Georgia, USA

Gilles Fénelon
Department of Neurology
GHU Albert-Chenevier
Henri-Mondor
Créteil, France

Joaquim J. Ferreira
Centro de Estudos Egas Moniz
Faculdade de Medicina de Lisboa
Lisbon, Portugal

Maria João Forjaz
National School of Public Health and
REDISSEC
Carlos III Institute of Health
Madrid, Spain

Clare J. Fowler
Department of Uro-Neurology
Institute of Neurology
National Hospital for Neurology and
Neurosurgery
London, UK

Birgit Frauscher
Department of Neurology
Innsbruck Medical University
Innsbruck, Austria

Joseph H. Friedman
NeuroHealth Parkinson's
Disease and Movement Disorders
Center
Warwick, Rhode Island, USA

Carles Gaig
Neurology Service
Hospital Clinic and Institut
d'Investigacio
Biomediques August Pi I Sunyer
(IDIBAPS)
Barcelona, Spain

David A. Gallagher
Royal Free Campus
Institute of Neurology
University College London
London, UK

Nir Giladi
Department of Neurology,
Tel-Aviv Sourasky Medical Center
and Sackler School of Medicine,
Tel Aviv University
Tel Aviv, Israel

Christopher G. Goetz
Departments of Neurological
Sciences and Pharmacology
Rush University Medical Center
Chicago,
Illinois, USA

Sharon Hassin-Baer
Parkinson's Disease and Movement
Disorders Clinic
Department of Neurology
Sheba Medical Center, Tel Hashomer
and Sackler School of Medicine,
Tel Aviv University
Tel Aviv, Israel

Birgit Herting
Department of Neurology
University of Dresden
Dresden, Germany

Alex Iranzo
Neurology Service
Hospital Clinic and Institut d'Investigacio
Biomediques August Pi I Sunyer
(IDIBAPS)
Barcelona, Spain

Joseph Jankovic
Parkinson's Disease Center and
Movement Disorders Clinic
Department of Neurology, Baylor College
of Medicine
Houston, Texas, USA

Julia Johnson
Speech and Language Therapy
Movement Disorders Unit
King's College Hospital
London, UK

Meike Kasten
Department of Psychiatry and
Psychotherapy
University of Lübeck
Lübeck, Germany

Regina Katzenschlager
Department of Neurology and
Karl Landsteiner Institute for
Neuroimmunological and
Neurodegenerative Disorders

Donauspital/Danube Hospital
Vienna, Austria

Horacio Kaufmann
Departments of Neurology, Medicine and
Pediatrics
New York University School of
Medicine;
Director, Dysautonomia Research
Laboratory
New York University Medical Center
New York, New York, USA

Christine Klein
Institute of Neurogenetics
University of Lübeck
Lübeck, Germany

Benzi M. Kluger
University of Florida
Gainesville, Florida, USA

Anthony E. Lang
Division of Neurology University of
Toronto and
The Morton and Gloria Shulman
Movement Disorders Centre and
The Edmond J. Safra Program in
Parkinson's Disease
Toronto Western Hospital
Toronto, Ontario, Canada

Shen-Yang Lim
Division of Neurology
University of Malaya
Kuala Lumpur, Malaysia

Douglas G. MacMahon
Royal Cornwall Hospitals NHS Trust
Camborne-Redruth Hospital
Redruth, UK

Graeme J. A. MacPhee
Department of Medicine for the Elderly
Southern General Hospital
Glasgow, UK

Pablo Martinez-Martin
National Centre of Epidemiology and
CIBERNED
Carlos III Institute of Health
Madrid, Spain

J. Carsten Möller
Department of Neurology
Philipps University
Marburg, Germany

Orna Moore
Memory and Attention Disorders Center
Department of Neurology
Tel-Aviv Sourasky Medical Center
Tel Aviv, Israel

E. Mori
Department of Behavioral Neurology
Tohoku University Graduate School of
Medicine
Sendai, Japan

Elena Moro
Movement Disorders Unit
Department of Psychiatry and Neurology
Joseph Fourier University
Centre Hospitalier Universitaire de
Grenoble
Grenoble, France

Giovanni Mostile
Department GF Ingrassia, Section of
Neurosciences
University of Catania
Catania, Italy

Per Odin
Department of Neurology, Lund
University Hospital,
Sweden

Wolfgang H. Oertel
Department of Neurology
Philipps University
Marburg, Germany

William G. Ondo
University of Texas Health Science Center
Houston
Texas, USA

Nicola Pavese
Neurology Group
MRC Clinical Sciences Centre and Division
of Neurosciences and Mental Health
Faculty of Medicine
Imperial College London
Hammersmith Hospital
London, UK

Jean Pelleprat
Department of Clinical Pharmacology and
Department of Neurosciences
INSERM U825
University Hospital
Toulouse, France

Santiago Perez-Lloret
Laboratory of Clinical Pharmacology and
Epidemiology
Medicine School
Catholic University
Buenos Aires, Argentina

Werner Poewe
Department of Neurology
Innsbruck Medical University
Innsbruck, Austria

Niall Quinn
Institute of Neurology
University College London
National Hospital for Neurology and
Neurosurgery
London, UK

Olivier Rascol
Clinical Investigation Center (CIC 1436)
and Departments of Clinical Pharmacolgy
and Neurosciences, University Hospital
of Toulouse, INSERM and University of
Toulouse 3, Toulouse, France

Prashant Reddy
Movement Disorders Unit
National Parkinson Foundation Centre of
Excellence
King's College Hospital
London, UK

Heinz Reichmann
Department of Neurology
University of Dresden
Dresden, Germany

María Verónica Rey
Laboratory of Clinical Pharmacology and
Epidemiology
Medicine School
Catholic University
Buenos Aires, Argentina

Vincent Ries
Department of Neurology
Philipps University
Marburg, Germany

Carmen Rodriguez-Blazquez
Applied Epidemiology Area
National Center for Epidemiology and
CIBERNED
Carlos III Institute of Health
Madrid, Spain

David B. Rye
Department of Neurology
Emory University School of
Medicine
Atlanta, Georgia, USA

Ryuji Sakakibara
Neurology Division
Department of Internal Medicine
Sakura Medical Centre
Toho University
Sakura, Japan

Joan Santamaria
Neurology Service
Hospital Clinic and Institut d'Investigacio

Biomediques August Pi I Sunyer
(IDIBAPS)
Barcelona, Spain

Anthony H. V. Schapira
Department of Clinical Neurosciences
Institute of Neurology
University College of London
National Hospital for Neurology and
Neurosurgery
London, UK

Anette Schrag
Royal Free Campus, Institute of Neurology
University College London
London, UK

Fabrizio Stocchi
Department of Neurology
IRCCS San Raffaele
Rome, Italy

A. Takeda
Department of Neurology
Tohoku University Graduate School
of Medicine
Sendai, Japan

Ai Huey Tan
Division of Neurology
University of Malaya
Kuala Lumpur, Malaysia

Eduardo Tolosa
Neurology Service
Institute Clinic of Neurosciences
Hospital Clinic Universitari
Centro de Investigación Biomédica en
Red Enfermedades Neurodegenerativas
(CIBERNED)
University of Barcelona
Barcelona, Spain

Margherita Torti
Department of Neurology
IRCCS San Raffaele
Rome, Italy

Lynn Marie Trotti
Department of Neurology
Emory University School of Medicine
Atlanta, Georgia, USA

Marcus M. Unger
Department of Neurology
Saarland University
Homburg, Germany

Daisy L. Whitehead
Department of Psychology
King's College London

MRC Centre for Neurodegeneration
Research
Psychology Department
Institute of Psychiatry
London, UK

Alison J. Yarnall
Institute for Ageing and Health
Newcastle University
Newcastle upon Tyne, UK

Section 1

Non-motor symptoms: general concepts

Chapter 1

What are the non-motor symptoms of Parkinson's disease?

K. Ray Chaudhuri and Niall Quinn

Non-motor symptoms (NMS) have emerged as a key component of Parkinson's disease (PD); their importance ranges from acting as clinical biomarkers in the pre-motor phase of PD to a range of symptoms that accompany the whole journey of a person with PD. The overall burden of NMS has now been shown to be one of the defining determinants of the health-related quality of life (QoL) of people with PD. In addition, NMS also substantially increase the overall cost of care in PD and lead to increased hospitalization and also institutionalization in the late stage of the disease. However, there is as yet no effective evidence-based treatment of NMS, and this poses one of the biggest challenges in PD. In the clinic, NMS are often overshadowed by the dominance of motor symptoms and low awareness of NMS among treating healthcare professionals [1,2]. The NMS of PD were recognized by James Parkinson himself. In his 'Essay on the shaking palsy' in 1817, he referred to sleep disturbance, constipation, dysarthria, dysphonia, dysphagia, sialorrhoea, urinary incontinence and 'at the last, constant sleepiness with slight delirium' [3]. Since then, numerous studies have indicated that NMS are a frequent accompaniment to PD, affecting memory, the bladder and bowel and sleep, among others. In recent times, the heterogeneity of the concept of NMS in PD has been recognized, and classifications such as the one in Table 1.1 have been proposed.

NMS can be progressive or static in terms of their natural history. A list of individual NMS in PD is provided in Table 1.2. These NMS significantly impair QoL and may precipitate hospitalization [4–6]. While some, such as depression, dementia, dysautonomia and sleep problems, are well known, others, such as dysphagia, dribbling of saliva (sialorrhoea), weight changes, sexual problems and diplopia, are less well recognized. Some NMS can be precipitated by dopaminergic treatment of PD itself—the commonest examples would be the dopamine dysregulation syndrome, drug-induced hallucinations or psychosis and postural hypotension. Others occur particularly when the level of central dopaminergic stimulation is falling, when the patient is wearing off, or 'off' [7].

However, although common, the NMS of PD are not well recognized in clinical practice. One study in the United States showed that existing depression, anxiety and fatigue are not identified by neurologists in over 50% of consultations, and existing sleep disturbance is not recognized in over 40% [7]. Another recent study attempted to retrospectively examine

Table 1.1 A classification of the types of NMS in PD (Todorova et al. [21])

Related to the disease process or pathophysiology:
  dopaminergic origin
  non-dopaminergic origin

Related to a partial non-motor origin (usually autonomic, with a motor end result, such as constipation or diplopia)

Related to non-motor fluctuations (cognitive, autonomic and sensory):
  fluctuating
  constant (only 'off' related)

Related to drug therapy of PD:
  specific symptom (e.g. hallucinations, delirium)
  as part of syndromes (impulse control disorders, dopamine agonist withdrawal syndrome, Parkinson hyperpyrexia syndrome)

Possibly genetically determined:
  development of dementia in PD cases with glucocerebrocidase mutation
  depression and sleep disorders in cases with *LRRK-2* mutation

the documented frequency of NMS in PD at presentation after clinico-pathological confirmation of a diagnosis of PD [8]. Some 21% of patients had NMS at presentation, including pain, anxiety, urinary dysfunction and depression. It is notable that these patients were more likely to be misdiagnosed initially and to have inappropriate medical interventions.

In the Sydney Multicentre study, Hely et al. [4] reported that non-levodopa-responsive NMS were the most disabling, ahead of levodopa-induced dyskinesias, in a prospective study of PD patients followed up for 15–18 years. Other studies have reported the critical role played by NMS such as depression and sleep problems in predicting health-related QoL in PD [9,10].

A common misconception is that NMS only occur in late or advanced PD. However, they can first present at any stage of the disease. Prospective data based on studies including the Honolulu–Asia Aging Study suggest that several NMS of PD, such as olfactory problems, constipation, depression and erectile dysfunction, may pre-date the motor signs, symptoms and diagnosis of PD by a number of years [1,11]. These data indicate that NMS may appear early in the course of PD and become prominent as the disease progresses, often dominating the later stages of the disease. It is likely that some NMS such as olfactory dysfunction, in combination with other symptoms such as rapid eye movement (REM) sleep behavioural disorder (RBD) or constipation, may be suitable for inclusion in a battery of tests to identify a population 'at risk of PD', which will be particularly important if and when neuroprotective therapies become available. These issues are discussed in later chapters.

Stacy et al. [12] found that NMS were common in patients within 5 years of (motor) disease onset, and that they were captured much more frequently with the use of a patient-completed questionnaire than simply in the course of a routine clinic appraisal, including the questions in the original Unified Parkinson's Disease Rating Scale (UPDRS). More

Table 1.2 A list of the range of NMS that occur in PD

Symptom		Related to Parkinson's disease pathophysiology	Related to drug therapy	Contribution from both
Cognitive and neuropsychiatric symptoms	Cognitive impairment (ranging from mild cognitive impairment to frank dementia)	++	−	−
	Anxiety	+/−	++	+
	Major depression	++	+/−	+/−
	Apathy	++	−	−
	Delirium	+/−	++	+/−
	Hallucinations, delusions, illusions	+	++	+
	Panic attacks (could be 'off' period related)	+	++	+
Sleep disorders and dysfunctions	Excessive daytime somnolence, sudden onset of sleep (narcolepsy without cataplexy)	++	++	++
	Insomnia (onset and maintenance)	++	+	+
	Non-rapid eye movement parasomnias (confusional wondering, sleep talking)	++	−	−
	Rapid eye movement sleep behaviour disorder	++	−	−
	Restless legs syndrome	+	+	+
	Periodic leg movements	+	+	+
	Sleep-disordered breathing	++	−	−
Autonomic dysfunction	Bladder urgency, frequency, nocturia	++	+/−	+/−
	Orthostatic hypotension	++	+	++
	Post-prandial hypotension	++	+/−	+/−
	Sexual dysfunction	++($\downarrow$)	++($\uparrow$)	++
	Erectile dysfunction	+	−	−
	Thermoregulatory abnormalities (hyperhidrosis)	++	+	+

Table 1.2 (continued) A list of the range of NMS that occur in PD

Symptom		Related to Parkinson's disease pathophysiology	Related to drug therapy	Contribution from both
Gastrointestinal symptoms	Dribbling of saliva	++	+/–	+/–
	Dysphagia	++	+/–	+/–
	Ageusia (change in taste sensation)	++	+/–	+/–
	Constipation	++	+/–	+/–
	Faecal incontinence	++	+/–	+/–
	Nausea	+/–	++	+/–
	Reflux	+/–	++	+/–
	Vomiting	+/–	++	+/–
Other non-motor symptoms	Central fatigue	++	+/–	+/–
	Functional anosmia or hyposmia	++	–	–
	Visual disturbances (blurred vision, transient diplopia, impaired contrast-sensitivity, colour vision)	++	+/–	+/–
	Weight gain (could be related to impulse control disorders)	++	+	+
	Weight loss	++	+/–	+/–

Reproduced with permission from: Sauerbier A, Chaudhuri KR. Non motor symptoms: the core of multi-morbid Parkinson's disease. Brit J Hosp Med 2013; 74:696–703.

+ +, strong likelihood; +, possible likelihood; –, weak or no relationship.

recently, two important studies have identified the overwhelming importance of NMS in untreated PD—the DeNoPa study and the Icicle PD study. The DeNoPa study suggested that the use of the PD NMS Questionnaire (NMSQuest) along with an autonomic questionnaire coupled with a 'test' such as olfactory testing or transcranial ultrasound may emerge as a strong 'biomarker' for PD [13,14].

Recent studies using NMSQuest have highlighted the significant occurrence of a range of 30 different NMS in PD in comparison with an age-matched control group [15,16] (Fig. 1.1). These occurred across a range of PD patients from those with early to those with advanced disease, but correlating strongly with advancing disease. In particular many NMS, such as dribbling of saliva, dysphagia, sexual problems and pain, had not been discussed with a doctor before being flagged up by NMSQuest. The study also highlighted that, irrespective of country of study and disease stage, most PD patients are likely to flag up nine to twelve different NMS in NMSQuest at a clinic visit [16]. Additionally, further

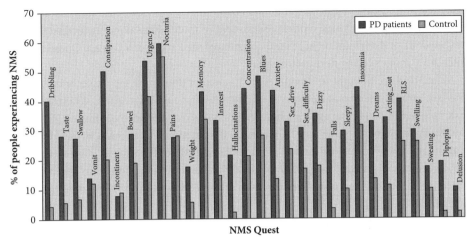

Fig. 1.1 NMS as recorded by NMSQuest in a control population and a PD population.

Reproduced with permission from Chaudhuri KR, Martinez-Martin P, Schapira AHV, et al. An international multicentre pilot study of the the first comprehensive self-completed non motor symptoms questionnaire for Parkinson's disease: The NMSQuest study. Mov Disord 2006; 21: 916–23.

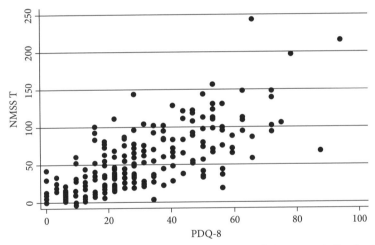

Fig. 1.2 Significant relationship between non-motor symptoms of PD as recorded by the PD Non-motor Scale Total (NMSS T) and health-related QoL in PD (recorded by PDQ-8).

Reproduced with permission from: Chaudhuri KR, Martinez-Martin P, Brown RG, et al. The metric properties of a novel non-motor symptoms scale for Parkinson's disease: results from an international pilot study. Mov Disord 2007; 22: 1901–11.

studies validating the first dedicated scale for the NMS of PD, the PD Non-motor Symptom Scale (NMSS), also indicated a strong relationship between the burden of NMS in PD and health-related QoL [17] (Fig. 1.2). The higher the burden of NMS as a whole, the worse the health-related QoL. The PDLIFE study, published in 2013, reported a serial and progressive deterioration in the self-reported health status of drug-naïve PD patients who were left untreated by clinicians at 9 and 18 months' review [18]. The decision to delay treatment was probably based on an assessment of motor state alone, as further analysis revealed major deterioration in several domains of the Parkinson's Disease Questionnaire (PDQ-39) influenced by non-motor issues.

Most NMS are thought to be refractory to current dopaminergic treatments, but this has not formally been assessed and is an idea that is being increasingly challenged. For example, some dopamine agonists have been reported to improve depression, RBD and nocturia, and apomorphine may help erectile dysfunction and anismus in PD [1,6]. Dopaminergic agents can alleviate 'off' period-related NMS of PD such as pain, anxiety and depressed mood. In particular, the rapid and reliable onset of action of an apomorphine injection or booster can transform the lives of subjects whose 'off' NMS dominate their lives [19].

However, many NMS may need specific targeted non-dopaminergic treatment, and the development of successful therapies for NMS will depend upon an accurate, reproducible and robust means of quantification and an understanding of their prevalence and evolution with disease progression and their effect on QoL. The development of tools such as NM-SQuest and NMSS alongside the revamped International Parkinson and Movement Disorder Society (MDS)-UPDRS [20], which includes a specific non-motor domain, will help refine research and therapy to improve the recognition and management of NMS of PD.

It is hoped that these developments will allow a more complete assessment of individuals who participate in therapeutic trials and will see NMS aspects included as secondary endpoints for the first time—and also, as with QoL scores, as a primary endpoint in some trials.

References

1 **Chaudhuri KR, Healy D, Schapira AHV.** The non-motor symptoms of Parkinson's disease. Diagnosis and management. Lancet Neurol 2006; **5**: 235–45.

2 **Schrag A, Jahanshahi M, Quinn N.** What contributes to quality of life in patients with Parkinson's disease? J Neurol Neurosurg Psychiatry 2000; **69**: 308–12.

3 **Parkinson J.** An essay on the shaking palsy. London: Sherwood, Neely and Jones, 1817.

4 **Hely MA, Morris JGL, Reid WGJ, Trafficante R.** Sydney multicenter study of Parkinson's disease: non-L-dopa-responsive problems dominate at 15 years. Mov Disord 2005; **20**: 190–9.

5 **Aarsland D, Larsen JP, Tandberg E, Laake K.** Predictors of nursing home placement in Parkinson's disease: a population-based, prospective study. J Am Geriatr Soc 2000; **48**: 938–42.

6 **Muzerengi S, Lewis H, Edwards M, et al.** Non-motor symptoms in Parkinson's disease: an underdiagnosed problem. Ageing Health 2006; **2**: 967–82.

7 **Shulman LM, Taback RL, Rabinstein AA, Weiner WJ.** Non-recognition of depression and other non-motor symptoms in Parkinson's disease. Parkinsonism Relat Disord 2002; **8**: 193–7.

8 **O'Sullivan SS, Williams DR, Gallagher DA, et al.** Nonmotor symptoms as presenting complaints in Parkinson's disease: a clinicopathological study. Mov Disord 2008; **23**: 101–6.

9 **Global Parkinson's Disease Survey Steering Committee.** Factors impacting on quality of life in Parkinson's disease: results from an international survey. Mov Disord 2002; **17**: 60–7.

10 **Findley L, Aujla M, Bain PG, et al.** Direct economic impact of Parkinson's disease: a research survey in the United Kingdom. Mov Disord 2003; **18**: 1139–45.

11 Tolosa E, Compta Y, Gaig C. The premotor phase of Parkinson's disease. Parkinsonism Relat Disord 2007; **13**(Suppl): S2–S7.

12 Stacy M, Bowron A, Guttman M, et al. Identification of motor and non-motor wearing off in Parkinson's disease: comparison of a patient questionnaire versus a clinician assessment. Mov Disord 2005; **20**: 726–33.

13 Mollenhauer B, Trautmann E, Sixel-Döring F, et al. Nonmotor and diagnostic findings in subjects with de novo Parkinson disease of the DeNoPa cohort. Neurology 2013; **81**: 1–9.

14 Khoo TK, Yarnall AJ, Duncan GW, et al. The spectrum of nonmotor symptoms in early Parkinson disease. Neurology 2013; **80**: 276–81.

15 Chaudhuri KR, Martinez-Martin P, Schapira AHV, et al. An international multicentre pilot study of the first comprehensive self-completed non-motor symptoms questionnaire for Parkinson's disease: the NMSQuest study. Mov Disord 2006; **21**: 916–23.

16 Martinez-Martin P, Schapira AHV, Stocchi F, et al. Prevalence of non-motor symptoms in Parkinson's disease in an international setting; study using non-motor symptoms questionnaire in 545 patients. Mov Disord 2007; **22**: 1623–9.

17 Chaudhuri KR, Martinez-Martin P, Brown RG, et al. The metric properties of a novel non-motor symptoms scale for Parkinson's disease: results from an international pilot study. Mov Disord 2007; **22**: 1901–11.

18 Grosset D, Taurah L, Burn DJ, et al. A multicentre longitudinal observational study of changes in self-reported health status in people with Parkinson's disease left untreated at diagnosis. J Neurol Neurosurg Psychiatry 2007; **78**: 465–9.

19 Quinn NP. Classification of fluctuations in patients with Parkinson's disease. Neurology 1998; **51**(Suppl 2): S25–S29.

20 Goetz CG, Tilley BC, Shaftman SR, et al. Movement Disorder Society-sponsored revision of the Unified Parkinson's disease Rating Scale (MDS-UPDRS): scale presentation and clinimetric testing results. Mov Disord 2008; **23**: 2129–70.

21 Todorova A, Jenner P, Ray Chaudhuri K. Non-motor Parkinson's: integral to motor Parkinson's, yet often neglected. Pract Neurol 2014; doi:10.1136/practneurol–2013–000741

Chapter 2

Non-motor symptoms and pre-motor diagnosis of Parkinson's disease

David A. Gallagher and Anthony H. V. Schapira

Introduction

Non-motor symptoms occur frequently in Parkinson's disease (PD) and are often under-recognized by treating physicians, yet they have a significant impact on disability and health-related quality of life, particularly in advanced disease [1]. Autopsy studies in PD have given us important insights into the potential pathological basis of these non-motor features. Clinical symptoms that precede development of the characteristic motor symptoms of PD have also been recognised, and in combination with functional neuroimaging or other non-clinical biomarkers (e.g. genetic testing) may aid early or pre-motor diagnosis of PD and distinguish it from other extrapyramidal disorders. Early and accurate diagnosis of PD is important so that appropriate treatment can be initiated, and this may have particular implications with the advent of potential disease-modifying therapies, given that the greatest rate of nigrostriatal dopaminergic depletion is likely to occur in the pre-motor and early motor phases.

Neuropathology of Parkinson's disease

The classical motor features of idiopathic PD—tremor, rigidity, bradykinesia and early gait disturbance—result from depletion of dopaminergic neurons in the substantia nigra pars compacta (SNc). Pathologically, PD is also characterized by the presence of α-synuclein-containing inclusions, Lewy bodies (LBs) and Lewy neurites, which can occur at a number of extra-nigral locations and involve non-dopaminergic neurotransmitter systems [2]. The pathogenesis of PD is complex and involves the ubiquitin proteasome system and mitochondrial dysfunction, oxidative stress and free radical-mediated neuronal damage, excitotoxic cell damage, oligodendrocytic interaction and the depletion of nerve trophic factor [3]. Over 70 molecular constituents have been identified in LBs, including α-synuclein, microtubule-associated proteins, cell cycle proteins, kinases and components of the ubiquitin proteasome system [4]; however, α-synuclein has received the most attention and α-synuclein immunohistochemistry has become an integral part of the neuropathological diagnosis of PD. The exact role of LBs in the pathogenesis of PD, whether toxic, neuroprotective or an epiphenomenon, remains unclear. Nonetheless, autopsy studies of the topographic distribution of α-synuclein pathology provide important insights into the neuroanatomical correlates of non-motor symptoms in PD and their temporal relationship to the onset of motor symptomatology. Braak and colleagues [2] have proposed a sequential staging of LB pathology in PD. Stage 1 involves the anterior olfactory structures and dorsal motor nucleus of the vagus (lower medulla); these have been proposed as neuropathological correlates for olfactory impairment and autonomic dysfunction (particularly gastrointestinal), respectively, which are common in early PD and during the pre-motor phase of the disease. Stage 2 involves the deposition of LBs in a number of brainstem nuclei, including the locus coeruleus, lower raphe nuclei and reticular formation, but confined to the medulla and pontine tegmentum. These pathological changes have been implicated in the development of rapid eye movement (REM) sleep behavioural disorder (RBD) and affective disorders in early PD. It is only during Stages 3 to 4 that LBs appear in the SNc and motor symptoms become a prominent feature of the disease. In more advanced disease (Stages 5 to 6) diffuse deposition of LBs can occur in neocortical structures. Re-examination of the caudal–rostral Braak concept in several detailed neuropathological studies reveals that this hypothesis accounts for only half of autopsied PD in some series [4] and other patterns of LB distribution can be found, including neocortical involvement in early disease. It is also notable that the first area to suffer actual neuronal cell loss is the SNc.

Pre-motor clinical features of Parkinson's disease

Non-motor symptoms occur throughout the course of PD and have a significant impact on quality of life. It is being increasingly recognized that non-motor symptoms can occur early (olfactory loss, RBD, depression and constipation) in the pre-motor phase of PD. In a large (433 cases) retrospective case-note analysis of pathologically proven PD, 21% of patients had exclusively non-motor symptoms at presentation to their general practitioner, and of these 53% presented with pain, 16.5% with urinary problems, 12.1% with affective disorders, 5.5% with non-specific cognitive impairment without functional limitation and 4.4% with fatigue [5]. A number of patients in this study had inappropriate specialist referrals (orthopaedics, rheumatology, psychiatry and urology) leading to unnecessary diagnostic and therapeutic interventions and delayed diagnosis of PD.

Sleep disorders and restless legs syndrome

RBD is a parasomnia that is common in PD and is characterized by dream enactment and loss of muscle atony during REM sleep. Insights into the pathophysiology of RBD have been gained from structural brainstem lesions in humans, post-mortem autopsy studies and animal models. RBD has been described in case reports in association with demyelination of the dorsal pontine tegmentum, an ischaemic pontine lesion, a ponto-mesencephalic cavernoma and brainstem neurinoma [6]. Incidental brainstem LB pathology has been demonstrated in an autopsied case of idiopathic RBD (iRBD) [8]. The proposed anatomical loci of RBD in humans, extrapolated from animal models, include the pre-coeruleus, sublaterodorsal nucleus and lateral pontine tegmentum [6]. These topographical locations correspond to regions of the brainstem that are involved before the development of striatal LB pathology (Stages 1 to 2) according to the Braak hypothesis. This may provide an explanation for the high prevalence of RBD in PD and its common occurrence prior to motor impairment.

There have been a number of epidemiological studies showing an association between RBD and the development of PD or other neurodegenerative disorders. For example, in one study of 44 patients presenting to a sleep centre with iRBD confirmed by polysomnography, 20/44 (45%) subsequently developed a neurodegenerative disorder [PD in nine, dementia with Lewy bodies (DLB) in six, and multisystem atrophy (MSA) in one] at a mean of 11.5 years after symptom onset and 5.1 years after formal diagnosis of RBD [8]. In a second study, 57% of patients presenting to a sleep clinic with RBD had an underlying neurological disorder, and of those with PD, 52% had symptoms of RBD that preceded the development of motor symptoms [9]. However, in a recent prospective study of iRBD, detailed annual motor assessments were made and subtle motor deficits were evident even at an early stage in those patients subsequently diagnosed with PD [10], suggesting subclinical nigral loss at this stage.

Several imaging studies in iRBD have demonstrated early pre-motor changes in the basal ganglia. An imaging study assessing pre-synaptic dopamine transporter (DAT) using ^{123}I-IPT single-photon emission computed tomography (SPECT) has revealed significantly reduced striatal uptake in patients with iRBD compared with controls, but less than in symptomatic PD [11]. ^{13}C-Dihydrotetrabenazine positron emission tomography (PET) in patients with iRBD has demonstrated reduced binding in all striatal nuclei, particularly the posterior putamen [12], and a cerebral perfusion study [^{99}Tc^m ethylene cysteinate dimer (ECD) SPECT] in iRBD has shown increased perfusion bilaterally in the pons and putamen with reduced perfusion of the frontal and temporo-parietal cortices, a metabolic picture consistent with that found in idiopathic PD [13].

These studies suggest that there is a predisposition to future development of PD in patients with iRBD and that early metabolic changes may already be present in the striatum and cortex, even years before the appearance of motor symptoms or clinical presentation of PD. Other sleep disorders may also predict subsequent development of PD. A large population-based study (the Honolulu–Asia Aging Study, $n = 3078$ [14]) revealed that excessive daytime somnolence was a risk factor [odds ratio (OR) 2.8, $P = 0.014$] for the development of PD.

Restless legs syndrome (RLS) is prevalent in PD, and in a proportion of patients it precedes motor involvement [15]. Given this epidemiological association and the documented response of idiopathic RLS (IRLS) to dopaminergic agents a common pathogenesis has been postulated, and it has been suggested that IRLS can predict future development of PD. However, there are clinical and neuroimaging differences between IRLS and RLS in the context of PD (PD/RLS). For example, in a study of PD patients with RLS ($n = 63$), PD/RLS occurred at an older age of onset, was less likely to be associated with a family history and was associated with significantly lower ferritin levels than IRLS [15]. A comparison of patients with RLS in the early stages of PD with IRLS patients using ^{123}I-IPT SPECT showed no pre-synaptic dopaminergic neuronal loss in IRLS, and no difference was found versus controls [16]. In another study using transcranial sonography (TCS), IRLS showed hypo-echogenicity of the substantia nigra (indicative of iron depletion) compared with hyper-echogenicity (a characteristic finding of dopaminergic depletion in PD) in PD/RLS [17]. These studies may indicate differences in the pathogenesis of IRLS and PD/RLS and the possibility that RLS in PD represents a secondary phenomenon. Although RLS is common in the pre-motor phase of PD it is also common in the general population, and there is currently insufficient evidence, particularly from prospective studies, that development of RLS in earlier life predicts subsequent development of PD.

Neuropsychiatric illness and cognitive impairment

Deposition of LBs occurs in brainstem loci implicated in affective disorders, such as the noradrenergic locus coeruleus and serotoninergic dorsal raphe nuclei, and this can precede basal midbrain involvement. This may explain the high prevalence of depression in early PD, often preceding the development of motor symptoms [18]. In a systematic review of psychiatric illness preceding motor symptoms in PD [19], two cohort studies, one nested case–control study and six case–control studies were identified for depression and PD. Five of six case–control studies, both cohort studies and the NCC showed a statistically significant association between a history of depression and subsequent development of PD. These studies included a large retrospective cohort study $n = 105$) [20] using a general practice based register, which found that at diagnosis of PD 9.2% of patients had a history of depression compared with 4.0% of controls [OR 2.4, 95% confidence interval (CI) 2.1–2.7].

The retrospective cohort study by Schuurman and colleagues found that, compared with controls, depressed subjects had a relative risk (RR) of 3.13 (95% CI 1.95–5.01) of subsequently developing PD [21]. Meanwhile, a similar study to assess the likelihood of developing PD found that depressed subjects had a relative risk of 2.20 (95% CI 1.70–2.84) and 2.24 (95% CI 1.72–2.93) compared with a diabetes cohort and osteoarthritis cohort, respectively [22]. A case–control study identified an increased prevalence of pre-morbid anxiety disorders in PD compared with controls [18], and in a large prospective study ($n = 35\,815$) using the Crown–Crisp index of phobic anxiety there was an increased risk of developing PD (RR 1.5, 95% CI 1.0–2.1) in those with highest level of anxiety at baseline [23].

Therefore, depression and anxiety may be predictive of future development of PD. Several functional imaging studies in PD have demonstrated signal change in the brainstem (corresponding to loci of early LB deposition), which correlate with clinimetric indices of mood. For example, in a study using ^{123}I-βCIT SPECT, dorsal midbrain binding, reflecting serotoninergic function was significantly correlated with Unified Parkinson's Disease Rating Scale (UPDRS) mood and mentation scores but not motor function [24]. Additionally, TCS has shown hypo-echogenicity of the dorsal raphe in PD patients in whom depression preceded motor symptoms [25]. These imaging studies suggest that degeneration of serotoninergic and noradrenergic brainstem nuclei can occur in parallel or precede degeneration of the substantia nigra, leading to affective disorders in the early and pre-motor phase of PD.

Development of dementia is common in PD, particularly in the later stages. However, a number of studies using detailed neuropsychological assessments, including tests sensitive to frontal lobe function, have revealed that cognitive impairment, particularly dysexecutive impairment, can occur early in PD [26]. PD dementia (PDD) and DLB are distinguished by whether dementia occurs within a year of onset of motor symptoms, but this is perhaps an arbitrary distinction given the common neuropathology (deposition of LBs containing α-synuclein) and overlapping non-motor symptomatology of the two diseases. Imaging studies in PD have revealed that disruption of frontal–striatal dopaminergic connections can occur early in PD and is associated with abnormalities in frontal executive cognitive function. In a study using ^{18}F-fluorodopa PET in patients with early PD (mean disease duration 1.3 years) fluorodopa uptake was, as expected, decreased in the striatum compared with controls [27]. However, in PD there was also increased cortical fluorodopa activity and uptake in the right dorsolateral prefrontal cortex (DLPFC), which was correlated with tests of sustained attention (vigilance test), and increased uptake in the medial frontal and anterior cingulate cortices, which was negatively correlated with the Stroop test. In a functional magnetic resonance imaging (fMRI) study comparing early PD patients with and without selective executive impairment [28], significantly more hypo-activation in the DLPFC, ventrolateral PFC and putamen during working memory testing was demonstrated in the executively impaired group. These cognitive changes may in part be levodopa responsive, given their association with striatal changes on functional imaging, the association of cognitive and attentional deficits with 'on'/'off' motor fluctuations in some patients and evidence of exacerbation of executive dysfunction secondary to levodopa withdrawal in some studies [29]. In the Honolulu–Asia Aging Study, overall cognitive scores were not associated with increased risk of developing PD, but there was a trend for higher risk based on executive function subscore (verbal fluency and judgment-related questions) [30]. The association of cognitive impairment with striatal dopamine depletion and impairment of striato-frontal cortical projections suggests that executive dysfunction may be an early or pre-motor feature of PD.

Olfaction

Several epidemiological studies have suggested that impaired olfaction is an early marker of idiopathic PD. In the Honolulu–Asia Aging Study, 2267 participants had olfactory testing at baseline and those in the lowest quartile of olfaction had a significantly increased age-adjusted risk of subsequently developing PD (OR 5.2, 95% CI 1.5–25.6) compared with the top two quartiles [31]. In a 2-year longitudinal study of first-degree relatives of patients with PD, olfactory testing was used to select normosmic and hyposmic individuals who then underwent DAT SPECT [32]. At 2 years, 10% of the hyposmic group who had shown markedly reduced DAT binding on SPECT imaging at baseline had developed clinical PD. In the remainder of the hyposmic group, despite no clinical evidence of parkinsonism, DAT binding had decreased more than in normosmic controls. In a further study of 30 subjects with idiopathic hyposmia, 11 demonstrated hyper-echogenicity of the substantia nigra on TCS (a potential diagnostic tool for early dopamine depletion in PD), yet the majority had no motor features or signs suggestive of PD. Despite this, DAT SPECT was abnormal in five and had borderline binding ratios in two [33], suggestive of possible pre-motor PD.

The University of Pennsylvania Smell Identification Test (UPSIT), a 40-item odour identification test, has been extensively used in PD studies. In a study of early PD (mean Hoehn and Yahr Stage 1.4), a strong correlation between UPSIT scores and DAT SPECT imaging indices in the striatum as a whole (regression coefficient 0.66, $P = 0.001$), and particularly the putamen (0.74, $P < 0.001$) [34], was demonstrated. Extrapolation of these findings into the pre-motor phase of PD is consistent with epidemiological studies of smell loss antecedent to clinical PD, is supported by the topographical distribution of LB in anterior olfactory structures in autopsy studies of early PD and suggests a potential role for smell testing in the early diagnosis of PD.

The use of self-administered smell identification kits (such as UPSIT) in the diagnosis of early or pre-motor PD, to differentiate PD from other extrapyramidal disorders and to differentiate tremor-dominant PD from essential tremor, has undergone extensive research. For example, olfactory function has been used to distinguish vascular parkinsonism (diagnosis based on localization of MRI lesions and vascular risk factors) and idiopathic PD [35]. UPSIT scores were significantly lower in PD than in both vascular parkinsonism and controls. In a study where olfaction in PD was compared with atypical parkinsonian syndromes [36], UPSIT scores were normal in progressive supranuclear palsy (PSP) and corticobasal degeneration (CBD) compared with controls, and there was only mild impairment in MSA. However, UPSIT scores were markedly reduced in the PD group and demonstrated good sensitivity (77%) and specificity (85%) in differentiating PD from atypical parkinsonism. Smell testing can be used to differentiate essential tremor and tremor-dominant PD, particularly in the early stages when other akinetic–rigid extrapyramidal features are not present [37].

Methods of smell testing include smell identification (such as the UPSIT), threshold detection, smell discrimination and odour memory [38]. Olfactory identification tests may have reduced diagnostic utility in those with cognitive impairment or depression, features which can occur commonly in early PD. Additionally, local nasal disease should be actively sought (tests do not discriminate between conductive and sensorineural olfactory loss), as should lifestyle factors such as smoking history. Olfactory loss also occurs in the context of other neurodegenerative disorders such as Alzheimer's disease [38]. Nonetheless, given these caveats, olfactory testing may provide an important screening tool in PD to allow risk stratification in combination with other pre-motor symptoms and direct use of diagnostic imaging (DAT SPECT scanning, TCS).

Autonomic dysfunction

Early and prominent autonomic dysfunction in the context of an akinetic–rigid syndrome (particularly if pyramidal or cerebellar features are also present) raises the possibility of

MSA. However, autonomic features occur commonly in PD and often pre-date the onset of motor features. Epidemiological evidence suggests that constipation in particular may be an early pre-motor feature of PD. In the Honolulu Heart Program, 6790 subjects were questioned about their bowel habits and in a 24-year follow-up period less than one bowel movement per day was associated with greater risk of developing PD (RR 4.1, 95% CI 1.7–9.6, $P = 0.001$) compared with those whose bowels were opened twice per day [39]. In a retrospective study, 44.6% of respondents described onset of constipation preceding motor symptoms, with a mean latency of 18.7 years [40].

Sexual dysfunction is common in PD, and includes difficulties with sexual arousal, reduced libido, erectile dysfunction and anorgasmia [41]. In a large retrospective epidemiological study (32 616 participants), men with erectile dysfunction had increased risk of subsequently developing PD (RR 3.8, 95% CI 2.4–6.0, $P < 0.0001$) [42]. In another study, 23.3% of men and 21.9% of women reported that pre-morbid sexual dysfunction contributed to cessation of sexual activity following diagnosis of PD [41]. In a large retrospective analysis of patients with pathologically proven PD [5], 3.5% of patients initially presented with urinary symptoms but without motor features of PD.

Orthostatic hypotension is common in PD, particularly in later disease, and can be exacerbated by dopaminergic medication. However, in a study of patients with a clinical diagnosis of PD, in whom MSA had been excluded by imaging of myocardial sympathetic function (cardiac ^{18}F-fluorodopa SPECT), orthostatic hypotension was of early onset (within 1 year of onset of motor symptoms) in 60% and in 13% preceded motor involvement [43]. Autopsy examinations have revealed early involvement (LB deposition) of central (medulla oblongata) and peripheral (sympathetic and parasympathetic) neurons that control autonomic function in PD, which may represent a pathological basis for early autonomic symptoms [44].

Sensory disturbance and pain syndromes

Pain is a common and often early feature of PD. Of the 21% of PD patients that manifest with non-motor symptoms [5], 53% presented to their general practitioner with pain syndromes which were often attributed to degenerative joint or spinal disease [5], and a number had unnecessary surgical interventions. An autopsy study has demonstrated immunoreactive α-synuclein inclusion bodies in the spinal cord lamina I neurons in PD, and these changes can occur early in the disease [44]. These neurons are important in the transmission of painful sensations and may represent a pathological basis for this pre-motor symptom. In addition, the emerging increase in tone that denotes SNc cell loss often leads to pain, typically presenting as a 'frozen shoulder'.

Non-clinical biomarkers

A number of gene mutations have been implicated in the pathogenesis of PD, including the autosomal dominant α-synuclein, leucine-rich repeat kinase (*LRRK2*) and the autosomal recessive parkin (*PARK2*), PTEN-induced putative kinase (*PINK1*) and *DJ1* genes [45]. Genetic testing for monogenic forms of parkinsonism in susceptible family members in well-documented pedigrees allows pre-motor diagnosis of PD. However, there is clinical heterogeneity in both genetic and non-genetic forms of parkinsonism. For example, olfaction is relatively preserved in *PARK2* disease [46] and RLS and RBD are uncommon in polysomnographic studies in *PINK1* disease [47]. The non-motor symptom complex in monogenic forms of parkinsonism may differ from idiopathic PD and requires further elucidation. Therefore the role of genetic testing in individuals with early onset pre-motor features (RBD, olfactory loss, autonomic failure) is currently unclear. Other genetic polymorphisms, such as glucocerebrosidase mutations, have been implicated in the development of PD and may have a role in pre-motor diagnosis [48]. Patients with heterozygous glucocerebrosidase mutations may have more severe non-motor features and brainstem non-dopaminergic involvement (brainstem raphe on TCS) than sporadic PD [49]. Other potential diagnostic tools used in a research setting, including α-synuclein and neuromelanin antibodies [50] and cerebrospinal fluid biomarkers, will require further evaluation but are currently of uncertain use.

The use of neuroimaging in the pre-motor diagnosis of Parkinson's disease

All of the pre-motor symptoms identified in PD are also prevalent in the general population and are associated with a wide range of other medical disorders, limiting specificity. Population-based studies have revealed that olfactory and gustatory loss are common in the general population, mainly in association with upper respiratory and chronic nasal or paranasal disease [51]. In a UK prevalence study of depression in the elderly (>65 years old, 2640 participants), depression occurred in 8.7%, increasing to 9.7% in those with co-morbid dementia [52]. Autonomic dysfunction, including orthostatic hypotension [53] and constipation [54], occurs frequently, particularly in the geriatric population. While the presence of characteristic early non-motor features is insufficient to make a diagnosis of PD, pre-motor symptoms may have the potential to allow stratification for risk of future development of neurodegenerative disorders and to direct the appropriate use of imaging techniques to allow diagnosis of PD in the pre-motor phase or when there are as yet insufficient motor symptoms to fulfil current diagnostic criteria [55].

SPECT imaging using ligands (^{123}I-βCIT and ^{123}I-FP-CIT) which bind to pre-synaptic DAT is widely used in clinical practice to help diagnose PD. However, DAT SPECT does not easily differentiate nigrostriatal dopaminergic depletion in PD from other atypical parkinsonian syndromes (PSP, CBD or MSA) [56]. ^{18}F-fluorodopa PET is less often clinically available, but it is a marker of pre-synaptic function and shows asymmetrically reduced uptake in PD [56]. ^{18}F-fluorodopa PET and DAT SPECT have both been used as markers of dopaminergic cell loss and neuroprotection in prospective drug trials. However, the sensitivity of DAT SPECT and ^{18}F-fluorodopa may be limited, given that some studies have suggested that up to 10% of patients with a clinical diagnosis of PD have normal DAT or fluorodopa activity [57,58]. Whether this is related to clinical misdiagnosis or lack of sensitivity of the diagnostic test remains unresolved. Nonetheless, the patients participating in these trials were considered by their treating neurologist to fulfil diagnostic criteria for PD and this would suggest that in the pre-motor phase with no or few motor symptoms sensitivity could be reduced.

In current clinical practice, DAT SPECT is generally used in patients who have already developed at least one motor feature (e.g. differentiating essential tremor and tremor-dominant PD) but in the pre-motor phase of PD more subtle dopaminergic depletion would be expected, making diagnostic sensitivity problematic. Additionally, accurate quantitative analysis of DAT uptake, as used in the research studies, is not available in the clinical setting and subjective interpretation is made by nuclear medicine physicians.

TCS has also been used, but mainly as a research tool in the diagnosis of PD. Hyper-echogenicity of the substantia nigra on sonography has been demonstrated as an early marker of PD and is present in monogenetic forms of PD in the pre-clinical phase [59]. However, hyper-echogenicity of the substantia nigra has been shown in up to 10% of normal subjects, limiting the diagnostic utility of the test [59].

Cardiac sympathetic denervation is a feature of LB disorders, and extra-striatal imaging modalities, such as metaiodobenzylguanidine (MIBG) SPECT, have been demonstrated to be abnormal in early PD [60]. Further refinement of imaging techniques will be required to determine the true diagnostic sensitivity and specificity of neuroimaging in pre-motor PD.

The importance of early diagnosis in Parkinson's disease

There are several reasons why early diagnosis of PD is important. Misdiagnosis is common in cases where non-motor symptoms predominate or where there are only subtle extrapyramidal features, and this can lead to unnecessary diagnostic and therapeutic interventions [5]. Also, research is ongoing into the potential disease-modifying action of the currently available dopaminergic and non-dopaminergic medications, as well as novel molecules in PD [61]. While there is currently no agent that can be considered definitively neuroprotective in PD, the identification of subjects at an earlier stage of PD (including the pre-motor phase) may provide a more appropriate *in vivo* neurobiological substrate for assessing the disease-modifying action of pharmacotherapies.

It is estimated from autopsy studies that at motor presentation of PD at least 50% of dopaminergic neurons in the substantia nigra will have been lost and that there is a negative exponential progression of the disease [62]. This has been extrapolated to suggest a pre-symptomatic phase of approximately 5 years. The non-linear pattern of dopaminergic cell loss is consistent with clinical and imaging studies. In a longitudinal study using ^{18}F-fluorodopa PET, change in the fluorodopa signal was inversely related to the duration of PD at baseline [63]. In a prospective study using UPDRS as a clinical marker of disease progression, deterioration in motor scores decreased with advancing disease duration [64]. Given the rapid rate of depletion of dopamine in the substantia nigra in the pre-motor phase, it could be inferred that to derive most benefit any potential disease-modulating therapy should be started before the onset of motor symptoms. This requires early and accurate diagnosis, which is currently not possible in pre-motor PD.

Pharmacological interventions in PD have traditionally been delayed for as long as possible due to the inevitable development of motor fluctuations and dyskinesias, and uncertainty as to the influence of medication on underlying disease progression and the potential for neurotoxic effects. However, some studies of dopaminergic medication using a 'delayed start' protocol (the monoamine oxidase B inhibitor rasagiline in the TEMPO [65] and ADAGIO [66] studies) or comparison of placebo and active treatment groups following 'washout' (levodopa versus placebo in the ELLDOPA study [67]) have suggested that the early use of PD medication may have long-term benefits on disease progression or delay the requirement for additional dopaminergic therapy [68]. Other studies using functional imaging as a surrogate marker of dopamine depletion have been interpreted as suggesting that the use of a dopamine agonist may reduce the rate of disease progression compared with levodopa (ropinirole versus levodopa, using ^{18}F-fluorodopa PET in the REAL-PET study [58], and pramipexole versus levodopa, using ^{123}I-βCIT SPECT [57]). However, the role of imaging as a marker of neuroprotection in PD is unclear and requires clarification. There is often poor correlation between clinical and imaging parameters; for example, in the ELLDOPA study [67] ^{123}I-βCIT SPECT suggested greater dopaminergic loss in the levodopa group—completely opposite results to the clinical markers of disease progression (UPDRS) in the same study. The results of the delayed start study using pramipexole were published in 2013, and showed that at 1.5 mg there was no benefit in motor function at 15 months for those patients who began the drug 6–9 months earlier [69]. That study also used SPECT and showed that there was no difference in the rate of decline in DAT between early and later treatment initiation groups. These results imply that the changes seen in the levodopa/dopamine agonist imaging studies were related to levodopa effects and not to any protection by dopamine agonists. Several other non-dopaminergic agents (e.g. co-enzyme Q10 [70] and the anti-apoptotic agent TCH346 [71]) have been studied to determine if they have any disease-modifying potential, but none have proven efficacy. The emergence of disease-modifying agents will necessitate early and accurate diagnosis in PD.

Conclusion

Olfactory loss, autonomic dysfunction, affective disorders and RBD can occur in the pre-motor phase of PD. Neuropathological loci implicated in the development of these non-motor symptoms correspond to areas affected by the deposition of LBs in autopsy studies and in the temporal sequence predicted by the Braak hypothesis [2] and functional imaging studies in PD. The presence of early non-motor symptoms in combination with characteristic changes in neuroimaging (DAT SPECT, PET, TCS) may allow a diagnosis of PD before the emergence of motor symptoms. This will be of particular importance when or if pharmacological agents that modify disease progression become available.

References

1 **Chaudhuri KR, Healy DG, Schapira AH**. Non-motor symptoms of Parkinson's disease: diagnosis and management. Lancet Neurol 2006; **5**: 235–45.

2 **Braak H, Bohl JR, Müller CM, et al**. Stanley Fahn Lecture 2005: the staging procedure for the inclusion body pathology associated with sporadic Parkinson's disease reconsidered. Mov Disord 2006; **21**: 2042–51.

3 **Olanow CW**. The pathogenesis of cell death in Parkinson's disease. Mov Disord 2007; **22**(Suppl 17): S335–S342.

4 **Wakabayashi K, Tanji K, Mori F, Takahashi H**. The Lewy body in Parkinson's disease: molecules implicated in the formation and degradation of alpha-synuclein aggregates. Neuropathology 2007; **27**: 494–506.

5 **O'Sullivan SS, Williams DR, Gallagher DA, et al**. Nonmotor symptoms as presenting complaints in Parkinson's disease: a clinicopathological study. Mov Disord 2008; **23**: 101–6.

6 **Boeve BF, Silber MH, Saper CB, et al**. Pathophysiology of REM sleep behaviour disorder and relevance to neurodegenerative disease. Brain 2007; **130**: 2770–88.

7 **Uchiyama M, Isse K, Tanaka K, et al**. Incidental Lewy body disease in a patient with REM sleep behavior disorder. Neurology 1995; **45**: 709–12.

8 **Iranzo A, Molinuevo JL, Santamaría J, et al**. Rapid-eye-movement sleep behaviour disorder as an early marker for a neurodegenerative disorder: a descriptive study. Lancet Neurol 2006; **5**: 572–7.

9 **Olson EJ, Boeve BF, Silber MH**. Rapid eye movement sleep behaviour disorder: demographic, clinical and laboratory findings in 93 cases. Brain 2000; **123**: 331–9.

10 **Postuma RB, Lang AE, Gagnon JF, Pelletier A, Montplaisir JY**. How does parkinsonism start? Prodromal parkinsonism motor changes in idiopathic REM sleep behaviour disorder. Brain 2012; **135**: 1860–70.

11 **Eisensehr I, Linke R, Noachtar S, et al**. Reduced striatal dopamine transporters in idiopathic rapid eye movement sleep behaviour disorder. Comparison with Parkinson's disease and controls. Brain 2000; **123**: 1155–60.

12 **Albin RL, Koeppe RA, Chervin RD, et al**. Decreased striatal dopaminergic innervation in REM sleep behavior disorder. Neurology 2000; **55**: 1410–12.

13 **Mazza S, Soucy JP, Gravel P, et al**. Assessing whole brain perfusion changes in patients with REM sleep behavior disorder. Neurology 2006; **67**: 1618–22.

14 **Abbott RD, Ross GW, White LR, et al**. Excessive daytime sleepiness and subsequent development of Parkinson disease. Neurology 2005; **65**: 1442–6.

15 **Ondo WG, Vuong KD, Jankovic J**. Exploring the relationship between Parkinson disease and restless legs syndrome. Arch Neurol 2002; **59**: 421–4.

16 **Linke R, Eisensehr I, Wetter TC, et al**. Presynaptic dopaminergic function in patients with restless legs syndrome: are there common features with early Parkinson's disease? Mov Disord 2004; **19**: 1158–62.

17 **Schmidauer C, Sojer M, Seppi K, et al**. Transcranial ultrasound shows nigral hypoechogenicity in restless legs syndrome. Ann Neurol 2005; **58**: 630–4.

18 **Shiba M, Bower JH, Maraganore DM, et al**. Anxiety disorders and depressive disorders preceding Parkinson's disease: a case-control study. Mov Disord 2000; **15**: 669–77.

19 **Ishihara L, Brayne C**. A systematic review of depression and mental illness preceding Parkinson's disease. Acta Neurol Scand 2006; **113**: 211–20.

20 **Leentjens AF, Van den Akker M, Metsemakers JF, et al**. Higher incidence of depression preceding the onset of Parkinson's disease: a register study. Mov Disord 2003; **18**: 414–18.

21 **Schuurman AG, van den Akker M, Ensinck KT, et al**. Increased risk of Parkinson's disease after depression: a retrospective cohort study. Neurology 2002; **58**: 1501–4.

22 Nilsson FM, Kessing LV, Bolwig TG. Increased risk of developing Parkinson's disease for patients with major affective disorder: a register study. Acta Psychiatr Scand 2001; **104**: 380–6.

23 Weisskopf MG, Chen H, Schwarzschild MA, et al. Prospective study of phobic anxiety and risk of Parkinson's disease. Mov Disord 2003; **18**: 646–51.

24 Murai T, Müller U, Werheid K, et al. *In vivo* evidence for differential association of striatal dopamine and midbrain serotonin systems with neuropsychiatric symptoms in Parkinson's disease. J Neuropsychiatry Clin Neurosci 2001; **13**: 222–8.

25 Walter U, Hoeppner J, Prudente-Morrissey L, et al. Parkinson's disease-like midbrain sonography abnormalities are frequent in depressive disorders. Brain 2007; **130**: 1799–807.

26 Lees AJ, Smith E. Cognitive deficits in the early stages of Parkinson's disease. Brain 1983; **106**: 257–70.

27 Brück A, Aalto S, Nurmi E, et al. Cortical 6-[18F]fluoro-L-dopa uptake and frontal cognitive functions in early Parkinson's disease. Neurobiol Aging 2005; **26**: 891–8.

28 Lewis SJ, Dove A, Robbins TW, et al. Cognitive impairments in early Parkinson's disease are accompanied by reductions in activity in frontostriatal neural circuitry. J Neurosci 2003; **23**: 6351–6.

29 Lange KW, Paul GM, Robbins TW, Marsden CD. L-dopa and frontal cognitive function in Parkinson's disease. Adv Neurol 1993; **60**: 475–8.

30 Ross GW, Abbott RD, Petrovitch H, Tanner CM, White LR. Pre-motor features of Parkinson's disease: the Honolulu-Asia Aging Study experience. Parkinsonism Relat Disord 2012; **18**(Suppl 1): S199–S202.

31 Ross GW, Petrovitch H, Abbott RD, et al. Association of olfactory dysfunction with risk for future Parkinson's disease. Ann Neurol 2008; **63**: 167–73.

32 Ponsen MM, Stoffers D, Booij J, van Eck-Smit BL, Wolters ECh, Berendse HW. Idiopathic hyposmia as a preclinical sign of Parkinson's disease. Ann Neurol 2004; **56**: 173–81.

33 Sommer U, Hummel T, Cormann K, et al. Detection of presymptomatic Parkinson's disease: combining smell tests, transcranial sonography, and SPECT. Mov Disord 2004; **19**: 1196–202.

34 Siderowf A, Newberg A, Chou KL, et al. [99mTc]TRODAT-1 SPECT imaging correlates with odor identification in early Parkinson disease. Neurology 2005; **64**: 1716–20.

35 Katzenschlager R, Zijlmans J, Evans A, et al. Olfactory function distinguishes vascular parkinsonism from Parkinson's disease. J Neurol Neurosurg Psychiatry 2004; **75**: 1749–52.

36 Wenning GK, Shephard B, Hawkes C, et al. Olfactory function in atypical parkinsonian syndromes. Acta Neurol Scand 1995; **91**: 247–50.

37 Ondo WG, Lai D. Olfaction testing in patients with tremor-dominant Parkinson's disease: is this a distinct condition? Mov Disord 2005; **20**: 471–5.

38 Hawkes C. Olfaction in neurodegenerative disorder. Mov Disord 2003; **18**: 364–72.

39 Abbott RD, Petrovitch H, White LR, et al. Frequency of bowel movements and the future risk of Parkinson's disease. Neurology 2001; **57**: 456–62.

40 Ueki A, Otsuka M. Life style risks of Parkinson's disease: association between decreased water intake and constipation. J Neurol 2004; **251**(Suppl 7): vII18–23.

41 Bronner G, Royter V, Korczyn AD, Giladi N. Sexual dysfunction in Parkinson's disease. J Sex Marital Ther 2004; **30**: 95–105.

42 Gao X, Chen H, Schwarzschild MA, et al. Erectile function and risk of Parkinson's disease. Am J Epidemiol 2007; **166**: 1446–50.

43 Goldstein DS. Orthostatic hypotension as an early finding in Parkinson's disease. Clin Auton Res 2006; **16**: 46–54.

44 Braak H, Sastre M, Bohl JR, de Vos RA, Del Tredici K. Parkinson's disease: lesions in dorsal horn layer I, involvement of parasympathetic and sympathetic pre- and postganglionic neurons. Acta Neuropathol 2007; **113**: 421–9.

45 **Gasser T**. Update on the genetics of Parkinson's disease. Mov Disord 2007; **22**(Suppl 17): S343–S350.

46 **Khan NL, Katzenschlager R, Watt H, et al**. Olfaction differentiates parkin disease from early-onset parkinsonism and Parkinson disease. Neurology 2004; **62**: 1224–6.

47 **Tuin I, Voss U, Kessler K, et al**. Sleep quality in a family with hereditary parkinsonism (PARK6). Sleep Med 2008; **9**: 684–8.

48 **Mata IF, Samii A, Schneer SH, et al**. Glucocerebrosidase gene mutations: a risk factor for Lewy body disorders. Arch Neurol 2008; **65**: 379–82.

49 **Brockmann K, Srulijes K, Hauser AK, et al**. GBA-associated PD presents with nonmotor characteristics. Neurology. 2011; **77**: 276–80.

50 **Gerlach M, Hendrich A, Hueber R, et al**. Early detection of Parkinson's disease: unmet needs. Neurodegener Dis 2008; **5**: 137–9.

51 **Deems DA, Doty RL, Settle RG, et al**. Smell and taste disorders, a study of 750 patients from the University of Pennsylvania Smell and Taste Center. Arch Otolaryngol Head Neck Surg 1991; **117**: 519–28.

52 **McDougall FA, Kvaal K, Matthews FE, et al**. Prevalence of depression in older people in England and Wales: the MRC CFA study. Psychol Med 2007; **37**: 1787–95.

53 **Atli T, Keven K**. Orthostatic hypotension in the healthy elderly. Arch Gerontol Geriatr 2006; **43**: 313–17.

54 **Choung RS, Locke GR 3rd, Schleck CD, et al**. Cumulative incidence of chronic constipation: a population-based study 1988–2003. Aliment Pharmacol Ther 2007; **26**: 1521–8.

55 **Jankovic J**. Parkinson's disease: clinical features and diagnosis. J Neurol Neurosurg Psychiatry 2008; **79**: 368–76.

56 **Tolosa E, Wenning G, Poewe W**. The diagnosis of Parkinson's disease. Lancet Neurol 2006; **5**: 75–86.

57 **Parkinson Study Group**. Dopamine transporter brain imaging to assess the effects of pramipexole vs levodopa on Parkinson disease progression. J Am Med Assoc 2002; **287**: 1653–61.

58 **Whone AL, Watts RL, Stoessl AJ, et al**. Slower progression of Parkinson's disease with ropinirole versus levodopa: the REAL-PET study. Ann Neurol 2003; **54**: 93–101.

59 **Berg D**. Transcranial sonography in the early and differential diagnosis of Parkinson's disease. J Neural Transm Suppl 2006; **70**: 249–54.

60 **Suzuki M, Kurita A, Hashimoto M, et al**. Impaired myocardial ^{123}I-metaiodobenzylguanidine uptake in Lewy body disease: comparison between dementia with Lewy bodies and Parkinson's disease. J Neurol Sci 2006; **240**: 15–19.

61 **Schapira AH, Olanow CW**. Neuroprotection in Parkinson disease: mysteries, myths, and misconceptions. J Am Med Assoc 2004; **291**: 358–64.

62 **Greffard S, Verny M, Bonnet AM, et al**. Motor score of the Unified Parkinson Disease Rating Scale as a good predictor of Lewy body-associated neuronal loss in the substantia nigra. Arch Neurol 2006; **63**: 584–8.

63 **Hilker R, Schweitzer K, Coburger S, et al**. Nonlinear progression of Parkinson disease as determined by serial positron emission tomographic imaging of striatal fluorodopa F18 activity. Arch Neurol 2005; **62**: 378–82.

64 **Schrag A, Dodel R, Spottke A, et al**. Rate of clinical progression in Parkinson's disease. A prospective study. Mov Disord 2007; **22**: 938–45.

65 **Parkinson Study Group**. A controlled, randomized, delayed-start study of rasagiline in early Parkinson disease. Arch Neurol 2004; **61**: 561–6.

66 **Rascol O, Fitzer-Attas CJ, Hauser R, et al**. A double-blind, delayed-start trial of rasagiline in Parkinson's disease (the ADAGIO study): prespecified and post-hoc analyses of the need for additional therapies, changes in UPDRS scores, and non-motor outcomes. Lancet Neurol 2011; **10**: 415–23.

67 **Fahn S, and the Parkinson Study Group**. Does levodopa slow or hasten the rate of progression of Parkinson's disease? J Neurol 2005; **252**(Suppl 4): IV37–IV42.

68 **Schapira AH, Obeso J**. Timing of treatment initiation in Parkinson's disease: a need for reappraisal? Ann Neurol 2006; **59**: 559–62.

69 **Schapira AH, McDermott MP, Barone P, et al**. Pramipexole in patients with early Parkinson's disease (PROUD): a randomised delayed-start trial. Lancet Neurol 2013 **12**: 747–55.

70 **Shults CW, Oakes D, Kieburtz K, et al**. Effects of coenzyme Q10 in early Parkinson disease: evidence of slowing of the functional decline. Arch Neurol 2002; **59**: 1541–50.

71 **Olanow CW, Schapira AH, LeWitt PA, et al**. TCH346 as a neuroprotective drug in Parkinson's disease: a double-blind, randomised, controlled trial. Lancet Neurol 2006; **5**: 1013–20.

Chapter 3

Non-motor symptoms in the early motor stages of Parkinson's disease

Eduardo Tolosa, Carles Gaig, Joan Santamaria and Yaroslau Compta

Introduction

Dysautonomia, sleep, neuropsychiatric and cognitive disturbances are non-motor symptoms (NMS) that are frequently prominent in the mid and late stages of Parkinson's disease (PD). However, NMS can also occur in the early stages of PD at the time of diagnosis, and some even pre-date the onset of the classical motor signs. It is indeed not uncommon that when they initially present to the doctor patients describe symptoms that are seemingly unrelated to the motor system and which may have been present for some time. Symptoms occurring in this early and prodromal phase include depression, nightmares, fatigue, pain, difficulties with concentration or prominent constipation.

Most NMS that occur in early PD are currently thought to reflect the involvement of early PD-related lesions of nervous system structures other than the dopaminergic nigrostriatal pathway. These structures include the lower brainstem, olfactory and limbic structures and the peripheral autonomic nervous system (Table 3.1). However, some NMS in early PD are mostly related to drug treatment. The drugs most frequently used in early PD are anticholinergics and amantadine, monoamine oxidase-B inhibitors, dopamine agonists and levodopa; all of these can produce non-motor side effects or potentiate PD-related NMS. Acknowledgement of this is important, because manipulation of the treatment regime can greatly alleviate some of these symptoms. Examples of NMS induced or aggravated by medications in early PD are orthostatic hypotension (OH), hallucinations, excessive daytime sleepiness (EDS) or insomnia associated with dopaminergic treatment, and memory problems caused by the anticholinergics.

Non-motor complaints in early PD are frequently under-reported by patients—who do not consider them to be related to the neurological problem. Both patients and clinicians frequently put these symptoms aside and focus on the motor signs that have actually brought the patient to the neurologist, constitute the basis for diagnosis and are the target for existing treatments. The frequency and the extent to which these NMS are disabling at the time of diagnosis, when treatment is usually initiated, or even in the initial months post-diagnosis has only been infrequently investigated.

Table 3.1 Non-motor symptoms in early PD and the proposed neuropathological substrate

Non-motor symptoms	Presumed underlying brain structures	Documented in the pre-motor phase	Corresponding Braak stage
Smell loss			
Impairments in odour detection, identification and discrimination	Olfactory bulb, anterior olfactory nucleus, amygdala, perirhinal cortex	Hyposmia	1
Autonomic dysfunction			
Gastrointestinal disturbances: gastroparesis, constipation Urinary dysfunction: urinary frequency and urgency, nocturia, urinary incontinence Sexual dysfunction: (men) impaired erection and ejaculation dysfunction; (women) impaired vaginal lubrication, problems in reaching orgasm Orthostatic and post-prandial hypotension	Amygdala, dorsal nucleus of the vagus, intermediolateral column of the spinal cord, sympathetic ganglia, enteric plexus neurons	Constipation, genito-urinary dysfunction	1
Sleep disturbances			
REM sleep behaviour disorder, excessive daytime sleepiness, insomnia	Nucleus subcoeruleus, pedunculopontine nucleus, thalamus; hypothalamus	REM behaviour disorder, excessive daytime sleepiness	2, 2–3
Behavioural/emotional dysfunction			
Depression, anxiety	Locus ceruleus, raphe nuclei, amygdala, mesolimbic and mesocortical cortex	Depression, anxiety	2–3

In the rest of this chapter emphasis will be placed upon NMS occurring in early PD when motor symptoms are mild (Hoehn and Yahr Stages 1 and 2), which is the case for most patients at the time of diagnosis. Emphasis will also be placed on those NMS that are considered to be an intrinsic part of the PD process. Infrequent NMS, and particularly those NMS mostly related to treatment, such as impulse control disorders associated with dopaminergic treatment, are listed in Table 3.2. Others, such as apathy and memory loss, are extensively reviewed elsewhere in this book. NMS occurring in the pre-motor phase of PD are discussed elsewhere.

Table 3.2 Other non-motor symptoms that can occur in early PD

Neuropsychiatric disturbances
- Apathy
- Anhedonia without depression
- As adverse event of antiparkinsonian (dopaminergic agonists) therapy: hallucinations and dopaminergic psychosis; impulse control disorder (pathological gambling, hypersexuality and others)

Sweating disturbances
- Hyperhidrosis (more frequent)
- Hypohidrosis

Cutaneous disturbances
- Facial seborrhoea (seborrhoeic dermatitis) (related to autonomic dysfunction?)

As adverse event of antiparkinsonian therapy:
- Amantadine-induced livedo reticularis
- Leg oedema (dopamine agonists)
- Erythromelalgia-like (dopamine agonists)

Ocular disturbances
- Dry eyes (xerostomia, related to autonomic dysfunction)
- Diplopia
- Blurred vision

Other disturbances
- Drug-induced nausea
- Weight loss
- Weight gain (possibly drug-induced)
- Rhinorrhoea
- Hypersalivation (dysautonomia? swallowing difficulties?), dry mouth
- Dysgeusia

Olfactory dysfunction

Olfactory dysfunction is a common feature of PD. Patients with PD rarely mention smell loss spontaneously, but when specifically asked between 22 and 70% may indicate subjective smell loss [1–3], and when formally tested hyposmia is detected in 70–100% of cases [1,4–6]. Olfactory dysfunction in PD involves several features, such as impairments in odour detection, identification and discrimination. These deficits are pronounced in PD but are milder or not observed at all in other types of parkinsonism [6]. Smell loss in PD is already present in the earliest stages of the disease. It occurs independently of disease severity and duration, is present in untreated PD patients with only mild motor symptoms and does not seem to vary with the use of dopaminergic treatment or between 'on' and 'off' states. In addition, hyposmia occurs bilaterally, even when motor signs are asymmetrical or unilateral [1,2,4–6].

The lack of association between olfactory dysfunction and the severity or duration of disease suggests that olfactory deficits reach a maximum early in the course of PD. This idea is supported by an imaging study in PD patients in the earliest stage of the disease, which found a significant positive correlation between odour identification scores and dopamine transporter (DAT) binding on ^{99}Tc^{m}-TRODAT-1 single-photon emission computed tomography (SPECT) in the putamen but no correlation between DAT binding and motor function or symptom duration [7]. Other studies conducted in early PD have found abnormalities in the olfactory tract and in central olfactory areas evaluated by diffusion-weighted magnetic resonance imaging. These abnormalities correlated with reduced ability to smell and were not related to motor symptoms, indicating that the time course of the neuropathological processes in the olfactory tract does not correlate with the temporal profile of motor dysfunction [8–10]. In some studies olfactory deficits have been reported to occur differently in different subtypes of PD (i.e. tremor-dominant PD presents better odour scores than non-tremor-dominant PD) [11,12].

The observation that hyposmia is present in the early stages of disease (when motor symptoms appear) and does not seem to worsen with disease progression led to the consideration that smell loss is a possible pre-motor symptom of PD. Several epidemiological studies, and studies in subjects with idiopathic hyposmia or in asymptomatic relatives of patients with either familial or sporadic forms of PD, have added strong support for the proposal that hyposmia can be a pre-motor symptom of PD [13–16]. Although it is still unclear exactly when the olfactory loss starts, available data from several studies suggest that it may start between 2 and 7 years before a diagnosis of PD [14–17].

Smell loss in PD causes little disability but it is relevant because olfactory testing is easy to perform; therefore hyposmia could be useful in the differentiation of PD from other parkinsonian syndromes. Furthermore, as smell loss can be an early pre-motor symptom of PD, olfactory evaluation is likely to have a role as a biomarker in future strategies aimed at detecting subjects at risk of developing PD who are in the pre-motor phase of the disease.

Neuropsychiatric and cognitive disturbances

The neuropsychiatric disturbances most frequently observed in the early stage of the disease are depression and anxiety [18]. Apathy is also common and is reported to occur in about 40% of patients(see Chapter 9). Apathetic patients suffer diminished goal-directed behaviour, cognition or emotion. There is overlap between apathy and depression, but apathy can occur independently. Patients with apathy do not express a sad mood or the cognitive features of depression such as helplessness or feelings of guilt. Patients rarely complain of lack of motivation, which is brought to the attention of doctors by caregivers. Other psychiatric disturbances that can occur in early PD are hallucinations, psychosis and impulse control disorders such as pathological gambling or hypersexuality [19–22] mostly related to dopaminergic treatment.

A systematic review of the various studies assessing the prevalence of depressive syndromes in PD found an average prevalence of major depressive disorder in PD of 17%, while minor depression was present in 22% and dysthymia in 13% of PD patients [23]. There is evidence to support the concept that depression in PD has a biological basis rather than being a pure psychological reaction to having a disabling disease [24].

The occurrence of depression in PD has been suggested to have a bimodal pattern with an initial peak at onset and a second peak in the advanced stages of the disease [25,26].

Santamaria et al. [27] found that depression was present at the time of evaluation in 32% of patients with PD of recent onset. In 67% of these patients, there was a past history of depression and, interestingly, in 44% of them depression preceded the motor manifestation of PD by several years. Depression in these patients with PD of recent onset was usually moderate in intensity and either dysthymia or major depression. It was also observed that depressed patients were younger and had milder parkinsonian motor signs than the non-depressed ones [27]. However, another study in newly diagnosed PD patients found that depressive symptoms were more common in patients with an intermediate age of onset (in their sixth decade) than those with a younger or older onset [28].

Recent studies indicate that depression can occur in 8–44% of PD patients during the early stages of the disease [29–33]. Ravina and co-workers [30] assessed the presence of depression in 413 subjects with early untreated PD who had been enrolled in two clinical trials; they found that 27.6% of these subjects had clinically significant, but generally mild, depressive symptoms. It is possible that the overlap between mild depressive symptoms and motor and other non-motor aspects of PD, such as apathy, fatigue or anhedonia, may have made it difficult to detect minor depression in these patients during the early stage of the disease [30]. A recent study found that the frequency of depressive symptoms, present in up to 44% of untreated and newly diagnosed PD patients, was significantly reduced (by up to 21%) 2 years later, and once dopaminergic therapy had been initiated [33].

The presence of depressive symptoms in PD of recent onset is associated with clinically important impairment in activities of daily living and increases the likelihood of starting antiparkinsonian treatment [30,34]. Furthermore, mood disturbances seem to be a main determinant of quality of life in mild to moderate PD [31]. Depression in early PD does not correlate with the presence of cognitive impairment or apathy [29,31,35], but the presence of mild depressive symptoms has been associated with gait abnormalities in patients newly diagnosed with PD [36].

Anxiety disorders are also common in early as well as in advanced PD, and frequently co-occur with depression. Anxiety disorders, including generalized anxiety disorder, panic disorder, agoraphobia and social phobia, have been reported in 20–43% of patients with PD [18,37–39]. Anxiety symptoms can be present in 17–63% of PD patients in the early stages [32,40]. In a recent study, anxiety was among the most common NMS along with excessive salivation, forgetfulness, urinary urgency, hyposmia and constipation [41]. As with depression, anxiety does not seem to correlate with disease duration, severity of motor symptoms, dose of levodopa treatment or degree of disability, and it could have a bimodal distribution with an initial peak at onset of PD and a second peak in the advanced stages [42,43]. In addition, and similar to what is seen with depression, the frequency of anxiety appears to lessen in the 2 years following the diagnosis of PD and onset of dopamine replacement therapy [33]. It has also been suggested that PD patients who are of intermediate age at disease onset (in their sixth decade) may have more anxiety disorders than those patients with a younger or older age at onset [28]. Anxiety has a similar effect to depression on quality of life in mild to moderate PD [31].

Depression and anxiety are also common pre-motor features of PD. In some PD patients, depression and/or anxiety can precede the development of motor manifestations by several years, especially during the 3–6 years before a diagnosis of PD [27,44–47]. Several studies have shown that subjects with depression or anxiety disorders have a 2.2 to 3.2 times higher risk of developing PD than non-depressed or non-anxious subjects [27,44–47].

Dementia in PD usually occurs late in the course of the disease, but it can occasionally occur early. Such patients are conventionally diagnosed with dementia with Lewy bodies (DLB) [27,28,48,49] event though the pathological features of DLB are identical to those of advanced PD. Subtle cognitive dysfunction, predominantly in the domains of memory and executive functions, can be detected in the early stages of PD, especially in those patients with an older age of disease onset [29,50–53]. The concept from mild cognitive impairment (MCI), as used in the field of Alzheimer's, is now frequently applied to subjects with early PD to describe a state of cognitive decline that is not sufficient in its severity of impact to warrant a dementia diagnosis. In some studies of early untreated PD up to 20% of subjects have been considered to have MCI [54]. Both dementia and cognitive changes occurring in non-demented patients are extensively reviewed in Chapters 8 and 10.

Dysautonomia

Some autonomic disturbances are frequent in PD at the time of diagnosis [55]. Such early autonomic involvement in PD can be understood by considering the proposed caudal–rostral ascending pattern of pathological involvement starting at lower brainstem nuclei with autonomic function [56], and the finding of α-synuclein pathology in autonomic nuclei in the thoracic spinal cord, the sacral parasympathetic spinal cord nuclei, the myenteric plexus of the oesophagus, the sympathetic ganglia and the vagus nerve in up to 17% of neurologically unimpaired elderly subjects [24,55].

Increasing attention is being paid to dysautonomia in early disease stages because it may be as disabling as motor symptoms, particularly in young patients. The use of a validated and structured questionnaire, the SCOPA-AUT [58], has shown that almost all the PD-related dysautonomic complaints are frequent in patients during the early stages of PD [59]. Furthermore, a recent case–control study testing the discriminant power of a number of non-motor features in early PD has shown visual dysfunction, hyposmia and dysautonomia to have a significant and independent ability to discriminate early PD cases from controls, with the combination of visual deficits and dysautonomia reaching an optimal sensitivity and specificity [60].

Gastrointestinal disturbances

The role of autonomic nuclei of the brainstem and the enteric nervous system in the control of gastrointestinal function explains the early involvement of this function in PD [61]. Gastroparesis characterized by symptoms such as post-prandial bloating or abdominal discomfort, early satiety, nausea and weight loss has been shown to occur in up to 43% of untreated early PD patients [62]. The mean time to empty half of the gastric contents was shown to be 15 minutes longer in 28 untreated patients with PD compared with a group of healthy controls [63]. Gastroparesis can be also relevant for levodopa pharmacokinetics as delayed gastric emptying and retention of levodopa may lead to erratic intestinal absorption of levodopa and subsequent motor fluctuations at an earlier stage than expected [64]. Decreased bowel movement resulting in constipation is the best known gastrointestinal symptom related to PD. Lengthening of the colon transit time has been recorded in early untreated PD patients [65]. Although most interest in PD-related constipation has in recent years focused on it being a pre-motor symptom of PD [66,67], gastrointestinal complaints are frequent in early PD patients, as shown in a study using the SCOPA-AUT questionnaire in which more than 40% of patients at Hoehn and Yahr Stages 1 and 2 had early abdominal fullness and constipation [59].

Urinary dysfunction

Patients with PD frequently complain of urinary frequency and urgency, incomplete bladder emptying, double micturition and urge incontinence. Although some authors have found a correlation of urinary dysfunction in PD with neurological disability [68] as well as disease stage [69], and urogenital failure is a classical late feature of PD, with a mean latency of 144 months in PD versus 12 months in multiple system atrophy (MSA) [70], different studies have challenged this view. Urinary complaints that are present during early disease stages range from nocturia to urinary urgency, as recorded using specific questionnaires [71] and shown in a clinico-pathological survey of 433 pathologically confirmed PD cases; urinary dysfunction was among the commonest non-motor presenting complaints of the disease [72]. Using the SCOPA-AUT questionnaire, more than 80% of PD patients at Hoehn and Yahr Stages 1 and 2 have been shown to suffer from urinary frequency and nocturia, nearly 60% from urinary urgency and up to 43% from urinary incontinence [59]. Similar figures have been reported using a urinary questionnaire and urodynamic testing in early PD cases, with detrusor overactivity in more than half of cases but none with sphincter denervation [73].

Sexual dysfunction

Sexual dysfunction, in particular erectile and ejaculatory failure in men, can be present in PD at the time of diagnosis in young-onset cases [74]. Sexual dysfunction has also been recorded in Hoehn and Yahr Stage 1 and 2 patients, with 53% of men having impaired erection and 39% ejaculatory dysfunction, and 39% of women showing impaired vaginal lubrication and 25% problems with orgasm [59]. As in the case of gastrointestinal complaints, PD-related sexual dysfunction is now being considered as a putative pre-motor feature of PD [75].

Orthostatic and post-prandial hypotension

OH and post-prandial hypotension are defined as a drop of more than 20 mmHg in systolic pressure or 10 mmHg in diastolic pressure from lying to standing and after meals, respectively [76,77]. Clinically they present with similar symptoms, such as somnolence, light-headedness, coat-hanger neck pain and syncope [78,79]. OH and post-prandial hypotension have been considered late-stage non-motor features of PD, but there is growing evidence that they can occur early in the disease course [59,80]. Reduced metaiodobenzylguanidine (MIBG) uptake indicative of sympathetic heart denervation [81] and the reduction of tyrosine-hydroxylase immunoreactive fibres in the epicardium in the absence of neuronal loss in the sympathetic ganglia and the dorsal nucleus of the vagus in cases with incidental Lewy body disease [82] support early involvement of the sympathetic nervous system in PD. OH can also be the consequence of the use of antiparkinsonian drugs, chiefly levodopa and dopamine agonists. In one study using the SCOPA-AUT questionnaire, up to 56% of PD patients at Hoehn and Yahr Stage 1 and 2 felt light-headed after standing up, although only 2% had had syncopes [59]. Goldstein et al. [83] studied 35 patients with PD and OH (defined in that study as a drop of more than 20 mmHg in systolic pressure and 5 mmHg in diastolic pressure from lying to standing). Among those patients, 21 (60%) had documentation of OH developing before, concurrently with or within 1 year after onset of symptomatic parkinsonism [83]. In four such patients, OH dominated the early clinical picture. Additionally, OH may be accompanied and aggravated by recumbent hypertension, defined as systolic blood pressure ≥ 150 mmHg and diastolic blood pressure ≥ 90 mmHg [84]; this is usually asymptomatic but may sometimes result in 'head-fullness' or headache. Impaired baroreflex, residual sympathetic activity [85] and drugs used to reverse OH are potential mechanisms accounting for recumbent hypertension, which may in turn lead to increased risk of ventricular hypertrophy, renal failure and brain haemorrhage.

Sleep disturbances

Sleep disturbances are 1.5 to 3.5 times more common in PD patients than in healthy controls of a similar age or in patients with other chronic disorders [86–90]. The most frequently reported nocturnal problems in PD are sleep fragmentation, nocturia, inability to turn over in bed, early awakening or vivid dreams and nightmares [91].

Several studies have shown, however, that there are minimal differences in sleep quality between untreated PD patients and age-matched healthy controls [86,91–93], other than slight increases in electromyogram (EMG) activity during rapid eye movement (REM) sleep [93]. Only when the disease advances do sleep disturbances become more common. Exceptions to this, however, are the early occurrence of REM sleep behaviour disorder (RBD), a parasomnia that may pre-date the diurnal motor symptoms of PD by several years [94–96], and the presence of EDS ('feeling sleepy most of the day') or of increased daytime napping ('napping more than one hour per day'), which in two large epidemiological studies were found significantly more frequent in healthy elderly men [97] or men and women [98] who later developed PD than in those who did not. Finally, in some forms of familial parkinsonism abnormal sleep may be an early disease feature [99].

Insomnia, motor restlessness and sleep quality

While sleep structure is preserved in early untreated PD, the use of dopaminergic treatments in early PD, and in particular selegiline or amantadine, may have an alerting effect at night. Restless legs syndrome (RLS) and depression may also produce insomnia in PD patients. In an 8-year follow-up longitudinal study of a cohort of patients with PD, Gjerstad et al. [100] showed that the prevalence of insomnia (defined as sleep fragmentation, difficulties in falling asleep, waking up too early or using hypnotic pills) was of 59%. The mean age of patients on entry to the study was 73 years, with a Hoehn and Yahr Stage of 2.9 and disease duration of 8–10 years. Interestingly, the prevalence of insomnia did not appear to change throughout the 8 years of follow-up, although the patients affected by the problem at each follow-up visit were different, indicating that this symptom disappears in some patients and appears later in others. Duration of the disease, female gender and the presence of depression were factors more often associated with insomnia. In contrast, the prevalence of hypersomnia in the same study population increased during follow-up from 15.1% at baseline to 44.9% 8 years later [100].

Motor restlessness, defined as an urge to move the legs without worsening at night—therefore not fulfilling all the criteria for RLS—was found in 50 out of 200 untreated PD patients and in 15 out of 173 age- and gender matched controls in an epidemiological study in Norway. Typical RLS, however was not statistically different in patients (31/200) and controls (16/173). Motor restlessness was associated with reduction in sleep quality [101].

REM sleep behaviour disorder

RBD consists of recurrent episodes of sudden, abnormally vigorous body, head or limb movements that appear during REM sleep, usually associated with dreams in which the patient defends against a threat of aggression (e.g. by people or animals). In the most severe form, patients may injure themselves or their bed partner, resulting in fractures, lacerations or contusions of varying degrees. There are, however, patients with milder forms of RBD who may not mention the sleep problems to the physician if not specifically asked. Other patients, particularly those who sleep alone, may not be aware of the parasomnia [94]. RBD has been found to occur less often in the tremor-predominant subtype of PD.

The prevalence of RBD in early PD, at the time of diagnosis or when the motor symptoms develop, is not known. Gagnon and colleagues [102] found that in established PD at least 30% of the cases had clinically or polysomnographic findings suggestive of RBD, but this figure is probably conservative because patients treated with antidepressants or hypnotics or those with cognitive changes were excluded. In one-fifth of patients with PD and RBD, the reported onset of RBD pre-dates that of parkinsonism by several years [103]. In one series of PD patients with RBD, the parasomnia only preceded PD when parkinsonism appeared after the age of 50 years [104,105].

It can be inferred from these studies that, in early PD, RBD probably occurs in around one-fifth of patients. There is insufficient information regarding the natural course of RBD in PD. In the only longitudinal study available [105], the authors reported that the prevalence of probable RBD (diagnosed by a specific questionnaire stating: 'Are you restless/agitated/or physically active while sleeping during the night?') was 34/231 (14.7%) at initial examination, 39/143 (27.3%) 4 years later but only 13/90 (14.6%) after 8 years of follow-up. Only three patients were considered to have probable RBD at all three evaluations, while the rest changed. Interestingly, in 16 patients (18%) probable RBD disappeared between the second and third evaluations. The presence of RBD in PD has been associated with a higher frequency of OH and minimal cognitive impairment and with an increased risk of developing dementia in the follow-up [106,107].

Zarranz et al. [99] reported a family harbouring a novel mutation in the α-synuclein gene (*E46K*) that segregated with a phenotype of parkinsonism or DLB. Two affected members presented with abnormal sleep behaviours very suggestive of RBD years before parkinsonism, although when studied in the sleep laboratory these behaviours could not be recorded. In less affected patients or in asymptomatic carriers, a reduction in sleep efficiency was already present, and in one excessive EMG activity was recorded during REM sleep [99].

Excessive daytime sleepiness

EDS has been under-recognized in PD, and although initially considered a side effect of non-ergot D2/D3 agonists [108] it is not restricted to a specific class of dopaminomimetic agents. Sleepiness occurs either as a constant feeling that the patient is aware of or as episodes of 'sudden, irresistible, overwhelming sleepiness without awareness of falling asleep' (sleep 'attacks'). Sleep attacks usually occur against a background of relaxed wakefulness and mostly while doing sedentary activities. The frequency of EDS in PD depends upon the study, but ranges between 15% and 71% of patients or between 1.5 to 15 times that found in healthy controls [86–90,109–112]. Despite these studies, the prevalence and clinical characteristics of sleepiness in early PD have not been well documented.

Fabbrini and collaborators [86] did not find a significantly increased prevalence of EDS in untreated PD patients compared with an age-matched healthy control group, whereas EDS was more frequent in treated patients, suggesting that the progression of the disease, the treatment or a combination of both may be critical in the development of this symptom. The degree of nocturnal sleep disruption does not seem to be related to EDS in most studies [113–115], although other authors have found the opposite [116]. Several factors have been associated with EDS in PD—severity of motor impairment, amount of dopaminergic treatment (all the different drugs), cognitive impairment [117], Epworth Sleepiness Scale score or the Inappropriate Sleep Composite Score [111]—without universal agreement on which of them is more relevant. In addition, the presence of sleep attacks has been linked to an abnormally high Epworth Sleepiness Scale score, duration of the disease and the use of dopaminergic drugs (mostly dopamine agonists) but is not associated with cognitive or motor impairment.

Dopamine agonists widely used for the management of PD in the early stages significantly increase the risk of sudden uncontrollable somnolence in a dose-related manner, and attention to this potentially serious adverse event is important when prescribing dopamine agonists in early onset patients. Drug agencies such as the US Food and Drug

Administration and the European Medicines Agency have issued recommendations for the patient leaflets accompanying these drugs, indicating that patients must be informed of this potential side effect and be advised to exercise caution while driving or operating machinery during treatment with these drugs. Furthermore, a reduction in the dosage or termination of therapy must be seriously considered in patients who have experienced somnolence or sleep attacks.

Gjerstad and co-workers studied the development of EDS over time in a group of 142 PD patients followed over a 4-year period and found that the 11 patients who had EDS at the beginning of the study continued to present with it at follow-up and showed more cognitive impairment than the others, whereas 30 patients developed EDS for the first time during the follow-up, suggesting that EDS correlates with more advanced disease and dementia [117]. Finally, an epidemiological study has suggested that the presence of EDS (defined as 'being sleepy most of the day') in asymptomatic elderly men increases their risk of developing PD by three times [97], even when adjusted for other features like insomnia, depression, coffee drinking or cigarette smoking.

Decreased sleep latency and two or more REM sleep onset episodes in the Multiple Sleep Latency Test (MSLT), typical of narcolepsy, have been described in 30, 22 or 29% of PD patients evaluated for EDS [113,115,118]. This fact has created speculation about the presence of a subtype of PD patients with a narcoleptic phenotype due to degeneration of specific brain areas. Hypocretin cell loss in the brains of patients with PD has been described in two different studies [119,120], but studies measuring hypocretin-1 levels in the cerebrospinal fluid in PD have found low [121] or normal values [122,123].

Other NMS in early Parkinson's disease: fatigue, pain and other sensory disturbances

PD patients often show greater physical and mental fatigue than normal controls [123]. Although fatigue may be a consequence of the motor impairment or secondary to NMS such as depression, anxiety, EDS, cognitive dysfunction or apathy, it seems to also be a primary symptom of PD, relatively independent of these other co-morbidities [124]. Fatigue can be a major problem in PD and can be present in untreated early PD patients: it frequently develops early in the course of the disease, and when present it seems to be a persistent symptom that worsens as the disease advances [125,126]. In a recent study, clinically significant fatigue was present in 55% of patients with incident PD [127]. On the other hand, a third of early PD patients enrolled in the ELLDOPA clinical trial, who were untreated, non-demented and non-depressed, suffered from fatigue at baseline, and at follow-up, nearly 1 year later, fatigue was present in half of these patients [128]. In this study, fatigue showed a partial response to dopaminergic treatment and did not correlate with striatal binding on ^{123}I-βCIT SPECT, suggesting that dopaminergic pathways are moderately involved in the pathogenesis of fatigue [128].

Pain and sensory complaints in PD are common, with percentages of patients with sensory symptoms ranging from 10 to 70%, with a median value of about 40%. Generally, patients with pain have more advanced disease than those without, but there is only an approximate relationship between sensory symptoms and the severity of motor signs [129–132]. In early PD, pain and sensory complaints are present in as many as 34–37% [41,133] and these symptoms can be among the most troublesome after the three classical motor symptoms of slowness, tremor and stiffness [134]. It has been estimated that pain can herald the disease in about 10% of patients [129]. Quinn [130], for example, classified one type of pain associated with PD as 'pain preceding diagnosis of Parkinson disease' and 9% of the 43 PD patients with sensory symptoms studied by Snider et al. [129] had aching, tingling or numbness for weeks or months before the onset of overt parkinsonism. Similarly, in four of the 19 patients with sensory complaints studied by Koller [131], the sensory symptoms started either before or at the same time as the motor symptoms. O'Sullivan et al. [72] have also described pathologically proven PD cases with pain as the presenting complaint. When sensory symptoms precede a diagnosis of parkinsonism, diagnostic difficulties can occur because patients are often first referred to other specialists, such as rheumatologists and orthopaedic surgeons, and PD is frequently misdiagnosed as frozen shoulder or degenerative spinal disease [135].

Sensory symptoms including pain in the early stages of PD are usually transient and occur most often in the most bradykinetic or rigid limb, on the side where the motor symptoms first appeared [132,136]. Not uncommonly, intensity varies during the day even though these patients do not have levodopa-related fluctuations. Medications such as levodopa or the anticholinergics can ameliorate pain in PD, but the response to medication is not always predictable and at times antiparkinsonian drugs can cause sensory symptoms to worsen.

In early PD, back and neck pain may result from stiff shoulders or neck rigidity, and pain may also result from dystonia [130–132,136]. Pain in the leg from dystonia when walking (kinesigenic foot dystonia) is a not uncommon presentation of young-onset PD. Frozen shoulder constitutes another painful manifestation of PD. It was the first symptom of PD in at least 8% of cases in a survey of 150 patients, and occurred 0–2 years prior to the onset of more commonly recognized motor features of the disease [137]. Akathisia or akathisia-like symptoms may also occur before dopaminergic treatment has been started [138]. Finally, RLS can be considered a pain-like symptom that has been reported in as many as 24% of PD patients [139]. However, the frequency of RLS can be overestimated in PD as a consequence of the difficulties in differentiating sensory complaints of PD from typical RLS [140]. A recent study found that the frequency of motor restlessness in the leg was increased in early PD compared with controls, while the prevalence of true RLS was similar [101].

Conclusions

Evidence from everyday clinical practice and results from studies such as those reviewed in this chapter [141] indicate that symptoms of dysautonomia, sleep, sensory abnormalities, mood and cognition are not uncommon in early PD. The reported prevalence of the various symptoms has varied, probably reflecting the different assessment methods, and only a few studies have compared their prevalence with that in controls. Various comprehensive investigations studying NMS in cohorts of early PD patients at the time of diagnosis have shown, for example, that excessive salivation, hyposmia, constipation, forgetfulness or urinary frequency are common in early PD compared with controls [41,133], with a greater number of NMS occurring in patients with higher motor scores and the so-called postural instability gait phenotype.

Generally, NMS in early untreated PD tend to be mild with only a slight influence on daily activities [133]. But, as with the motor symptoms, in some instances they can be disabling for the patient (e.g. urinary urgency) or their caregivers (e.g. apathy) Those NMS generally reported to have a greater impact on patients' quality of life have been depression and sleep problems [142].

In some patients, an NMS such as shoulder pain, urinary urgency or depressive mood prompts a first visit to the doctor [143]. This is another reason why NMS in early PD are important. In these instances such symptoms not infrequently lead to an erroneous diagnosis and to extensive and unnecessary diagnostic investigations and a delayed diagnosis of PD.

Some NMS present in the early stages of motor PD; they are thought to be part of the disease process can partially improve with levodopa or other dopaminergic drugs. Because of its mostly non-dopaminergic substrate, though, drugs used to treat the motor symptoms are generally not useful for the management of NMS. Modern treatments can nonetheless be of remarkable help (see the chapters on specific NMS in Section 2), as exemplified by the use of clonazepam for the treatment of RBD. Accordingly an appropriate search for the most common PD-related NMS seems desirable in patients with recently diagnosed early PD. Informing the patient about the nature of these symptoms is also useful. Follow-up of these symptoms so as to initiate treatment later if needed is also recommended. The various medicines currently used to treat early PD frequently have non-motor side effects which can at times be just as disabling as the classical motor signs of the illness. These side effects have not been the focus of the present chapter, but attention to them is essential for the proper management of PD as many can be prevented or minimized if appropriately identified.

References

1 **Doty RL, Stern MB, Pfeiffer C, Gollomp SM, Hurtig HI**. Bilateral olfactory dysfunction in early stage treated and untreated idiopathic Parkinson's disease. J Neurol Neurosurg Psychiatry 1992; **55**: 138–42.

2 **Muller A, Mungersdorf M, Reichmann H, Strehle G, Hummel T**. Olfactory function in Parkinsonian syndromes. J Clin Neurosci 2002; **9**: 521–4.

3 **Henderson JM, Lu Y, Wang S, Cartwright H, Halliday GM**. Olfactory deficits and sleep disturbances in Parkinson's disease: a case-control survey. J Neurol Neurosurg Psychiatry 2003; **74**: 956–8.

4 **Doty RL, Deems DA, Stellar S**. Olfactory dysfunction in parkinsonism: a general deficit unrelated to neurologic signs, disease stage, or disease duration. Neurology 1988; **38**: 1237–44.

5 **Hawkes CH, Shephard BC, Daniel SE**. Olfactory dysfunction in Parkinson's disease. J Neurol Neurosurg Psychiatry 1997; **62**: 436–46.

6 Katzenschlager R, Lees AJ. Olfaction and Parkinson's syndromes: its role in differential diagnosis. Curr Opin Neurol 2004; **17**: 417–23.

7 Siderowf A, Newberg A, Chou KL, et al. [99mTc]TRODAT-1 SPECT imaging correlates with odor identification in early Parkinson disease. Neurology 2005; **64**: 1716–20.

8 Scherfler C, Schocke MF, Seppi K, et al. Voxel-wise analysis of diffusion weighted imaging reveals disruption of the olfactory tract in Parkinson's disease. Brain 2006; **129**: 538–42.

9 Ibarretxe-Bilbao N, Junque C, Marti MJ, et al. Olfactory impairment in Parkinson's disease and white matter abnormalities in central olfactory areas: a voxel-based diffusion tensor imaging study. Mov Disord 2010; **25**: 1888–94.

10 Rolheiser TM, Fulton HG, Good KP, et al. Diffusion tensor imaging and olfactory identification testing in early-stage Parkinson's disease. J Neurol 2011; **258**: 1254–60.

11 Stern MB, Doty RL, Dotti M, et al. Olfactory function in Parkinson's disease subtypes. Neurology 1994; **44**: 266–8.

12 Ondo WG, Lai D. Olfaction testing in patients with tremor-dominant Parkinson's disease: is this a distinct condition? Mov Disord 2005; **20**: 471–5.

13 Ross GW, Abbott RD, Petrovitch H, et al. Association of olfactory dysfunction with incidental Lewy bodies. Mov Disord 2006; **21**: 2062–7.

14 Ross GW, Petrovitch H, Abbott RD, et al. Association of olfactory dysfunction with risk for future Parkinson's disease. Ann Neurol 2008; **63**: 167–73.

15 Ponsen MM, Stoffers D, Booij J, van Eck-Smit BL, Wolters E, Berendse HW. Idiopathic hyposmia as a preclinical sign of Parkinson's disease. Ann Neurol 2004; **56**: 173–81.

16 Sommer U, Hummel T, Cormann K, et al. Detection of presymptomatic Parkinson's disease: combining smell tests, transcranial sonography, and SPECT. Mov Disord 2004; **19**: 1196–202.

17 Marras C, Goldman S, Smith A, et al. Smell identification ability in twin pairs discordant for Parkinson's disease. Mov Disord 2005; **20**: 687–93.

18 Aarsland D, Larsen JP, Lim NG, et al. Range of neuropsychiatric disturbances in patients with Parkinson's disease. J Neurol Neurosurg Psychiatry 1999; **67**: 492–6.

19 Voon V, Hassan K, Zurowski M, et al. Prospective prevalence of pathologic gambling and medication association in Parkinson disease. Neurology 2006; **66**: 1750–2.

20 Grosset KA, MacPhee G, Pal G, et al. Problematic gambling on dopamine agonists: not such a rarity. Mov Disord 2006; **21**: 2206–8.

21 Pontone G, Williams JR, Bassett SS, Marsh L. Clinical features associated with impulse control disorders in Parkinson disease. Neurology 2006; **67**: 1258–61.

22 Gallagher DA, O'Sullivan SS, Evans AH, Lees AJ, Schrag A. Pathological gambling in Parkinson's disease: risk factors and differences from dopamine dysregulation. An analysis of published case series. Mov Disord 2007; **22**: 1757–63.

23 Reijnders JS, Ehrt U, Weber WEJ, et al. A systematic review of prevalence studies of depression in Parkinson's disease. Mov Disord 2008; **23**: 183–9.

24 Leentjens AF. Depression in Parkinson's disease: conceptual issues and clinical challenges. J Geriatr Psychiatry Neurol 2004; **17**: 120–6.

25 Schrag A, Jahanshahi M, Quinn NP. What contributes to depression in Parkinson's disease? Psychol Med 2001; **31**: 65–73.

26 Brown R, Jahanshahi M. Depression in Parkinson's disease: a psychosocial viewpoint. Adv Neurol 1995; **65**: 61–84.

27 Santamaria J, Tolosa E, Valles A. Parkinson's disease with depression: a possible subgroup of idiopathic parkinsonism. Neurology 1986; **36**: 1130–3.

28 Post B, Speelman JD, de Haan RJ. Clinical heterogeneity in newly diagnosed Parkinson's disease. J Neurol 2008; **255**: 716–22.

29 Foltynie T, Brayne CE, Robbins TW, Barker RA. The cognitive ability of an incident cohort of Parkinson's patients in the UK. The CamPaIGN study. Brain 2004; **127**: 550–60.

30 Ravina B, Camicioli R, Como PG, et al. The impact of depressive symptoms in early Parkinson disease. Neurology 2007; **69**: 342–7.

31 Muslimovic D, Post B, Speelman JD, Schmand B, de Haan RJ. Determinants of disability and quality of life in mild to moderate Parkinson disease. Neurology 2008; **70**: 2241–7.

32 Aarsland D, Bronnick K, Alves G, et al. The spectrum of neuropsychiatric symptoms in patients with early untreated Parkinson's disease. J Neurol Neurosurg Psychiatry 2009; **80**: 928–30.

33 Erro R, Picillo M, Vitale C, et al. Non-motor symptoms in early Parkinson's disease: a 2-year follow-up study on previously untreated patients. J Neurol Neurosurg Psychiatry 2013; **84**: 14–17.

34 Grosset D, Taurah L, Burn DJ, et al. A multicentre longitudinal observational study of changes in self reported health status in people with Parkinson's disease left untreated at diagnosis. J Neurol Neurosurg Psychiatry 2007; **78**: 465–9.

35 Dujardin K, Sockeel P, Devos D, et al. Characteristics of apathy in Parkinson's disease. Mov Disord 2007; **22**: 778–84.

36 Lord S, Galna B, Coleman S, Burn D, Rochester L. Mild depressive symptoms are associated with gait impairment in early Parkinson's disease. Mov Disord 2013; **28**: 634–9.

37 Walsh K, Bennett G. Parkinson's disease and anxiety. Postgrad Med J 2001; **77**: 89–93.

38 Shulman LM, Taback RL, Bean J, Weiner WJ. Comorbidity of the nonmotor symptoms of Parkinson's disease. Mov Disord 2001; **16**: 507–10.

39 Pontone GM, Williams JR, Anderson KE, et al. Prevalence of anxiety disorders and anxiety subtypes in patients with Parkinson's disease. Mov Disord 2009; **24**: 1333–8.

40 Borroni B, Turla M, Bertasi V, Agosti C, Gilberti N, Padovani A. Cognitive and behavioral assessment in the early stages of neurodegenerative extrapyramidal syndromes. Arch Gerontol Geriatr 2008; **47**: 53–61.

41 Khoo TK, Yarnall AJ, Duncan GW, et al. The spectrum of nonmotor symptoms in early Parkinson disease. Neurology 2013; **80**: 276–81.

42 Stein MB, Heuser IJ, Juncos JL, Uhde TW. Anxiety disorders in patients with Parkinson's disease. Am J Psychiatry 1990; **147**: 217–20.

43 Mondolo F, Jahanshahi M, Grana A, Biasutti E, Cacciatori E, Di Benedetto P. Evaluation of anxiety in Parkinson's disease with some commonly used rating scales. Neurol Sci 2007; **28**: 270–5.

44 Shiba M, Bower JH, Maraganore DM, et al. Anxiety disorders and depressive disorders preceding Parkinson's disease: a case-control study. Mov Disord 2000; **15**: 669–77.

45 Nilsson FM, Kessing LV, Bolwig TG. Increased risk of developing Parkinson's disease for patients with major affective disorder: a register study. Acta Psychiatr Scand 2001; **104**: 380–6.

46 Nilsson FM, Kessing LV, Sorensen TM, Andersen PK, Bolwig TG. Major depressive disorder in Parkinson's disease: a register-based study. Acta Psychiatr Scand 2002; **106**: 202–11.

47 Leentjens AF, Van den Akker M, Metsemakers JF, Lousberg R, Verhey FR. Higher incidence of depression preceding the onset of Parkinson's disease: a register study. Mov Disord 2003; **18**: 414–18.

48 Emre M, Aarsland D, Brown R, et al. Clinical diagnostic criteria for dementia associated with Parkinson's disease. Mov Disord 2007; 22: 1689–707 [quiz 1837].

49 Lippa CF, Duda JE, Grossman M, et al. DLB and PDD boundary issues: diagnosis, treatment, molecular pathology, and biomarkers. Neurology 2007; **68**: 812–19.

50 Marinus J, Visser M, Verwey NA, et al. Assessment of cognition in Parkinson's disease. Neurology 2003; **61**: 1222–8.

51 Muslimovic D, Post B, Speelman JD, Schmand B. Cognitive profile of patients with newly diagnosed Parkinson disease. Neurology 2005; **65**: 1239–45.

52 Williams-Gray CH, Foltynie T, Brayne CE, Robbins TW, Barker RA. Evolution of cognitive dysfunction in an incident Parkinson's disease cohort. Brain 2007; **130**: 1787–98.

53 Verbaan D, Marinus J, Visser M, et al. Cognitive impairment in Parkinson's disease. J Neurol Neurosurg Psychiatry 2007; **78**: 1182–7.

54 Aarsland D, Bronnick K, Larsen JP, Tysnes OB, Alves G. Cognitive impairment in incident, untreated Parkinson disease: the Norwegian ParkWest study. Neurology 2009; **72**: 1121–6.

55 Awerbuch GI, Sandyk R. Autonomic functions in the early stages of Parkinson's disease. Int J Neurosci 1994; **74**: 9–16.

56 Braak H, Del Tredici K, Rub U, de Vos RA, Jansen Steur EN, Braak E. Staging of brain pathology related to sporadic Parkinson's disease. Neurobiol Aging 2003; **24**: 197–211.

57 Bloch A, Probst A, Bissig H, Adams H, Tolnay M. Alpha-synuclein pathology of the spinal and peripheral autonomic nervous system in neurologically unimpaired elderly subjects. Neuropathol Appl Neurobiol 2006; **32**: 284–95.

58 Visser M, Marinus J, Stiggelbout AM, Van Hilten JJ. Assessment of autonomic dysfunction in Parkinson's disease: the SCOPA-AUT. Mov Disord 2004; **19**: 1306–12.

59 Verbaan D, Marinus J, Visser M, van Rooden SM, Stiggelbout AM, van Hilten JJ. Patient-reported autonomic symptoms in Parkinson disease. Neurology 2007; **69**: 333–41.

60 Diederich NJ, Pieri V, Hipp G, Rufra O, Blyth S, Vaillant M. Discriminative power of different nonmotor signs in early Parkinson's disease. A case-control study. Mov Disord 2010; **25**: 882–7.

61 Pfeiffer RF. Gastrointestinal dysfunction in Parkinson's disease. Lancet Neurol 2003; **2**: 107–16.

62 Edwards LL, Pfeiffer RF, Quigley EM, Hofman R, Balluff M. Gastrointestinal symptoms in Parkinson's disease. Mov Disord 1991; **6**: 151–6.

63 Sulla M, Hardoff R, Giladi N, et al. Gastric emptying time and gastric motility in patients with untreated Parkinson's disease [abstract]. Mov Disord 1996; **11**(Suppl 1): 167.

64 Kurlan R, Rothfield KP, Woodward WR, et al. Erratic gastric emptying of levodopa may cause 'random' fluctuations of parkinsonian mobility. Neurology 1988; **38**: 419–21.

65 Jost WH, Schrank B. Defecatory disorders in de novo Parkinsonians—colonic transit and electromyogram of the external anal sphincter. Wien Klin Wochenschr 1998; **110**: 535–7.

66 Abbott RD, Petrovitch H, White LR, et al. Frequency of bowel movements and the future risk of Parkinson's disease. Neurology 2001; **57**: 456–62.

67 Ueki A, Otsuka M. Life style risks of Parkinson's disease: association between decreased water intake and constipation. J Neurol 2004; 251(Suppl 7): vII18–23.

68 Araki I, Kuno S. Assessment of voiding dysfunction in Parkinson's disease by the International Prostate Symptom Score. J Neurol Neurosurg Psychiatry 2000; **68**: 429–33.

69 Sakakibara R, Shinotoh H, Uchiyama T, et al. Questionnaire-based assessment of pelvic organ dysfunction in Parkinson's disease. Auton Neurosci 2001; **92**: 76–85.

70 Wenning GK, Scherfler C, Granata R, et al. Time course of symptomatic orthostatic hypotension and urinary incontinence in patients with postmortem confirmed parkinsonian syndromes: a clinicopathological study. J Neurol Neurosurg Psychiatry 1999; **67**: 620–3.

71 Lemack GE, Dewey RB, Jr, Roehrborn CG, O'Suilleabhain PE, Zimmern PE. Questionnaire-based assessment of bladder dysfunction in patients with mild to moderate Parkinson's disease. Urology 2000; **56**: 250–4.

72 O'Sullivan SS, Williams DR, Gallagher DA, Massey LA, Silveira-Moriyama L, Lees AJ. Nonmotor symptoms as presenting complaints in Parkinson's disease: a clinicopathological study. Mov Disord 2008; **23**: 101–6.

73 **Uchiyama T, Sakakibara R, Yamamoto T, et al**. Urinary dysfunction in early and untreated Parkinson's disease. J Neurol Neurosurg Psychiatry 2011; **82**: 1382–6.

74 **Wermuth L, Stenager E**. Sexual problems in young patients with Parkinson's disease. Acta Neurol Scand 1995; **91**: 453–5.

75 **Gao X, Chen H, Schwarzschild MA, et al**. Erectile function and risk of Parkinson's disease. Am J Epidemiol 2007; **166**: 1446–50.

76 The Consensus Committee of the American Autonomic Society and the American Academy of Neurology. Consensus statement on the definition of orthostatic hypotension, pure autonomic failure, and multiple system atrophy. Neurology 1996; **46**: 1470.

77 **O'Mara G, Lyons D**. Postprandial hypotension. Clin Geriatr Med 2002; **18**: 307–21.

78 **Bleasdale-Barr KM, Mathias CJ**. Neck and other muscle pains in autonomic failure: their association with orthostatic hypotension. J R Soc Med 1998; **91**: 355–9.

79 **Oka H, Yoshioka M, Onouchi K, et al**. Characteristics of orthostatic hypotension in Parkinson's disease. Brain 2007; **130**: 2425–32.

80 **Cavallini A, Micieli G, Martignoni E, Blandini F, Fariello R, Nappi G**. Cardiopressor effects of short-term treatment with cabergoline in L-dopa stable responder parkinsonian patients: relevance of postprandial hypotension. Clin Neuropharmacol 1991; **14**: 343–51.

81 **Takatsu H, Nishida H, Matsuo H, et al**. Cardiac sympathetic denervation from the early stage of Parkinson's disease: clinical and experimental studies with radiolabeled MIBG. J Nucl Med 2000; **41**: 71–7.

82 **Orimo S, Takahashi A, Uchihara T, et al**. Degeneration of cardiac sympathetic nerve begins in the early disease process of Parkinson's disease. Brain Pathol 2007; **17**: 24–30.

83 **Goldstein DS**. Orthostatic hypotension as an early finding in Parkinson's disease. Clin Auton Res 2006; **16**: 46–54.

84 **Goldstein DS, Pechnik S, Holmes C, Eldadah B, Sharabi Y**. Association between supine hypertension and orthostatic hypotension in autonomic failure. Hypertension 2003; **42**: 136–42.

85 **Shannon JR, Jordan J, Diedrich A, et al**. Sympathetically mediated hypertension in autonomic failure. Circulation 2000; **101**: 2710–15.

86 **Fabbrini G, Barbanti P, Aurilia C, Vanacore N, Pauletti C, Meco G**. Excessive daytime sleepiness in de novo and treated Parkinson's disease. Mov Disord 2002; **17**: 1026–30.

87 **Tandberg E, Larsen JP, Karlsen K**. A community-based study of sleep disorders in patients with Parkinson's disease. Mov Disord 1998; **13**: 895–9.

88 **van Hilten JJ, Weggeman M, van der Velde EA, Kerkhof GA, van Dijk JG, Roos RA**. Sleep, excessive daytime sleepiness and fatigue in Parkinson's disease. J Neural Transm Park Dis Dement Sect 1993; **5**: 235–44.

89 **Factor SA, McAlarney T, Sanchez-Ramos JR, Weiner WJ**. Sleep disorders and sleep effect in Parkinson's disease. Mov Disord 1990; **5**: 280–5.

90 **Kumar S, Bhatia M, Behari M**. Sleep disorders in Parkinson's disease. Mov Disord 2002; **17**: 775–81.

91 **Carter J, Carroll VS, Lannon MCJ**. Sleep disruption in untreated Parkinson's disease. Neurology 1990; **40**(Suppl 1): 220–5.

92 **Ferini-Strambi L, Franceschi M, Pinto P, Zucconi M, Smirne S**. Respiration and heart rate variability during sleep in untreated Parkinson patients. Gerontology 1992; **38**: 92–8.

93 **Diederich NJ, Rufra O, Pieri V, Hipp G, Vaillant M**. Lack of polysomnographic non-REM sleep changes in early Parkinson's disease. Mov Disord 2013; **28**: 1443–6.

94 **Schenck CH, Mahowald MW**. REM sleep behavior disorder: clinical, developmental, and neuroscience perspectives 16 years after its formal identification in SLEEP. Sleep 2002; **25**: 120–38.

95 Iranzo A, Molinuevo JL, Santamaria J, et al. Rapid-eye-movement sleep behaviour disorder as an early marker for a neurodegenerative disorder: a descriptive study. Lancet Neurol 2006; **5**: 572–7.

96 Iranzo A, Tolosa E, Gelpi E, et al. Neurodegenerative disease status and post-mortem pathology in idiopathic rapid-eye-movement sleep behaviour disorder: an observational cohort study. Lancet Neurol 2013; **12**: 443–53.

97 Abbott RD, Ross GW, White LR, et al. Excessive daytime sleepiness and subsequent development of Parkinson disease. Neurology 2005; **65**: 1442–6.

98 Gao J, Huang X, Park Y, et al. Daytime napping, nighttime sleeping, and Parkinson disease. Am J Epidemiol 2011; **173**: 1032–8.

99 Zarranz JJ, Fernandez-Bedoya A, Lambarri I, et al. Abnormal sleep architecture is an early feature in the E46K familial synucleinopathy. Mov Disord 2005; **20**: 1310–15.

100 Gjerstad MD, Wentzel-Larsen T, Aarsland D, Larsen JP. Insomnia in Parkinson's disease: frequency and progression over time. J Neurol Neurosurg Psychiatry 2007; **78**: 476–9.

101 Gjerstad MD, Tysnes OB, Larsen JP. Increased risk of leg motor restlessness but not RLS in early Parkinson disease. Neurology 2011; **77**: 1941–6.

102 Gagnon JF, Bedard MA, Fantini ML, et al. REM sleep behavior disorder and REM sleep without atonia in Parkinson's disease. Neurology 2002; **59**: 585–9.

103 Iranzo A, Santamaria J, Rye DB, et al. Characteristics of idiopathic REM sleep behavior disorder and that associated with MSA and PD. Neurology 2005; **65**: 247–52.

104 Kumru H, Santamaria J, Tolosa E, Iranzo A. Relation between subtype of Parkinson's disease and REM sleep behavior disorder. Sleep Med 2007; **8**: 779–83.

105 Gjerstad MD, Boeve B, Wentzel-Larsen T, Aarsland D, Larsen JP. Occurrence and clinical correlates of REM sleep behaviour disorder in patients with Parkinson's disease over time. J Neurol Neurosurg Psychiatry 2008; **79**: 387–91.

106 Nomura T, Inoue Y, Kagimura T, Nakashima K. Clinical significance of REM sleep behavior disorder in Parkinson's disease. Sleep Med 2013; **14**: 131–5.

107 Postuma RB, Bertrand JA, Montplaisir J, et al. Rapid eye movement sleep behavior disorder and risk of dementia in Parkinson's disease: a prospective study. Mov Disord 2012; **27**: 720–6.

108 Frucht S, Rogers JD, Greene PE, Gordon MF, Fahn S. Falling asleep at the wheel: motor vehicle mishaps in persons taking pramipexole and ropinirole. Neurology 1999; **52**: 1908–10.

109 Tan EK, Lum SY, Fook-Chong SM, et al. Evaluation of somnolence in Parkinson's disease: comparison with age- and sex-matched controls. Neurology 2002; **58**: 465–8.

110 Brodsky MA, Godbold J, Roth T, Olanow CW. Sleepiness in Parkinson's disease: a controlled study. Mov Disord 2003; **18**: 668–72.

111 Hobson DE, Lang AE, Martin WR, Razmy A, Rivest J, Fleming J. Excessive daytime sleepiness and sudden-onset sleep in Parkinson disease: a survey by the Canadian Movement Disorders Group. J Am Med Assoc 2002; **287**: 455–63.

112 Verbaan D, van Rooden SM, Visser M, Marinus J, van Hilten JJ. Nighttime sleep problems and daytime sleepiness in Parkinson's disease. Mov Disord 2008; **23**: 35–41.

113 Rye DB, Bliwise DL, Dihenia B, Gurecki P. FAST TRACK: daytime sleepiness in Parkinson's disease. J Sleep Res 2000; **9**: 63–9.

114 Young A, Home M, Churchward T, Freezer N, Holmes P, Ho M. Comparison of sleep disturbance in mild versus severe Parkinson's disease. Sleep 2002; **25**: 573–7.

115 Roth T, Rye DB, Borchert LD, et al. Assessment of sleepiness and unintended sleep in Parkinson's disease patients taking dopamine agonists. Sleep Med 2003; **4**: 275–80.

116 Stevens S, Cormella CL, Stepanski EJ. Daytime sleepiness and alertness in patients with Parkinson disease. Sleep 2004; **27**: 967–72.

117 Gjerstad MD, Aarsland D, Larsen JP. Development of daytime somnolence over time in Parkinson's disease. Neurology 2002; **58**: 1544–6.

118 Arnulf I, Konofal E, Merino-Andreu M, et al. Parkinson's disease and sleepiness: an integral part of PD. Neurology 2002; **58**: 1019–24.

119 Thannickal TC, Lai YY, Siegel JM. Hypocretin (orexin) cell loss in Parkinson's disease. Brain 2007; **130**: 1586–95.

120 Fronczek R, Overeem S, Lee SY, et al. Hypocretin (orexin) loss and sleep disturbances in Parkinson's disease. Brain 2008; **131**: e88.

121 Drouot X, Moutereau S, Nguyen JP, et al. Low levels of ventricular CSF orexin/hypocretin in advanced PD. Neurology 2003; **61**: 540–3.

122 Baumann C, Ferini-Strambi L, Waldvogel D, Werth E, Bassetti CL. Parkinsonism with excessive daytime sleepiness—a narcolepsy-like disorder? J Neurol 2005; **252**: 139–45.

123 van Hilten JJ, Hoogland G, van der Velde EA, Middelkoop HA, Kerkhof GA, Roos RA. Diurnal effects of motor activity and fatigue in Parkinson's disease. J Neurol Neurosurg Psychiatry 1993; **56**: 874–7.

124 Friedman JH, Brown RG, Comella C, et al. Fatigue in Parkinson's disease: a review. Mov Disord 2007; **22**: 297–308.

125 Friedman JH, Friedman H. Fatigue in Parkinson's disease: a nine-year follow-up. Mov Disord 2001; **16**: 1120–2.

126 Alves G, Wentzel-Larsen T, Larsen JP. Is fatigue an independent and persistent symptom in patients with Parkinson disease? Neurology 2004; **63**: 1908–11.

127 Herlofson K, Ongre SO, Enger LK, Tysnes OB, Larsen JP. Fatigue in early Parkinson's disease. Minor inconvenience or major distress? Eur J Neurol 2012; **19**: 963–8.

128 Schifitto G, Friedman JH, Oakes D, et al. Fatigue in levodopa-naive subjects with Parkinson disease. Neurology 2008; **71**: 481–5.

129 Snider SR, Fahn S, Isgreen WP, Cote LJ. Primary sensory symptoms in parkinsonism. Neurology 1976; **26**: 423–9.

130 Quinn NP. Parkinson's disease: clinical features. Baillieres Clin Neurol 1997; **6**: 1–13.

131 Koller WC. Sensory symptoms in Parkinson's disease. Neurology 1984; **34**: 957–9.

132 Quinn NP, Koller WC, Lang AE, Marsden CD. Painful Parkinson's disease. Lancet 1986; **1**: 1366–9.

133 Muller B, Larsen JP, Wentzel-Larsen T, Skeie GO, Tysnes OB. Autonomic and sensory symptoms and signs in incident, untreated Parkinson's disease: frequent but mild. Mov Disord 2011; **26**: 65–72.

134 Politis M, Wu K, Molloy S, P GB, Chaudhuri KR, Piccini P. Parkinson's disease symptoms: the patient's perspective. Mov Disord 2010; **25**: 1646–51.

135 Williams DR, Lees AJ. How do patients with parkinsonism present? A clinicopathological study. Intern Med J 2009; **39**: 7–12.

136 Quittenbaum BH, Grahn B. Quality of life and pain in Parkinson's disease: a controlled cross-sectional study. Parkinsonism Relat Disord 2004; **10**: 129–36.

137 Riley D, Lang AE, Blair RD, Birnbaum A, Reid B. Frozen shoulder and other shoulder disturbances in Parkinson's disease. J Neurol Neurosurg Psychiatry 1989; **52**: 63–6.

138 Lang AE, Johnson K. Akathisia in idiopathic Parkinson's disease. Neurology 1987; **37**: 477–81.

139 Peralta CM, Frauscher B, Seppi K, et al. Restless legs syndrome in Parkinson's disease. Mov Disord 2009; **24**: 2076–80.

140 Moller JC, Unger M, Stiasny-Kolster K, Oertel WH. Restless legs syndrome (RLS) and Parkinson's disease (PD)-related disorders or different entities?. J Neurol Sci 2010; **289**: 135–7.

141 Barone P, Antonini A, Colosimo C, et al. The PRIAMO study: a multicenter assessment of nonmotor symptoms and their impact on quality of life in Parkinson's disease. Mov Disord 2009; **24**: 1641–9.

142 Martinez-Martin P, Rodriguez-Blazquez C, Kurtis MM, Chaudhuri KR. The impact of non-motor symptoms on health-related quality of life of patients with Parkinson's disease. Mov Disord 2011; **26**: 399–406.

143 Gallagher DA, Lees AJ, Schrag A. What are the most important nonmotor symptoms in patients with Parkinson's disease and are we missing them? Mov Disord 2010; **25**: 2493–500.

Chapter 4

Non-motor symptoms in advanced Parkinson's disease

Miguel Coelho and Joaquim J. Ferreira

Introduction

Parkinson's disease (PD) is a progressive neurodegenerative disorder typically associated with neuronal loss of the dopaminergic neurons of the substantia nigra pars compacta [1], but the cholinergic, noradrenergic and serotonergic systems are also affected [2]. Clinically, the cardinal motor manifestations of PD are characterized by the slowly progressive onset of bradykinesia, rest tremor and rigidity [3,4]. However, non-motor symptoms (NMS) of PD, such as dementia, depression, psychosis or dysautonomia, are now recognized as important features of the disease and a major source of disability, and they have been changing the way we conceive the progression of PD [5]. Pathologically, most NMS seem to derive from cell loss outside the dopaminergic nigrostriatal system [1]. There is an increase in the severity and extent of extra-nigral degeneration with advancing disease, as well as an accompanying increase in the frequency and severity of NMS [6].

Recent advances in the field of PD, such as the growing importance of NMS and the advent of deep brain stimulation (DBS), have contributed to the effort to properly define 'advanced stage PD' [5]. As a progressive disorder, attempts have been made to assign severity stages to PD [4]. The Hoehn and Yahr (HY) staging scale [4] was proposed in 1967 and remains the most widely used system to stage PD severity today. Originally designed as a five-point scale, the HY scale combines physical impairments (deficit in a bodily function or structure) and disability (the functional consequence of an impairment) [4]. It was designed on the assumption that the severity of parkinsonism and the independence of parkinsonian patients is mostly related to the severity of motor symptoms and loss of balance [4]. Reaching HY Stage 3 (loss of balance) is of critical importance, as it has been associated with a higher risk of dementia and mortality [4]. Nevertheless, advanced PD based on the HY scale has usually been defined as Stages 4 and 5 (loss of physical independence) [7]. In another attempt to assign stages to PD, the terms *early*, *intermediate* or *moderate* and *advanced stage* have been used to categorize patients according to the severity of motor symptoms, the overall benefit from antiparkinsonian drugs and the emergence of levodopa-induced motor complications [8]. Most PD patients under dopaminergic therapy will develop levodopa-induced motor complications after an initial phase of sustained and smooth response to dopaminergic drugs [9]. Based on this staging system, patients are usually classified as advanced stage once they start motor complications, or alternatively when motor complications become severe enough to impair the quality of life (QoL) and the ability of patients to independently perform the activities of daily living [8]. More recently, Tolosa and Katzenschlager [10] defined patients with advanced stage PD as those manifesting the cardinal motor symptoms of PD associated with motor and non-motor complications, either disease-related (e.g. freezing) or drug-induced (e.g. fluctuations or hallucinations). Although different definitions of advanced stage might exist they are mainly anchored on the severity of motor symptoms, the presence of postural instability and the emergence of levodopa-induced motor complications. Thus, as a rule these staging systems do not capture other features of PD such as NMS [7].

Indeed, NMS in advanced stages of PD may not only dominate the clinical picture but may also have a stronger impact on disability than motor symptoms and levodopa-induced motor complications, emerging as the strongest independent predictors of nursing home placement [6,11–15]. On the other hand, DBS has been a major breakthrough in the treatment of levodopa-induced motor complications, and it has considerably changed the natural history and the phenotype of advanced PD [5]. However, DBS does not avoid the progression of neurodegeneration or the emergence in the long term of treatment-resistant axial, cognitive and behavioural symptoms that ultimately determine the disability of patients in later stages [6,15–17]. Taken together, these data suggest that the concept of disease staging in advanced PD is complex and difficult to categorize in a simple manner [7]. At least a subgroup of these advanced stage patients will progress to a later phase, when severe motor and NMS resistant to levodopa dominate the phenotype and are the major determinants of disability, whereas levodopa-induced motor complications, albeit frequent, are less disabling [6,15,17,18]. Overall, NMS should be incorporated in the current definitions of advanced stage in order to capture the most disabling symptoms in advanced PD [5].

For the present review, we tried to be as inclusive and broad as possible, and defined *advanced stage* as occurring in those PD patients with levodopa-induced motor complications or HY Stage 4/5 or those whose clinical picture is dominated by symptoms resistant to levodopa.

Epidemiology

NMS are present across all disease stages of PD and even before motor onset [6,15,17,19–26]. However, their frequency and severity increase with disease progression [11,19,22,23], and in conjunction with motor axial symptoms they constitute the main determinants of disability and poor QoL in the more advanced stages [6,14,15,17–19,27–31]. Indeed, NMS tend to progress together with axial symptoms [3,20,32] and it has been shown that the association of cognitive impairment, psychosis, depression, daytime sleepiness, autonomic dysfunction and axial symptoms are strongly correlated with PD progression [33].

Cross-sectional studies

Cross-sectional data show that patients with advanced PD according to HY staging report a high frequency of NMS [15,19,22,34–36]. Two cross-sectional studies using the NMS screening questionnaire (NMSQuest) showed that the frequency of NMS increased with disease severity based on HY staging [34,35]. In one of the studies, the authors assessed the prevalence of NMS in 525 patients using NMSQuest [34]. Patients in all HY stages were included, though most gathered around HY Stages 2/3 (70.7%), while those in Stages 4/5 represented 8.8% of the total [34]. Results showed that the prevalence of NMS increased significantly with an onset of PD at age >50 years, disease duration and severity defined according to HY staging [34]. Only 8 (1.6%) patients reported no NMS. The domain pertaining to urine was the one with the highest number of registered problems, followed by depression or anxiety and then the domains of apathy, attention and memory [34]. Chaudhuri et al. [36] reported similar findings using the NMS Scale in a cross-sectional, multicentre study of 242 PD patients with a mean disease duration of 6.4 years. Only one patient reported no NMS, and the authors also identified a significant association between the frequency and severity of NMS and the severity of PD based on the HY scale, as well as a significant correlation with the severity of levodopa-induced motor complications [36]. An Italian multicentre hospital-based study enrolled 1072 PD patients (49 in HY Stages 4/5), and found that 98.6% of them reported the presence of NMS [19]. Similar to previous studies, the frequency of NMS correlated with disease severity, either defined by HY stage or the Unified Parkinson's Disease Rating Scale (UPDRS) motor score [19]. The most frequent reported NMS were psychiatric (66.8%), sleep (64.1%), gastrointestinal and pain (61%), fatigue (58.1%), urinary (57.3%) and attention/memory (44.7%), whereas the single most frequent symptoms were fatigue (58.1%) and anxiety (55.8%) [19]. In a community-based study assessing neuropsychiatric symptoms in 1449 PD patients (17% in HY Stages 4/5), 71% reported at least one neuropsychiatric symptom, of which the most frequent were insomnia (49%) followed by depression (23.8%) and anxiety (19.6%) [22]. Higher HY staging was again associated with a higher frequency of neuropsychiatric symptoms [22]. In a cross-sectional study of 50 late-stage PD patients recruited on the basis of motor disability (HY Stage 4/5 in the 'on' state), all had NMS [15]. The most frequent belonged to the cognition, mood and behaviour domain (100%), closely followed by dysautonomia (96%). Even in the pre-levodopa era, Martin et al. found that in a sample of 100 parkinsonian patients (44 in HY Stages 4/5), those in later HY stages had more frequent and severe cognitive decline [3] (Table 4.1).

Substantial transverse data show that patients with advanced PD, as defined by the presence of levodopa-induced motor complications, have a high frequency of NMS [15,36–40]. In a cross-sectional study of 50 PD patients with motor fluctuations, Witjas et al. found that all had NMS [37]. These findings were further established by the same group in a cohort of 40 patients selected for DBS [38]. In both studies, the most frequent NMS belonged to the psychic (54–66%) and dysautonomic (40–64%) domains [37,38]. In a recent study of 100 patients with levodopa-induced motor complications, all patients had at least two

Table 4.1 Non-motor symptoms in advanced Parkinson's disease[a]

(1) Disease- related
Dementia
Depression
Orthostatic hypotension
Urinary dysfunction
Pain and sensory symptoms
(2) Drug-related
Non-fluctuating
Hallucinations
Delirium
Hypersexuality
Fluctuating
Drenching sweats
Anxiety
Slowness of thinking
Fatigue
Akathisia

Adapted from Tolosa and Katzenschlager [10].

[a] Some symptoms are both disease and drug-related (e.g. orthostatic hypotension and pain).

and a median of 12 NMS [39]. The most frequent was fatigue (88%), followed by problems with concentration/attention (67%) [39]. However, Hillen et al. found a lower frequency (17%) of NMS among 130 PD patients with motor fluctuations, but similarly the most frequent symptoms were cognitive, psychiatric and dysautonomic [41] (Table 4.2).

Longitudinal studies

Prospective studies have added further evidence that NMS increase in frequency and severity with advancing disease, and that ultimately they dominate the clinical manifestations of PD in advanced disease [6,17]. In a prospective cohort of 149 patients followed

Table 4.2 The most frequent non-motor fluctuations in advanced Parkinson's disease

	Hillen et al. [41] ($n = 130$)	Witjas et al.[37] ($n = 50$)	Witjas et al. [38] ($n = 40$)
Drenching sweats, n (%)	2 (1.5)	32 (64)	35 (87.5)
Fatigue, n (%)	–	28 (56)	27 (67.5)
Akathisia, n (%)	–	27 (54)	27 (67.5)
Anxiety, n (%)	4 (3)	33 (66)	23 (57)
Slowness of thinking, n (%)	–	29 (58)	18(45)
Irritability, n (%)	–	26 (52)	17 (42.5)
Dyspnoea, n (%)	4 (3)	20 (40)	–
Panic attacks, n (%)	4 (3)	9 (18)	–

Table 4.3 Frequency of selected non-motor symptoms in advanced Parkinson's disease

	Hely et al. [6] (n = 52)	Hely et al. [17] (n = 30)	Martin et al. [3] (n = 100)	Coelho et al. [15] (n = 50)	Hillen et al. [41] (n = 130)	Witjas et al. [37] (n = 50)	Witjas et al. [38] (n = 40)
Study design	Prospective	Prospective	Cross-sectional	Cross-sectional	Cross-sectional	Cross-sectional	Prospective
Age, mean ± SD (years)	71 ± 7.9	74 ± 7.9	60.2	74.1 ± 7.0	–	66.2 ± 8.5	59 ± 8
Duration of disease, mean ± SD (years)	17.6 ± 0.7	19.8 to 20	–	17.9 ± 6.3	–	12.7 ± 5.4	12.4 ± 4.5
Hoehn and Yahr stage score, mean	4.1 ('off')	4.6 ('off')	3.4	4.4 ('on')	–	3.8 ('off')	2.8 ('off')
Neuropsychiatric dysfunction (total), n (%)	–	–	4 (4)	50 (100)	11 (8.5)	50 (100)	7.1 (21)d
Depression/sadness, n (%)	22 (54% of those tested)	–	2 (2)	31 (62)	3 (2.3)	19 (38)	–
Hallucinations, n (%)	26 (50)	23 (74)	1 (1)	22 (44)	–	24 (49)	–
Dementia, n (%)	25 (48)	25 (83)	23 (23)a	25 (50)	–	–	–
Dysautonomic dysfunction (total), n (%)	–	–	–	48 (96)	15 (11.5)	–b	6.2 (26)d
Symptomatic orthostatic hypotension, n (%)	18 (35)	15 (48)	Patients excluded if they had orthostatic hypotension	13 (26)	–	0 (0)c	–
Urinary dysfunction, n (%)	22 (41)	22 (71)	–	32 (64)	2 (1.5)	17 (35)	–
Pain and sensory symptoms, n (%)	–	–	–	12 (24)	8 (6.1)	–	1.7 (7)d

a This number represents the patients classified with moderate and severe cognitive impairment in this study; a diagnosis of dementia was not applied to the patients.

b Total number of patients with dysautonomia not given; drenching sweats, the most frequent dysautonomic symptom, occurred in 28 patients (56%).

c Assumed to be 0, because orthostatic hypotension is not specifically stated in the report, although patients were asked about an extensive list of dysautonomic symptoms.

d This study reported the effects of deep brain stimulation on non-motor fluctuations 1 year after surgery; the values given in this table are the mean number of symptoms, for each category of non-motor fluctuation, reported by patients before surgery. The numbers in brackets are the total number of non-motor symptoms, for each category that patients were asked about during the interview.

Table 4.4 Time course of non-motor symptoms in the Sydney Multicentre Study [6,17] of Parkinson's disease

Symptom	Time to onset (years)
Symptomatic postural hypotension	10 [6]
Hallucinations	10.7 [6]
Urinary incontinence	14 [6]
Dementia	15.1 [6]; 10.9 [17]
Depression	Not given

for more than 15 years, the clinical picture in the 52 surviving patients was dominated by falls (81%), visual hallucinations (50%), dementia (48%), urinary incontinence (41%) and symptomatic postural hypotension (35%) [6]. Mean HY stage was 3.8 'on' and 4.1 'off'; 95% of the 52 patients had experienced levodopa-induced motor complications, consolidating the results in cross-sectional studies showing an association of motor complications with NMS [6]. Notably, for such a long-term cohort, dementia was not an inevitable outcome for all surviving patients. Several studies of the Norwegian ParkWest project addressing single NMS, such as psychosis, cognitive impairment, apathy, depression and anxiety, have found that more advanced stages of PD were correlated with an increase in the frequency and severity of NMS [29,42–45]. Recently, a prospective Chinese cohort including 171 patients at baseline with a mean follow-up of 11 years have confirmed that more advanced motor disease is associated with the development of levodopa-resistant NMS [46]. Even patients submitted to DBS show an increase in the development of NMS with the progression of motor disease [47]. Merola et al., reporting on a cohort of 19 PD patients submitted to DBS with a mean age at disease onset of 38 years and a mean disease duration of 30 years, found that although NMS were associated with motor progression, their onset was much later in the disease course than usually reported—hallucinations at 31 years, dementia and mood depression at 32 years [47]. The prevalence of NMS may differ between community- and clinic-based samples of PD patients [11]. In a clinic-based sample, patients with more advanced disease had higher rates of falls and hallucinations, as well as worse scores on the Mini Mental State Examination (MMSE) and Beck Depression Inventory (BDI) compared with those with less severe disease [11]. In contrast, community-based patients with more advanced disease had higher rates of falls and worse MMSE and BDI scores than those in less advanced stages, but not greater rates of hallucinations [11] (Tables 4.3 and 4.4).

Clinical aspects of NMS in advanced PD

Clinical suspicion

NMS are often under-diagnosed and overlooked in clinical practice [23,48–50]. A prospective study of 101 PD patients compared the clinical impression of the treating neurologist regarding the presence or absence of depression, anxiety, fatigue and sleep problems with the results of a brief screening questionnaire and specific rating scales given to patients [48]. The results showed that the diagnostic accuracy of neurologists for the presence of depression, anxiety and fatigue was less than 50% (25–42%) and for sleep problems 60% [48]. In another hospital-based sample of 89 PD patients, a mean of 11 NMS were reported by patients whereas a mean of only 4.8 were documented in the clinical notes, a detection rate of 44% [23]. Cognitive and neuropsychiatric NMS were generally well registered in medical charts, in contrast to autonomic symptoms, especially sexual dysfunction, and problems in the domains of apathy/memory/attention and sleep [23]. In a community-based sample of 202 patients, rating scales were used to diagnose the presence of dementia, depression, anxiety and excessive daytime sleepiness, and then compared with the medical charts for accuracy of diagnosis [50]. At least one NMS was present in 151 patients but in only 29.1% of the cases were they recognized by physicians [50]. On the other hand, patients fail many times to declare their NMS to physicians, as shown by Chaudhuri et al. [49]. In this study of 242 patients, NMSQuest was used to screen for NMS; 42.8% of the symptoms were not declared by the patients to their physicians, and among these the most frequently non-declared symptoms were delusions (65.2%), daytime sleepiness (52.4%), intense and vivid dreaming (52.4%) and dizziness (50%) [49].

Fluctuation of NMS in advanced PD

NMS may fluctuate with levodopa response, in a similar manner to levodopa-induced motor fluctuations. Non-motor fluctuations (NMF) are frequent in patients with levodopa-induced motor fluctuations [15,36–39]. In two studies of PD patients with levodopa-induced motor fluctuations, Witjas et al. found that NMF are frequent as well as disabling to patients [37,38]. Assessing the presence of NMF in three domains (autonomic, cognitive/psychiatric and sensory/pain) in 50 PD patients, the authors found that all patients had at least one type of NMF, of which most occurred in the 'off' state, and that the overall number of NMF correlated with motor disability [37]. The most frequent NMF were anxiety (66%), drenching sweats (64%), slowness of thinking (58%), fatigue (56%), and akathisia (54%) [37]. One-third of the patients reported that NMF were more disabling than motor fluctuations [37]. The same authors assessed NMF in 40 PD patients selected for DBS [38]. Similarly, most NMF (82%) occurred in the 'off' state, while euphoria and hyperactivity occurred in the 'on' state; the most frequent NMS were drenching sweats (87.5%), akathisia (67.5%), fatigue (67.5%), anxiety (57%) and slowness of thinking (42%), and in contrast to the previous study, only 17.5% reported NMF as more disabling than motor fluctuations [38]. In a recent study of 100 PD patients with levodopa-induced motor complications, all patients had at least two NMS [39]. All NMS were more frequent in 'off' compared with 'on', with the exception of dysphagia, bladder urgency and excessive sweating, and only 3–10% of patients had more frequent symptoms in 'on' [39]. For most NMS, comparable percentages of patients had symptoms only in 'off' and in both 'off' and 'on', with the exception of fatigue and psychiatric symptoms; indeed, anxiety and fatigue were the symptoms with the largest change in frequency between 'off' and 'on' [39]. Regarding severity, all NMS except excessive sweating were more severe in 'off'. However, a high percentage of patients reported no significant change in severity between 'off' and 'on', while 18–76% complained that symptoms were significantly worse in 'off' [39]. Interestingly, the demographic and clinical features of PD correlated neither with frequency and severity of NMS nor with the difference in severity of NMS in 'off' and 'on' [39]. One study by Hillen et al. [41] found a smaller frequency (17%) of NMS in 130 PD patients with levodopa-induced motor fluctuations, but this finding may be explained due to the fact that patients were asked an open question about symptoms that they associated with the 'off' state. The symptoms most reported in 'off' were autonomic, followed by cognitive/psychiatric and then sensory [41]. In a study recruiting PD patients in HY Stage 4/5 in the 'on' state, 78% had levodopa-induced motor complications while 66% had NMF; the most frequent fluctuating NMS were neuropsychiatric (48%), autonomic (22%) and sensory (16%) [15].

Relative frequency and clustering of NMS in advanced PD

Although NMS are common in advanced PD, their relative frequency and severity differ, and both longitudinal and cross-sectional studies give overall similar hierarchical order of the frequency of NMS. In the Sydney cohort at 15 years follow-up, the most frequent NMS were cognitive impairment in 84% of patients, with dementia in 48%, followed by excessive daytime sleepiness in 79%, hallucinations and depression in 50%, urinary incontinence in 41% and postural hypotension in 35% of the patients [6]. In the same cohort assessed at 20 years, dementia was present in 83% of the patients, hallucinations in 74%, urinary incontinence in 71%, excessive daytime sleepiness in 70% and symptomatic postural hypotension affected 48% of the patients [17]. In another study in late-stage PD, the most frequent NMS were constipation (82%), drooling (70%), urinary dysfunction (64%), depression (62%), apathy (56%), slowness of thinking, anxiety and dementia in 50%, and hallucinations in 44% of the patients [15]. In studies recruiting patients with levodopa-induced motor complications, the most frequent NMS in two studies from the same group were either anxiety (57–66%) or drenching sweats (64–87.5%), followed by fatigue (56–67.5%) and akathisia (54–67.5%), and slowness of thinking (42–58%) [37,38], while in the study by Storch et al. [39] the most frequent NMS were fatigue, concentration/attention, inner restlessness, pain, bladder urgency and depression.

Risk factors for NMS in advanced PD

The progression of PD, either as a function of disease duration, UPDRS motor score, HY staging or development of levodopa-induced motor complications, is a risk factor for the emergence of NMS in advanced PD [4,6,15,17,19,22,23,37–39]. Moreover, axial motor symptoms per se have been identified as an independent risk factor for the occurrence of major NMS in advanced stages of PD, such as psychosis, dementia and dysautonomia [51,52]. Interestingly, some NMS are even risk factors for the emergence of others. Fatigue was found to be correlated with more advanced disease [53] and with the presence of depression [53,54], anxiety [53,54], apathy [54] and sleep disorders [53]. Psychosis is a strong independent predictor of dementia, and apathy has also been associated with the presence of dementia [42,52,55–57]. Even NMS that may be present before motor onset, such as hyposmia and rapid eye movement sleep behavioural disorder (RBD), seem to increase the risk of dementia or cognitive impairment and dysautonomia [58–64]. Increasing evidence has associated the presence of hypo/anosmia with the presence of cognitive impairment or dementia [58,59,61] and one study [59] has found an increased risk for psychosis in hyposmic patients. In a prospective study of 42 PD patients, the presence of RBD at baseline significantly predicted the occurrence of dementia, hallucinations and cognitive fluctuations [62]. The presence of RBD was also found to be associated with a higher frequency of freezing and falls [65], and both hyposmia and RBD were found to increase the risk of dysautonomia, in particular orthostatic hypotension [60,65]. Recently, some genetic forms of PD have been associated with a higher or lower frequency of NMS. One study comparing young-onset PD (onset at age <45 years) with or without homozygous or compound heterozygote parkin mutations versus late-onset PD (onset at age >45 years) suggested that NMS, with the exception of anxiety, were less frequent in parkin patients [66]. A clinico-pathological study of 5 parkin disease patients found no case of cognitive impairment or dementia [67]. Marras et al. compared *LRRK2* (G2019S mutation) with *LRRK2*-negative PD patients and found that *LRRK2* PD was associated with worse depression scores and worse colour discrimination, although they had better olfaction than patients with idiopathic PD [68]. On the other hand, the presence of mutations in the glucocerebrosidase gene (*GBA*) seems to be associated with a higher frequency of dementia, neuropsychiatric symptoms and dysautonomia in PD patients [69–72].

Disability, disability milestones and mortality

In advanced PD, NMS contribute significantly to patients' disability [6,14,15,17,31]. After disease durations of 15 and 20 years, the results from the Sydney cohort showed that the major sources of disability were falls and NMS such as autonomic dysfunction, neuropsychiatric symptoms and dementia [6,17]. In a cohort of late-stage PD patients from Barcelona and Lisbon, the symptoms causing an extreme or severe impact on patients' perceived health status were axial symptoms such as falls, postural instability, freezing, speech problems and dysphagia, as well as NMS belonging to the domains of dysautonomia (sweats, urinary incontinence and constipation), cognition/mood/behaviour (dementia, depression, anxiety and apathy) and pain [15]. The study by Schrag et al., reporting on a community- and a hospital-based sample of PD patients, found that increased disability in more advanced stages was mostly due to levodopa-induced motor complications, falls and NMS such as hallucinations, memory impairment, depression and bladder symptoms, and not due to the decline in motor scores [11]. NMS that fluctuate with levodopa response are also a major source of disability [37–39] and 17.5 to 30% of patients consider NMF more disabling than motor fluctuations [37,38]. Several studies on the QoL, usually including patients in all disease stages, show that NMS have a strong impact on QoL [39,73,74]. Although the NMS with the strongest impact on QoL may differ slightly between studies and according to disease stages, depression is almost always identified as one of the strongest predictors of worse QoL [31,39]. In studies including more advanced stage PD patients, the symptoms that more robustly contribute to QoL are dementia, depression, fatigue, daytime somnolence, gastrointestinal symptoms, orthostatic hypotension and urinary incontinence [23]. The disability from NMS in advanced PD may also impact on motor function [51]. In a cohort of 232 patients with a mean disease duration of 9 years at baseline and followed up over 8 years, excessive daytime somnolence and cognitive impairment at baseline were strong predictors of greater impairment in motor function and higher HY stage, respectively [51].

Disability milestones were defined by Kempster et al. [75] as symptoms of disease progression requiring additional medical attention. In two clinico-pathological studies, Kempster et al. found that four disability milestones (visual hallucinations, falls, dementia and institutionalization) clustered together in the later phase of PD, preceding death by 5 years on average [14,75]. This sequence of events appeared to be independent of age at PD onset, disease duration or age at death [14,75]. The authors found that visual hallucinations, falls, dementia and nursing home placement preceded death by 5.1, 4.1, 3.3 and 3.3 years, respectively [14].

Other studies have found that the strongest independent predictors of nursing home placement and death are postural instability and falls, dementia and hallucinations [6,13,28,29]. Concerning mortality, the symptoms most consistently correlated with an increased risk of death are dementia and postural instability [76,77]. More recently, a prospective study in PD with dementia and dementia with Lewy bodies found that persistent orthostatic hypotension was an independent predictor of shorter survival, and those with urinary incontinence and/or constipation had a poorer prognosis than patients with isolated orthostatic hypotension [78]. In a retrospective study, Willis et al. identified that, in addition to dementia, white men had an increased risk of death compared with female, Hispanic or Asian patients [76]. In a community-based study with 166 patients, demented patients with younger age at disease onset (55–74 years) had a shorter life expectancy than demented patients with older age at disease onset (>75 years) [77].

Caregiver burden

Caregivers of PD patients in the advanced stage report a high burden and a decreased QoL [79–81]. The presence of NMS is highly correlated with greater burden and worse QoL in caregivers [79–86]. A study of 80 patients and their caregivers (30 patients in HY Stage 3 or higher) found that the main predictors of caregiver burden were the caregiver's psychological well-being, patient mood, disability level and severity of PD, and QoL in both patients and caregivers [79]. The results of a postal survey of 123 caregivers (mean HY stage of patients = 2.6) showed that caregiver burden increased with the disability level of patients and the presence of depression, hallucinations, delirium and falls [81]. In addition to depression, the presence of cognitive impairment and dementia in patients was also correlated with higher psychosocial and total burden in caregivers [80,82,83,86]. In a somewhat different study assessing pre-death grief in the caregivers of PD patients, grief was significantly higher in caregivers whose relative had a more severe disease, and the presence of NMS had a slightly higher contribution to grief than motor symptoms [87].

Conclusion

Currently, the most widely accepted definition of advanced PD is based on the severity of motor symptoms, namely the onset of levodopa-induced motor complications. This definition does not take into account the incidence and severity of NMS, which have emerged as the main contributors to disability in advanced PD and should be incorporated into future staging classifications of PD. Moreover, NMS, and in particular hallucinations and dementia, have been consistently reported as strong predictors of hard outcomes in advanced disease, such as nursing home placement and mortality. In addition, NMS are among the major determinants of caregiver burden and poor QoL in advanced disease.

References

1 Braak H, Del Tredici K, Rub U, de Vos RA, Jansen Steur EN, Braak E. Staging of brain pathology related to sporadic Parkinson's disease. Neurobiol Aging 2003; **24**: 197–211.

2 Brooks DJ. Imaging non-dopaminergic function in Parkinson's disease. Mol Imaging Biol 2007; **9**: 217–22.

3 Martin WE, Loewenson RB, Resch JA, Baker AB. Parkinson's disease. Clinical analysis of 100 patients. Neurology 1973; **23**: 783–90.

4 Hoehn MM, Yahr MD. Parkinsonism: onset, progression and mortality. Neurology 1967; **17**: 427–42.

5 Coelho M, Ferreira JJ. Late-stage Parkinson disease. Nat Rev Neurol 2012; **8**: 435–42.

6 Hely MA, Morris JG, Reid WG, Trafficante R. Sydney Multicenter Study of Parkinson's disease: non-L-dopa-responsive problems dominate at 15 years. Mov Disord 2005; **20**: 190–9.

7 Goetz CG, Poewe W, Rascol O, et al. Movement Disorder Society Task Force report on the Hoehn and Yahr staging scale: status and recommendations. Mov Disord 2004; **19**: 1020–8.

8 Obeso JA, Rodriguez-Oroz MC, Chana P, Lera G, Rodriguez M, Olanow CW. The evolution and origin of motor complications in Parkinson's disease. Neurology 2000; **55**: S13–S20 [discussion S21–S23].

9 Schrag A, Quinn N. Dyskinesias and motor fluctuations in Parkinson's disease. A community-based study. Brain 2000; **123**: 2297–305.

10 Tolosa E, Katzenschlager K. Pharmacological management of Parkinson's disease. In: Jankovic J and Tolosa E (ed.) Parkinson's disease and movement disorders, pp. 110–45. Philadelphia: Lippincott Williams & Wilkins, 2007.

11 Schrag A, Dodel R, Spottke A, Bornschein B, Siebert U, Quinn NP. Rate of clinical progression in Parkinson's disease. A prospective study. Mov Disord 2007; **22**: 938–45.

12 Aarsland D, Larsen JP, Tandberg E, Laake K. Predictors of nursing home placement in Parkinson's disease: a population-based, prospective study. J Am Geriatr Soc 2000; **48**: 938–42.

13 Goetz CG, Stebbins GT. Risk factors for nursing home placement in advanced Parkinson's disease. Neurology 1993; **43**: 2227–9.

14 Kempster PA, O'Sullivan SS, Holton JL, Revesz T, Lees AJ. Relationships between age and late progression of Parkinson's disease: a clinico-pathological study. Brain 2010; **133**: 1755–62.

15 Coelho M, Marti MJ, Tolosa E, et al. Late-stage Parkinson's disease: the Barcelona and Lisbon cohort. J Neurol 2010; **257**: 1524–32.

16 Castrioto A, Lozano AM, Poon YY, Lang AE, Fallis M, Moro E. Ten-year outcome of subthalamic stimulation in Parkinson disease: a blinded evaluation. Arch Neurol 2011; **68**: 1550–6.

17 Hely MA, Reid WG, Adena MA, Halliday GM, Morris JG. The Sydney multicenter study of Parkinson's disease: the inevitability of dementia at 20 years. Mov Disord 2008; **23**: 837–44.

18 Papapetropoulos S, Mash DC. Motor fluctuations and dyskinesias in advanced/end stage Parkinson's disease: a study from a population of brain donors. J Neural Transm 2007; **114**: 341–5.

19 Barone P, Antonini A, Colosimo C, et al. The PRIAMO study: a multicenter assessment of nonmotor symptoms and their impact on quality of life in Parkinson's disease. Mov Disord 2009; **24**: 1641–9.

20 Khoo TK, Yarnall AJ, Duncan GW, et al. The spectrum of nonmotor symptoms in early Parkinson disease. Neurology 2013; **80**: 276–81.

21 Muller B, Larsen JP, Wentzel-Larsen T, Skeie GO, Tysnes OB. Autonomic and sensory symptoms and signs in incident, untreated Parkinson's disease: frequent but mild. Mov Disord 2011; **26**: 65–72.

22 Riedel O, Klotsche J, Spottke A, et al. Frequency of dementia, depression, and other neuropsychiatric symptoms in 1,449 outpatients with Parkinson's disease. J Neurol 2010; **257**: 1073–82.

23 Gallagher DA, Lees AJ, Schrag A. What are the most important nonmotor symptoms in patients with Parkinson's disease and are we missing them? Mov Disord 2010; **25**: 2493–500.

24 Berg D. Biomarkers for the early detection of Parkinson's and Alzheimer's disease. Neurodegener Dis 2008; **5**: 133–6.

25 Iranzo A, Molinuevo JL, Santamaria J, et al. Rapid-eye-movement sleep behaviour disorder as an early marker for a neurodegenerative disorder: a descriptive study. Lancet Neurol 2006; **5**: 572–7.

26 Postuma RB, Gagnon JF, Rompre S, Montplaisir JY. Severity of REM atonia loss in idiopathic REM sleep behavior disorder predicts Parkinson disease. Neurology 2010; **74**: 239–44.

27 Schrag A, Jahanshahi M, Quinn N. How does Parkinson's disease affect quality of life? A comparison with quality of life in the general population. Mov Disord 2000; **15**: 1112–18.

28 Forsaa EB, Larsen JP, Wentzel-Larsen T, Alves G. What predicts mortality in Parkinson disease?: a prospective population-based long-term study. Neurology 2010; **75**: 1270–6.

29 Buter TC, van den Hout A, Matthews FE, Larsen JP, Brayne C, Aarsland D. Dementia and survival in Parkinson disease: a 12-year population study. Neurology 2008; **70**: 1017–22.

30 Goetz CG, Stebbins GT. Mortality and hallucinations in nursing home patients with advanced Parkinson's disease. Neurology 1995; **45**: 669–71.

31 Hinnell C, Hurt CS, Landau S, Brown RG, Samuel M. Nonmotor versus motor symptoms: how much do they matter to health status in Parkinson's disease? Mov Disord 2012; **27**: 236–41.

32 Factor SA, Steenland NK, Higgins DS, et al. Disease-related and genetic correlates of psychotic symptoms in Parkinson's disease. Mov Disord 2011; **26**: 2190–5.

33 van Rooden SM, Visser M, Verbaan D, Marinus J, van Hilten JJ. Patterns of motor and non-motor features in Parkinson's disease. J Neurol Neurosurg Psychiatry 2009; **80**: 846–50.

34 Martinez-Martin P, Schapira AH, Stocchi F, et al. Prevalence of nonmotor symptoms in Parkinson's disease in an international setting; study using nonmotor symptoms questionnaire in 545 patients. Mov Disord 2007; **22**: 1623–9.

35 Chaudhuri KR, Martinez-Martin P, Schapira AH, et al. International multicenter pilot study of the first comprehensive self-completed nonmotor symptoms questionnaire for Parkinson's disease: the NMSQuest study. Mov Disord 2006; **21**: 916–23.

36 Chaudhuri KR, Martinez-Martin P, Brown RG, et al. The metric properties of a novel non-motor symptoms scale for Parkinson's disease: results from an international pilot study. Mov Disord 2007; **22**: 1901–11.

37 **Witjas T, Kaphan E, Azulay JP, et al**. Nonmotor fluctuations in Parkinson's disease: frequent and disabling. Neurology 2002; **59**: 408–13.

38 **Witjas T, Kaphan E, Regis J, et al**. Effects of chronic subthalamic stimulation on nonmotor fluctuations in Parkinson's disease. Mov Disord 2007; **22**: 1729–34.

39 **Storch A, Schneider CB, Wolz M, et al**. Nonmotor fluctuations in Parkinson disease: severity and correlation with motor complications. Neurology 2013; **80**: 800–9.

40 **Hwynn N, Haq IU, Malaty IA, et al**. The frequency of nonmotor symptoms among advanced Parkinson patients may depend on instrument used for assessment. Parkinsons Dis 2011; 2011: art. 290195.

41 **Hillen ME, Wagner ML, Sage JI**. 'Subclinical' orthostatic hypotension is associated with dizziness in elderly patients with Parkinson disease. Arch Phys Med Rehabil 1996; **77**: 710–12.

42 **Pedersen KF, Alves G, Aarsland D, Larsen JP**. Occurrence and risk factors for apathy in Parkinson disease: a 4-year prospective longitudinal study. J Neurol Neurosurg Psychiatry 2009; **80**: 1279–82.

43 **Aarsland D, Larsen JP, Cummins JL, Laake K**. Prevalence and clinical correlates of psychotic symptoms in Parkinson disease: a community-based study. Arch Neurol 1999; **56**: 595–601.

44 **Aarsland D, Larsen JP, Lim NG, et al**. Range of neuropsychiatric disturbances in patients with Parkinson's disease. J Neurol Neurosurg Psychiatry 1999; **67**: 492–6.

45 **Aarsland D, Marsh L, Schrag A**. Neuropsychiatric symptoms in Parkinson's disease. Mov Disord 2009; **24**: 2175–86.

46 **Auyeung M, Tsoi TH, Mok V, et al**. Ten year survival and outcomes in a prospective cohort of new onset Chinese Parkinson's disease patients. J Neurol Neurosurg Psychiatry 2012; **83**: 607–11.

47 **Merola A, Zibetti M, Angrisano S, et al**. Parkinson's disease progression at 30 years: a study of subthalamic deep brain-stimulated patients. Brain 2011; **134**: 2074–84.

48 **Shulman LM, Taback RL, Rabinstein AA, Weiner WJ**. Non-recognition of depression and other non-motor symptoms in Parkinson's disease. Parkinsonism Relat Disord 2002; **8**: 193–7.

49 **Chaudhuri KR, Prieto-Jurcynska C, Naidu Y, et al**. The nondeclaration of nonmotor symptoms of Parkinson's disease to health care professionals: an international study using the nonmotor symptoms questionnaire. Mov Disord 2010; **25**: 697–701.

50 **Hu M, Cooper J, Beamish R, et al**. How well do we recognise non-motor symptoms in a British Parkinson's disease population? J Neurol 2011; **258**: 1513–17.

51 **Alves G, Wentzel-Larsen T, Aarsland D, Larsen JP**. Progression of motor impairment and disability in Parkinson disease: a population-based study. Neurology 2005; **65**: 1436–41.

52 **Aarsland D, Andersen K, Larsen JP, et al**. The rate of cognitive decline in Parkinson disease. Arch Neurol 2004; **61**: 1906–11.

53 **Metta V, Logishetty K, Martinez-Martin P, et al**. The possible clinical predictors of fatigue in Parkinson's disease: a study of 135 patients as part of international nonmotor scale validation project. Parkinsons Dis 2011; 2011: art. 125271.

54 **Saez-Francas N, Hernandez-Vara J, Corominas Roso M, Alegre Martin J, Casas Brugue M**. The association of apathy with central fatigue perception in patients with Parkinson's disease. Behav Neurosci 2013; **127**: 237–44.

55 **Aarsland D, Andersen K, Larsen JP, Lolk A, Kragh-Sorensen P**. Prevalence and characteristics of dementia in Parkinson disease: an 8-year prospective study. Arch Neurol 2003; **60**: 387–92.

56 **Forsaa EB, Larsen JP, Wentzel-Larsen T, et al**. A 12-year population-based study of psychosis in Parkinson disease. Arch Neurol 2010; **67**: 996–1001.

57 **Dujardin K, Sockeel P, Delliaux M, Destee A, Defebvre L**. Apathy may herald cognitive decline and dementia in Parkinson's disease. Mov Disord 2009; **24**: 2391–7.

58 Damholdt MF, Borghammer P, Larsen L, Ostergaard K. Odor identification deficits identify Parkinson's disease patients with poor cognitive performance. Mov Disord 2011; **26**: 2045–50.

59 Morley JF, Weintraub D, Mamikonyan E, Moberg PJ, Siderowf AD, Duda JE. Olfactory dysfunction is associated with neuropsychiatric manifestations in Parkinson's disease. Mov Disord 2011; **26**: 2051–7.

60 Goldstein DS, Sewell L, Holmes C. Association of anosmia with autonomic failure in Parkinson disease. Neurology 2010; **74**: 245–51.

61 Baba T, Kikuchi A, Hirayama K, et al. Severe olfactory dysfunction is a prodromal symptom of dementia associated with Parkinson's disease: a 3 year longitudinal study. Brain 2012; **135**: 161–9.

62 Postuma RB, Bertrand JA, Montplaisir J, et al. Rapid eye movement sleep behavior disorder and risk of dementia in Parkinson's disease: a prospective study. Mov Disord 2012; **27**: 720–6.

63 Ratti PL, Terzaghi M, Minafra B, et al. REM and NREM sleep enactment behaviors in Parkinson's disease, Parkinson's disease dementia, and dementia with Lewy bodies. Sleep Med 2012; **13**: 926–32.

64 Boot BP, Boeve BF, Roberts RO, et al. Probable rapid eye movement sleep behavior disorder increases risk for mild cognitive impairment and Parkinson disease: a population-based study. Ann Neurol 2012; **71**: 49–56.

65 Romenets SR, Gagnon JF, Latreille V, et al. Rapid eye movement sleep behavior disorder and subtypes of Parkinson's disease. Mov Disord 2012; **27**: 996–1003.

66 Kagi G, Klein C, Wood NW, et al. Nonmotor symptoms in Parkin gene-related parkinsonism. Mov Disord 2010; **25**: 1279–84.

67 Doherty KM, Silveira-Moriyama L, Parkkinen L, et al. Parkin disease: a clinicopathologic entity? JAMA Neurol 2013; **70**: 571–9.

68 Marras C, Schule B, Munhoz RP, et al. Phenotype in parkinsonian and nonparkinsonian LRRK2 G2019S mutation carriers. Neurology 2011; **77**: 325–33.

69 Nalls MA, Duran R, Lopez G, et al. A multicenter study of glucocerebrosidase mutations in dementia with Lewy bodies. JAMA Neurol 2013; **70**: 727–35.

70 Brockmann K, Srulijes K, Hauser AK, et al. GBA-associated PD presents with nonmotor characteristics. Neurology 2011; **77**: 276–80.

71 Winder-Rhodes SE, Evans JR, Ban M, et al. Glucocerebrosidase mutations influence the natural history of Parkinson's disease in a community-based incident cohort. Brain 2013; **136**: 392–9.

72 Alcalay RN, Caccappolo E, Mejia-Santana H, et al. Cognitive performance of GBA mutation carriers with early-onset PD: the CORE-PD study. Neurology 2012; **78**: 1434–40.

73 Slawek J, Derejko M, Lass P. Factors affecting the quality of life of patients with idiopathic Parkinson's disease—a cross-sectional study in an outpatient clinic attendees. Parkinsonism Relat Disord 2005; **11**: 465–8.

74 Schrag A, Jahanshahi M, Quinn N. What contributes to quality of life in patients with Parkinson's disease? J Neurol Neurosurg Psychiatry 2000; **69**: 308–12.

75 Kempster PA, Williams DR, Selikhova M, Holton J, Revesz T, Lees AJ. Patterns of levodopa response in Parkinson's disease: a clinico-pathological study. Brain 2007; **130**: 2123–8.

76 Willis AW, Schootman M, Kung N, Evanoff BA, Perlmutter JS, Racette BA. Predictors of survival in patients with Parkinson disease. Arch Neurol 2012; **69**: 601–7.

77 Hobson P, Meara J, Ishihara-Paul L. The estimated life expectancy in a community cohort of Parkinson's disease patients with and without dementia, compared with the UK population. J Neurol Neurosurg Psychiatry 2010; **81**: 1093–8.

78 Stubendorff K, Aarsland D, Minthon L, Londos E. The impact of autonomic dysfunction on survival in patients with dementia with Lewy bodies and Parkinson's disease with dementia. PLoS One 2012; **7**: e45451.

79 **Martinez-Martin P, Forjaz MJ, Frades-Payo B, et al.** Caregiver burden in Parkinson's disease. Mov Disord 2007; 22: 924–31 [quiz 1060].

80 **Thommessen B, Aarsland D, Braekhus A, Oksengaard AR, Engedal K, Laake K.** The psychosocial burden on spouses of the elderly with stroke, dementia and Parkinson's disease. Int J Geriatr Psychiatry 2002; 17: 78–84.

81 **Schrag A, Hovris A, Morley D, Quinn N, Jahanshahi M.** Caregiver-burden in Parkinson's disease is closely associated with psychiatric symptoms, falls, and disability. Parkinsonism Relat Disord 2006; 12: 35–41.

82 **Leroi I, McDonald K, Pantula H, Harbishettar V.** Cognitive impairment in Parkinson disease: impact on quality of life, disability, and caregiver burden. J Geriatr Psychiatry Neurol 2012; 25: 208–14.

83 **Shin H, Youn J, Kim JS, Lee JY, Cho JW.** Caregiver burden in Parkinson disease with dementia compared to Alzheimer disease in Korea. J Geriatr Psychiatry Neurol 2012; 25: 222–6.

84 **Cupidi C, Realmuto S, Lo Coco G, et al.** Sleep quality in caregivers of patients with Alzheimer's disease and Parkinson's disease and its relationship to quality of life. Int Psychogeriatr 2012; 24: 1827–35.

85 **O'Connor EJ,.McCabe MP.** Predictors of quality of life in carers for people with a progressive neurological illness: a longitudinal study. Qual Life Res 2011; 20: 703–11.

86 **Stella F, Banzato CE, Quagliato EM, Viana MA, Christofoletti G.** Psychopathological features in patients with Parkinson's disease and related caregivers' burden. Int J Geriatr Psychiatry 2009; 24: 1158–65.

87 **Carter JH, Lyons KS, Lindauer A, Malcom J.** Pre-death grief in Parkinson's caregivers: a pilot survey-based study. Parkinsonism Relat Disord 2012; 18(Suppl 3): S15–S18.

Chapter 5

Assessment tools for non-motor symptoms of Parkinson's disease in the clinical setting

Pablo Martinez-Martin, Carmen Rodriguez-Blazquez and Maria João Forjaz

Background

Parkinson's disease (PD) is a complex neurodegenerative disease traditionally characterized as a motor disorder with bradykinesia, rigidity, tremor and gait and postural abnormalities. However, more recently, non-motor symptoms (NMS) have emerged as an important part of the clinical spectrum of PD. NMS of PD may precede the onset of motor features and tend to become more prevalent with advancing disease.

In PD, the range of NMS includes neuropsychiatric (dementia, depression, apathy, compulsive behaviour), sleep-related (insomnia, vivid dreaming, daytime hypersomnia), autonomic (gastrointestinal, bladder, sexual, cardiovascular, thermoregulatory dysfunction) and sensory (pain, paraesthesias, restless legs syndrome, anosmia, visual disturbances) symptoms [1]. Over time, NMS make an important contribution to disability and restrict the patient's social role and activities, therefore affecting health-related quality of life.

For decades, research has focused on the motor disturbances, but recent awareness of the importance of NMS in PD has attracted increasing interest from researchers. If research is to develop in this area there is a need for sound clinimetric instruments to detect and evaluate NMS in PD.

Clinimetric characteristics of measurement instruments

The selection of a measurement instrument is an important step in the design of a study and may even determine the chance of success. Prior to using a measurement or screening instrument in PD research, information on validity and reliability for its use in this setting should be available. The clinimetric qualities of a scale have important implications for the sample size, the assessment tools and costs associated with a study.

To obtain accurate information using a measurement instrument, it needs to fulfil certain clinimetric requirements. Although such attributes as acceptability, scaling assumptions and precision should be taken into account, the most important criteria are validity, reliability and responsiveness. Validity is the extent to which an instrument measures what it is purported to measure. Reliability is the extent to which a measurement instrument is free from measurement error. Responsiveness relates to an instrument's sensitivity to detect changes.

To determine the quality of screening tools, sensitivity, specificity and predictive values should be tested.

Developments in instruments for assessing NMS in Parkinson's disease

Previously, non-specific measures were used to assess some NMS domains (such as sleep, mood and cognition), unsupported by appropriate validation studies in people with PD. In the last decade, however, several initiatives [Scales for Outcomes in PD (SCOPA); Non-Motor Symptoms Group (NMSG); and the Movement Disorder Society (MDS), with the MDS-sponsored Unified Parkinson's Disease Rating Scale (MDS-UPDRS)] have developed a set of specific measures of NMS for application in clinical practice and research.

This chapter aims to briefly review the most relevant instruments that have been used in PD and to provide information about their clinimetric properties in this population.

Assessment instruments for NMS in Parkinson's disease

Screening questionnaires

The NMSG (<http://www.pdnmg.com>) has developed the NMS Questionnaire (NM-SQuest), a self-administered screening tool to detect the presence of NMS and initiate further investigation [1]. It consists of 30 items, in nine domains [2], derived from experiences of the members of the NMSG and nurse specialists, published literature, patient group responses, results from a survey of over 1000 patients and caregivers carried out in the UK and a hospital-based survey. The instrument has demonstrated good feasibility and validity in an international scenario and can be used during routine consultations to flag symptoms needing attention. In addition, it may be useful for epidemiological studies [2].

A MDS Task Force for revision of the UPDRS has developed a new format for the evaluation of PD [3]. The new MDS-UPDRS includes a section for assessment of the non-motor experiences of daily life. This section is mainly intended to screen for the presence of NMS and not for a detailed assessment of NMS. When NMS are identified, the use of specific scales that can properly assess this topic is recommended.

The NMS Scale

The NMS Scale is a specific scale for comprehensive evaluation of NMS developed by the NMSG [4,5]. It is a 30-item instrument, clinician-rated by interview, that explores nine domains (cardiovascular, sleep/fatigue, mood/cognition, perceptual problems/hallucinations, attention/memory, gastrointestinal, urinary, sexual and miscellaneous). Items are scored for frequency and severity, and a total sum may be obtained for the domain and for the whole scale. The results of its clinimetric testing were satisfactory, and the correlation between NMSQuest and the NMS Scale was high [4,5].

Domain-specific rating scales

Cognitive impairment and dementia

In PD, cognitive impairment may occur early in the disease course and is a predictor of dementia. Prevalence data for dementia have varied between 20 and 40%, underscoring that dementia in PD is more frequent than in the general population [6,7]. Consensus regarding the characteristics and criteria of dementia [7] and mild cognitive impairment [8] associated with PD has been reached. The most characteristic cognitive disturbances associated with PD (PDD) include: impaired attention, memory and verbal fluency; executive and visuospatial dysfunction; and personality change and behavioural disorders.

A wide diversity of tests has been used for assessment of cognition in PD, with two different aims: (1) to screen and globally evaluate cognitive impairment; (2) to evaluate the impairment in specific neuropsychological areas. It is important to consider that, in general, instruments used to evaluate cognitive function in PD have a bias towards the more cortical functions and include items that are sensitive to the motor impairment of PD. Additionally, as motor fluctuations may influence cognitive functioning, it is recommended that tests to evaluate cognition in PD are administered during the 'on' phase.

Generic assessments

- The Mini-Mental State Examination (MMSE) [9], derived from previously existing cognitive instruments, is very frequently used for screening and evaluating the severity of cognitive dysfunction in PD, and has shown satisfactory results when applied in parallel with other measures. However, the MMSE is not a specific instrument for PDD and has been considered inappropriate for use in PD due to the high proportion of items focused on cortical cognitive aspects and the fact that two items are sensitive to motor impairments. Additionally, it does not adequately assess executive and visuospatial functions, which are typically deteriorated in PD.

- The Mattis Dementia Rating Scale (DRS) [10] was developed as a brief test to assess cognitive impairment caused by neurological disease. A revised version to clarify ambiguous scoring situations and to simplify the administration is preferred by many researchers [11]. It includes five subscales: attention, initiation/perseveration, construction, conceptualization and memory. The DRS is widely used in PD studies, a setting where it is considered very useful due to the inclusion of items exploring executive dysfunction. It is considered valid for screening of PDD.

- The Montreal Cognitive Assessment (MoCA) [12] aims to assess mild cognitive impairment in the general population. It is formed by 12 items, assessing short-term memory recall, visuospatial abilities, executive functions, attention, concentration and working memory, language and orientation. The MoCA has been considered the most suitable measure for cognitive screening in clinical trials of PD [13].

Disease-specific assessments

◆ The Parkinson's Disease Cognitive Rating Scale (PD-CRS) [14] was designed to assess the frontal-subcortical and instrumental cortical functions in PD at all levels of severity. It has good psychometric abilities, and it discriminates between intact cognition, mild cognitive impairment and dementia in PD patients. However, there is little information about the scale's responsiveness.

◆ Mini-Mental Parkinson (MMP) [15]. Derived from the Folstein MMSE, the MMP was specifically designed for the screening of cognitive disorders in PD. However, the scale has rarely been used and has not been independently validated. Several important metric properties (internal consistency, stability, responsiveness) have never been tested.

◆ Scales for Outcomes in Parkinson's Disease—Cognition (SCOPA-COG) [16]. This scale was specifically designed to assess the cognitive domains that are most vulnerable to PD (memory, attention, executive functions and visuospatial functions). The scale does not cover cortical aspects of cognition and is designed to measure the severity of cognitive impairment, not for screening or diagnostic purposes. In advanced dementia, the instrument has a limited usefulness. The scientific qualities of the SCOPA-COG have been established by independent studies. As with all instruments that assess cognition, age and education are important factors to take into account. In view of population differences, cutoff values have to be established against the background of the differences in educational levels.

SCOPA-COG is easy to apply and provides an evaluation of severity. The MoCA is recommended as a cognitive screening measure for clinical trials. DRS is valid for screening, but the length (36 items) may be an obstacle for use in daily practice. The MMSE may complete the evaluation of cortical aspects.

Impairment of specific neuropsychological areas

A variety of neuropsychological tests has been applied to PD patients in order to determine the impairment of specific areas which may be affected as a consequence of the structural and functional changes. A list of these instruments is displayed in Table 5.1.

Depression Rating scales for depression have been recently reviewed by the MDS Task Force [17]. This is a high-quality report and readers are therefore referred to this article and its complementary information, accessible from the corresponding website of the journal. The following are most commonly used:

◆ The Hamilton Depression Scale (Ham-D) [18] is administered by a clinician and is probably the most used measure to evaluate the severity of depression, but it covers DSM-IV criteria incompletely and contains a high proportion of somatic items which overlap with PD manifestations. There are several versions (17, 21 and 24 items). It has been used for evaluation of severity and screening of depression in PD.

◆ The Beck Depression Inventory (BDI) [19]. There are several versions of this widely used instrument. It may be administered by an interviewer but is more commonly used

Table 5.1 Some tests used for assessment of specific cognitive aspects in Parkinson's disease

Cognitive/functional area	Test
Pre-morbid estimate of intelligence	National Adult Reading Test (NART)
	Wechsler Test of Adult Reading (WTAR)
Language	Verbal Comprehensive Index of the Wechsler Adult Intelligence Scale (WAIS-III)
	Phoneme and category fluency
Attention/concentration/ working memory	Trail Making Test (Part A)
	Letter Number Sequencing from WAIS-III
	Stroop Colour and Word Test
Verbal memory	Rey Auditory Verbal Learning Test
	Buschke Selective Reminding Test
Visual-spatial memory	Benton Visual Retention Test
	Cambridge Neuropsychological Test Automated Battery (CANTAB)
Visual-spatial function	CANTAB
	Mental Rotations Test (MRT)
	Clock Drawing Test
	Procedural and Associative Learning (CANTAB)
Executive function	Trail Making Test (Part B)
	Controlled Oral Word Association test (COWA)
	CANTAB
	Delis–Kaplan Executive Function Scale (DKEFS)
Behavioural changes	Frontal Assessment Battery (FAB)
	Mach IV scale

for self-assessment. The most common version contains 21 items related to emotions, behaviour and somatic symptoms. It may be used for depression screening and for evaluation of severity, and is widely used in PD.

◆ The Zung Self-Rating Depression Scale (SDS) [20] is a 20-item self-administered scale which assesses the frequency with which respondents experience the symptoms or feelings related to affective, somatic, psychomotor and psychological disturbances. The SDS is used both for screening and for measurement of the severity of depression. Information about the use of SDS in dementia is not available. It is only partially validated for use in PD, but it has shown acceptable performance in this setting.

◆ The Montgomery–Åsberg Depression Rating Scale (MADRS) [21] is composed of 10 items. Administered by interview, it assesses the severity of depression and was specifically designed to be responsive. In PD it has been validated for screening. It contains some somatic and neurovegetative symptoms. The MADRS is a very commonly used measure in clinical trials for depression.

◆ The Hospital Anxiety and Depression Scale (HADS) [22] is a self-assessment scale that includes a seven-item subscale for the detection of depression. It is mainly focused on anhedonia, is relatively free of somatic symptoms, but does not include some important components of depression. This scale is best used for screening purposes.

Other scales including the Geriatric Depression Scale (GDS), the Cornell Scale for Depression in Dementia and the Centre for Epidemiologic Studies Depression Scale are potentially useful. The MDS Task Force recommendations are: selection of the scale is dependent on the objectives of the study; observer-rated scales are preferred; for screening purposes, the Ham-D, BDI, HADS, MADRS and GDS are considered appropriate; and for evaluation of severity, the Ham-D, MADRS, BDI and SDS are recommended [17].

Anxiety Instruments for detection and evaluation of anxiety in PD have been reviewed by the MDS Task Force [23]. That report forms the basis for comments in this section. Anxiety has not been extensively studied in PD but is almost as prevalent as depression. Panic disorder is the most frequent anxiety disorder in PD. Anxiety can overlap with depression and with physical symptoms of PD. Scales include:

- The Hamilton Anxiety Rating Scale (HARS) [24]. There are several versions of this clinician-rated scale, but the 14- and 15-item versions are most often used. Designed to measure the severity of anxiety, it contains a high proportion of somatic items. Psychic and somatic anxiety scores may be separately obtained. Some psychometric attributes have never been tested in PD patients.

- The Spielberger State Trait Anxiety Inventory (STAI) [25]. There are two versions, the original one (STAI-X) and the reviewed version (STAI-Y). It is a self-administered scale for evaluation of severity of anxiety. It contains two parts (state and trait), each containing 20 items addressing somatic, affective and cognitive aspects.

- The Zung Self-rating Anxiety Scale (SAS) and the Anxiety Status Inventory (ASI) [26] contain two parts, SAS (self-rated) and ASI (clinician-rated) which can be administered independently. Each scale consists of 20 items that are moderately correlated with each other. Some items overlap with somatic PD symptoms. It is an evaluative instrument, with acceptable psychometric properties.

- The HADS [22], a subscale for screening of anxiety, is self-administered and contains seven items (referring to panic and generalized anxiety). It does not include physical or cognitive symptoms of anxiety. This scale has been mainly used for screening purposes.

The MDS Task Force also reviewed the Beck Anxiety Inventory and item 5 (anxiety) of the Neuropsychiatric Inventory (NPI). The reviewed scales are not recommended due to the overlap with constructs different to anxiety, weak criterion-related validity, or lack of adequate clinimetric information [23].

Apathy Apathy is a frequent manifestation of PD, but it has received little attention, probably due to an overlap with depression, anhedonia and dementia. Nevertheless, some scales are available to assess apathy in PD and they were the object of a review of the MDS Task Force [27]:

- The Apathy Scale (AS) [28] is a version of the Apathy Evaluation Scale (AES) [29] specifically designed for screening and assessment of severity of apathy in PD patients. It is a 14-item scale that can be rated by the patient or the caregiver. It is easy to use, with satisfactory psychometric properties and sensitivity to change. A cutoff score of 14 or more indicates clinically meaningful apathy. The scale cannot be used in PD patients with dementia or low insight. The AS is a recommended instrument for the assessment of apathy in PD [27].

- The Lille Apathy Rating Scale (LARS) [30] was developed for screening and evaluation of severity of apathy in PD. The scale consists of 33 items, grouped in nine dimensions, and is administered by structured interview. A caregiver-based version has also been developed, with good psychometric characteristics and high correlation with the self-reported version. Although the LARS is the longest scale for apathy, it is applied in around 10 minutes on average. It has been validated in the recent years and applied to PD patients, even in advanced stages of the disease.

Other tools for assessing apathy in PD are the Apathy Inventory [31], which has been the object of a study of adaptation and validation, and item 7 (apathy) of the Neuropsychiatric Inventory.

Anhedonia Anhedonia is frequent in PD. It is mostly considered a symptom lacking a precise definition, and may be related to and confounded with depression and apathy. A review of the instruments applied to measure anhedonia in PD has been carried out by the MDS Task Force [27]:

- The Snaith–Hamilton Pleasure Scale (SHAPS) [32] is a self-administered, 14-item scale developed for rapid and simple evaluation of anhedonia. It has been used for assessment of anhedonia in PD, but has some overlap with symptoms of parkinsonism. The MDS Task Force considered that SHAPS may be suggested for use in PD. Since then, several studies have reported on psychometric properties in PD patients, but the information furnished in these studies is still insufficient to allow recommendation of the SHAPS in this setting.

The Chapman scales for physical and social anhedonia [33] were also reviewed but were found to be too complex and are not recommended in PD.

Psychotic symptoms Hallucinations and delusions are more frequent in older and severely affected patients. Hallucinations, mainly visual, are the most frequent manifestation and may be also present in earlier phases of disease. In this case, they might be associated with dopaminergic treatment. Psychotic symptoms are a consistent feature of PDD. A review of the scales for assessing psychosis in PD performed by the MDS Task Force has been published [34]. None of the reviewed scales adequately covered the full spectrum of PD psychosis:

- The Parkinson Psychiatric Rating Scale (PPRS) [35] is the first specific instrument to be developed for evaluation of the severity of psychotic manifestations related to PD. The quality of tested clinimetric attributes is satisfactory, but the scale exhibits problems with content validity and consistency of response options, and thus it has been designated as 'suggested' by the MDS Task Force.

- The SCOPA-Psychiatric Complications (SCOPA-PC) [36] questionnaire was developed to improve the items of the PPRS, adding an item on compulsive behaviour in PD to the latter scale. The SCOPA-PC is a reliable, valid, easily administered semi-structured questionnaire for both psychotic and compulsive complications in PD.

The MDS Task Force has recommended the use of several non-PD specific psychosis scales, such as the NPI, the Brief Psychiatric Rating Scale (BPRS), the Positive and Negative Syndrome Scale (PANSS) and the Schedule for Assessment of Positive Symptoms (SAPS). All of them have been applied in PD and have demonstrated good clinimetric characteristics. A 12-item specific scale, the Scale for Evaluation of Neuropsychiatric Disorders in PD (SEND-PD) [37] has been recently developed and validated with promising results, but there is a lack further studies confirming the findings.

Sleep disorders and excessive daytime sleepiness Nighttime sleep problems (NSP) may occur in up to 80% of patients with PD [38]. In PD, NSP mainly relate to difficulties with maintaining sleep, whereas problems with falling asleep generally are no different from elderly subjects without PD. Rapid eye movement (REM) sleep behaviour disorder (RBD), which is characterized by the loss of muscle atonia and the presence of complex motor behaviours during REM sleep, has received considerable attention. RBD has been found in 15–34% of PD patients [39]. Excessive daytime sleepiness (EDS) affects up to 50% of PD patients [40]. NSP and EDS have a significant influence on the well-being of patients and their partners.

There are many generic instruments available for assessing sleep disorders and EDS, two of which have been used regularly in PD: the Pittsburgh Sleep Quality Index (PSQI) and the Epworth Sleepiness Scale (ESS). More recently, two disease-specific sleep scales have become available (the Parkinson's Disease Sleep Scale and SCOPA-Sleep). The MDS Task Force has published its criticisms and recommended scales [41]:

- The PSQI [42] is a 19-item self-completed scale which evaluates the presence and severity of sleep disturbances over the previous month. Frequently used in PD, it has shown good psychometric properties. It is a recommended by the MDS Task Force as a screening tool for overall sleep impairment and as a measure of severity, although the PSQI has serious problems with content validity for its use in PD and is of limited usefulness in patients with dementia.

- The ESS [43] comprises eight items and is a commonly used self-rated scale that evaluates the chance of dozing off without actually having to have had experience with that particular situation. It has been validated in PD patients with good results, but some items may actually be experienced infrequently by the most severely affected or older patients. The MDS Task Force has recommended its use as a screening instrument.

- The Parkinson's Disease Sleep Scale (PDSS) [44] was the first specifically developed instrument for self-evaluation of nocturnal sleep in PD. The timeframe of assessment is the past week. The patient's response to each item is marked on a 10-cm visual analogue scale. All PDSS items are focused on nocturnal sleep disturbances, except item 15 which is about daytime sleepiness. The PDSS also includes questions concerning potential causes of sleep disturbances. Hence the total score reflects three constructs, namely sleep disturbance, its causes and daytime sleepiness. The reliability of the PDSS has been shown to be good [45]. It has been applied in several studies and independently validated, and thus is recommended by the MDS Task Force for the screening and assessment of severity of sleep disorders in PD. The PDSS has been revised and validated (PDSS-2) [46], and now includes an extended spectrum of nocturnal disabilities and a five-category response option.

◆ SCOPA-Sleep [47] was developed for clinical practice and research and consists of two parts. The NSP subscale addresses the past month and includes five items assessing sleep initiation, sleep fragmentation, sleep efficiency, sleep duration and early wakening. One additional question evaluates overall sleep quality and is used separately as a global measure of sleep quality. The Daytime Sleepiness (DS) subscale evaluates DS in the past month and includes six items. Subjects indicate how often they fell asleep unexpectedly, fell asleep in particular situations (while sitting peacefully, while watching television or reading, or while talking to someone), how often they had difficulty staying awake and whether falling asleep in the daytime was considered a problem. SCOPA-Sleep has a good validity and reliability and is recommended by the MDS Task Force.

Reliable detection of RBD is carried out by polysomnography. The RBD Screening Questionnaire (RBDSQ) [48] has been used in PD patients with RBD. It appears useful as a screening tool, but lacks an adequate validation study and poorly discriminates RBD from other disorders, such as sleepwalking or epilepsy.

Fatigue Fatigue is present in 33–58% of PD patients. It is a disabling symptom which has received relatively little attention until very recently. Assessment of fatigue is a difficult task because it is essentially subjective in nature and unspecific. It overlaps and is easily confounded with depression, apathy and sleepiness. The MDS Task Force review of fatigue rating scales [49] identified several tools for screening or severity rating:

◆ The Fatigue Severity Scale (FSS) [50] is a generic unidimensional scale with nine items assessing the functional impact of physical and mental fatigue. Its brevity and ease of administration, its applicability throughout the different disease stages, good clinimetric properties and sensitivity to change make it a recommended scale for screening and severity of fatigue in PD.

◆ The Multidimensional Fatigue Inventory (MFI) [51] is a generic 20-item self-reported instrument assessing the severity of physical and mental fatigue. Its usefulness in PD patients has been proved, with good clinimetric properties and sensitivity to change. It has been recommended by the MDS Task Force.

◆ The Functional Assessment of Chronic Illness Therapy-Fatigue Scale (FACIT-F) [52]. was originally developed for oncology patients. It has been used in PD studies, although further replication studies and more information on its sensitivity to change are needed. The MDS Task Force recommends its use as a screening tool.

- The Parkinson Fatigue Scale (PFS) [53] is the first specific measure for fatigue in PD. It is a 16-item scale focused on the physical aspects of fatigue and their impact on patient functioning. Its authors deliberately excluded emotional and cognitive features because they may occur independently of fatigue in the PD setting. In the original article, satisfactory clinimetric properties were found and cutoff points for the presence of and limitations due to fatigue are suggested. The MDS Task Force has classified the PFS as recommended for severity rating and screening purposes.

Other non-specific scales which have been applied for assessment of fatigue in PD are, for instance, the Fatigue Impact Scale for Daily Use (D-FIS), the Fatigue Assessment Inventory, the Rhoten Fatigue Scale and visual analogue scales. Some of these scales have not been validated for use in PD patients or the validation data are incomplete [54].

Autonomic dysfunction Symptoms and signs of autonomic dysfunction in PD may include cardiovascular, gastrointestinal, urinary, thermoregulatory, pupillomotor and sexual dysfunction. The reported prevalence of the various autonomic symptoms in PD varies greatly between studies (14–80%), and symptoms tend to increase with advancing disease. Several features of autonomic dysfunction are evaluated with specific objective tests (e.g. barium swallow videofluoroscopy in the case of dysphagia, oesophageal and anorectal manometry for gastrointestinal dysfunction, urodynamic assessment, etc.) and scales (Table 5.2), but it is beyond the scope of the present chapter to address all these tests. A review of scales for assessing of sialorrhoea, dysphagia and constipation [55] and orthostatic hypotension [56] has been carried out by the MDS Task Force:

- SCOPA-Autonomic (SCOPA-AUT) [57] was the first specific, reliable and valid instrument that covered the full spectrum of autonomic dysfunction in PD. It was designed after consulting medical specialists and patients. The questionnaire is self-completed by patients and addresses 25 items assessing the following domains: gastrointestinal, urinary, cardiovascular, thermoregulatory, pupillomotor and sexual dysfunction. Full validation studies, including Rasch analysis [58] have been published. The MDS Task Force has designed SCOPA-AUT as a recommended scale, although with some limitations [55,56].

Table 5.2 Some scales used for assessment of specific autonomic dysfunctions in Parkinson's disease (PD)

Autonomic domain	Instrument
Drooling/sialorrhoea	Extensive Drooling Questionnaire Sialorrhea Clinical Scale for PD
Dysphagia	Swallowing Disturbance Questionnaire
Pelvic organ dysfunction	Questionnaire on Pelvic Organ Function
Bladder dysfunction	Overactive Bladder Questionnaire Lower urinary tract symptoms
Constipation	Cleveland Constipation Score

◆ The Composite Autonomic Symptom Scale (COMPASS) [59] comprises nine domains of autonomic dysfunction. The orthostatic section, including nine items, has been reviewed by the MDS Task Force [56] and deemed as recommended with limitations.

The NMS Scale [4] and the NMS Questionnaire [1] contain several questions assessing a variety of autonomic symptoms. Both are recommended by the MDS Task Force [55]. Several scales have been used to evaluate a specific subdomain of autonomic dysfunction in PD (Table 5.2). However, these scales have rarely been subjected to elaborate clinimetric evaluation procedures for use in PD or have assessed only some aspects of reliability or validity.

Pain A pain prevalence of between 38 and 50% has been found in PD. Pain among PD patients may be primary (central) or associated with musculosketal or radicular/neuritic disorders or dystonic features. Although pain is a direct cause of suffering and deterioration in quality of life, it has received relatively little attention in PD. Studies in this setting have used generic measures, such as visual analogue scales, pain charts, the Brief Pain Inventory [60] or the McGill Pain Questionnaire [61]. To our knowledge, no validation studies have been carried out for the specific application of these scales in PD.

Future developments

A wide diversity of instruments has been used for the detection and evaluation of NMS. For many of these NMS, which are frequently present in non-PD patients (e.g. depression, anxiety, fatigue, pain, insomnia, restless legs), assessment instruments were available before they were applied to people with PD. Subsequently, these instruments were used in PD, frequently without a formal validation in this population. Mostly in the last decade researchers have assessed the validity of these measures or developed specific tools for the assessment of NMS in PD. In the coming years it is very likely that more valid instruments will be developed in response to the needs of clinical practice and research. Scales that broadly cover NMS as well as symptom-specific scales will allow the collection of valuable information about the course of NMS over time and determine the effect of therapies.

References

1 **Chaudhuri KR, Martinez-Martin P, Schapira AHV, et al**. International multicenter pilot study of the first comprehensive self-completed nonmotor symptoms questionnaire for Parkinson's disease: the NMSQuest study. Mov Disord 2006; **21**: 916–23.

2 **Martinez-Martin P, Schapira AHV, Stocchi F, et al**. Prevalence of nonmotor symptoms in Parkinson's disease in an international setting; study using nonmotor symptoms questionnaire in 545 patients. Mov Disord 2007; **22**: 1623–9.

3 **Goetz CG, Tilley BC, Shaftman SR, et al**. Movement Disorder Society-sponsored revision of the Unified Parkinson's Disease Rating Scale (MDS-UPDRS): scale presentation and clinimetric testing results. Mov Disord 2008; **23**: 2129–70.

4 **Chaudhuri KR, Martinez-Martin P, Brown RG, et al**. The metric properties of a novel non-motor symptoms scale for Parkinson's disease: results from an international pilot study. Mov Disord 2007; **22**: 1901–11.

5 Martinez-Martin P, Rodriguez-Blazquez C, Abe K, et al. International study on the psychometric attributes of the non-motor symptoms scale in Parkinson disease. Neurology 2009; **73**: 1584–91.

6 Aarsland D, Andersen K, Larsen JP, Lolk A, Nielsen H, Kragh-Sørensen P. Risk of dementia in Parkinson's disease: a community-based, prospective study. Neurology 2001; **56**: 730–6.

7 Emre M, Aarsland D, Brown R, et al. Clinical diagnostic criteria for dementia associated with Parkinson's disease. Mov Disord 2007; 22: 1689–707 [quiz 1837].

8 Litvan I, Goldman JG, Tröster AI, et al. Diagnostic criteria for mild cognitive impairment in Parkinson's disease: Movement Disorder Society Task Force guidelines. Mov Disord 2012; **27**: 349–56.

9 Folstein MF, Folstein SE, McHugh PR. «Mini-mental state». A practical method for grading the cognitive state of patients for the clinician. J Psychiatr Res 1975; **12**: 189–98.

10 Mattis S. Mental status examination for organic mental syndrome in the elderly patient. In: Geriatric psychiatry: a handbook for psychiatrists and primary care physicians, pp. 77–121. New York: Grune and Stratton, 1976.

11 Johnson-Greene D. Dementia Rating Scale-2 (DRS-2). Arch Clin Neuropsychol 2004; **19**: 145–7.

12 Nasreddine ZS, Phillips NA, Bédirian V, et al. The Montreal Cognitive Assessment, MoCA: a brief screening tool for mild cognitive impairment. J Am Geriatr Soc 2005; **53**: 695–9.

13 Chou KL, Amick MM, Brandt J, et al. A recommended scale for cognitive screening in clinical trials of Parkinson's disease. Mov Disord 2010; **25**: 2501–7.

14 Pagonabarraga J, Kulisevsky J, Llebaria G, García-Sánchez C, Pascual-Sedano B, Gironell A. Parkinson's disease-cognitive rating scale: a new cognitive scale specific for Parkinson's disease. Mov Disord 2008; **23**: 998–1005.

15 Mahieux F, Michelet D, Manifacier M-J, Boller F, Fermanian J, Guillard A. Mini-Mental Parkinson: first validation study of a new bedside test constructed for Parkinson's disease. Behav Neurol 1995; **8**: 15–22.

16 Marinus J, Visser M, Verwey NA, et al. Assessment of cognition in Parkinson's disease. Neurology 2003; **61**: 1222–8.

17 Schrag A, Barone P, Brown RG, et al. Depression rating scales in Parkinson's disease: critique and recommendations. Mov Disord 2007; **22**: 1077–92.

18 Hamilton M. A rating scale for depression. J Neurol Neurosurg Psychiatry 1960; **23**: 56–62.

19 Beck AT, Ward CH, Mendelson M, Mock J, Erbaugh J. An inventory for measuring depression. Arch Gen Psychiatry 1961; **4**: 561–71.

20 Zung WW. A self-rating depression scale. Arch Gen Psychiatry 1965; **12**: 63–70.

21 Montgomery SA, Åsberg M. A new depression scale designed to be sensitive to change. Br J Psychiatry 1979; **134**: 382–9.

22 Zigmond AS, Snaith RP. The hospital anxiety and depression scale. Acta Psychiatr Scand 1983; **67**: 361–70.

23 Leentjens AFG, Dujardin K, Marsh L, et al. Anxiety rating scales in Parkinson's disease: critique and recommendations. Mov Disord 2008; **23**: 2015–25.

24 Hamilton M. The assessment of anxiety states by rating. Br J Med Psychol 1959; **32**: 50–5.

25 Spielberger C, Gorsuch R, Lushene R. Manual for the state-trait inventory. Palo Alto, CA: Consulting Psychology Press, 1970.

26 Zung WW. A rating instrument for anxiety disorders. Psychosomatics 1971; **12**: 371–9.

27 Leentjens AFG, Dujardin K, Marsh L, et al. Apathy and anhedonia rating scales in Parkinson's disease: critique and recommendations. Mov Disord 2008; **23**: 2004–14.

28 Starkstein SE, Mayberg HS, Preziosi TJ, Andrezejewski P, Leiguarda R, Robinson RG. Reliability, validity, and clinical correlates of apathy in Parkinson's disease. J Neuropsychiatry Clin Neurosci 1992;4:134–9.

29 Marin RS, Biedrzycki RC, Firinciogullari S. Reliability and validity of the Apathy Evaluation Scale. Psychiatry Res 1991;**38**:143–62.

30 Sockeel P, Dujardin K, Devos D, Denève C, Destée A, Defebvre L. The Lille apathy rating scale (LARS), a new instrument for detecting and quantifying apathy: validation in Parkinson's disease. J Neurol Neurosurg Psychiatry 2006; **77**: 579–84.

31 Robert PH, Clairet S, Benoit M, et al. The apathy inventory: assessment of apathy and awareness in Alzheimer's disease, Parkinson's disease and mild cognitive impairment. Int J Geriatr Psychiatry 2002; **17**: 1099–105.

32 Snaith RP, Hamilton M, Morley S, Humayan A, Hargreaves D, Trigwell P. A scale for the assessment of hedonic tone the Snaith–Hamilton Pleasure Scale. Br J Psychiatry 1995; **167**: 99–103.

33 Chapman LJ, Chapman JP, Raulin ML. Scales for physical and social anhedonia. J Abnorm Psychol 1976; **85**: 374–82.

34 Fernandez HH, Aarsland D, Fénelon G, et al. Scales to assess psychosis in Parkinson's disease: critique and recommendations. Mov Disord 2008; **23**: 484–500.

35 Friedberg G, Zoldan J, Weizman A, Melamed E. Parkinson Psychosis Rating Scale: a practical instrument for grading psychosis in Parkinson's disease. Clin Neuropharmacol 1998; **21**: 280–4.

36 Visser M, Verbaan D, Van Rooden SM, Stiggelbout AM, Marinus J, Van Hilten JJ. Assessment of psychiatric complications in Parkinson's disease: the SCOPA-PC. Mov Disord 2007; **22**: 2221–8.

37 Martinez-Martin P, Frades-Payo B, Agüera-Ortiz L, Ayuga-Martinez A. A short scale for evaluation of neuropsychiatric disorders in Parkinson's disease: first psychometric approach. J Neurol 2012; **259**: 2299–308.

38 Caap-Ahlgren M, Dehlin O. Insomnia and depressive symptoms in patients with Parkinson's disease. Relationship to health-related quality of life. An interview study of patients living at home. Arch Gerontol Geriatr 2001; **32**: 23–33.

39 Gagnon JF, Postuma RB, Mazza S, Doyon J, Montplaisir J. Rapid-eye-movement sleep behaviour disorder and neurodegenerative diseases. Lancet Neurol 2006; **5**: 424–32.

40 Chaudhuri KR, Healy DG, Schapira AH. Non-motor symptoms of Parkinson's disease: diagnosis and management. Lancet Neurol 2006; **5**: 235–45.

41 Högl B, Arnulf I, Comella C, et al. Scales to assess sleep impairment in Parkinson's disease: critique and recommendations. Mov Disord 2010; **25**: 2704–16.

42 Buysse DJ, Reynolds CF, Monk TH, Berman SR, Kupfer DJ. The Pittsburgh Sleep Quality Index: a new instrument for psychiatric practice and research. Psychiatry Res 1989; **28**: 193–213.

43 Johns MW. A new method for measuring daytime sleepiness: the Epworth sleepiness scale. Sleep 1991; **14**: 540–5.

44 Chaudhuri KR, Pal S, Dimarco A, et al. The Parkinson's disease sleep scale: a new instrument for assessing sleep and nocturnal disability in Parkinson's disease. J Neurol Neurosurg Psychiatry 2002; **73**: 629–35.

45 Martínez-Martín P, Salvador C, Menéndez-Guisasola L, González S, Tobías A, Almazán J, Chaudhuri KR. Parkinson's Disease Sleep Scale: validation study of a Spanish version. Mov Disord 2004; **19**: 1226–32.

46 Trenkwalder C, Kohnen R, Högl B, et al. Parkinson's disease sleep scale-validation of the revised version PDSS-2. Mov Disord 2011; **26**: 644–52.

47 Marinus J, Visser M, Van Hilten JJ, Lammers GJ, Stiggelbout AM. Assessment of sleep and sleepiness in Parkinson disease. Sleep 2003; **26**: 1049–54.

48 Stiasny-Kolster K, Mayer G, Schäfer S, Möller JC, Heinzel-Gutenbrunner M, Oertel WH. The REM sleep behavior disorder screening questionnaire—a new diagnostic instrument. Mov Disord 2007; **22**: 2386–93.

49 Friedman JH, Alves G, Hagell P, et al. Fatigue rating scales critique and recommendations by the Movement Disorders Society task force on rating scales for Parkinson's disease. Mov Disord 2010; **25**: 805–22.

50 Krupp LB, LaRocca NG, Muir-Nash J, Steinberg AD. The fatigue severity scale. Application to patients with multiple sclerosis and systemic lupus erythematosus. Arch Neurol 1989; **46**: 1121–3.

51 Smets EM, Garssen B, Bonke B, De Haes JC. The Multidimensional Fatigue Inventory (MFI) psychometric qualities of an instrument to assess fatigue. J Psychosom Res 1995; **39**: 315–25.

52 Schwarz R, Krauss O, Hinz A. Fatigue in the general population. Onkologie 2003; **26**: 140–4.

53 Brown RG, Dittner A, Findley L, Wessely SC. The Parkinson fatigue scale. Parkinsonism Relat Disord 2005; **11**: 49–55.

54 Elbers RG, Rietberg MB, Van Wegen EEH, et al. Self-report fatigue questionnaires in multiple sclerosis, Parkinson's disease and stroke: a systematic review of measurement properties. Qual Life Res 2012; **21**: 925–44.

55 Evatt ML, Chaudhuri KR, Chou KL, et al. Dysautonomia rating scales in Parkinson's disease: sialorrhea, dysphagia, and constipation—critique and recommendations by movement disorders task force on rating scales for Parkinson's disease. Mov Disord 2009; **24**: 635–46.

56 Pavy-Le Traon A, Amarenco G, Duerr S, et al. The Movement Disorders task force review of dysautonomia rating scales in Parkinson's disease with regard to symptoms of orthostatic hypotension. Mov Disord 2011; **26**: 1985–92.

57 Visser M, Marinus J, Stiggelbout AM, Van Hilten JJ. Assessment of autonomic dysfunction in Parkinson's disease: the SCOPA-AUT. Mov Disord 2004; **19**: 1306–12.

58 Forjaz MJ, Ayala A, Rodriguez-Blazquez C, Frades-Payo B, Martinez-Martin P, on behalf of the Spanish-American Longitudinal PD Patient Study Group. Assessing autonomic symptoms of Parkinson's disease with the SCOPA-AUT: a new perspective from Rasch analysis. Eur J Neurol 2010; **17**: 273–9.

59 Suarez GA, Opfer-Gehrking TL, Offord KP, Atkinson EJ, O'Brien PC, Low PA. The Autonomic Symptom Profile: a new instrument to assess autonomic symptoms. Neurology 1999; **52**: 523–8.

60 Daut RL, Cleeland CS, Flanery RC. Development of the Wisconsin Brief Pain Questionnaire to assess pain in cancer and other diseases. Pain 1983; **17**: 197–210.

61 Melzack R. The McGill Pain Questionnaire: major properties and scoring methods. Pain 1975; **1**: 277–99.

Chapter 6

Imaging non-motor aspects of Parkinson's disease

David J. Brooks and Nicola Pavese

Background

Positron emission tomography (PET), single-photon emission computed tomography (SPECT) and magnetic resonance imaging (MRI) have contributed enormously to our understanding of the pathophysiological and pharmacological mechanisms underlying the motor complications of Parkinson's disease (PD) and other movement disorders. These neuroimaging techniques enable one to investigate *in vivo* the function of the basal ganglia, their cortical projection areas and other brainstem nuclei in both healthy subjects and patients. In PD, PET and SPECT have been employed to evaluate: (1) the patterns of change in cerebral metabolism related to the disease and dysfunction of pre-synaptic dopaminergic terminals; (2) the availability of post-synaptic dopaminergic receptors and changes in brain dopamine levels during akinesia and dyskinesia; and (3) the contribution of non-dopaminergic neurotransmitters to motor and non-motor complications of PD.

Several studies have reported a significant inverse correlation between putamen ^{18}F-fluorodopa uptake, a marker of striatal dopamine terminal dysfunction in PD, and the degree of motor disability [1–3]. Interestingly, decreases in putamen ^{18}F-fluorodopa correlate with the degree of rigidity and bradykinesia but not with the degree of tremor; this suggests that pathways other than the nigrostriatal pathway are implicated in the pathogenesis of this symptom [4]. ^{11}C-raclopride PET is a marker of increases in dopamine levels in the synaptic cleft during different behaviours or following pharmacological challenges, evidenced as decreases in D2 receptor availability [5]. This technique has been used to evaluate *in vivo* the relationship between clinical improvement of classical motor symptoms of PD, rated with motor sub-items from the Unified Parkinson's Disease Rating Scale (UPDRS), and increases in synaptic dopamine after a single oral dose of levodopa. It was found that individual improvements in rigidity and bradykinesia, but not in tremor or axial symptoms, correlated with dopamine increases in the putamen, suggesting that neither tremor nor axial symptoms result from dopamine deficiency in the nigrostriatum [6].

MRI techniques including diffusion-weighted MRI and functional MRI (fMRI) also provide objective and unprecedented information about changes in brain size, function, metabolism and network integrity in patients with PD. Diffusion-weighted MRI can detect reduced directionality (fractional anisotropy) of water flow in the substantia nigra in

PD [7]. Resting fMRI using blood-oxygen-level dependent (BOLD) sequence acquisition has revealed reduced striatal–motor cortex and striatal–cerebellar connectivity in PD patients alongside increased striatal–association cortex connectivity [8,9].

Recently, PET, SPECT and MRI have been employed to elucidate the pathogenesis of non-motor symptoms of PD. The spectrum of non-motor symptoms in PD includes impaired cognition, dementia, mood disorders and psychosis, sleep disorders, hyposmia and autonomic dysfunction [10]. Lewy body pathology involves not only the central dopaminergic system, but also the noradrenergic, serotonergic and cholinergic systems. Dysfunction of all these projections may contribute to the onset of non-motor complications which can appear both early and late in the disease and even before the onset of the first motor symptoms.

This chapter will discuss the role that functional imaging has played in revealing the mechanisms underlying non-motor symptoms in PD. We will primarily focus on dementia, depression, fatigue and sleep disorders, as they are the most common symptoms reported by patients. However, other non-motor symptoms, including hyposmia and cardiac sympathetic denervation, will also be discussed.

Imaging dementia in Parkinson's disease

The prevalence of dementia in patients with PD is as high as 80% across different series, but averages at around 40%. The incidence of dementia is about six times higher than that in age-matched healthy people and increases exponentially with age [11]. Dementia in PD patients is characterized by a dysexecutive syndrome along with impairment of visuospatial capacities, attentional control and short-term memory. Compared with Alzheimer's disease (AD), language is relatively preserved. Many of these cognitive deficits are thought to be associated with degeneration of the medial substantia nigra and ventral tegmental area and subsequent loss of mesolimbic and mesocortical dopaminergic projections. However, reported pathological changes in PD patients with dementia also include direct involvement of the cortex by Lewy body pathology, which targets the cingulate and association areas, cholinergic cell loss in the nucleus basalis of Meynert, microglial activation and the occurrence of neuroinflammation and incidental AD or vascular pathology. Neuroimaging techniques are helping to clarify the role of these factors in the development of dementia in PD.

Metabolic studies

^{18}F-deoxyglucose (FDG) PET is a marker of hexokinase activity and so reveals resting patterns of regional cerebral glucose metabolism (rCMRGlc) in humans. In AD, PET shows a consistent pattern of reduced rCMRGlc, beginning in posterior cingulate, parietal and temporal association regions, and later spreading to the prefrontal cortex [12]. Reduced parietal and lateral temporal rCMRGlc has also been observed in elderly asymptomatic carriers of a single copy of the apolipoprotein ε4 allele, the major known genetic risk for AD. Interestingly, the pattern of reduced cerebral glucose metabolism in these subjects predicted subsequent cognitive decline during 2 years of longitudinal follow-up [13]. Similarly, FDG PET in PD patients who develop dementia one or more years after diagnosis (PD dementia, PDD) has demonstrated reduced glucose metabolism in frontal and temporoparietal association areas [14–16].

Dementia with Lewy bodies (DLB) is characterized by dementia, parkinsonism, visual hallucinations, psychosis and fluctuating confusion. The dementia is present at onset or within the first year of PD diagnosis. Yong and colleagues [17] compared patterns of glucose metabolism in PD patients with and without dementia and patients fulfilling the consensus criteria for DLB. Statistical comparisons between groups were performed at a voxel level using statistical parametric mapping (SPM). Compared with normal controls, both PDD and DLB patients showed significant metabolic decreases in the parietal lobe, occipital lobe, temporal lobe, frontal lobe and anterior cingulate. When DLB patients and PDD patients were compared with PD patients without dementia, both dementia groups showed relative reductions of glucose metabolism in the inferior and medial frontal lobes bilaterally and the right parietal lobe. These metabolic deficits were greater in DLB patients. A direct comparison between DLB and PDD showed a relative metabolic decrease in the anterior cingulate in patients with DLB. Interestingly, metabolic deficits in the anterior cingulate are known to be associated with delusions and psychosis in patients with AD. In summary, these findings support the concept that PD with later dementia and DLB have a similar underlying pattern of cortical dysfunction reminiscent of AD, although the anterior cingulate and occipital lobe are more involved in DLB.

Temporoparietal cortical hypometabolism can also be observed in around one-third of non-demented PD patients with established disease. Hu and colleagues [18] have used SPM to localize significant decreases in glucose metabolism in PD patients without dementia. Reductions in mean rCMRGlc were observed in the posterior temporal and parietal cortex of PD patients compared with controls. Individual volume of interest analysis showed that one-third of PD patients had either right or left posterior parietal rCMRGlc values that fell more than two standard deviations below the normal mean. The temporoparietal dysfunction in PD patients without dementia could reflect the presence of occult primary cortical pathology or be secondary to a loss of cholinergic or monoaminergic input. Glucose hypometabolism in PD patients without dementia could be a predictive factor for later onset of dementia. In a recently published longitudinal PET study [19], 23 PD patients without dementia had a FDG scan at baseline and again after 3.9 years' follow-up. At the end of follow-up, six patients (26.1%) had developed dementia. The analysis of baseline scans based on final diagnosis showed that patients who developed PDD had significant hypometabolism in the occipital cortex including the visual association cortex, the posterior cingulate and the caudate nucleus compared with the controls, whereas those who did not only had mild hypometabolism in the primary occipital cortex. A further 2-year follow-up in five of the PPD patients showed widespread metabolic reductions in both subcortical and cortical regions, including the mesiofrontal lobe. Taken together these findings suggest that early metabolic changes in visual association and the posterior cingulate cortex might be a useful biomarker of progression to PDD.

Dopaminergic function

^{123}I-FP-CIT SPECT, an *in vivo* marker of dopamine transporter (DAT) binding, has been used to discriminate PD and DLB from AD during life based on the detection of dysfunction of striatal dopamine terminals. Walker and colleagues [20] assessed the integrity of nigrostriatal metabolism in patients with PD, AD and DLB and reported that the DLB and PD patients had a significantly lower striatal uptake of ^{123}I-FP-CIT than controls and patients with AD. Autopsy data subsequently became available for ten of the dementia subjects investigated with SPECT. All four cases proven to have DLB at post mortem showed reduced striatal ^{123}I-FP-CIT uptake. Four of five autopsy-proven AD cases showed normal striatal ^{123}I-FP-CIT uptake, while the fifth, who had been diagnosed as DLB in life, had concomitant small vessel disease and reduced DAT binding. SPECT therefore provided a sensitivity of 100% and a specificity of 83% for DLB and performed far better than clinical impression, as only four of nine DLB cases were correctly diagnosed in life.

O'Brien et al. [21] also used ^{123}I-FP-CIT SPECT to assess the extent and pattern of dopamine transporter loss in patients with DLB compared with other dementias, including PDD. There were no differences in striatal ^{123}I-FP-CIT between AD patients and healthy controls, whereas transporter loss in patients with DLB was of a similar magnitude to that seen in PD. Interestingly, the group of patients with PDD had the greatest reduction in striatal ^{123}I-FP-CIT binding. Compared with PD patients, where a selective involvement of the putamen was observed, DLB patients and PDD patients showed a more global striatal reduction in ^{123}I-FP-CIT binding with loss of caudate–putamen gradient. Additionally, a significant correlation between the Mini Mental State Examination scores and ^{123}I-FP-CIT binding was observed in PDD patients, supporting the hypothesis that striatal dopaminergic loss may contribute to the cognitive impairment of these patients. No such correlation was found in patients with DLB.

While striatal dopamine terminal dysfunction is a hallmark of DLB and PDD, it is unlikely to explain fully the presence of the dementia. The role of the mesolimbic and mesocortical dopaminergic projections in PDD has been investigated with ^{18}F-fluorodopa PET. Regional ^{18}F-fluorodopa uptake, measured as an influx-constant K_i, mainly reflects the pre-synaptic decarboxylation of the radiotracer by aromatic amino acid decarboxylase (AADC) and the density of the axonal terminal plexus. Measurements of ^{18}F-fluorodopa uptake in dopaminergic areas in PD will therefore reflect the function of the remaining dopamine terminals. Using ^{18}F-fluorodopa PET and SPM, Ito and colleagues [22] assessed changes in dopaminergic function in PD patients with and without later dementia matched for age, disease duration and disease severity. Compared with the PD patients without dementia, the PDD patients showed additional reductions in ^{18}F-fluorodopa uptake in the right caudate and bilaterally in the ventral striatum and the anterior cingulate. These findings therefore add support to the concept that PDD is associated with impaired mesolimbic, mesocortical and caudate dopaminergic function.

Cholinergic function

The SPECT tracer ^{123}I-iodobenzovesamicol (^{123}I-BVM), an acetylcholine vesicle transporter marker, has been employed to assess the association of cholinergic deficiency in patients with PDD. PD patients without dementia showed selectively reduced binding of ^{123}I-BVM in the parietal and occipital cortex, whereas PDD and AD patients had globally reduced cortical binding [23]. More recently, cortical acetylcholinesterase (AChE) activity in PD with and without dementia has been investigated with the PET ligands ^{11}C-MP4A and ^{11}C-PMP, acetylcholine analogues that serve as selective substrates for AChE hydrolysis [24,25]. Global cortical ^{11}C-MP4A binding was reduced by 30% in PDD but only by 11% in PD. The PDD group had significantly lower parietal ^{11}C-MP4A uptake than the PD patients and loss of frontal and temporoparietal ^{11}C-MP4A binding correlated with striatal reduction of ^{18}F-fluorodopa uptake. The authors concluded that PDD is associated with a parallel reduction in both dopaminergic and cholinergic function [24]. Using ^{11}C-PMP PET, a significant correlation was reported between cortical AChE activity in a combined group of PD and PDD patients and performances on the WAIS-III Digit Span, a test of working memory and attention, and other tests of attentional and executive functions, such as the Trail Making and Stroop Color Word tests. Interestingly, cortical AChE deficiency did not correlate with motor symptoms [25]. In conclusion, degeneration of the cholinergic system is associated with significant cognitive decline in PD and imaging findings support the use of AChE inhibitors in PDD.

Muscarinic acetylcholine receptor availability has also been assessed in PD. Asahina and colleagues [26] reported that binding of the muscarinic receptor PET ligand ^{11}C-NMPB was significantly higher in the frontal cortex of PD patients. One of the PD patients in this study had dementia in addition to the highest binding in frontal and temporal areas. The authors suggested that the increased availability of muscarinic receptor in the frontal cortex in PD reflected denervation hypersensitivity caused by loss of ascending cholinergic input to the cortex. Conversely, in another study, where muscarinic acetylcholine receptor binding was measured with ^{123}I-iodo-quinuclidinyl-benzilate (QNB) SPECT, PDD patients showed significantly reduced tracer uptake in the frontal regions and temporal lobes bilaterally. Interestingly, however, both PDD and DLB patients showed significant elevation of ^{123}I-QNB binding in the occipital lobe. This last finding may help explain the visual disturbances that are frequent in both these disorders [27].

Amyloid deposition

Over the last few years, radiotracers have been developed to image β-amyloid plaques in dementia. β-Amyloid plaques and neurofibrillary tangles are pathological hallmarks of AD and post-mortem studies suggest that incidental β-amyloid deposition may occur years before the clinical symptoms of dementia. The PET ligand ^{11}C-PIB is a neutral thioflavin that in AD brain slices shows nanomolar affinity for neuritic β-amyloid plaques but low affinity towards amorphous diffuse β-amyloid deposits and intracellular neurofibrillary tangles and Lewy bodies [28].

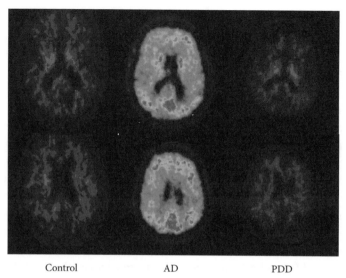

Control   AD   PDD

Fig. 6.1 Positron emission tomography images of ^{11}C-PIB uptake in the brain of a control subject, a patient with Alzheimer's disease (AD) and a patient with Parkinson's disease and later dementia (PDD). Increased ^{11}C-PIB uptake is visible in the AD patient.

[11]C-PIB PET studies have shown a twofold increase in tracer retention in the association areas of patients with AD compared with healthy controls. In a recent study [29], 17 of 19 clinically probable AD subjects (89%) revealed an increased β-amyloid plaque load as measured by ^{11}C-PIB PET. Compared with the controls, the AD group showed mean 2- to 2.5-fold increases in ^{11}C-PIB uptake in association cortical areas and cingulate gyri. This magnitude of increase in signal suggests that ^{11}C-PIB PET should prove a sensitive diagnostic marker for AD.

[11]C-PIB has also been used to assess the amyloid load associated with PD, PDD and DLB. While ^{11}C-PIB binding is increased in association cortical areas (mostly in the frontal and cingulate cortices) in the majority of DLB patients [30], that is not the case for PD and PDD patients who have normal or marginally increased levels of cortical ^{11}C-PIB binding [31–33] (Fig. 6.1). Recently, Gomperts and colleagues [34] reported that those PD cases with low levels of cortical amyloid show a faster rate of cognitive deterioration than patients who are amyloid free.

[18F]-florbetaben is a novel ^{18}F-labelled PET tracer for β-amyloid imaging. In agreement with the ^{11}C-PIB PET findings, none of five non-demented PD patients investigated in one series showed cortical retention of ^{18}F-florbetaben [35]. Taken together, these findings suggest that β-amyloid deposition does not seem to make a significant contribution to the pathogenesis of later dementia in PD.

Microglial activation

Microglial activation is a non-specific response to brain injury. Microglial cells are able to promote neuronal survival by releasing growth factors, walling off necrotic tissue and stripping and remodelling synapses [36]. However, there is cumulative evidence suggesting that in chronic neurodegenerative diseases activated microglia may also cause neuronal death and promote further neurodegeneration through the release of a variety of cytokines and other neurotoxic factors [37]. The isoquinoline ^{11}C-(R)-PK11195 PET is a selective *in vivo* marker of activated microglia. The 18-kDa translocator protein (TSPO) is expressed on the mitochondrial membranes of activated but not resting microglia and has a binding site for ^{11}C-(R)-PK11195 [38]. Two studies have reported significant increases in ^{11}C-(R)-PK11195 binding in both striatal and extra-striatal regions (mainly frontal and temporal cortices) in PD patients compared with normal controls [39,40]. More recently, Edison and colleagues [33] reported that PPD patients have more extensive microglial activation than PD patients, with a significant increase in ^{11}C-(R)-PK11195 binding in anterior and posterior cingulate, striatum, frontal, temporal, parietal and occipital cortical regions compared with normal controls. Additionally, in PDD, cortical microglial activation was inversely correlated with Mini Mental State Examination scores, suggesting that neuroinflammation may contribute to cognitive impairment in these patients.

Structural and functional MRI studies

Several MRI studies have revealed significant cortical atrophy in PDD patients which progresses over time [41–46]. In early MRI studies, where a traditional region-of-interest approach was used, the most common finding observed in PDD patients was atrophy of the hippocampus and amygdala. More recently, voxel based morphometry (VBM), a MRI technique that localizes significant changes in regional tissue volume or density between groups of subjects, has demonstrated that PDD is associated with structural changes in limbic areas and widespread neocortical atrophy, targeting hippocampus, parahippocampus, frontal regions, the cingulate gyrus and the medial temporal lobe [41–46]. In most of these regions, grey matter loss in PDD patients correlated with global cognitive score but not motor impairment [46]. Recently, it has been reported that changes in cortical volume can also be detected with VBM in non-demented PD patients. Loss of frontal volume correlated with poor performance on the Iowa gambling and facial expression recognition tasks [47].

Diffusion tensor imaging (DTI) measures the direction and magnitude of diffusivity of water molecules in tissues and provides an index of damage to neuronal tracts. DTI has been used to investigate PDD. Matsui and colleagues compared PD patients with and without dementia and found water flow abnormalities in the posterior cingulate in the latter [48]. In a recent DTI study, microstructural lesions characterized by increased mean diffusivity (MD) values were found in the hippocampus of PD patients without dementia having hippocampal size within the normal range. Interestingly, patients with high hippocampal MD values obtained low memory scores on neuropsychological tests, suggesting that memory impairment in patients with PD without dementia may be predicted by the rate of microstructural alterations in the hippocampus as detected by DTI [49].

Finally, fMRI has been employed to assess changes in connectivity in the default mode network (DMN) in PDD patients. BOLD MRI sequences were used to detect brain regions which are anatomically separated but show synchronized slow oscillations of oxygenation in the resting state. Compared with PD without cognitive impairment and healthy volunteers, PDD patients showed significant decreases of connectivity in the right inferior frontal gyrus [50]. However, in another study, decreased functional connectivity of the right medial temporal lobe and bilateral inferior parietal cortex within the DMN was also found in PD patients with no cognitive impairment [51]. It remains to be determined whether a dysfunction of DMN connectivity may have a role in the development of cognitive decline in these patients.

Imaging depression in Parkinson's disease

Depression is common in PD patients, having a reported prevalence that varies from 10 to 45% depending on the criteria used for diagnosis [52]. Symptoms of depression can precede the onset of motor symptoms in PD patients, but the precise pathophysiological substrates of affective symptoms in PD remain obscure. Although a pure reactive basis cannot be excluded, and may certainly play a significant role, it is also conceivable that depression in PD could be the result of damage to serotonergic and noradrenergic pathways along with loss of limbic dopaminergic neurotransmission.

Several neuroimaging studies have suggested an association between major depression and striatal function. Depressed patients have shown decreased DAT binding of the whole striatum [53] or of the left caudate nucleus only [54]. In PD patients with depression, Mayberg and colleagues [55] reported selective glucose hypometabolism in the caudate and orbital-inferior region of the frontal lobe compared with both non-depressed PD patients and control subjects. More recently, Weintraub and colleagues [56] showed associations between depression in PD and DAT binding in the left anterior putamen using $^{99}Tc^m$-TRODAT-1 SPECT. Taken together, these findings suggest that disruption of basal ganglia circuits involving the inferior region of the frontal lobe may affect the regulation of mood. MRI studies with VBM and DTI largely support this view. Feldmann and colleagues [57] reported VBM findings in a group of PD patients with and without depression. They found a decrease in grey matter in the bilateral orbitofrontal cortex, the right superior temporal pole and the limbic system of the depressed PD patients. However, Kostić and colleagues [58] found more severe white matter loss in the right frontal lobe, including the anterior cingulate bundle and the inferior orbitofrontal region in depressed PD patients compared with non-depressed patients but no differences in grey matter loss were observed between the two groups. The severity of depression in these patients significantly correlated with white matter loss in the right inferior orbitofrontal region. Differences in patient demographics, diagnostic criteria for depression and processing of MRI images could be responsible for the discrepancies between the two studies.

With DTI, Matsui and colleagues [59] found bilateral abnormalities in the anterior cingulate in depressed PD patients. More recently, compared with non-depressed PD patients, depressed patients were found to have reduced fractional anisotropy values in the bilateral mediodorsal (limbic) thalamic regions, which negatively correlated with the scores of depression severity [60].

Functioning of the serotonergic system has been investigated in PD patients with both PET and SPECT ligands. ^{11}C-DASB PET measures levels of the brain serotonin transporter

(SERT), a marker of serotonergic terminal function. In patients with advanced PD without overt depression, [11]C- DASB binding levels have been reported to be significantly lower than those in controls in all examined brain areas, including orbitofrontal cortex (−22%), caudate (−30%), putamen (−26%) and midbrain (−29%), suggesting that a modest, widespread loss of brain serotonergic innervation is a feature of advanced PD. Interestingly, a non-significant 7% reduction was also observed in the dorsolateral prefrontal cortex, an area implicated in major depression [61]. ^{123}I-β-CIT is a potent cocaine analogue which binds with nanomolar affinity to dopamine, noradrenaline and serotonin transporters. In both non-human primates and humans the tracer concentrates in striatal and midbrain regions. It has been demonstrated that striatal binding of the tracer 3–4 hours after intravenous injection reflects DAT binding, whereas midbrain binding 1 hour after intravenous injection reflects the availability of SERT [62,63]. Using ^{123}I-β-CIT SPECT, Kim and colleagues [64] found reduced striatal DAT binding in a cohort of 45 PD patients with early disease. By contrast, they found no reduction of ^{123}I-β-CIT binding in the brainstem of PD patients compared with normal subjects. PD patients with and without depression showed similar midbrain uptake of the radioligand at 1 hour, and there was no correlation between radiotracer binding in this region and Hamilton Depression Rating Scale scores.

[11]C-WAY 100635 is a PET ligand which binds to serotonin 5-HT$_{1A}$ receptors. These receptors are both pre-synaptic somatodendritic autoreceptors localized on 5-HT cell bodies in the midbrain raphe nuclei, where they inhibit serotonin release, and are also distributed post-synaptically on cortical pyramidal neurons and on glia. HT$_{1A}$ sites have the highest density in the hippocampus, a lower density in the striatum and are absent in the cerebellum. Our group has reported a 25% reduction of ^{11}C-WAY 100635 binding in midbrain raphe in PD patients compared with healthy controls (Fig. 6.2 and Plate 1). However, the magnitude of reduction was no different in PD patients with and without depression (Fig. 6.3 and Plate 2) [65]. The results from these ^{123}I-β-CIT SPECT and

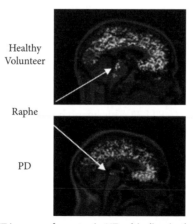

Healthy Volunteer

Raphe

PD

Fig. 6.2 ^{11}C-WAY 100635 PET images of serotonin HT$_{1A}$ binding in the brain of a control subject and a patient with Parkinson's disease (PD). Decreased ^{11}C-WAY 100635 binding in the median raphe is visible in the PD patient. (See also Plate 1)

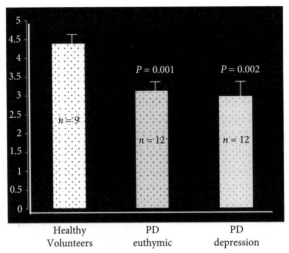

Fig. 6.3 Mean values of ^{11}C-WAY 100635 binding in the midbrain raphe of healthy volunteers, patients with Parkinson's disease without depression, and patients with Parkinson's disease and depression. The two PDD groups show similar reductions in HT_{1A} binding. (See also Plate 2)

[11]C-WAY 100635 PET studies therefore do not support the view that serotonergic loss contributes to depression in PD. These imaging findings are discordant with the finding that depressed PD patients have decreased concentrations of 5-hydroxyindoleacetic acid, a serotonin metabolite, in their cerebrospinal fluid [66]. More recently, the post-synaptic serotonergic system in PD patients with and without depression has been assessed with ^{18}F-MPPF, another selective 5-HT_{1A} receptor antagonist. Compared with non-depressed PD patients, depressed patients exhibited reduced tracer uptake in the left hippocampus, the right insula, the left superior temporal cortex and the orbitofrontal cortex. HT_{1A} sites are expressed by cortical pyramidal cells, and this finding suggests that depression in PD might be linked to dysfunction of neocortical regions as well as subcortical structures [67]. It should be noted, however, that a very small number of subjects were included in this study (four PD patients with depression and eight without depression). Further investigations are required to establish whether serotonergic neurotransmission in the neocortex is decreased in those patients with PD who have a major depressive disorder in order to provide a rationale for the widespread use of serotonin reuptake inhibitors.

The role of noradrenergic and dopaminergic dysfunction in PD depression has been investigated with PET and ^{11}C-RTI 32. This ligand binds with similar nanomolar affinities to the dopamine and noradrenaline transporters and with far lower affinity to the serotonin transporter. In PD there is a reduced binding of ^{11}C-RTI 32 in both striatal and extrastriatal areas. Remy and colleagues [68] compared ^{11}C-RTI 32 PET findings in PD patients with and without depression matched for age, disability, disease duration and doses of antiparkinsonian medications. Compared with those without depression, patients with depression showed a significant reduction of ^{11}C-RTI 32 binding in the noradrenergic locus coeruleus, the thalamus and several regions of the limbic system, including the amygdala, ventral striatum and anterior cingulate. The severity of anxiety in PD was inversely correlated with ^{11}C-RTI 32 binding in these regions, whereas apathy was inversely correlated with the radiotracer binding in the ventral striatum. These results suggest that depression and anxiety in PD are associated with a loss of noradrenaline innervation and a selective loss of dopaminergic projections to the limbic system.

Imaging fatigue in Parkinson's disease

In the PRIAMO study, the largest multicentre assessment of non-motor symptoms and their impact on quality of life in PD to date, fatigue occurred in 58.1% of a cohort of 1072 patients ranging from 37.7% in Hoehn and Yahr (HY) Stage 1 patients to 81.6% in Stages 4–5 [69].

Recent PET studies have shed light on the neurobiology of fatigue in PD. In a study among untreated PD patients, those who complained of fatigue had similar striatal dopamine transporter uptake to the patients without fatigue, suggesting that dopamine loss does per se does not cause fatigue in PD [70]. In a more recent study [71], PD patients with and without fatigue were assessed with ^{18}F-fluorodopa PET and ^{11}C-DASB PET to assess the integrity of dopaminergic and serotonergic pathways in the brains of these patients. PD patients with fatigue showed significantly lower SERT binding than patients without fatigue in ventral basal ganglia structures, cingulate and amygdala. Significant decreases in ^{18}F-fluorodopa K_i were also found in the cohort of PD patients with fatigue compared with patients without fatigue, but were limited to the caudate bilaterally and the left insula. These findings suggest that the presence of fatigue in PD is associated with relative serotonergic denervation in the basal ganglia and associated limbic circuits and provide the rationale for its treatment with strategies to increase the level of serotonin and serotonergic transmission in the brain.

Imaging sleep disorders in Parkinson's disease

Sleep disorders are very common in PD, occurring in up to 90% of patients, and are associated with significant morbidity as they have functional effects on the patient's work and social life [72]. Sleep disorders can be categorized as insomnia, excessive daytime somnolence and parasomnias including dreams/nightmares/somnambulism/rapid eye movement (REM) sleep behaviour disorder (RBD). Although dopaminergic drugs and age-related pathologies certainly play a part in the pathogenesis of these disorders, it has been suggested that degeneration of the neurons of the central nervous system in PD may affect central sleep regulatory centres which modulate wakefulness and REM sleep [73]. These centres include the noradrenergic locus ceruleus, the serotonergic dorsal raphe, the histaminergic tuberomammilary nucleus, the dopaminergic ventral tegmental area and the hypothalamus.

So far less attention has been paid to the pathology of sleep disturbances compared with other non-motor symptoms. Happe and colleagues [74] reported a significant inverse correlation between excessive daytime sleepiness, rated with the Epworth Sleepiness Scale (ESS), and striatal ^{123}I-FP-CIT binding in early PD. No correlation of the EES score with age, disease duration, UPDRS motor score or depression score was found. These data suggest that daytime sleepiness may be associated with dopaminergic nigrostriatal degeneration in early PD. In another study, Hilker and colleagues [75] measured striatal and midbrain ^{18}F-fluorodopa uptake in PD patients with a history of sleep disorders. They found a significant inverse correlation between mesopontine ^{18}F-fluorodopa uptake and REM sleep duration, as measured by polysomnography. The authors suggested that increased monoaminergic activity in the rostral brainstem might result in the suppression of nocturnal REM sleep in PD.

Our group has recently studied PD patients with and without excessive daytime sleepiness (EDS) with ^{18}F-fluorodopa PET and ^{11}C-DASB PET to assess the integrity of monoaminergic terminals function and the availability of serotonin transport in the main sleep regulatory centres. Compared with healthy volunteers, EDS patients had significant decreases in ^{11}C-DASB binding in thalamus, locus coeruleus, rostral raphe and hypothalamus and significantly reduced ^{18}F-fluorodopa uptake in the locus coeruleus, rostral raphe and ventral tegmental area. The same structures, except the locus coeruleus, were preserved in the PD group without EDS. Additionally, a direct comparison between PD patients with and without EDS showed a significant reductions in ^{11}C-DASB binding in thalamus, rostral raphe, frontal and insular cortices in the former [76]. These findings provide evidence that serotonergic and possibly noradrenergic dysfunction in the neuronal networks responsible for arousal contributes to EDS in PD.

MRI morphometry studies also support the occurrence of degeneration of brainstem sleep structures in PD patients with EDS. Gama and colleagues [77] found that PD patients with EDS had significantly more atrophy of the medial cerebellar peduncle than patients without this symptom.

Finally, Kotagal and colleagues [78] have recently reported that the presence of RBD in PD patients is associated with cholinergic system degeneration in neocortical, limbic cortical and thalamic areas.

There is growing evidence indicating that RBD is highly associated with α-synucleinopathies such as PD, DLB and multiple system atrophy, and it has been suggested that it may represent the first feature of neurodegeneration, and therefore an early marker of these disorders. Several studies have shown that more than 50% of the subjects diagnosed with RBD will develop PD or allied neurodegenerative disease within a time span of 5–12 years [79–81]. Serial SPECT scans have shown progressive nigrostriatal dysfunction before the onset of parkinsonism in RBD patients [82].

Imaging cardiac sympathetic denervation in Parkinson's disease

Several SPECT and PET studies have now reported that the majority of patients with idiopathic PD show a significant loss of sympathetic innervation of the heart and other organs, whereas this is not seen in atypical variants [83]. Decreased myocardial uptake of the sympathetic markers ^{123}I-metaiodobenzylguanidine (MIBG) and ^{18}F-fluorodopamine has been reported in PD patients even at early stages of the disease when cardiovascular reflexes are still intact. However, MIBG SPECT is not a sensitive marker of early PD as 50% of HY Stage 1 cases still show normal tracer binding [83,84]. Both ^{18}F-fluorodopamine and MIBG use the same metabolic pathway as norepinephrine, and their myocardial uptake reflects not only the density of post-ganglionic sympathetic neurons but also their functional integrity. A recent study with ^{11}C-meta-hydroxyephedrine PET suggests that there is a segmental pattern of cardiac sympathetic denervation in PD, with the proximal lateral left ventricular wall most severely affected and the anterior and proximal septal walls relatively preserved [85].

It has been suggested that cardiac sympathetic denervation contributes to symptoms of autonomic failure such as orthostatic hypotension [83]. Oka and colleagues [86] examined the association between myocardial ^{123}I-MIBG uptake and orthostatic hypotension, pulse and blood pressure changes during the Valsalva manoeuvre, and erect and supine plasma norepinephrine concentrations in PD patients. Mean myocardial ^{123}I-MIBG uptake was significantly lower in PD patients with orthostatic hypotension and an abnormal Valsalva response. However, no association was found between the fall in systolic blood pressure on head-up tilt and baroreflex sensitivity or plasma norepinephrine concentrations. These results indicate that cardiac sympathetic dysfunction is a primary cause of impaired cardiovascular reflexes in PD.

Imaging and olfactory function in Parkinson's disease

Olfactory dysfunction (hyposmia) is a frequent feature of PD, affecting up to 60% of patients and often preceding the motor symptoms by several years, providing a potential marker of subclinical disease. Using diffusion-weighted MRI, Scherfler and colleagues [87] have shown that PD patients show abnormal olfactory tract signals. In contrast, olfaction is normal in atypical PD and so olfactory function tests may be a useful tool for the differential diagnosis of parkinsonian syndromes.

PET and SPECT have been used to correlate the presence of olfactory and dopaminergic dysfunction in subjects with and at risk for PD. Siderowf and colleagues [88] evaluated the relationship between integrity of striatal DAT binding, measured with [99]Tc[m]-TRODAT-1 (TRODAT) SPECT, odour identification skills and motor function in patients with early PD. Olfactory testing was performed using the 40-odour University of Pennsylvania Smell Identification Test (UPSIT). UPSIT scores were strongly correlated with TRODAT uptake in the putamen.

Another study [89] has investigated the relationship between selective deficits in smell identification and nigrostriatal dopaminergic denervation as measured with ^{11}C-β-CFT PET in patients with PD. The total UPSIT scores were significantly lower in the PD patients than in the control subjects. Analysis of the individual smell scores identified three odours (banana, liquorice and dill pickle) with an accuracy of >0.75 for the diagnosis of PD. A PD-specific smell identification score (UPSIT-3) was therefore calculated for these three odours. Analysis of the patients' PET data demonstrated significant correlations between dorsal striatal ^{11}C-β-CFT uptake and both the UPSIT-3 and the total UPSIT scores. In a subsequent study where DAT binding was measured in several brain regions, the same authors observed that the more robust correlation between UPSIT-3 and DAT binding was found in the hippocampus, suggesting that the mesolimbic dopamine innervation of the hippocampus could play the main role in the development of selective hyposmia in PD [90].

The relationship between individual UPSIT scores and measures of motor disability (disease duration, stage and severity), non-motor function (cognitive function, depression, anxiety and sleep) and severity of nigrostriatal dysfunction has also been investigated in PD patients. UPSIT scores correlated positively with striatal DAT binding and negatively with years of disease duration, UPDRS motor score, severity of anxiety and depressive symptoms. Taken together these findings suggest that the olfactory impairment in PD may not be stationary in the early motor stages and continues to progress over time [91].

Finally, Haehner and colleagues [92] followed patients with idiopathic hyposmia over 4 years. At baseline, olfactory testing was combined with transcranial sonography of the substantia nigra and ^{123}I-FP-CIT SPECT. At follow-up, 7% of the individuals with idiopathic hyposmia had developed clinical PD and another 6% had soft motor abnormalities. Reduction of striatal ^{123}I-β-CIT binding has been reported in seven out of 40 (17.5%) hyposmic relatives of PD patients who had no parkinsonian symptoms. Four out of these seven (57%) subjects with reduced striatal ^{123}I-β-CIT binding converted to clinical PD over a 2-year follow-up [93]. In summary, findings from these studies suggest that a combination of olfactory testing and neuroimaging techniques may provide a screening tool for the risk of developing PD, although the sensitivity of these modalities is relatively low and will only become of real value when neuroprotective agents are available for PD.

Future developments

Recently, PET radioligands to image the cerebral cannabinoid receptor CB1 have become available. The endogenous cannabinoid system plays a role in controlling behaviour and emotions. Dysfunction of cannabinoid transmission has been associated with neuropsychiatric disorders including depression and psychosis. Interestingly, depression in PD patients seems to be related to a genetic polymorphism of the cannabinoid receptor gene [94]. Development of new radiotracers is therefore needed to explore the different non-dopaminergic brain pathways involved in the pathology of non-motor symptoms of PD. It is hoped that these new tracers will lead to a better understanding and treatment of these disabling complications. Further neuroimaging studies are also warranted to detect early neurotransmitter changes that could be predictive factors for later onset of depression, dementia or sleep disorders in non-complicated PD patients.

References

1 **Brooks DJ, Salmon EP, Mathias CJ, et al**. The relationship between locomotor disability, autonomic dysfunction, and the integrity of the striatal dopaminergic system in patients with multiple system atrophy, pure autonomic failure, and Parkinson's disease, studied with PET. Brain 1990; **113**: 1539–52.

2 Broussolle E, Dentresangle C, Landais P, et al. The relation of putamen and caudate nucleus 18F-Dopa uptake to motor and cognitive performances in Parkinson's disease. J Neurol Sci 1999; **166**: 141–51.

3 Vingerhoets FJ, Schulzer M, Calne DB, Snow BJ. Which clinical sign of Parkinson's disease best reflects the nigrostriatal lesion? Ann Neurol 1997; **41**: 58–64.

4 Otsuka M, Ichiya Y, Kuwabara Y, et al. Differences in the reduced 18F-Dopa uptakes of the caudate and the putamen in Parkinson's disease: correlations with the three main symptoms. J Neurol Sci 1996; **136**: 169–73.

5 Laruelle M. Imaging synaptic neurotransmission with in vivo binding competition techniques: a critical review. J Cereb Blood Flow Metab 2000; **20**: 423–51.

6 Pavese N, Evans AH, Tai YF, et al. Clinical correlates of levodopa-induced dopamine release in Parkinson disease: a PET study. Neurology 2006; **67**: 1612–17.

7 Vaillancourt DE, Spraker MB, Prodoehl J, et al. High-resolution diffusion tensor imaging in the substantia nigra of de novo Parkinson disease. Neurology 2009; **72**: 1378–84.

8 Hacker CD, Perlmutter JS, Criswell SR, Ances BM, Snyder AZ. Resting state functional connectivity of the striatum in Parkinson's disease. Brain 2012; **135**:3699–711.

9 Sharman M, Valabregue R, Perlbarg V, et al. Parkinson's disease patients show reduced cortical-subcortical sensorimotor connectivity. Mov Disord 2013; **28**: 447–54.

10 Chaudhuri KR, Healy DG, Schapira AH, National Institute for Clinical Excellence. Non-motor symptoms of Parkinson's disease: diagnosis and management. Lancet Neurol 2006; **5**: 235–45.

11 Emre M. Dementia associated with Parkinson's disease. Lancet Neurol 2003; **2**: 229–37.

12 Hoffman JM, Guze BH, Baxter LR, et al. [18F]-fluorodeoxyglucose (FDG) and positron emission tomography (PET) in aging and dementia. A decade of studies. Eur Neurol 1989; **29**(Suppl 3): 16–24.

13 Small GW, Ercoli LM, Silverman DH, et al. Cerebral metabolic and cognitive decline in persons at genetic risk for Alzheimer's disease. Proc Natl Acad Sci USA 2000; **97**: 6037–42.

14 Peppard RF, Martin WR, Carr GD, et al. Cerebral glucose metabolism in Parkinson's disease with and without dementia. Arch Neurol 1992; **49**: 1262–8.

15 Goto I, Taniwaki T, Hosokawa S, et al. Positron emission tomographic (PET) studies in dementia. J Neurol Sci 1993; **114**: 1–6.

16 Vander Borght T, Minoshima S, Giordani B, et al. Cerebral metabolic differences in Parkinson's and Alzheimer's diseases matched for dementia severity. J Nucl Med 1997; **38**: 797–802.

17 Yong SW, Yoon JK, An YS, Lee PH. A comparison of cerebral glucose metabolism in Parkinson's disease, Parkinson's disease dementia and dementia with Lewy bodies. Eur J Neurol 2007; **14**: 1357–62.

18 Hu MT, Taylor-Robinson SD, Chaudhuri KR, et al. Cortical dysfunction in non-demented Parkinson's disease patients: a combined (31)P-MRS and (18)FDG-PET study. Brain 2000; **123**: 340–52.

19 Bohnen NI, Koeppe RA, Minoshima S, et al. Cerebral glucose metabolic features of Parkinson disease and incident dementia: longitudinal study. J Nucl Med 2011; **52**: 848–55.

20 Walker Z, Costa DC, Walker RW, et al. Differentiation of dementia with Lewy bodies from Alzheimer's disease using a dopaminergic presynaptic ligand. J Neurol Neurosurg Psychiatry 2002; **73**: 134–40.

21 O'Brien JT, Colloby S, Fenwick J, et al. Dopamine transporter loss visualized with FP-CIT SPECT in the differential diagnosis of dementia with Lewy bodies. Arch Neurol 2004; **61**: 919–25.

22 Ito K, Nagano-Saito A, Kato T, et al. Striatal and extrastriatal dysfunction in Parkinson's disease with dementia: a 6-[18F]fluoro-L-dopa PET study. Brain 2002; **125**: 1358–65.

23 Kuhl DE, Minoshima S, Fessler JA, et al. In vivo mapping of cholinergic terminals in normal aging, Alzheimer's disease, and Parkinson's disease. Ann Neurol 1996; **40**: 399–410.

24 Hilker R, Thomas AV, Klein JC, et al. Dementia in Parkinson disease: functional imaging of cholinergic and dopaminergic pathways. Neurology 2005; **65**: 1716–22.

25 Bohnen NI, Kaufer DI, Hendrickson R, et al. Cognitive correlates of cortical cholinergic denervation in Parkinson's disease and parkinsonian dementia. J Neurol 2006; **253**: 242–7.

26 Asahina M, Suhara T, Shinotoh H, et al. Brain muscarinic receptors in progressive supranuclear palsy and Parkinson's disease: a positron emission tomographic study. J Neurol Neurosurg Psychiatry 1998; **65**: 155–63.

27 Colloby SJ, Pakrasi S, Firbank MJ, et al. In vivo SPECT imaging of muscarinic acetylcholine receptors using (R,R) 123I-QNB in dementia with Lewy bodies and Parkinson's disease dementia. Neuroimage 2006; **33**: 423–9.

28 Bacskai BJ, Frosch MP, Freeman SH, et al. Molecular imaging with Pittsburgh Compound B confirmed at autopsy: a case report. Arch Neurol 2007; **64**: 431–4.

29 Edison P, Archer HA, Hinz R, et al. Amyloid, hypometabolism, and cognition in Alzheimer disease: an [11C]PIB and [18F]FDG PET study. Neurology 2007; **68**: 501–8.

30 Rowe CC, Ng S, Ackermann U, et al. Imaging beta-amyloid burden in aging and dementia. Neurology 2007; **68**: 1718–25.

31 Edison P, Rowe CC, Rinne JO, et al. Amyloid load in Parkinson's disease dementia and Lewy body dementia measured with [11C]PIB positron emission tomography. J Neurol Neurosurg Psychiatry 2008; **79**: 1331–8.

32 Jokinen P, Scheinin N, Aalto S, et al. [(11)C]PIB-, [(18)F]FDG-PET and MRI imaging in patients with Parkinson's disease with and without dementia. Parkinsonism Relat Disord 2010; **16**: 666–70.

33 Edison P, Ahmed I, Fan Z, et al. Microglia, amyloid, and glucose metabolism in Parkinson's disease with and without dementia. Neuropsychopharmacology 2013; **38**: 938–49.

34 Gomperts SN, Locascio JJ, Rentz D, et al. Amyloid is linked to cognitive decline in patients with Parkinson disease without dementia. Neurology 2013; **80**: 85–91.

35 Villemagne VL, Ong K, Mulligan RS, et al. Amyloid imaging with (18)F-florbetaben in Alzheimer disease and other dementias. J Nucl Med 2011; **52**: 1210–17.

36 Kim SU, de Vellis J. Microglia in health and disease. J Neurosci Res 2005; **81**: 302–13.

37 Wilms H, Claasen J, Röhl C, Sievers J, Deuschl G, Lucius R. Involvement of benzodiazepine receptors in neuroinflammatory and neurodegenerative diseases: evidence from activated microglial cells in vitro. Neurobiol Dis 2003; **14**: 417–24.

38 Banati RB, Newcombe J, Gunn RN, et al. The peripheral benzodiazepine binding site in the brain in multiple sclerosis: quantitative in vivo imaging of microglia as a measure of disease activity. Brain 2000; **123**: 2321–37.

39 Ouchi Y, Yoshikawa E, Sekine Y, et al. Microglial activation and dopamine terminal loss in early Parkinson's disease. Ann Neurol 2005; **57**: 168–75.

40 Gerhard A, Pavese N, Hotton G, et al. In vivo imaging of microglial activation with [11C](R)-PK11195 PET in idiopathic Parkinson's disease. Neurobiol Dis 2006; **21**: 404–12.

41 Burton EJ, McKeith IG, Burn DJ, Williams ED, O'Brien JT. Cerebral atrophy in Parkinson's disease with and without dementia: a comparison with Alzheimer's disease, dementia with Lewy bodies and controls. Brain 2004; **127**: 791–800.

42 Summerfield C, Junqué C, Tolosa E, et al. Structural brain changes in Parkinson disease with dementia: a voxel-based morphometry study. Arch Neurol 2005; **62**: 281–5.

43 Ramírez-Ruiz B, Martí MJ, Tolosa E, et al. Longitudinal evaluation of cerebral morphological changes in Parkinson's disease with and without dementia. J Neurol 2005; **252**: 1345–52.

44 Nagano-Saito A, Washimi Y, Arahata Y, et al. Cerebral atrophy and its relation to cognitive impairment in Parkinson disease. Neurology 2005; **64**: 224–9.

45 Beyer MK, Janvin CC, Larsen JP, Aarsland D. A magnetic resonance imaging study of patients with Parkinson's disease with mild cognitive impairment and dementia using voxel-based morphometry. J Neurol Neurosurg Psychiatry 2007; **78**: 254–9.

46 Melzer TR, Watts R, MacAskill MR, et al. Grey matter atrophy in cognitively impaired Parkinson's disease. J Neurol Neurosurg Psychiatry 2012; **83**: 188–94.

47 Ibarretxe-Bilbao N, Junque C, Tolosa E, et al. Neuroanatomical correlates of impaired decision-making and facial emotion recognition in early Parkinson's disease. Eur J Neurosci 2009; **30**: 1162–71.

48 Matsui H, Nishinaka K, Oda M, Niikawa H, Kubori T, Udaka F. Dementia in Parkinson's disease: diffusion tensor imaging. Acta Neurol Scand 2007; **116**: 177–81.

49 Carlesimo GA, Piras F, Assogna F, Pontieri FE, Caltagirone C, Spalletta G. Hippocampal abnormalities and memory deficits in Parkinson disease: a multimodal imaging study. Neurology 2012; **78**: 1939–45.

50 Rektorova I, Krajcovicova L, Marecek R, Mikl M. Default mode network and extrastriate visual resting state network in patients with Parkinson's disease dementia. Neurodegener Dis 2012; **10**: 232–7.

51 Tessitore A, Esposito F, Vitale C, et al. Default-mode network connectivity in cognitively unimpaired patients with Parkinson disease. Neurology 2012; **79**: 2226–32.

52 Burn DJ. Beyond the iron mask: towards better recognition and treatment of depression associated with Parkinson's disease. Mov Disord 2002; **17**: 445–54.

53 Meyer JH, Kruger S, Wilson AA, et al. Lower dopamine transporter binding potential in striatum during depression. Neuroreport 2001; **12**: 4121–5.

54 Martinot M, Bragulat V, Artiges E, et al. Decreased presynaptic dopamine function in the left caudate of depressed patients with affective flattening and psychomotor retardation. Am J Psychiatry 2001; **158**: 314–16.

55 Mayberg HS, Starkstein SE, Sadzot B, et al. Selective hypometabolism in the inferior frontal lobe in depressed patients with Parkinson's disease. Ann Neurol 1990; **28**: 57–64.

56 Weintraub D, Newberg AB, Cary MS, et al. Striatal dopamine transporter imaging correlates with anxiety and depression symptoms in Parkinson's disease. J Nucl Med 2005; **46**: 227–32.

57 Feldmann A, Illes Z, Kosztolanyi P, et al. Morphometric changes of gray matter in Parkinson's disease with depression: a voxel-based morphometry study. Mov Disord 2008; **23**: 42–6.

58 Kostić VS, Agosta F, Petrović I, et al. Regional patterns of brain tissue loss associated with depression in Parkinson disease. Neurology 2010; **75**: 857–63.

59 Matsui H, Nishinaka K, Oda M, et al. Depression in Parkinson's disease. Diffusion tensor imaging study. J Neurol 2007; **254**: 1170–3.

60 Li W, Liu J, Skidmore F, Liu Y, Tian J, Li K. White matter microstructure changes in the thalamus in Parkinson disease with depression: A diffusion tensor MR imaging study. Am J Neuroradiol 2010; **31**: 1861–6.

61 Guttman M, Boileau I, Warsh J, et al. Brain serotonin transporter binding in non-depressed patients with Parkinson's disease. Eur J Neurol 2007; **14**: 523–8.

62 Laruelle M, Baldwin RM, Malison RT, et al. SPECT imaging of dopamine and serotonin transporters with [123I]beta-CIT: pharmacological characterization of brain uptake in nonhuman primates. Synapse 1993; **13**: 295–309.

63 Seibyl JP, Wallace E, Smith EO, et al. Whole-body biodistribution, radiation absorbed dose, and brain SPECT imaging with iodine-123-beta-CIT in healthy human subjects. J Nucl Med 1994; **35**: 764–70.

64 Kim SE, Choi JY, Choe YS, et al. Serotonin transporters in the midbrain of Parkinson's disease patients: a study with 123I-beta-CIT SPECT. J Nucl Med 2003; **44**: 870–6.

65 Doder M, Rabiner EA, Turjanski N, et al. Brain serotonin $5HT_{1A}$ receptor in Parkinson's disease with and without depression measured with positron emission tomography with 11C-WAY100635. Mov Disord 2000; **15**: 213.

66 Mayeux R, Stern Y, Cote L, Williams JB. Altered serotonin metabolism in depressed patients with Parkinson's disease. Neurology 1984; **34**: 642–6.

67 Ballanger B, Klinger H, Eche J, et al. Role of serotonergic 1A receptor dysfunction in depression associated with Parkinson's disease. Mov Disord 2012; **27**: 84–9.

68 Remy P, Doder M, Lees A, et al. Depression in Parkinson's disease: loss of dopamine and noradrenaline innervation in the limbic system. Brain 2005; **128**: 1314–22.

69 Barone P, Antonini A, Colosimo C, et al. The PRIAMO study: a multicenter assessment of nonmotor symptoms and their impact on quality of life in Parkinson's disease. Mov Disord 2009; **24**: 1641–9.

70 Schifitto G, Friedman JH, Oakes D, et al. Fatigue in levodopa-naive subjects with Parkinson disease. Neurology 2008; **71**: 481–5.

71 Pavese N, Metta V, Bose SK, Chaudhuri KR, Brooks DJ. Fatigue in Parkinson's disease is linked to striatal and limbic serotonergic dysfunction. Brain 2010; **133**: 3434–43.

72 Chaudhuri KR. Nocturnal symptom complex in PD and its management. Neurology 2003; **61**(Suppl 3): S17–S23.

73 Rye DB, Jankovic J. Emerging views of dopamine in modulating sleep/wake state from an unlikely source: PD. Neurology 2002; **58**: 341–6.

74 Happe S, Baier PC, Helmschmied K, et al. Association of daytime sleepiness with nigrostriatal dopaminergic degeneration in early Parkinson's disease. J Neurol 2007; **254**: 1037–43.

75 Hilker R, Razai N, Ghaemi M, et al. [18F]fluorodopa uptake in the upper brainstem measured with positron emission tomography correlates with decreased REM sleep duration in early Parkinson's disease. Clin Neurol Neurosurg 2003; **105**: 262–9.

76 Pavese N, Metta V, Simpson BS, et al. Sleep regulatory centres dysfunction in Parkinson's disease patients with excessive daytime sleepiness. An in vivo PET study. Parkinsonism Relat Disord 2012; **18**(Suppl 2): S24–S25.

77 Gama RL, Távora DG, Bomfim RC, Silva CE, de Bruin VM, de Bruin PF. Sleep disturbances and brain MRI morphometry in Parkinson's disease, multiple system atrophy and progressive supranuclear palsy—a comparative study. Parkinsonism Relat Disord 2010; **16**: 275–9.

78 Kotagal V, Albin RL, Müller ML, et al. Symptoms of rapid eye movement sleep behavior disorder are associated with cholinergic denervation in Parkinson disease. Ann Neurol 2012; **71**: 560–8.

79 Iranzo A, Molinuevo JL, Santamaría J, et al. Rapid-eye-movement sleep behaviour disorder as an early marker for a neurodegenerative disorder: a descriptive study. Lancet Neurol 2006; **5**: 572–7.

80 Postuma RB, Gagnon JF, Vendette M, Fantini ML, Massicotte-Marquez J, Montplaisir J. Quantifying the risk of neurodegenerative disease in idiopathic REM sleep behavior disorder. Neurology 2009; **72**: 1296–300.

81 Postuma RB, Gagnon JF, Rompré S, Montplaisir JY. Severity of REM atonia loss in idiopathic REM sleep behavior disorder predicts Parkinson disease. Neurology 2010; **74**: 239–44.

82 Iranzo A, Valldeoriola F, Lomeña F, et al. Serial dopamine transporter imaging of nigrostriatal function in patients with idiopathic rapid-eye-movement sleep behaviour disorder: a prospective study. Lancet Neurol 2011; **10**: 797–805.

83 Goldstein DS, Holmes CS, Dendi R, et al. Orthostatic hypotension from sympathetic denervation in Parkinson's disease. Neurology 2002; **58**: 1247–55.

84 Takatsu H, Nishida H, Matsuo H, et al. Cardiac sympathetic denervation from the early stage of Parkinson's disease: clinical and experimental studies with radiolabeled MIBG. J Nucl Med 2000; **41**: 71–7.

85 **Wong KK, Raffel DM, Koeppe RA, Frey KA, Bohnen NI, Gilman S.** Pattern of cardiac sympathetic denervation in idiopathic Parkinson disease studied with 11C hydroxyephedrine PET. Radiology 2012; **265**: 240–7.

86 **Oka H, Yoshioka M, Onouchi K, et al.** Characteristics of orthostatic hypotension in Parkinson's disease. Brain 2007; **130**: 2425–32.

87 **Scherfler C, Schocke MF, Seppi K, et al.** Voxel-wise analysis of diffusion weighted imaging reveals disruption of the olfactory tract in Parkinson's disease. Brain 2006; **129**: 538–42.

88 **Siderowf A, Newberg A, Chou KL, et al.** [99mTc]TRODAT-1 SPECT imaging correlates with odor identification in early Parkinson disease. Neurology 2005; **64**: 1716–20.

89 **Bohnen NI, Gedela S, Kuwabara H, et al.** Selective hyposmia and nigrostriatal dopaminergic denervation in Parkinson's disease. J Neurol 2007; **254**: 84–90.

90 **Bohnen NI, Gedela S, Herath P, Constantine GM, Moore RY.** Selective hyposmia in Parkinson disease: association with hippocampal dopamine activity. Neurosci Lett 2008; **447**: 12–16.

91 **Berendse HW, Roos DS, Raijmakers P, Doty RL.** Motor and non-motor correlates of olfactory dysfunction in Parkinson's disease. J Neurol Sci 2011; **310**: 21–4.

92 **Haehner A, Hummel T, Hummel C, et al.** Olfactory loss may be a first sign of idiopathic Parkinson's disease. Mov Disord 2007; **22**: 839–42.

93 **Ponsen MM, Stoffers D, Booij J, et al.** Idiopathic hyposmia as a preclinical sign of Parkinson's disease. Ann Neurol 2004; **56**: 173–81.

94 **Barrero FJ, Ampuero I, Morales B, et al.** Depression in Parkinson's disease is related to a genetic polymorphism of the cannabinoid receptor gene (CNR1). Pharmacogenomics J 2005; **5**: 135–41.

Chapter 7

Non-motor signs in genetic forms of Parkinson's disease

Meike Kasten and Christine Klein

Introduction

Parkinson's disease (PD) is clinically characterized by 'classical parkinsonism' that has been defined phenomenologically as the triad of bradykinesia, rigidity and rest tremor (not all features are mandatory) with a therapeutic response to levodopa, and the frequent development of motor complications [1]. The identification of several monogenic forms of classical parkinsonism that are frequently clinically indistinguishable from 'idiopathic' PD (IPD) has demonstrated that there are multiple known causes of parkinsonism. However, information on the genetic status is not usually available in the clinical setting. In this chapter, the term 'classical parkinsonism' or 'parkinsonism' for short will be employed for patients with the aforementioned classical clinical characteristics, irrespective of the aetiology.

Although not part of the aforementioned definition, non-motor signs (NMS) have increasingly been recognized as an important feature of classical parkinsonism [2] including both IPD and monogenic forms of parkinsonism. For example, psychiatric features may be part of the phenotypic spectrum conferred by *PINK1* mutations [3] and also appear to be more common in patients with *LRRK2* mutations than in non-mutation carriers and may be unrelated to dopaminergic medication [4,5]. In the present chapter, we will review current knowledge on NMS in monogenic forms of parkinsonism.

Overview of monogenic parkinsonism

About 5% of 'idiopathic' cases can currently be linked to a single genetic factor. However, this proportion may be significantly higher in selected populations; for example, about 40% of PD patients of North African Arab descent and about 20% of PD patients of Ashkenazi Jewish descent have been identified to carry the G2019S founder mutation in the *LRRK2* gene [6,7].

The genes and chromosomal loci linked to familial forms of parkinsonism have been designated as *PARK1–18*. Genes with a well-documented role in the pathogenesis of parkinsonism are summarized in Table 7.1 (for review see [8]). In this table genetic forms of parkinsonism for which information on NMS is available are given in bold type and those

Table 7.1 Monogenic forms of parkinsonism with known gene

Symbol (PARK locus)	Gene locus	Disorder	Inheritance	Gene	Status and remarks
PARK1	**4q21–22**	**Early-onset parkinsonism**	**AD**	**SNCA**	**Confirmed**
PARK2	**6q25.2–q27**	**Early-onset parkinsonism**	**AR**	**PARK2 encoding Parkin**	**Confirmed**
PARK3	2p13	Classical parkinsonism	AD	Unknown	Unconfirmed. May represent a risk factor. Gene not found since first described in 1998
PARK4	4q21–q23	Early-onset parkinsonism	AD	SNCA	Erroneous locus (identical to PARK1)
PARK5	4p13	Classical parkinsonism	AD	UCHL1	Unconfirmed (not replicated since described in 1998)
PARK6	**1p35–p36**	**Early-onset parkinsonism**	**AR**	**PINK1**	**Confirmed**
PARK7	**1p36**	**Early-onset parkinsonism**	**AR**	**PARK7 encoding DJ-1**	**Confirmed**
PARK8	**12q12**	**Classical parkinsonism**	**AD**	**LRRK2**	**Confirmed. Variations in LRRK2 gene include risk-conferring variants and disease-causing mutations**
PARK9	**1p36**	**Kufor–Rakeb syndrome. Atypical parkinsonism with dementia, spasticity and supranuclear gaze palsy**	**AR**	**ATP13A2**	**Confirmed**
PARK10	1p32	Classical parkinsonism	Risk factor	Unknown	Confirmed susceptibility locus. Gene unknown since first described in 2002
PARK11	2q36–27	Late-onset parkinsonism	AD	Unknown. Not G/GYF2	Not independently confirmed. May represent a risk factor. Gene not found since first described in 2002

Table 7.1 (continued) Monogenic forms of parkinsonism with known gene

Symbol (*PARK* locus)	Gene locus	Disorder	Inheritance	Gene	Status and remarks
PARK12	Xq21–q25	Classical parkinsonism	Risk factor	Unknown	Confirmed susceptibility locus. Represents maybe a risk factor. Gene not found since first described in 2003
PARK13	2p12	Classical parkinsonism	AD or risk factor	*HTRA2*	Unconfirmed
PARK14	22q13.1	Early-onset dystonia–parkinsonism	AR	*PLA2G6*	Confirmed. Vast majority of cases do not include parkinsonism
PARK15	22q12–q13	Early-onset parkinsonian–pyramidal syndrome	AR	*FBXO7*	Confirmed
PARK16	1q32	Classical parkinsonism	Risk factor	Unknown	Confirmed susceptibility locus
PARK17	**16q13**	**Classical parkinsonism**	**Causative gene**	***VPS35***	**Confirmed causative gene**
PARK18	3q27.1	Classical parkinsonism	Causative gene	*ELF4G1*	Unconfirmed

In this table genetic forms of parkinsonism for which information on NMS is available are given in bold type and are included in the present review.

AD, autosomal dominant; AR, autosomal recessive.

Table 7.2 Monogenic forms of parkinsonism with a known gene listed according to the latest classification.

New designation and phenotypic subgroup	Age at onset	Additional phenotypic notes	Inheritance pattern	Locus symbol
Classical parkinsonism				
PARK-SNCA	Variable. Duplications or triplications cause early onset	Missense mutations: classical parkinsonism. Duplication or triplication mutations in this gene: early onset parkinsonism with prominent dementia	AD	*PARK1*
PARK-LRRK2	Late onset	Classical parkinsonism	AD	*PARK8*
PARK-VPS35	Within the range of typical age of onset	Classical parkinsonism	AD	*PARK17*
PARK-PARKIN*	Early onset (30–40 years)	Relatively slow course, exquisite levodopa response	AR	*PARK2*
PARK-PINK1	Early onset (30–40 years)	Relatively slow course, exquisite levodopa response	AR	*PARK6*
PARK-DJ-1*	Early onset (30–40 years)	Classical parkinsonism	AR	*PARK7*
Susceptibility genes				
Glucocerebrosidase (*GBA*)	Within the range of typical age of onset	Heterozygous carriers classical parkinsonism	Uncertain	
Atypical parkinsonism or complex phenotypes				
PARK-ATP13A2	Early onset	Kufor–Rakeb syndrome	AR	*PARK9*

AD, autosomal dominant; AR, autosomal recessive.

* For these entries the gene has been identified but the HUGO Gene Nomenclature Committee (HGNC) has not yet provided a gene name. To make it clear that the gene has been identified we use the protein name in these locus symbols.

genetic forms are included in the present review. Table 7.2 gives monogenic forms of parkinsonism with a known gene listed according to the most recent classification.

In the following short overview of types of genetic parkinsonism for which information on NMS is available in the literature, monogenic forms of parkinsonism will be grouped according to their mode of inheritance. This is in agreement with functional findings that suggest a gain-of-function mechanism for dominant forms and a loss-of-function mechanism for recessive forms. However, in reality the situation may be more complex and this classification has been challenged by a remarkably reduced penetrance (the percentage of mutation carriers who actually develop the disease) in dominant forms and by a putative role of single heterozygous mutations in recessive forms (for review see [8]).

Alpha-synuclein (PARK1/4; dominant)

The *alpha-synuclein* (*SNCA*) gene was the first to be unequivocally associated with familial parkinsonism [9]. In addition to four point mutations, several families and individuals with parkinsonism were shown to carry duplications or triplications of the wild-type gene [10,11] (initially assigned as *PARK4*) [12]. However, *SNCA* mutations are overall extremely rare [13,14], and penetrance may be as low as 33% [10]. Interestingly, the severity of the phenotype appears to depend on gene dosage, and patients with *SNCA* duplications present clinically with classical parkinsonism more often than those with triplications. Although the phenotypic spectrum can be broad, the latter are often characterized by fast disease progression, marked dementia and a reduced lifespan [15,16]. To address the remarkable genotype–phenotype association for *SNCA* we present the data stratified by mutation type. For recent reviews see [17,18].

LRRK2 (PARK8; dominant)

Mutations in the *LRRK2 (leucine-rich repeat kinase 2)* gene [19,20] are considered the most common known genetic cause of classical parkinsonism; however, penetrance is reduced. *LRRK2* is a large gene that consists of 51 exons [19,20]. To date, more than 50 variants including at least 16 disease-causing mutations have been reported [21–31]. By far the most frequent and best studied mutation is the c.6055G>A (p.G2019S) substitution. Interestingly, at least 29 patients have been reported to carry this mutation in the homozygous state. However, there were no observable differences between homozygous and heterozygous carriers, thus arguing against a gene dosage effect [32]. *LRRK2* mutations are predominantly, but not exclusively [21,33,34], associated with a late-onset, classical parkinsonism phenotype [35].

VPS35 (PARK17; dominant)

This is the most recently discovered genetic cause for parkinsonism and the first identified via next-generation sequencing [36]. The vacuolar protein sorting 35 (VPS35) is involved in retromer-mediated transmembrane protein sorting, rescue and recycling, and disruptions in these processes may lead to neurodegeneration. The variant p.Asp620Asn was the first reported, has been confirmed in independent studies and its pathogenic relevance has been shown [37]. Thus, we include this variant and the p.Leu774Met variant, which has been reported in two independent studies, in our analyses but no other variants due to uncertainty about their pathogenic impact.

Parkin (PARK2; recessive)

Mutations in *Parkin* [38] are a common cause (10–20%) of early onset parkinsonism (variably defined across studies as an age of onset below 40–50 years) worldwide. Alterations in *Parkin* are spread over the entire gene and comprise deletions and duplications of one or more exons in more than 50% of reported cases [39,40]. Overall, *Parkin* mutation carriers present with classical parkinsonism but have an earlier age of onset, slower disease progression, a more symmetrical onset, more frequently dystonia as initial sign and hyperreflexia, and a tendency towards a better response to levodopa despite lower doses than patients without *Parkin* mutation [41].

PINK1 (PARK6; recessive)

The frequency of *PINK1* (*PTEN-induced kinase 1*) mutations [42] ranges from 1–8% in patients of different ethnicities [43–48]. *PINK1* mutation carriers are clinically indistinguishable from *Parkin* mutation carriers, with the possible exception of a higher rate of psychiatric symptoms [49–51].

DJ-1 (PARK7; recessive)

The *DJ-1* gene [52] is infrequently (<2%) associated with early onset parkinsonism and phenotypically closely resembles the *Parkin-* and *PINK1*-linked forms [53].

ATP13A2 (PARK9; recessive)

Homozygous and compound heterozygous mutations in a predominantly neuronal P-type ATPase gene (*ATP13A2*) have been demonstrated in the two identified families with Kufor–Rakeb syndrome (KRS), a form of recessively inherited atypical parkinsonism. KRS is clinically characterized by subacute, juvenile-onset, levodopa-responsive parkinsonism, pyramidal signs, dementia, a supranuclear gaze palsy, along with globus pallidus atrophy and later generalized brain atrophy [54,55]. Single heterozygous mutations in this gene may be associated with a phenotype of classical parkinsonism with an early age of onset [56].

Heterozgyous mutations in the Glucocerebrosidase gene (GBA)

Gaucher's disease is the most common of the lipidoses and among the most frequently inherited recessive disorders in Ashkenazi Jews. An association between Gaucher's disease and PD has been suggested by the co-occurrence of parkinsonism in rare cases on the one hand and by the identification of *Glucocerebrosidase* (*GBA*) mutations in probands with PD on the other [57,58]. As early as 1979 the observation of parkinsonian features in some patients with Gaucher's disease first suggested the unexpected link [59]. Intriguingly, both homozygous and heterozygous *GBA* mutations appear to predispose to PD, making *GBA* mutations the most important genetic susceptibility factor for PD in terms of effect size known to date [60]. This was almost unequivocally confirmed by a number of studies (see <http://www.pdgene.org/>) including a multiethnic analysis of *GBA* mutations in more than 10 000 patients and controls [61]. Intriguingly, a nationwide inquiry in Spain on co-morbidity of Gaucher's disease in 370 participants from 79 different families conducted in 2000 had identified both 'dementia' and 'PD' as the first two of a number of concurrent conditions of Gaucher's disease [62]. More recent studies have focused specifically on cognitive function and found dementia or various degrees of cognitive impairment to be common in *GBA* mutation carriers manifesting PD [63].

Digenic parkinsonism

Perhaps not surprisingly, a number of patients have been reported with mutations in more than one of the known PD genes, including one patient with heterozygous missense mutations in both *DJ-1* and *PINK1* [64]. Several patients carried combined mutations in *LRRK2* and *Parkin* [6,25,65,66]. Interestingly, these patients did not present with an earlier age at onset or a faster disease progression when compared with patients with a single *LRRK2* or *Parkin* mutation, thus not supporting a synergistic effect of *LRRK2* and *Parkin*.

Literature review of NMS in genetic parkinsonism

We searched the MEDLINE database (via PubMed, a service of the National Library of Medicine's National Center for Biotechnology Information, at <http://www.ncbi.nlm.nih.gov>) for publications from January 1966 to February 2013, using the search terms 'parkinson' and the name of known PD genes (e.g. 'Parkin parkinson', 'PINK1 parkinson' etc.). This resulted in 3740 citations. Based on the abstract or paper, we selected 852 publications that included genetic information on PD patients. We avoided double counts and included a total of 173 articles containing any information on any type of NMS (2295 cases; Table 7.3).

Table 7.3 Results of the literature review

Search term Parkinson and ...	Number of references		Articles with genetic information		Number of papers (cases) including information on non-motor symptoms
	2008	2013	2008	2013	
Synuclein/SNCA/PARK1	975	609	60	106	25 (117) [10,16,69,82,89,90,[93–111]
LRRK2/PARK8	189	462	97	232	66 (866) [4,5,25,26,28,29, 32–35,72,81,83,112–165]
VPS35	0	14	0	11	5 (39) [37,166–169]
Parkin/PARK2	449	421	79	114	33 (377) [41,46,67,85,140,141,146, 170–194]
PINK1/PARK6	79	261	28	64	19 (98) [43–45,47–49, 51,86,87,140,141,195–207]
DJ-1/PARK7	103	25	15	6	5 (12) [77–79,140,208–219]
ATP13A2/PARK9	3	53	2	18	3 (10) [56,212,213]
Glucocerebrosidase/GBA	27	70	20	30	17 (776) [61,63,77–79, 214–225]
Total	1825	1915	301	581	173 (2295)
	3740		882		

Methods of studies reporting any type of NMS in patients with genetic parkinsonism

Overall, the methods were variable, as were the study aims. Naturally, the majority of identified studies primarily addressed genetic questions such as types, frequency, penetrance and pathogenicity of mutations. In these studies, the clinical information was often kept to a minimum. However, articles often featured tables summarizing the clinical information and the recognition of the impact of NMS led to the partial inclusion of NMS information in those overview tables.

Relatively few studies specifically addressed NMS in genetic PD (e.g. cognitive function [63,67]; psychiatric disturbances [3]; rapid eye movement (REM) sleep behaviour disorder (RBD) [68]; cardiac denervation [69]; olfaction [70,71]) or listed assessment of NMS as one of their main aims (olfactory function [72]; neuropsychological and neuropsychiatric function [5]). Furthermore, even between those studies addressing NMS, the assessment methods and the spectrum of NMS covered were variable, leading to problems with comparability. Among studies not focused on NMS, only a minority provided detailed clinical information on NMS. Most papers simply reported on 'absence of dementia', frequently without further mention of how this was assessed. A subgroup of the remaining studies described more detailed information on several features of NMS including psychiatric, autonomic, sleep, sensory disturbances and decreased sense of smell.

Before presenting the data, we would like to point out several caveats that need to be kept in mind when interpreting the results:

- Data were extracted from all selected articles, although methods and study subjects differed widely between studies.

- The diagnostic definitions for NMS varied across articles; for example, some but not all studies used DSM IV criteria for dementia.

- Information on the severity of, for example, dementia or depression was rarely given, which impacts on the frequency estimates.

- Diagnostic procedures differed between articles; for example, many but not all used the Mini Mental State Examination (MMSE) as a diagnostic procedure. Furthermore, different cutoff scores were used for the diagnosis of dementia, ranging from 16/30 to 24/30.

- Examination methods ranged from in-person specialist examination to history taking or chart review. Some authors screened for NMS, others only reported treatments for certain NMS, such as depression, yielding highly variable symptom frequencies.

- In examinations and screenings, for example with the Beck Depression Inventory (BDI), a point prevalence of the symptom is assessed. Chart reviews or medical history usually assess the lifetime prevalence up to the time of examination.

- It was impossible to account for all of these differences: in many articles the information about the assessment of NMS was not detailed enough to distinguish all of the listed differences; often the diagnostic criteria and diagnostic procedures were not stated in detail. This can mostly be explained by the fact that we tried to extract this information from work that was never designed to answer these questions.

◆ Most reported genetic cases were identified in tertiary care centres, in clinic series or sometimes as single cases that were screened for mutations, mostly in highly selected subgroups, for instance young-onset patients with dystonia as a presenting symptom to be screened for *Parkin* mutations. Another large group of cases was identified via family studies. Both ascertainment methods are prone to bias and possibly not representative of all monogenic PD patients.

◆ The cases differed widely in age at onset, disease duration, ethnicity, treatment, co-morbidity and many other factors that cannot be accounted for in this chapter.

◆ Only articles with information on at least one NMS of interest were selected for review. The numbers and percentages of cases labelled as 'without information' on the respective NMS correspond to the cases in this subset of the literature only. Our aim in presenting the numbers and percentages of cases without available information is to provide a clear 'red flag' that the percentage of cases presenting with the symptom of interest needs to be interpreted with care.

◆ The overview on how many cases have been identified since 2008 (the date of the version of this chapter in the first edition) refers only to articles fulfilling our inclusion criteria.

Methods of evaluating the selected studies

Whenever a paper stated that 'x' patients had depression, the remaining 'y' patients were counted as having no depression, unless the authors made a comment that not all patients were available for examination. Whenever the presence of any NMS was reported, this information was entered in the summary tables even if no details about the diagnostic procedure were available. For example, a BDI score above the cutoff, a history of depression upon interview or chart review or a treatment for depression all counted as 'depression present'. We did not distinguish between anxiety and panic attacks, which was impossible because of lack of detailed information and small number of cases; they were therefore combined as 'anxiety present'. 'Hallucinations' represent an assortment of all types of hallucinations disregarding their frequency, type and severity (e.g. rare visual hallucinations counted as 'present'), and this 'label' may also extend to psychiatrically different but related domains such as psychosis, paranoia and delusion. We defined dementia based on a MMSE cutoff of <24 for all cases with a MMSE available; therefore, in a small number of cases we counted dementia as present, although the article stated, for example, 'no dementia, MMSE 21'. In addition, cognitive impairment, memory loss, confusion, recall of 0/3 words and lack of orientation were all counted as dementia if no MMSE score was given. Autonomic symptoms comprised any of the following: urinary frequency/urgency/incontinence, constipation and orthostatic hypotension. 'Sleep problems' included restless legs syndrome (RLS), RBD, daytime sleepiness or any statement of 'sleep disturbance'. However, we decided not to count every person without RBD as 'no sleep problem', as RBD is less common than

Table 7.4 Overview of frequency of symptoms and availability of information in the selected articles

Symptom	Frequency of symptom	Availability of information
Depression	282/933 (30%)	933/2295 (41%)
Anxiety	106/530 (20%)	530/2295 (23%)
Hallucinations	202/924 (22%)	924/2295 (40%)
Dementia	269/1199 (22%)	1199/2295 (52%)
Autonomic	136/461 (30%)	461/2295 (20%)
Sleep	124/256 (48%)	256/2295 (11%)

most other sleep disturbances. Finally, some articles stated 'psychological disturbances' or 'behavioural problems' which were not further specified and thus could not be assigned to any of the described categories and were therefore counted as 'without information' in the tables (for overview, see Table 7.4).

Despite all the aforementioned uncertainties, we tried to assemble all available information but need to emphasize that the listed numbers are fraught with methodological challenges and cannot be considered as prevalences of NMS in representative populations. Therefore we refrained from the presentation of confidence intervals for the frequency counts, although the numbers would mostly be sufficient, as we felt that may indicate a false sense of certainty and precision.

Frequency of non-motor signs by gene

Table 7.5–7.13 and the following short paragraphs summarize published data on the presence of depression, anxiety, hallucinations, dementia, autonomic dysfunction and sleep problems for each of the genes with available information. The information density is different for each of these features, as well as across genes. Overall, within the reviewed articles, hallucinations and dementia were most frequently commented on, followed by depression and anxiety. Little information was given on autonomic symptoms and sleep problems. Of further note, the numbers of cases reviewed differ widely across genes. This is due to the variable frequency of mutations in the genes under study and the fact that some of the genes have been discovered only recently. Finally, different (types of) mutations in the various genes may have variable effects on the phenotype. For example, as previously mentioned, a *SNCA* duplication tends to result in a phenotype more reminiscent of that of iPD, whereas triplications are associated with a more rapidly progressive disease course and more prominent cognitive features. Apart from *SNCA*, different mutation types were not accounted for when compiling information for the tables.

Overall, for *SNCA* mutation carriers, depression, hallucinations, dementia and autonomic symptoms were frequently assessed, resulting in a relatively large amount of information being available. Dementia was the most frequently described NMS, followed by depression, autonomic symptoms and hallucinations, each in about a quarter of the

Table 7.5 *SNCA* missense mutations

Symptom	Frequency of symptom	Availability of information
Depression	11/28 (39%)	28/54 (52%)
Anxiety	0	0
Hallucinations	6/17 (35%)	17/54 (31%)
Dementia	17/35 (49%)	35/54 (65%)
Autonomic	13/35 (37%)	35/54 (65%)
Sleep	1 Insomnia, 1 EDS	2/54 (4%)
Other/comments	E46K family diagnosed as DLB A53T: three cases with central hypoventilation [90] 1 patient cocaine abuse 1 patient pathological gambling and stealing	Substance abuse and impulse control disorders not systematically examined but two severe cases identified

EDS, excessive daytime sleepiness; DLB, dementia with Lewy bodies.

Table 7.6 *SNCA* multiplications (36 cases with duplication, 27 with triplications including two with homozygous duplications)

Symptom	Frequency of symptom		Availability of information	
	Duplication	Triplication	Duplication	Triplication
Depression	7/15 (47%)	13/13 (100%)	15/36 (42%)	13/27 (48%)
Anxiety	2	1	2/36 (6%)	1/27 (15%)
Hallucinations	10/17 (59%)	13/13 (100%)	17/36 (47%)	13/27 (48%)
Dementia	12/24 (50%)	13/13 (100%)	24/36 (67%)	13/27 (48%)
Autonomic	3/7 (43%)	13/13 (100%)	7/36 (19%)	13/27 (48%)
Sleep	na	2 RBD, 1 insomnia, 1 parasomnia	na	4/27 (15%)
Other/comments	AAO of dementia: 57 ± 11 years Time PD to dementia: 6 ± 4 years	AAO of dementia: 39 ± 4 years Time PD to dementia: 5 ± 5 years		Other symptoms mentioned: severe weight loss, fatigue (initial symptom), myoclonus (in course of disease)

na, not applicable; AAO, average age of onset; RBD, rapid eye movement (REM) sleep behavioural disorder; PD, Parkinson's disease.

patients. However, the systematic evaluation of the 117 published *SNCA* mutation carriers with NMS information confirmed a mutation (type)-specific clinical expression, which appears to be rather unique to *SNCA* mutations compared with other PD genes. The A53T mutation is associated with an age of onset about 10 years earlier than the other three known missense mutations, including the new H50Q mutation [18]. Similarly, *SNCA* triplication carriers have an age of onset about 10 years earlier and a more rapid disease course than duplication carriers, who overall closely resemble iPD patients. Furthermore, higher-order SNCA multiplications are associated with additional neurological features, such as myoclonus. Similarly, the frequencies of NMS differ markedly by mutation type. However, for the non-motor features, their mere frequency appears less striking than their severity, with an early age of onset of depression or dementia, suicidal ideation and multi-modal hallucinations. Thus, we conclude that a differential view of *SNCA* mutations and variants may allow important pathophysiological inferences even beyond monogenic PD and is warranted in the context of clinical counselling. Although in comparison with iPD, *SNCA* duplication carriers seem to have the most similar disease course, even for duplication carriers the frequencies of dementia, hallucinations and depression seem higher than in iPD. Dementia is a particularly important NMS, but also the NMS for which mere frequency counts seem to be insufficient to deduce clinically relevant information. The cumulative prevalence of dementia in IPD is estimated to be 75% [73], while the point prevalence is reported as 30% [74]. These two figures alone demonstrate that the time from the onset of parkinsonism to the onset of dementia is crucial information. This information, however, could be extracted for the comparison of *SNCA* duplications versus triplications only and in this case shows important differences.

Although the total number of cases described for *LRRK2*-associated parkinsonism was large, overall only limited information was available on NMS, with dementia being the most commonly assessed sign (49%). Furthermore, the availability of information tended to decrease from 2008 to 2013, for example with information available for dementia in 65% of the mutation carriers in 2008 and 49% in 2013. Sleep problems appeared to be the most commonly present but least commonly assessed NMS, and were described in 61% of the patients. The second most common NMS was depression, present in almost 35% of the mutation carriers. However, this number does not differ from the described prevalence of depression in iPD [75]. Despite this similar frequency of depression, this syndrome is of particular interest as there are indications that *LRRK2* carriers may suffer from severe depression more frequently than patients with other types of parkinsonism, with two completed suicides reported and several descriptions of severe, recurrent major depression. In contrast, the occurrence of dementia in 17% of the *LRRK2* mutation carriers is lower than

Table 7.7 *LRRK2*

Symptom	Frequency of symptom	Availability of information
Depression	127/363 (35%)	363/866 (42%)
Anxiety	60/210 (29%)	210/866 (24%)
Hallucinations	58/354 (16%)	354/866 (41%)
Dementia	71/425 (17%)	425/866 (49%)
Autonomic	55/224 (25%)	224/866 (26%)
Sleep	106/174 (61%)	174/866 (20%)
Other/comments	Two completed suicides reported, one in the context of severe recurrent depression	

that reported in a systematic review of iPD (25–30%) [74]. This is in line with the indication that *LRRK2* mutation carriers have an overall slightly more benign course of disease than iPD cases. Of note, the patients listed in our Table 7.7 harbour different types of mutations, although the G2019S mutation is by far the most common. The data for different *LRRK2* mutations are comparable, and even between heterozygous and the rare homozygous mutations no striking clinical differences have been reported, arguing against a genotype–phenotype correlation within subtypes of *LRRK2* mutations. In summary, the extracted information supports the notion that *LRRK2*-linked parkinsonism is clinically indistinguishable from iPD.

Although the NMS information for *VPS35* carriers seems rather complete at first glance, the summary presented in Table 7.8 is based on few reports and within these the NMS information was mainly 'NMS present' or 'NMS absent' without further specification as to method of assessment and NMS included. Thus, this information needs to be viewed with some caution.

Overall, the frequencies of NMS in patients with *Parkin* mutations seem relatively low, but unfortunately only limited information is available. In particular the frequency of

Table 7.8 *VPS35*

Symptom	Frequency of symptom	Availability of information
Depression	1/31 (3%)	31/39 (79%)
Anxiety	0/31 (0%)	31/39 (79%)
Hallucinations	1/17 (6%)	17/39 (44%)
Dementia	2/22 (9%)	22/39 (56%)
Autonomic	2/2 (100%)	2/39 (5%)
Sleep	1/1 (100%)	1/39 (3%)
Other/comments	One impulse control behaviour	

Table 7.9 *Parkin*

Symptom	Frequency of symptom	Availability of information
Depression	35/248 (14%)	248/377 (66%)
Anxiety	16/194 (8%)	194/377 (51%)
Hallucinations	7/226 (3%)	226/377 (60%)
Dementia	5/104 (5%)	104/377 (28%)
Autonomic	7/41 (17%)	41/377 (11%)
Sleep	5/14 (36%)	14/377 (4%)
Other/comments	53 tested [70,71,179,192,193], 22/30 normal test result, in others mean scores reported, all show less impairment than in IPD	

IPD, idiopathic Parkinson's disease.

dementia is well below the frequencies reported in iPD and matches the frequency in the general population above the age of 65 years. This may be influenced by the young age of most patients with *Parkin* mutations but holds true even for cases with disease durations over 20 years and could thus be helpful information for patients in genetic counselling. Taken together, these data support the notion that *Parkin*-associated parkinsonism is less frequently complicated by NMS than iPD and probably also compared with other genetic forms of parkinsonism.

Compared with the combined *Parkin* mutation carriers, psychiatric symptoms are more common in *PINK1*-associated disease, although the age of onset is comparable. When comparing *PINK1* mutation carriers with all genetic parkinsonism (Table 7.4), depression was similarly common, anxiety was twice as frequent, hallucinations and dementia were less common as were autonomic and sleep disturbances. The difference in frequency of depression compared with *Parkin* mutation carriers is particularly interesting in light of the postulated pathophysiological similarities between the two entities. This difference might even be larger than represented in our tables, since in *PINK1* mutation carriers DSM IV diagnostic criteria were more frequently applied than in patients with other genetic forms of parkinsonism. For example, the diagnosis of a major depression according to DSM IV

Table 7.10 *PINK1*

Symptom	Frequency of symptom	Availability of information
Depression	28/80 (35%)	80/98 (82%)
Anxiety	18/44 (41%)	44/98 (45%)
Hallucinations	11/71 (15%)	71/98 (72%)
Dementia	6/75 (8%)	75/98 (77%)
Autonomic	7/55 (13%)	55/98 (56%)
Sleep	4/19 (21%)	19/98 (19%)
Other/comments	Ten manifesting carriers tested for olfactory function, less impaired than IPD [70]	

IPD, idiopathic Parkinson's disease.

Table 7.11 *DJ-1* (total number of cases reviewed: 12)

Symptom	Frequency of symptom	Availability of information
Depression	0/2	2/10
Anxiety	2/4	2/10
Hallucinations	0/2	2/10
Dementia	0/1	1/10
Autonomic	0/2	2/10
Sleep	1/1	1/10
Other/comments	One case with normosmia [71]	

requires a certain severity and duration of symptoms that do not have to be fulfilled in order to screen positive on the BDI or Hamilton Depression Scale. On the other hand, application of DSM criteria via a structured clinical interview usually yields lifetime prevalences which may in turn differ considerably from point prevalences (e.g. the last 4 weeks in most questionnaires) for an episodic disorder such as depression.

To give a complete overview of the currently available information, we included tables on *DJ-1* and *ATP13A2*-associated parkinsonism (Table 7.11 and 7.12). However, due to the scarcity of published data, we cannot draw any meaningful conclusions on NMS in these forms of genetic parkinsonism.

Similar to *ATP13A2*-linked disease, *GBA*-associated parkinsonism in homozygous carriers is often accompanied by atypical clinical signs such as supranuclear gaze palsy, pyramidal signs, metabolic disorders and a less prominent response to levodopa. However, heterozygous mutations in *GBA* and in *ATP13A2* have been associated with clinically more typical parkinsonism. In both conditions, an increased frequency of dementia has been suggested, although to date no obvious differences in the prevalence of dementia have been shown compared with IPD. Of interest, an autopsy study on nine *GBA* mutation carriers established a neuropathological diagnosis of dementia with Lewy bodies/

Table 7.12 *ATP13A2*

Symptom	Frequency of symptom	Availability of information
Depression	3/10	10/10
Anxiety	2/2	2/10
Hallucinations	6/10	10/10
Dementia	5/10	10/10
Autonomic	2/6	6/10
Sleep	1/4	4/10
Other/Comments	None	

Table 7.13 *GBA* (35 of the cases carry two *GBA* mutations)

Symptom	Frequency of symptom	Availability of information
Depression	57/143 (40%)	143/776 (18%)
Anxiety	6/43 (14%)	43/776 (6%)
Hallucinations	90/197 (46%)	197/776 (25%)
Dementia	138/490 (28%)	490/776 (63%)
Autonomic	34/76 (45%)	76/776 (10%)
Sleep	5/42 (12%)	42/776 (5%)
Other/comments	Several reports of lower mean scores in cognitive tests in *GBA* PD than IPD	

PD, Parkinson's disease; IPD, idiopathic PD.

Alzheimer's disease in eight of the nine cases, whereas only one patient received a post mortem diagnosis of PD [58].

Anheim et al. [76] systematically addressed the penetrance of *GBA* mutation for parkinsonism. Their study was based on 525 familial PD cases including 24 *GBA* carriers estimated penetrance rates of 7.6, 13.7, 21.4 and 29.7% at ages 50, 60, 70 and 80 years, respectively, under a dominant model. Thus, *GBA* may be considered a dominant causal gene for parkinsonism with reduced penetrance and be taken into account in genetic counselling accordingly. Furthermore, there are indications of a genotype–phenotype correlation [77–79] based on the classification of *GBA* mutations into mild and severe mutations according to the grouping specified by researchers studying Gaucher's disease [80]. To date, the data on genotype–phenotype correlations are limited and partly conflicting, comparisons being hampered by the lack of systematic assessments and the variability of methods, reports and available information.

Additional information on different NMS

Another important and intriguing non-motor symptom is olfactory dysfunction. It has been postulated that autosomal dominant forms of monogenic parkinsonism exhibit more severe olfactory impairment than the recessive forms. In particular, for *Parkin* mutation-associated parkinsonism a largely preserved sense of smell has been reported by different groups with a total of 53 manifesting carriers tested. Similar observations have been made for *PINK1* (10 cases tested) and *DJ-1* (1 case reported with normosmia). Furthermore, differences between carriers of one versus two mutations in the *Parkin* or *PINK1* gene have been shown, with those with one mutation having more severe olfactory impairment and thus being more similar to idiopathic cases in this regard. However, for *LRRK2* mutation carriers less severe olfactory impairment compared with IPD has also been reported [81].

Some of the reviewed articles provided more detailed data than are listed in the tables. In addition, sometimes data on the severity and impact of the different NMS were also included. For example, for a *SNCA* mutation carrier from a French family severe depressive episodes were reported and the patient committed suicide [82]. Similarly, severe depression and suicide have been reported in two *LRRK2* mutation carriers [83]. In addition, *LRRK2* mutations were associated with claustrophobia and alcohol and levodopa addiction, respectively, in one case each [72]. In general, no systematic report on impulse controls disorders in genetic parkinsonism has come to our attention despite the increased interest in this particular NMS. However, several reports on patients with different forms of monogenic parkinsonism mention various forms and severities of impulse control disorders, e.g. in a carrier of a *SNCA* triplication where the patient was even arrested for stealing [84]. Certain *Parkin* mutation carriers were reported to have obsessive compulsive disorder (OCD; *n* = 2) [41,85], verbal aggressiveness (*n* = 1), hypersexuality (*n* = 2), hysterical episodes and conversional symptoms (*n* = 1) [41]. One study specifically addressed the association of mutations in the *PINK1* gene with psychiatric disorders in a large family [50]. Of note, all of the 11 heterozygous mutation carriers were asymptomatic regarding motor symptoms, but six of them showed signs of probable or possible parkinsonism upon neurological examination [86]. Six of the heterozygotes had a lifetime diagnosis of affective schizophrenia spectrum disorder pre-dating the diagnosis of probable or possible parkinsonism: bipolar I disorder with psychotic symptoms ($n = 2$), non-psychotic major depression ($n = 1$), schizotypal personality disorder ($n = 3$). One homozygous and one heterozygous carrier additionally suffered from an anxiety disorder; another two had an adjustment disorder and obsessive compulsive personality disorder [50]. All diagnoses were established by psychiatrist examination using DSM IV criteria. Another study reported two *PINK1* mutation carriers with anxiety and somatoform disorder and anxiety and OCD, respectively [87]. *ATP13A2* mutations have been linked to severe psychosis with delusional episodes, aggressive behaviour requiring hospitalization ($n = 1$) and OCD ($n = 1$) [56]. However, as these symptoms or co-morbidities are reported only for individual cases and no information on the presence or absence of these symptoms is available for a larger number of cases or within systematic assessment, no prevalence rates can be calculated and compared with IPD or the general population.

Autonomic symptoms listed in the tables comprised urinary urgency, frequency or incontinence, and orthostatic hypotension or dizziness. Additional autonomic symptoms were reported in one *SNCA* mutation carrier with excessive drooling [88]; three patients with *SNCA* mutations had signs of cardiac denervation upon cardial scintigraphy [69,89]. Furthermore, the autonomic symptoms in *SNCA* mutation carriers were often severe, such as orthostatic hypotension requiring medication or even precluding the patients from standing. In a family carrying the A53T mutation reported by Spira et al. [90], all affected carriers exhibited central hypoventilation.

Comparison of symptom frequency across genes

While the previous section focused mainly on the NMS profile of each gene with only some mention of similarities between genes, Table 7.14–7.19 are designed to facilitate comparison across genes (except *DJ-1* and *ATP13A2* which were omitted because of the small case numbers) by NMS.

Table 7.14 Depression in different forms of genetic parkinsonism

Gene	Cases with symptom/cases with information (% with symptom)	Cases with/without information (% with information)
SNCA	31/56 (55%)	56/117 (37%)
LRRK2	127/363 (35%)	363/866 (42%)
VPS35	1/31 (3%)	31/39 (79%)
Parkin	35/248 (14%)	248/377 (66%)
PINK1	28/80 (35%)	80/98 (82%)
GBA	57/143 (40%)	143/776 (18%)

Note: because of the small case numbers we omitted the counts for *DJ-1* and *ATP13A2*.

Table 7.15 Anxiety in different forms of genetic parkinsonism

Gene	Cases with symptom/cases with information (% with symptom)	Cases with/without information (% with information)
SNCA	3/3 (100%)	3/117 (3%)
LRRK2	60/210 (29%)	210/866 (24%)
VPS35	0/31 (0%)	31/39 (79%)
Parkin	16/194 (8%)	194/377 (51%)
PINK1	18/44 (41%)	44/98 (45%)
GBA	6/43 (14%)	43/776 (6%)

Table 7.16 Hallucinations in different forms of genetic parkinsonism

Gene	Cases with symptom/cases with information (% with symptom)	Cases with/without information (% with information)
SNCA	29/47 (62%)	47/117 (40%)
LRRK2	58/354 (16%)	354/866 (41%)
VPS35	1/17 (6%)	17/39 (44%)
Parkin	7/226 (3%)	226/377 (60%)
PINK1	11/71 (15%)	71/98 (72%)
GBA	90/197 (46%)	197/776 (25%)

Table 7.17 Dementia in different forms of genetic parkinsonism

Gene	Cases with symptom/cases with information (% with symptom)	Cases with/without information (% with information)
SNCA	42/72 (58%)	72/117 (62%)
LRRK2	71/425 (17%)	425/866 (49%)
VPS35	2/22 (9%)	22/39 (56%)
Parkin	5/104 (5%)	104/377 (28%)
PINK1	6/75 (8%)	75/98 (77%)
GBA	138/490 (28%)	490/776 (63%)

Table 7.18 Autonomic dysfunction in different forms of genetic parkinsonism

Gene	Cases with symptom/cases with information (% with symptom)	Cases with/without information (% with information)
SNCA	29/55 (53%)	55/117 (47%)
LRRK2	55/224 (25%)	224/866 (26%)
VPS35	2/2 (100%)	2/39 (5%)
Parkin	7/41 (17%)	41/377 (11%)
PINK1	7/55 (13%)	55/98 (56%)
GBA	34/76 (45%)	76/776 (10%)

Table 7.19 Sleep problems in different forms of genetic parkinsonism

Gene	Cases with symptom/cases with information (% with symptom)	Cases with/without information (% with information)
SNCA	6/6 (100%)	6/117 (5%)
LRRK2	106/174 (61%)	174/866 (20%)
VPS35	1/1	1/39 (3%)
Parkin	5/14 (36%)	14/377 (4%)
PINK1	4/19 (21%)	19/98 (19%)
GBA	5/42 (12%)	42/776 (5%)

Conclusions and perspectives

In conclusion, there are still limited data on NMS in genetic forms of parkinsonism. The frequent lack of a clear definition of symptoms and signs, a broad spectrum of study designs, predominance of convenience samples and the overall absence of systematic evaluations for all NMS in one patient sample render comparisons difficult and prone to bias. Overall, the frequency of NMS in patients with genetic parkinsonism, apart from SNCA mutations, does not appear to be higher and may even be lower than in iPD. An interesting difference from IPD is the preserved sense of smell in Parkin and possibly PINK1 mutation carriers. Other intriguing information is the difference in frequency of NMS and in particular psychiatric symptoms between Parkin and PINK1 mutation carriers despite the comparable age at onset of parkinsonism and the postulated pathophysiological overlap. These observations need to be verified in larger studies and, if confirmed, may help to differentiate between the otherwise clinically similar forms of genetic parkinsonism at the group, but most likely not at the individual patient, level.

NMS should be considered as important and often treatable concomitant features of genetic parkinsonism. A better understanding of the pathophysiology of the individual genetic forms may, in the future, lead to the development of more specific therapies not only for the motor syndrome but also for NMS. Validated questionnaires on NMS in PD are available, providing screening tools for the urgently needed systematic, large-scale assessment of NMS in genetic parkinsonism with the aim of improving the diagnosis and management of NMS [91,92]. Furthermore, the Movement Disorder Society has provided several reviews summarizing the basic clinimetric data on common scales and endorsing several scales for most of the relevant symptoms. From the reviewed articles it seems that agreement on the scales used is increasing. However, the observation that the amount of information on NMS is decreasing in more recent articles, as seems to be the case in the reports on LRRK2 and GBA mutation carriers, often in the context of increasing study and sample size, is alarming. Research into monogenic PD will always depend on an ability to pool data and review vast numbers of individual cases due to the rarity of these disorders. This calls for a minimal data set consisting of recommended scales which is then included in each publication in a small but uniform reporting format (such as a table). On the individual patient level, screening for relevant NMS, which are often treatable, should be part of the standard clinical assessment, and cases such as the reported cases of suicide in the context of severe depression only underline this necessity. In recent years, studies on quality of life have repeatedly demonstrated the impact on NMS on patients' lives.

Acknowledgement

Christine Klein is supported the Hermann and Lilly Schilling Foundation, NGFN-plus and MEFOPA; Meike Kasten received grant support from the German Research Foundation (DFG KA 3179/2–1) and an intramural career development grant from the University of Lübeck.

References

1 Galpern WR, Lang AE. Interface between tauopathies and synucleinopathies: a tale of two proteins. Ann Neurol 2006; **59**: 449–58.

2 Lang AE, Obeso JA. Challenges in Parkinson's disease: restoration of the nigrostriatal dopamine system is not enough. Lancet Neurol 2004; **3**: 309–16.

3 Steinlechner S, Stahlberg J, Volkel B, et al. Co-occurrence of affective and schizophrenia spectrum disorders with PINK1 mutations. J Neurol Neurosurg Psychiatry 2007; **78**: 532–5.

4 Tomiyama H, Li Y, Funayama M, et al. Clinicogenetic study of mutations in LRRK2 exon 41 in Parkinson's disease patients from 18 countries. Mov Disord 2006; **21**: 1102–8.

5 Goldwurm S, Zini M, Di Fonzo A, et al. LRRK2 G2019S mutation and Parkinson's disease: a clinical, neuropsychological and neuropsychiatric study in a large Italian sample. Parkinsonism Relat Disord 2006; **12**: 410–19.

6 Lesage S, Durr A, Tazir M, et al. LRRK2 G2019S as a cause of Parkinson's disease in North African Arabs. N Engl J Med 2006; **354**: 422–3.

7 Ozelius LJ, Senthil G, Saunders-Pullman R, et al. LRRK2 G2019S as a cause of Parkinson's disease in Ashkenazi Jews. N Engl J Med 2006; **354**: 424–5.

8 Kumar KR, Lohmann K, Klein C. Genetics of Parkinson disease and other movement disorders. Curr Opin Neurol 2012; **25**: 466–74.

9 Polymeropoulos MH, Lavedan C, Leroy E, et al. Mutation in the alpha-synuclein gene identified in families with Parkinson's disease. Science 1997; **276**: 2045–7.

10 Nishioka K, Hayashi S, Farrer MJ, et al. Clinical heterogeneity of alpha-synuclein gene duplication in Parkinson's disease. Ann Neurol 2006; **59**: 298–309.

11 Singleton AB, Farrer M, Johnson J, et al. Alpha-synuclein locus triplication causes Parkinson's disease. Science 2003; **302**: 841.

12 Farrer M, Gwinn-Hardy K, Muenter M, et al. A chromosome 4p haplotype segregating with Parkinson's disease and postural tremor. Hum Molec Genet 1999; **8**: 81–5.

13 Berg D, Niwar M, Maass S, et al. Alpha-synuclein and Parkinson's disease: implications from the screening of more than 1,900 patients. Mov Disord 2005; **20**: 1191–4.

14 Williams-Gray CH, Goris A, Foltynie T, et al. No alterations in alpha-synuclein gene dosage observed in sporadic Parkinson's disease. Mov Disord 2006; **21**: 731–2.

15 Golbe LI, Di Iorio G, Sanges G, et al. Clinical genetic analysis of Parkinson's disease in the Contursi kindred. Ann Neurol 1996; **40**: 767–75.

16 Fuchs J, Nilsson C, Kachergus J, et al. Phenotypic variation in a large Swedish pedigree due to SNCA duplication and triplication. Neurology 2007; **68**: 916–22.

17 Devine MJ, Gwinn K, Singleton A, Hardy J. Parkinson's disease and alpha-synuclein expression. Mov Disord 2011; **26**:2160–8.

18 Kasten M, Klein C. The many faces of alpha-synuclein. Mov Disord 2013; **28**: 697–701.

19 Zimprich A, Biskup S, Leitner P, et al. Mutations in LRRK2 cause autosomal-dominant parkinsonism with pleomorphic pathology. Neuron 2004; **44**: 601–7.

20 Paisan-Ruiz C, Jain S, Evans EW, et al. Cloning of the gene containing mutations that cause PARK8-linked Parkinson's disease. Neuron 2004; **44**: 595–600.

21 Hedrich K, Winkler S, Hagenah J, et al. Recurrent LRRK2 (Park8) mutations in early-onset Parkinson's disease. Mov Disord 2006; **21**: 1506–10.

22 Funayama M, Hasegawa K, Ohta E, et al. An LRRK2 mutation as a cause for the parkinsonism in the original PARK8 family. Ann Neurol 2005; **57**: 918–21.

23 Zabetian CP, Samii A, Mosley AD, et al. A clinic-based study of the LRRK2 gene in Parkinson disease yields new mutations. Neurology 2005; **65**: 741–4.

24 Farrer M, Stone J, Mata IF, et al. LRRK2 mutations in Parkinson disease. Neurology 2005; **65**: 738–40.

25 Paisan-Ruiz C, Lang AE, Kawarai T, et al. LRRK2 gene in Parkinson disease: mutation analysis and case control association study. Neurology 2005; **65**: 696–700.

26 Mata IF, Kachergus JM, Taylor JP, et al. LRRK2 pathogenic substitutions in Parkinson's disease. Neurogenetics 2005; **6**: 171–7.

27 Kachergus J, Mata IF, Hulihan M, et al. Identification of a novel LRRK2 mutation linked to autosomal dominant parkinsonism: evidence of a common founder across European populations. Am J Hum Genet 2005; **76**: 672–80.

28 Lesage S, Ibanez P, Lohmann E, et al. G2019S LRRK2 mutation in French and North African families with Parkinson's disease. Ann Neurol 2005; **58**: 784–7.

29 Berg D, Schweitzer K, Leitner P, et al. Type and frequency of mutations in the LRRK2 gene in familial and sporadic Parkinson's disease. Brain 2005; **128**: 3000–11.

30 Di Fonzo A, Tassorelli C, De Mari M, et al. Comprehensive analysis of the LRRK2 gene in sixty families with Parkinson's disease. Eur J Hum Genet 2006; **14**: 322–31.

31 Tomiyama H, Li Y, Funayama M, et al. Clinicogenetic study of mutations in LRRK2 exon 41 in Parkinson's disease patients from 18 countries. Mov Disord 2006; **21**: 1102–8.

32 Ishihara L, Warren L, Gibson R, et al. Clinical features of Parkinson disease patients with homozygous leucine-rich repeat kinase 2 G2019S mutations. Arch Neurol 2006; **63**: 1250–4.

33 Kay DM, Zabetian CP, Factor SA, et al. Parkinson's disease and LRRK2: frequency of a common mutation in U.S. movement disorder clinics. Mov Disord 2006; **21**: 519–23.

34 Goldwurm S, Di Fonzo A, Simons EJ, et al. The G6055A (G2019S) mutation in LRRK2 is frequent in both early and late onset Parkinson's disease and originates from a common ancestor. J Med Genet 2005; **42**: e65.

35 Marongiu R, Ghezzi D, Ialongo T, et al. Frequency and phenotypes of LRRK2 G2019S mutation in Italian patients with Parkinson's disease. Mov Disord 2006; **21**: 1232–5.

36 Vilarino-Guell C, Wider C, Ross OA, et al. VPS35 mutations in Parkinson disease. Am J Hum Genet 2011; **89**: 162–7.

37 Sharma M, Ioannidis JP, Aasly JO, et al. A multi-centre clinico-genetic analysis of the VPS35 gene in Parkinson disease indicates reduced penetrance for disease-associated variants. J Med Genet 2012; **49**: 721–6.

38 Kitada T, Asakawa S, Hattori N, et al. Mutations in the parkin gene cause autosomal recessive juvenile parkinsonism. Nature 1998; **392**: 605–8.

39 Hedrich K, Eskelson C, Wilmot B, et al. Distribution, type, and origin of Parkin mutations: review and case studies. Mov Disord 2004; **19**: 1146–57.

40 Grünewald A, Kasten M, Ziegler A, Klein C. Next generation phenotyping using the Parkin example: time to catch up with genetics. J Am Med Assoc 2013; **70**: 1186–91.

41 Lohmann E, Periquet M, Bonifati V, et al. How much phenotypic variation can be attributed to parkin genotype? Ann Neurol 2003; **54**: 176–85.

42 Valente EM, Abou-Sleiman PM, Caputo V, et al. Hereditary early-onset Parkinson's disease caused by mutations in PINK1. Science 2004; **304**: 1158–60.

43 Healy DG, Abou-Sleiman PM, Gibson JM, et al. PINK1 (PARK6) associated Parkinson disease in Ireland. Neurology 2004; **63**: 1486–8.

44 Rogaeva E, Johnson J, Lang AE, et al. Analysis of the PINK1 gene in a large cohort of cases with Parkinson disease. Arch Neurol 2004; **61**: 1898–904.

45 Li Y, Tomiyama H, Sato K, et al. Clinicogenetic study of PINK1 mutations in autosomal recessive early-onset parkinsonism. Neurology 2005; **64**: 1955–7.

46 Klein C, Djarmati A, Hedrich K, et al. PINK1, Parkin, and DJ-1 mutations in Italian patients with early-onset parkinsonism. Eur J Hum Genet 2005; **13**: 1086–93.

47 Bonifati V, Rohe CF, Breedveld GJ, et al. Early-onset parkinsonism associated with PINK1 mutations: frequency, genotypes, and phenotypes. Neurology 2005; **65**: 87–95.

48 Tan EK, Yew K, Chua E, et al. PINK1 mutations in sporadic early-onset Parkinson's disease. Mov Disord 2006; **21**: 789–93.

49 Abou-Sleiman PM, Muqit MM, McDonald NQ, et al. A heterozygous effect for PINK1 mutations in Parkinson's disease? Ann Neurol 2006; **60**: 414–19.

50 Steinlechner S, Stahlberg J, Voelkel B, et al. Co-occurrence of affective and schizophrenia spectrum disorders with PINK1 mutations. J Neurol Neurosurg Psychiatry 2007; **78**: 532–5.

51 Criscuolo C, Volpe G, De Rosa A, et al. PINK1 homozygous W437X mutation in a patient with apparent dominant transmission of parkinsonism. Mov Disord 2006; **21**: 1265–7.

52 Bonifati V, Rizzu P, van Baren MJ, et al. Mutations in the DJ-1 gene associated with autosomal recessive early-onset parkinsonism. Science 2003; **299**: 256–9.

53 Pankratz N, Pauciulo MW, Elsaesser VE, et al. Mutations in DJ-1 are rare in familial Parkinson disease. Neurosci Lett 2006; **408**: 209–13.

54 Williams DR, Hadeed A, al-Din AS, Wreikat AL, Lees AJ. Kufor–Rakeb disease: autosomal recessive, levodopa-responsive parkinsonism with pyramidal degeneration, supranuclear gaze palsy, and dementia. Mov Disord 2005; **20**: 1264–71.

55 Najim al-Din AS, Wriekat A, Mubaidin A, Dasouki M, Hiari M. Pallido-pyramidal degeneration, supranuclear upgaze paresis and dementia: Kufor–Rakeb syndrome. Acta Neurol Scand 1994; **89**: 347–52.

56 Di Fonzo A, Chien HF, Socal M, et al. ATP13A2 missense mutations in juvenile parkinsonism and young onset Parkinson disease. Neurology 2007; **68**: 1557–62.

57 Aharon-Peretz J, Rosenbaum H, Gershoni-Baruch R. Mutations in the glucocerebrosidase gene and Parkinson's disease in Ashkenazi Jews. N Engl J Med 2004; **351**: 1972–7.

58 Goker-Alpan O, Giasson BI, Eblan MJ, et al. Glucocerebrosidase mutations are an important risk factor for Lewy body disorders. Neurology 2006; **67**: 908–10.

59 Neil JF, Glew RH, Peters SP. Familial psychosis and diverse neurologic abnormalities in adult-onset Gaucher's disease. Arch Neurol 1979; **36**: 95–9.

60 Klein C, Krainc D. Glucocerebrosidase mutations: tipping point toward Parkinson disease and dementia? JAMA Neurol 2013: **70**: 686–8.

61 Sidransky E, Nalls MA, Aasly JO, et al. Multicenter analysis of glucocerebrosidase mutations in Parkinson's disease. N Engl J Med 2009; **361**: 1651–61.

62 Perez-Calvo J, Bernal M, Giraldo P, et al. Co-morbidity in Gaucher's disease results of a nationwide enquiry in Spain. Eur J Med Res 2000; **5**: 231–5.

63 Alcalay RN, Caccappolo E, Mejia-Santana H, et al. Cognitive performance of GBA mutation carriers with early-onset PD: the CORE-PD study. Neurology 2012; **78**: 1434–40.

64 Tang B, Xiong H, Sun P, et al. Association of PINK1 and DJ-1 confers digenic inheritance of early-onset Parkinson's disease. Hum Molec Genet 2006; **15**: 1816–25.

65 Dachsel JC, Mata IF, Ross OA, et al. Digenic parkinsonism: investigation of the synergistic effects of PRKN and LRRK2. Neurosci Lett 2006; **410**: 80–4.

66 Ferreira JJ, Guedes LC, Rosa MM, et al. High prevalence of LRRK2 mutations in familial and sporadic Parkinson's disease in Portugal. Mov Disord 2007; **22**: 1194–201.

67 Benbunan BR, Korczyn AD, Giladi N. Parkin mutation associated parkinsonism and cognitive decline, comparison to early onset Parkinson's disease. J Neural Transm 2004; **111**: 47–57.

68 Kumru H, Santamaria J, Tolosa E, et al. Rapid eye movement sleep behavior disorder in parkinsonism with parkin mutations. Ann Neurol 2004; **56**: 599–603.

69 Singleton A, Gwinn-Hardy K, Sharabi Y, et al. Association between cardiac denervation and parkinsonism caused by alpha-synuclein gene triplication. Brain 2004; **127**: 768–72.

70 Kertelge L, Bruggemann N, Schmidt A, et al. Impaired sense of smell and color discrimination in monogenic and idiopathic Parkinson's disease. Mov Disord 2010; **25**: 2665–9.

71 Verbaan D, Boesveldt S, van Rooden SM, et al. Is olfactory impairment in Parkinson disease related to phenotypic or genotypic characteristics? Neurology 2008; **71**: 1877–82.

73 Aarsland D, Kurz MW. The epidemiology of dementia associated with Parkinson disease. J Neurol Sci 2010; **289**: 18–22.

74 Aarsland D, Zaccai J, Brayne C. A systematic review of prevalence studies of dementia in Parkinson's disease. Mov Disord 2005; **20**: 1255–63.

75 Schrag A, Schott JM. Epidemiological, clinical, and genetic characteristics of early-onset parkinsonism. Lancet Neurol 2006; **5**: 355–63.

76 Anheim M, Elbaz A, Lesage S, et al. Penetrance of Parkinson disease in glucocerebrosidase gene mutation carriers. Neurology 2012; **78**: 417–20.

77 Gan-Or Z, Giladi N, Orr-Urtreger A. Differential phenotype in Parkinson's disease patients with severe versus mild GBA mutations. Brain 2009; **132**: e125.

78 Gan-Or Z, Giladi N, Rozovski U, et al. Genotype-phenotype correlations between GBA mutations and Parkinson disease risk and onset. Neurology 2008; **70**: 2277–83.

79 Neumann J, Bras J, Deas E, et al. Glucocerebrosidase mutations in clinical and pathologically proven Parkinson's disease. Brain 2009; **132**: 1783–94.

80 Beutler E, Gelbart T, Scott CR. Hematologically important mutations: Gaucher disease. Blood Cells Mol Dis 2005; **35**: 355–64.

81 Saunders-Pullman R, Stanley K, Wang C, et al. Olfactory dysfunction in LRRK2 G2019S mutation carriers. Neurology 2011; **77**: 319–24.

82 Chartier-Harlin MC, Kachergus J, Roumier C, et al. Alpha-synuclein locus duplication as a cause of familial Parkinson's disease. Lancet 2004; **364**: 1167–9.

83 Puschmann A, Englund E, Ross OA, et al. First neuropathological description of a patient with Parkinson's disease and LRRK2 p.N1437H mutation. Parkinsonism Relat Disord 2012; **18**: 332–8.

84 Sekine T, Kagaya H, Funayama M, et al. Clinical course of the first Asian family with Parkinsonism related to SNCA triplication. Mov Disord 2010; **25**: 2871–5.

85 Wu RM, Bounds R, Lincoln S, et al. Parkin mutations and early-onset parkinsonism in a Taiwanese cohort. Arch Neurol 2005; **62**: 82–7.

86 Hedrich K, Hagenah J, Djarmati A, et al. Clinical spectrum of homozygous and heterozygous PINK1 mutations in a large German family with Parkinson disease: role of a single hit? Arch Neurol 2006; **63**: 833–8.

87 Zadikoff C, Rogaeva E, Djarmati A, et al. Homozygous and heterozygous PINK1 mutations: considerations for diagnosis and care of Parkinson's disease patients. Mov Disord 2006; **21**: 875–9.

88 Papadimitriou A, Veletza V, Hadjigeorgiou GM, Patrikiou A, Hirano M, Anastasopoulos I. Mutated alpha-synuclein gene in two Greek kindreds with familial PD: incomplete penetrance? Neurology 1999; **52**: 651–4.

89 Obi T, Nishioka K, Ross OA, et al. Clinicopathologic study of a SNCA gene duplication patient with Parkinson disease and dementia. Neurology 2008; **70**: 238–41.

90 Spira PJ, Sharpe DM, Halliday G, Cavanagh J, Nicholson GA. Clinical and pathological features of a Parkinsonian syndrome in a family with an Ala53Thr alpha-synuclein mutation. Ann Neurol 2001; **49**: 313–19.

91 Chaudhuri KR, Martinez-Martin P, Brown RG, et al. The metric properties of a novel non-motor symptoms scale for Parkinson's disease: results from an international pilot study. Mov Disord 2007; **22**: 1901–11.

92 Chaudhuri KR, Healy DG, Schapira AH. Non-motor symptoms of Parkinson's disease: diagnosis and management. Lancet Neurol 2006; **5**: 235–45.

93 Langston JW, Sastry S, Chan P, Forno LS, Bolin LM, Di Monte DA. Novel alpha-synuclein-immunoreactive proteins in brain samples from the Contursi kindred, Parkinson's, and Alzheimer's disease. Exp Neurol 1998; **154**: 684–90.

94 Schweitzer KJ, Brussel T, Leitner P, et al. Transcranial ultrasound in different monogenetic subtypes of Parkinson's disease. J Neurol 2007; **254**: 613–16.

95 Fuchs J, Tichopad A, Golub Y, et al. Genetic variability in the SNCA gene influences alpha-synuclein levels in the blood and brain. FASEB J 2008; **22**: 1327–34.

96 Perani D, Garibotto V, Hadjigeorgiou GM, Papadimitriou D, Fazio F, Papadimitriou A. Positron emission tomography changes in PARK1 mutation. Mov Disord 2006; **21**: 127–30.

97 Papapetropoulos S, Ellul J, Paschalis C, Athanassiadou A, Papadimitriou A, Papapetropoulos T. Clinical characteristics of the alpha-synuclein mutation (G209A)-associated Parkinson's disease in comparison with other forms of familial Parkinson's disease in Greece. Eur J Neurol 2003; **10**: 281–6.

98 Papapetropoulos S, Paschalis C, Athanassiadou A, et al. Clinical phenotype in patients with alpha-synuclein Parkinson's disease living in Greece in comparison with patients with sporadic Parkinson's disease. J Neurol Neurosurg Psychiatry 2001; **70**: 662–5.

99 Bostantjopoulou S, Katsarou Z, Papadimitriou A, Veletza V, Hatzigeorgiou G, Lees A. Clinical features of parkinsonian patients with the alpha-synuclein (G209A) mutation. Mov Disord 2001; **16**: 1007–13.

100 Kojovic M, Sheerin UM, Rubio-Agusti I, et al. Young-onset parkinsonism due to homozygous duplication of alpha-synuclein in a consanguineous family. Mov Disord 2012; **27**: 1827–9.

101 Sironi F, Trotta L, Antonini A, et al. alpha-Synuclein multiplication analysis in Italian familial Parkinson disease. Parkinsonism Relat Disord 2010; **16**: 228–31.

102 Mutez E, Lepretre F, Le Rhun E, et al. SNCA locus duplication carriers: from genetics to Parkinson disease phenotypes. Hum Mutat 2011; **32**: E2079–E2090.

103 Nishioka K, Ross OA, Ishii K, et al. Expanding the clinical phenotype of SNCA duplication carriers. Mov Disord 2009; **24**: 1811–19.

104 Kruger R, Kuhn W, Leenders KL, et al. Familial parkinsonism with synuclein pathology: clinical and PET studies of A30P mutation carriers. Neurology 2001; **56**: 1355–62.

105 **Kruger R, Kuhn W, Muller T, et al**. Ala30Pro mutation in the gene encoding alpha-synuclein in Parkinson's disease. Nat Genet 1998; **18**: 106–8.

106 **Ahn TB, Kim SY, Kim JY, et al**. Alpha-synuclein gene duplication is present in sporadic Parkinson disease. Neurology 2008; **70**: 43–9.

107 **Muenter MD, Forno LS, Hornykiewicz O, et al**. Hereditary form of parkinsonism—dementia. Ann Neurol 1998; **43**: 768–81.

108 **Shin CW, Kim HJ, Park SS, Kim SY, Kim JY, Jeon BS**. Two Parkinson's disease patients with alpha-synuclein gene duplication and rapid cognitive decline. Mov Disord 2010; **25**: 957–9.

109 **Uchiyama T, Ikeuchi T, Ouchi Y, et al**. Prominent psychiatric symptoms and glucose hypometabolism in a family with a SNCA duplication. Neurology 2008; **71**: 1289–91.

110 **Itokawa K, Sekine T, Funayama M, et al**. A case of alpha-synuclein gene duplication presenting with head-shaking movements. Mov Disord 2013; **28**: 384–7.

111 **Gwinn K, Devine MJ, Jin LW, et al**. Clinical features, with video documentation, of the original familial Lewy body parkinsonism caused by alpha-synuclein triplication (Iowa kindred). Mov Disord 2011; **26**: 2134–6.

112 **Papapetropoulos S, Singer C, Ross OA, et al**. Clinical heterogeneity of the LRRK2 G2019S mutation. Arch Neurol 2006; **63**: 1242–6.

113 **Illarioshkin SN, Shadrina MI, Slominsky PA, et al**. A common leucine-rich repeat kinase 2 gene mutation in familial and sporadic Parkinson's disease in Russia. Eur J Neurol 2007; **14**: 413–17.

114 **Lesage S, Janin S, Lohmann E, et al**. LRRK2 exon 41 mutations in sporadic Parkinson disease in Europeans. Arch Neurol 2007; **64**: 425–30.

115 **Goldstein DS, Imrich R, Peckham E, et al**. Neurocirculatory and nigrostriatal abnormalities in Parkinson disease from LRRK2 mutation. Neurology 2007; **69**: 1580–4.

 72 **Khan NL, Jain S, Lynch JM, et al**. Mutations in the gene LRRK2 encoding dardarin (PARK8) cause familial Parkinson's disease: clinical, pathological, olfactory and functional imaging and genetic data. Brain 2005; **128**: 2786–96.

116 **Infante J, Rodriguez RL, Combarros O, et al**. LRRK2 G2019S is a common mutation in Spanish patients with late-onset Parkinson's disease. Neurosci Lett 2006; **395**: 224–6.

117 **Gaig C, Ezquerra M, Marti MJ, Munoz E, Valldeoriola F, Tolosa E**. LRRK2 mutations in Spanish patients with Parkinson disease: frequency, clinical features, and incomplete penetrance. Arch Neurol 2006; **63**: 377–82.

118 **Williams-Gray CH, Goris A, Foltynie T, et al**. Prevalence of the LRRK2 G2019S mutation in a UK community based idiopathic Parkinson's disease cohort. J Neurol Neurosurg Psychiatry 2006; **77**: 665–7.

119 **Zabetian CP, Morino H, Ujike H, et al**. Identification and haplotype analysis of LRRK2 G2019S in Japanese patients with Parkinson disease. Neurology 2006; **67**: 697–9.

120 **Scholz S, Mandel RJ, Fernandez HH, et al**. LRRK2 mutations in a clinic-based cohort of Parkinson's disease. Eur J Neurol 2006; **13**: 1298–301.

121 **Giordana MT, D'Agostino C, Albani G, et al**. Neuropathology of Parkinson's disease associated with the LRRK2 Ile1371Val mutation. Mov Disord 2007; **22**: 275–8.

122 **Wu T, Zeng Y, Ding X, et al**. A novel P755L mutation in LRRK2 gene associated with Parkinson's disease. Neuroreport 2006; **17**: 1859–62.

123 **Gaig C, Marti MJ, Ezquerra M, Rey MJ, Cardozo A, Tolosa E**. G2019S LRRK2 mutation causing Parkinson's disease without Lewy bodies. J Neurol Neurosurg Psychiatry 2007; **78**: 626–8.

124 **Squillaro T, Cambi F, Ciacci G, et al**. Frequency of the LRRK2 G2019S mutation in Italian patients affected by Parkinson's disease. J Hum Genet 2007; **52**: 201–4.

125 **Tan EK, Zhao Y, Tan L, et al**. Analysis of LRRK2 Gly2385Arg genetic variant in non-Chinese Asians. Mov Disord 2007; **22**: 1816–18.

126 Civitelli D, Tarantino P, Nicoletti G, et al. LRRK2 G6055A mutation in Italian patients with familial or sporadic Parkinson's disease. Clin Genet 2007; **71**: 367–70.

127 Johnson J, Paisan-Ruiz C, Lopez G, et al. Comprehensive screening of a North American Parkinson's disease cohort for LRRK2 mutation. Neurodegener Dis 2007; **4**: 386–91.

128 Bras JM, Guerreiro RJ, Ribeiro MH, et al. G2019S dardarin substitution is a common cause of Parkinson's disease in a Portuguese cohort. Mov Disord 2005; **20**: 1653–5.

129 Pchelina SN, Yakimovskii AF, Ivanova ON, Emelianov AK, Zakharchuk AH, Schwarzman AL. G2019S LRRK2 mutation in familial and sporadic Parkinson's disease in Russia. Mov Disord 2006; **21**: 2234–6.

130 Clark LN, Wang Y, Karlins E, et al. Frequency of LRRK2 mutations in early- and late-onset Parkinson disease. Neurology 2006; **67**: 1786–91.

131 Punia S, Behari M, Govindappa ST, et al. Absence/rarity of commonly reported LRRK2 mutations in Indian Parkinson's disease patients. Neurosci Lett 2006; **409**: 83–8.

132 Cossu G, van Doeselaar M, Deriu M, et al. LRRK2 mutations and Parkinson's disease in Sardinia—a Mediterranean genetic isolate. Parkinsonism Relat Disord 2007; **13**: 17–21.

133 Pankratz N, Pauciulo MW, Elsaesser VE, et al. Mutations in LRRK2 other than G2019S are rare in a north American-based sample of familial Parkinson's disease. Mov Disord 2006; **21**: 2257–60.

134 Gosal D, Lynch T, Ross OA, Haugarvoll K, Farrer MJ, Gibson JM. Global distribution and reduced penetrance: LRRK2 R1441C in an Irish Parkinson's disease kindred. Mov Disord 2007; **22**: 291–2.

135 Di Fonzo A, Rohe CF, Ferreira J, et al. A frequent LRRK2 gene mutation associated with autosomal dominant Parkinson's disease. Lancet 2005; **365**: 412–15.

136 Ishihara L, Gibson RA, Warren L, et al. Screening for LRRK2 G2019S and clinical comparison of Tunisian and North American Caucasian Parkinson's disease families. Mov Disord 2007; **22**: 55–61.

137 Hernandez DG, Paisan-Ruiz C, McInerney-Leo A, et al. Clinical and positron emission tomography of Parkinson's disease caused by LRRK2. Ann Neurol 2005; **57**: 453–6.

138 Aasly JO, Toft M, Fernandez-Mata I, et al. Clinical features of LRRK2-associated Parkinson's disease in central Norway. Ann Neurol 2005; **57**: 762–5.

139 Gosal D, Ross OA, Wiley J, et al. Clinical traits of LRRK2-associated Parkinson's disease in Ireland: a link between familial and idiopathic PD. Parkinsonism Relat Disord 2005;**11**: 349–52.

140 Macedo MG, Verbaan D, Fang Y, et al. Genotypic and phenotypic characteristics of Dutch patients with early onset Parkinson's disease. Mov Disord 2009; **24**: 196–203.

141 Camargos ST, Dornas LO, Momeni P, et al. Familial Parkinsonism and early onset Parkinson's disease in a Brazilian movement disorders clinic: phenotypic characterization and frequency of SNCA, PRKN, PINK1, and LRRK2 mutations. Mov Disord 2009; **24**: 662–6.

142 Rizzo G, Marconi S, Capellari S, Scaglione C, Martinelli P. Benign tremulous parkinsonism in a patient with dardarin mutation. Mov Disord 2009; **24**: 1399–401.

143 Marti-Masso JF, Ruiz-Martinez J, Bolano MJ, et al. Neuropathology of Parkinson's disease with the R1441G mutation in LRRK2. Mov Disord 2009; **24**: 1998–2001.

144 Covy JP, Yuan W, Waxman EA, Hurtig HI, Van Deerlin VM, Giasson BI. Clinical and pathological characteristics of patients with leucine-rich repeat kinase-2 mutations. Mov Disord 2009; **24**: 32–9.

145 Bardien S, Marsberg A, Keyser R, et al. LRRK2 G2019S mutation: frequency and haplotype data in South African Parkinson's disease patients. J Neural Transm 2010; **117**: 847–53.

146 Chan DK, Ng PW, Mok V, et al. LRRK2 Gly2385Arg mutation and clinical features in a Chinese population with early-onset Parkinson's disease compared to late-onset patients. J Neural Transm 2008; **115**: 1275–7.

147 **De Rosa A, Criscuolo C, Mancini P, et al.** Genetic screening for LRRK2 gene G2019S mutation in Parkinson's disease patients from southern Italy. Parkinsonism Relat Disord 2009; **15**: 242–4.

148 **Mata IF, Cosentino C, Marca V, et al.** LRRK2 mutations in patients with Parkinson's disease from Peru and Uruguay. Parkinsonism Relat Disord 2009; **15**: 370–3.

149 **Lohmann E, Leclere L, De Anna F, et al.** A clinical, neuropsychological and olfactory evaluation of a large family with LRRK2 mutations. Parkinsonism Relat Disord 2009; **15**: 273–6.

150 **Johansen KK, Hasselberg K, White LR, Farrer MJ, Aasly JO.** Genealogical studies in LRRK2-associated Parkinson's disease in central Norway. Parkinsonism Relat Disord 2010; **16**: 527–30.

151 **Gao L, Gomez-Garre P, Diaz-Corrales FJ, et al.** Prevalence and clinical features of LRRK2 mutations in patients with Parkinson's disease in southern Spain. Eur J Neurol 2009; **16**: 957–60.

152 **Floris G, Cannas A, Solla P, et al.** Genetic analysis for five LRRK2 mutations in a Sardinian parkinsonian population: importance of G2019S and R1441C mutations in sporadic Parkinson's disease patients. Parkinsonism Relat Disord 2009; **15**: 277–80.

153 **Criscuolo C, De Rosa A, Guacci A, et al.** The LRRK2 R1441C mutation is more frequent than G2019S in Parkinson's disease patients from southern Italy. Mov Disord 2011; **26**: 1733–6.

154 **Ruiz-Martinez J, Gorostidi A, Goyenechea E, et al.** Olfactory deficits and cardiac 123I-MIBG in Parkinson's disease related to the LRRK2 R1441G and G2019S mutations. Mov Disord 2011; **26**: 2026–31.

155 **Shanker V, Groves M, Heiman G, et al.** Mood and cognition in leucine-rich repeat kinase 2 G2019S Parkinson's disease. Mov Disord 2011; **26**: 1875–80.

156 **Valldeoriola F, Gaig C, Muxi A, et al.** 123I-MIBG cardiac uptake and smell identification in parkinsonian patients with LRRK2 mutations. J Neurol 2011; **258**: 1126–32.

157 **Belarbi S, Hecham N, Lesage S, et al.** LRRK2 G2019S mutation in Parkinson's disease: a neuropsychological and neuropsychiatric study in a large Algerian cohort. Parkinsonism Relat Disord 2010; **16**: 676–9.

158 **Hashad DI, Abou-Zeid AA, Achmawy GA, Allah HM, Saad MA.** G2019S mutation of the leucine-rich repeat kinase 2 gene in a cohort of Egyptian patients with Parkinson's disease. Genet Testing Molec Biomarkers 2011; **15**: 861–6.

159 **Ben Sassi S, Nabli F, Hentati E, et al.** Cognitive dysfunction in Tunisian LRRK2 associated Parkinson's disease. Parkinsonism Relat Disord 2012; **18**: 243–6.

160 **Healy DG, Falchi M, O'Sullivan SS, et al.** Phenotype, genotype, and worldwide genetic penetrance of LRRK2-associated Parkinson's disease: a case-control study. Lancet Neurol 2008; **7**: 583–90.

161 **Brockmann K, Groger A, Di Santo A, et al.** Clinical and brain imaging characteristics in leucine-rich repeat kinase 2-associated PD and asymptomatic mutation carriers. Mov Disord 2011; **26**: 2335–42.

162 **Kim JS, Cho JW, Shin H, et al.** A Korean Parkinson's disease family with the LRRK2 p.Tyr1699Cys mutation showing clinical heterogeneity. Mov Disord 2012; **27**: 320–4.

163 **Lorenzo-Betancor O, Samaranch L, Ezquerra M, et al.** LRRK2 haplotype-sharing analysis in Parkinson's disease reveals a novel p.S1761R mutation. Mov Disord 2012; **27**: 146–51.

164 **Marras C, Schule B, Munhoz RP, et al.** Phenotype in parkinsonian and nonparkinsonian LRRK2 G2019S mutation carriers. Neurology 2011; **77**: 325–33.

165 **Abdalla-Carvalho CB, Santos-Reboucas CB, Guimaraes BC, et al.** Genetic analysis of LRRK2 functional domains in Brazilian patients with Parkinson's disease. Eur J Neurol 2010; **17**: 1479–81.

166 **Kumar KR, Weissbach A, Heldmann M, et al.** Frequency of the D620N mutation in VPS35 in Parkinson disease. Arch Neurol 2012; **69**: 1360–4.

167 **Lesage S, Condroyer C, Klebe S, et al.** Identification of VPS35 mutations replicated in French families with Parkinson disease. Neurology 2012; **78**: 1449–50.

168 Sheerin UM, Charlesworth G, Bras J, et al. Screening for VPS35 mutations in Parkinson's disease. Neurobiol Aging 2012; **33**: 838.e1–5.

169 Zimprich A, Benet-Pages A, Struhal W, et al. A mutation in VPS35, encoding a subunit of the retromer complex, causes late-onset Parkinson disease. Am J Hum Genet 2011; **89**: 168–75.

170 Sasaki S, Shirata A, Yamane K, Iwata M. Parkin-positive autosomal recessive juvenile Parkinsonism with alpha-synuclein-positive inclusions. Neurology 2004; **63**: 678–82.

171 Lesage S, Magali P, Lohmann E, et al. Deletion of the parkin and PACRG gene promoter in early-onset parkinsonism. Hum Mutat 2007; **28**: 27–32.

172 Chung EJ, Ki CS, Lee WY, Kim IS, Kim JY. Clinical features and gene analysis in Korean patients with early-onset Parkinson disease. Arch Neurol 2006; **63**: 1170–4.

173 Biswas A, Gupta A, Naiya T, et al. Molecular pathogenesis of Parkinson's disease: identification of mutations in the Parkin gene in Indian patients. Parkinsonism Relat Disord 2006; **12**: 420–6.

174 Deng H, Le WD, Hunter CB, et al. Heterogeneous phenotype in a family with compound heterozygous parkin gene mutations. Arch Neurol 2006; **63**: 273–7.

175 Chien HF, Rohe CF, Costa MD, et al. Early-onset Parkinson's disease caused by a novel parkin mutation in a genetic isolate from north-eastern Brazil. Neurogenetics 2006; **7**: 13–19.

176 Madegowda RH, Kishore A, Anand A. Mutational screening of the parkin gene among South Indians with early onset Parkinson's disease. J Neurol Neurosurg Psychiatry 2005; **76**: 1588–90.

177 Ohsawa Y, Kurokawa K, Sonoo M, et al. Reduced amplitude of the sural nerve sensory action potential in PARK2 patients. Neurology 2005; **65**: 459–62.

178 Djarmati A, Hedrich K, Svetel M, et al. Detection of Parkin (PARK2) and DJ1 (PARK7) mutations in early-onset Parkinson disease: Parkin mutation frequency depends on ethnic origin of patients. Hum Mutat 2004; **23**: 525.

179 Khan NL, Katzenschlager R, Watt H, et al. Olfaction differentiates parkin disease from early-onset parkinsonism and Parkinson disease. Neurology 2004; **62**: 1224–6.

180 Lincoln S, Wiley J, Lynch T, et al. Parkin-proven disease: common founders but divergent phenotypes. Neurology 2003; **60**: 1605–10.

181 Thobois S, Ribeiro MJ, Lohmann E, et al. Young-onset Parkinson disease with and without parkin gene mutations: a fluorodopa F 18 positron emission tomography study. Arch Neurol 2003; **60**: 713–18.

182 Khan NL, Brooks DJ, Pavese N, et al. Progression of nigrostriatal dysfunction in a parkin kindred: an [18F]dopa PET and clinical study. Brain 2002; **125**: 2248–56.

183 Wu RM, Shan DE, Sun CM, et al. Clinical, 18F-dopa PET, and genetic analysis of an ethnic Chinese kindred with early-onset parkinsonism and parkin gene mutations. Mov Disord 2002; **17**: 670–5.

184 Alvarez V, Guisasola LM, Moreira VG, Lahoz CH, Coto E. Early-onset Parkinson's disease associated with a new parkin mutation in a Spanish family. Neurosci Lett 2001; **313**: 108–10.

185 Ruffmann C, Zini M, Goldwurm S, et al. Lewy body pathology and typical Parkinson disease in a patient with a heterozygous (R275W) mutation in the Parkin gene (PARK2). Acta Neuropathol 2012; **123**: 901–3.

186 Koentjoro B, Park JS, Ha AD, Sue CM. Phenotypic variability of parkin mutations in single kindred. Mov Disord 2012; **27**: 1299–303.

187 Bilgic B, Bayram A, Arslan AB, et al. Differentiating symptomatic Parkin mutations carriers from patients with idiopathic Parkinson's disease: contribution of automated segmentation neuroimaging method. Parkinsonism Relat Disorders 2012; **18**: 562–6.

188 Lohmann E, Dursun B, Lesage S, et al. Genetic bases and phenotypes of autosomal recessive Parkinson disease in a Turkish population. Eur J Neurol 2012; **19**: 769–75.

189 Hassin-Baer S, Hattori N, Cohen OS, Massarwa M, Israeli-Korn SD, Inzelberg R. Phenotype of the 202 adenine deletion in the parkin gene: 40 years of follow-up. Mov Disord 2011; **26**: 719–22.

190 **Dogu O, Johnson J, Hernandez D, et al.** A consanguineous Turkish family with early-onset Parkinson's disease and an exon 4 parkin deletion. Mov Disord 2004; **19**: 812–16.

191 **Mellick GD, Siebert GA, Funayama M, et al.** Screening PARK genes for mutations in early-onset Parkinson's disease patients from Queensland, Australia. Parkinsonism Relat Disord 2009; **15**: 105–9.

192 **Zhang BR, Hu ZX, Yin XZ, et al.** Mutation analysis of parkin and PINK1 genes in early-onset Parkinson's disease in China. Neurosci Lett 2010; **477**: 19–22.

193 **Alcalay RN, Siderowf A, Ottman R, et al.** Olfaction in Parkin heterozygotes and compound heterozygotes: the CORE-PD study. Neurology 2011; **76**: 319–26.

194 **Hayashi S, Wakabayashi K, Ishikawa A, et al.** An autopsy case of autosomal-recessive juvenile parkinsonism with a homozygous exon 4 deletion in the parkin gene. Mov Disord 2000; **15**: 884–8.

195 **Doostzadeh J, Tetrud JW, Allen-Auerbach M, Langston JW, Schule B.** Novel features in a patient homozygous for the L347P mutation in the PINK1 gene. Parkinsonism Relat Disord 2007; **13**: 359–61.

196 **Marongiu R, Brancati F, Antonini A, et al.** Whole gene deletion and splicing mutations expand the PINK1 genotypic spectrum. Hum Mutat 2007; **28**: 98.

197 **Chishti MA, Bohlega S, Ahmed M, et al.** T313M PINK1 mutation in an extended highly consanguineous Saudi family with early-onset Parkinson disease. Arch Neurol 2006; **63**: 1483–5.

198 **Leutenegger AL, Salih MA, Ibanez P, et al.** Juvenile-onset Parkinsonism as a result of the first mutation in the adenosine triphosphate orientation domain of PINK1. Arch Neurol 2006; **63**: 1257–61.

199 **Djarmati A, Hedrich K, Svetel M, et al.** Heterozygous PINK1 mutations: a susceptibility factor for Parkinson disease? Mov Disord 2006; **21**: 1526–30.

200 **Gandhi S, Muqit MM, Stanyer L, et al.** PINK1 protein in normal human brain and Parkinson's disease. Brain 2006; **129**: 1720–31.

201 **Fung HC, Chen CM, Hardy J, Singleton AB, Lee-Chen GJ, Wu YR.** Analysis of the PINK1 gene in a cohort of patients with sporadic early-onset parkinsonism in Taiwan. Neurosci Lett 2006; **394**: 33–6.

202 **Albanese A, Valente EM, Romito LM, Bellacchio E, Elia AE, Dallapiccola B.** The PINK1 phenotype can be indistinguishable from idiopathic Parkinson disease. Neurology 2005; **64**: 1958–60.

203 **Hatano Y, Sato K, Elibol B, et al.** PARK6-linked autosomal recessive early-onset parkinsonism in Asian populations. Neurology 2004; **63**: 1482–5.

204 **Kumazawa R, Tomiyama H, Li Y, et al.** Mutation analysis of the PINK1 gene in 391 patients with Parkinson disease. Arch Neurol 2008; **65**: 802–8.

205 **Cazeneuve C, San C, Ibrahim SA, et al.** A new complex homozygous large rearrangement of the PINK1 gene in a Sudanese family with early onset Parkinson's disease. Neurogenetics 2009; **10**: 265–70.

206 **Tuin I, Voss U, Kessler K, et al.** Sleep quality in a family with hereditary parkinsonism (PARK6). Sleep Med 2008; **9**: 684–8.

207 **Prestel J, Gempel K, Hauser TK, et al.** Clinical and molecular characterisation of a Parkinson family with a novel PINK1 mutation. J Neurol 2008; **255**: 643–8.

208 **Hedrich K, Djarmati A, Schafer N, et al.** DJ-1 (PARK7) mutations are less frequent than Parkin (PARK2) mutations in early-onset Parkinson disease. Neurology 2004; **62**: 389–94.

209 **Hague S, Rogaeva E, Hernandez D, et al.** Early-onset Parkinson's disease caused by a compound heterozygous DJ-1 mutation. Ann Neurol 2003; **54**: 271–4.

210 **Abou-Sleiman PM, Healy DG, Quinn N, Lees AJ, Wood NW.** The role of pathogenic DJ-1 mutations in Parkinson's disease. Ann Neurol 2003; **54**: 283–6.

211 **van Duijn CM, Dekker MC, Bonifati V, et al**. Park7, a novel locus for autosomal recessive early-onset parkinsonism, on chromosome 1p36. Am J Hum Genet 2001; **69**: 629–34.

212 **Ramirez A, Heimbach A, Grundemann J, et al**. Hereditary parkinsonism with dementia is caused by mutations in ATP13A2, encoding a lysosomal type 5 P-type ATPase. Nat Genet 2006; **38**: 1184–91.

213 **Park JS, Mehta P, Cooper AA, et al**. Pathogenic effects of novel mutations in the P-type ATPase ATP13A2 (PARK9) causing Kufor–Rakeb syndrome, a form of early-onset parkinsonism. Hum Mutat 2011; **32**: 956–64.

214 **Toft M, Pielsticker L, Ross OA, Aasly JO, Farrer MJ**. Glucocerebrosidase gene mutations and Parkinson disease in the Norwegian population. Neurology 2006; **66**: 415–17.

215 **Goker-Alpan O, Schiffmann R, LaMarca ME, Nussbaum RL, McInerney-Leo A, Sidransky E**. Parkinsonism among Gaucher disease carriers. J Med Genet 2004; **41**: 937–40.

216 **Tayebi N, Callahan M, Madike V, et al**. Gaucher disease and parkinsonism: a phenotypic and genotypic characterization. Mol Genet Metab 2001; **73**: 313–21.

217 **Sun QY, Guo JF, Wang L, et al**. Glucocerebrosidase gene L444P mutation is a risk factor for Parkinson's disease in Chinese population. Mov Disord 2010; **25**: 1005–11.

218 **Goker-Alpan O, Lopez G, Vithayathil J, Davis J, Hallett M, Sidransky E**. The spectrum of parkinsonian manifestations associated with glucocerebrosidase mutations. Arch Neurol 2008; **65**: 1353–7.

219 **Mata IF, Samii A, Schneer SH, et al**. Glucocerebrosidase gene mutations: a risk factor for Lewy body disorders. Arch Neurology 2008; **65**: 379–82.

220 **Huang CL, Wu-Chou YH, Lai SC, et al**. Contribution of glucocerebrosidase mutation in a large cohort of sporadic Parkinson's disease in Taiwan. Eur J Neurol 2011; **18**: 1227–32.

221 **Lesage S, Anheim M, Condroyer C, et al**. Large-scale screening of the Gaucher's disease-related glucocerebrosidase gene in Europeans with Parkinson's disease. Hum Molec Genet 2011; **20**: 202–10.

222 **Brockmann K, Srulijes K, Hauser AK, et al**. GBA-associated PD presents with nonmotor characteristics. Neurology 2011; **77**: 276–80.

223 **Mitsui J, Mizuta I, Toyoda A, et al**. Mutations for Gaucher disease confer high susceptibility to Parkinson disease. Arch Neurol 2009; **66**: 571–6.

224 **Nichols WC, Pankratz N, Marek DK, et al**. Mutations in GBA are associated with familial Parkinson disease susceptibility and age at onset. Neurology 2009; **72**: 310–16.

225 **Gan-Or Z, Bar-Shira A, Mirelman A, et al**. LRRK2 and GBA mutations differentially affect the initial presentation of Parkinson disease. Neurogenetics 2010; **11**: 121–5.

Specific non-motor symptoms of Parkinson's disease

Chapter 8

Cognitive dysfunction in Parkinson's disease

Daisy L. Whitehead and Richard. G. Brown

Introduction

In this chapter we consider both the 'typical' cognitive profile of Parkinson's disease (PD) patients without dementia as well as the heterogeneity in cognitive change noted in several community samples. We describe neuroimaging studies that have demonstrated changes in brain metabolism and structure associated with specific cognitive deficits, and genetic studies that have aimed to identify a basis for differing levels of cognitive impairment within people with PD. The possible biological mechanisms underlying these changes are discussed. We consider the clinical and pathophysiological bases of mild cognitive impairment (MCI) in PD, which may indicate risk of further decline and clinically relevant dementia, and discuss issues surrounding neuropsychological assessment in PD.

The cognitive 'profile' of Parkinson's disease

The most prominent and prevalent cognitive deficits in PD concern executive function, that is, the ability to plan, organize, monitor and regulate goal-directed behaviour. Deficits have been described in planning, problem-solving, rule and set formation, and set maintenance and shifting, and the term 'dysexecutive' syndrome is often applied to PD [1,2]. The frontal lobes are thought to underlie many key executive processes, and so frontal dysfunction is the likely basis for much of the cognitive change in PD. However, whereas patients with frontal lobe injury tend to demonstrate perseverative behaviour (i.e. a lack of mental flexibility and inability to adapt responses to environmental change), the impairment in PD is characterized by difficulty in ignoring or suppressing non-relevant stimuli or processes during cognition (i.e. difficulty in maintaining an adaptive response against competing alternatives) [1,2].

Attentional deficits have been described in PD patients without dementia, particularly when selective attention is required. During divided attention tasks, PD patients have difficulty ignoring distractors, and are also prone to interference in tasks which involve the active suppression of responses and redirection of attention, such as the Stroop task [3,4]. Purer measures of attention without an executive component, such as vigilance or sustained attention, appear to be better preserved, although these may later become impaired in PD dementia [2,4].

PD patients without dementia show specific impairment in free recall, with relatively preserved recognition, learning and long-term retention, suggesting that memory storage and consolidation are intact but that retrieval processes are in some way impaired. Memory paradigms requiring manipulation of to-be-remembered items, such as conditional associate learning, or temporal or spatial ordering, also produce deficits in PD, as they recruit executive and attentional processes [1,2,4]. Some authors have argued that all deficits in PD stem from problems with basic executive processes [1]. For example, the free recall deficit in PD can be largely overcome by cueing, that is, providing the subject with cues to help focus the recall process, thus overriding the need for internal generation of retrieval strategies.

Visuospatial and visuoperceptual function in PD without dementia show a range of impairments, including difficulties with body-spatial orientation, visual attention, construction and visual memory, line orientation and object recognition [5], although some authors argue that once the executive and motor components of visual tasks are removed little deficit remains [1].

Mild cognitive impairment in Parkinson's disease

Derived originally from the area of Alzheimer's disease, the concept of MCI describes a state of cognitive decline that is not sufficient in severity of impact to warrant a diagnosis of dementia with a range of different cognitive profiles suggested [6] (see Fig. 8.1). The concept of PD-MCI is increasingly recognized, although the definition and diagnosis remain subjects of debate [7]. Until recently the lack of diagnostic criteria for PD-MCI has hampered research, including efforts to estimate prevalence, with studies using different methods of assessment and different criteria for definition of impairment [e.g. 1.0, 1.5 or 2.0 standard deviations (SDs) below population norms]. In 2012, the Movement Disorder Society published a set of diagnostic criteria and guidelines for future research [8] (see Box 8.1). Recommendations are also offered for assessments able to provide either Level I evidence [using validated cognitive screening cutoffs (see Screening and assessment) or brief neuropsychological assessment] or Level II evidence (based on extensive neuropsychological assessment across a range of domains).

Although pre-dating the publication of these criteria, a study of 86 PD patients without dementia reported a prevalence of 21% PD-MCI applying a cutoff of >1.5 SD below population norms in at least one cognitive 'domain' [9]. Controlling for the effects of advanced disease and the presence of medication, a population study of early, untreated PD patients (the ParkWest study) [10], found a prevalence of 18.9% using a 1.5 SD cutoff. More recently, a large pooled study of 1346 patients at varying stages of PD applied a cutoff of 1.5 SD across the eight datasets included and found a overall prevalence of 25.8% PD-MCI [11]. In summary, it is clear that a sizeable proportion of PD patients can be classified as having MCI, and the section 'Cognitive impairment and dementia risk' later in this chapter addresses whether PD-MCI confers a greater risk of full-blown dementia.

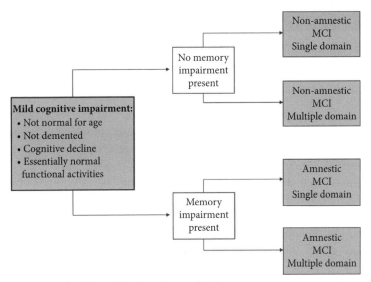

Fig. 8.1 Classification of mild cognitive impairment (MCI).

Adapted from Winblad B, Palmer K, Kivipelto M, et al. Mild cognitive impairment—beyond controversies, towards a consensus: report of the International Working Group on Mild Cognitive Impairment. J Intern Med 2004; 256: 240–6.

Box 8.1 Criteria for diagnosis of PD-MCI

I. Inclusion criteria:

◆ Diagnosis of Parkinson's disease as based on the UK PD Brain Bank Criteria

◆ Gradual decline, in the context of established PD, in cognitive ability reported by either the patient or informant, or observed by the clinician

◆ Cognitive deficits on either formal neuropsychological testing or a scale of global cognitive abilities (detailed in section III)

◆ Cognitive deficits are not sufficient to interfere significantly with functional independence, although subtle difficulties on complex functional tasks may be present

II. Exclusion criteria:

◆ Diagnosis of PD dementia based on MDS Task Force proposed criteria

◆ Other primary explanations for cognitive impairment (e.g. delirium, stroke, major depression, metabolic abnormalities, adverse effects of medication or head trauma)

◆ Other PD-associated co-morbid conditions (e.g. motor impairment or severe anxiety, depression, excessive daytime sleepiness or psychosis) that, in the opinion of the clinician, significantly influence cognitive testing

---

Box 8.1 Criteria for diagnosis of PD-MCI *(continued)*

III. Specific guidelines for PD-MCI Level I and Level II categories:

A. Level I (abbreviated assessment)

+ Impairment on a scale of global cognitive abilities validated for use in PD

or

+ Impairment on at least two tests, when a limited battery of neuropsychological tests is performed (i.e. the battery includes less than two tests within each of the five cognitive domains, or less than five cognitive domains are assessed)

B. Level II (comprehensive assessment)

+ Neuropsychological testing that includes two tests within each of the five cognitive domains (i.e. attention and working memory, executive, language, memory and visuospatial)

+ Impairment on at least two neuropsychological tests, represented by either two impaired tests in one cognitive domain or one impaired test in two different cognitive domains

+ Impairment on neuropsychological tests may be demonstrated by: Performance approximately 1 to 2 SDs below appropriate norms or significant decline demonstrated on serial cognitive testing or significant decline from estimated pre-morbid levels

IV. Subtype classification for PD-MCI (optional, requires two tests for each of the five cognitive domains assessed and is strongly suggested for research purposes):

+ PD-MCI single-domain—abnormalities on two tests within a single cognitive domain (specify the domain), with other domains unimpaired

or

+ PD-MCI multiple-domain—abnormalities on at least one test in two or more cognitive domains (specify the domains)

Reproduced with permission from Litvan I, Goldman JG, Troster AI, Schmand BA, Weintraub D, Petersen RC, et al. Diagnostic criteria for mild cognitive impairment in Parkinson's disease: Movement Disorder Society Task Force guidelines. Mov Disord 2012 Mar; 27(3): 349–56.

Heterogeneity and cognitive 'subtypes'

Studies of cognitive change in PD suggest the deficits are primarily in the executive domain, and so would fit into the single-domain non-amnestic MCI category (see Fig. 8.1). However, a number of PD patients also show deficits in visuospatial or mnemonic function and some show a pattern of widespread or 'global' cognitive decline. In the study by Caviness et al. [9], 39% of the PD sample showed a single-domain MCI in the executive domain,

22% a single-domain amnestic impairment, 22% a multiple-domain non-amnestic pattern and 11% multiple-domain MCI including amnestic impairment. Other studies of MCI have used a different classification of cognitive profiles, identifying specific categories of executive dysfunction, memory impairment, visuospatial/visuoperceptual impairment and a 'global' pattern of cognitive impairment [3,12]. A study of 128 PD-MCI patients attending a movement disorder centre identified 47.7% as non-amnestic single domain (predominantly attentional/executive or visuosptial), 24.2% amnestic multiple domain, 18.8% amnestic single domain and 9.5% non-amnestic single domain [13]. There is therefore a significant degree of heterogeneity in terms of cognitive profile within the PD population without dementia, with an executive profile being common but not universal.

It is likely that these different profiles have different underlying pathologies and may also have different prognostic implications: many PD patients experience dysfunction of frontostriatal pathways, resulting in specific executive impairments, some have hippocampal or temporal damage, resulting in a more amnestic type of impairment [14], and others may experience changes to posterior brain areas, which deal with visuospatial and visuoperceptual function. Although executive impairments remain the most prevalent finding throughout the disease process, the presence of deficits in other domains may also be important in determining the progression of cognitive change [15].

Another way of defining cognitive subtypes within PD is to consider the profile of motor symptoms. Those individuals with a tremor-dominant form of PD appear to be at *less* risk of developing cognitive decline than those with a postural instability and gait dominant (PIGD) profile [16,17]. PD patients with the PIGD subtype display greater levels of postural instability, stooped posture, speech and gait difficulties and little tremor [17], and appear to be particularly impaired in executive function, specifically on the Tower of London (TOL) task, which assesses planning ability [16]. Similar results have been shown with PD-MCI subtypes, with greater gait and postural problems in patients presenting with a multiple-domain non-amnestic profile [13]. As these motor signs are thought to originate from organic change outside the basal ganglia (i.e. extra-striatal damage), it is thought that non-dopaminergic mechanisms underlie cognitive dysfunction in this group [2,17]. Identifying phenotypes within the PD population may improve our knowledge of which individuals are likely to develop more severe cognitive decline and therefore may benefit from regular neuropsychological assessment, and the targeting of education, support and other resources.

Models of cognitive dysfunction in Parkinson's disease

Pathological models

PD falls within a range of diseases known as the α-synucleinopathies. The pathological hallmark of PD is the presence of Lewy bodies (α-synuclein deposits) in the nigrostriatal pathway. Autopsy studies have found that Lewy bodies are often more widespread than the basal ganglia, and Braak has proposed a staging system whereby Lewy bodies first arise in the brainstem (before the motor symptoms of PD emerge), then spread to the basal ganglia (causing the onset of motor symptoms) and later onto limbic and neocortical areas [18], that are in turn linked to cognitive decline [19]. There is also evidence that some PD patients display Alzheimer-like pathological changes at autopsy, including senile plaques and neurofibrillary tangles, in both cortical and subcortical regions [2]. A growing number of studies have used *in vivo* magnetic resonance imaging (MRI) to assess cortical and white matter (WM) changes associated with PD-MCI (see [20] for review), and suggest that alterations in critical WM tracts precede cortical hypoperfusion and atrophy in the development of PD-MCI [21]. This suggests that MRI may provide valuable biomarkers of early risk for cognitive decline, such as evidence that hippocampal degeneration precedes PD dementia [22]. Studies have revealed early changes in cortical thickness and surface area in both frontal and posterior cortical areas, with consistent evidence of WM abnormalities in PD-MCI. For example, Kandiah et al. [23] found increased periventricular and deep-subcortical WM hyperintensities (WMH), and also regionally in the frontal parietal and occipital areas. Increasing WMH was associated with worse cognitive performance. PD-MCI patients, however, also had more prevalent diabetes, hypertension and hyperlipidia, emphasizing the importance of assessing other important physical co-morbidities that could possibly contribute to cognitive decline.

Pathophysiological models

PD is characterized by a loss of dopaminergic function in the nigrostriatal pathways, which in turn leads to excessive inhibition of the striatum and associated motor pathways. It is thought that the striatum is compartmentalized in terms of function and that the *motoric* effects of PD are expressed primarily through the putamen and associated motor circuits, whereas the *cognitive* changes are driven by loss of function in the caudate and ascending corticostriatal pathways [1,2]. Alterations in brain metabolism and dopa uptake have been demonstrated at the site of cortical targets of the striatum, for example in the prefrontal cortex [24,25]. The fact that deficits in planning and working memory may be ameliorated by the use of dopaminergic therapy offers some evidence for the hypothesized role of dopamine [1,26].

However, *in vivo* imaging studies have shown neurochemical changes beyond dopaminergic loss, particularly in acetylcholine (ACh), noradrenaline (NE) and serotonin (5-HT) [27]. Based on knowledge of neurotransmitter function and associated cognitive performance in healthy individuals, a hypothesis has been put forward whereby executive, attentional and mnemonic dysfunction in PD are based on dopaminergic, noradrenaline and cholinergic losses, respectively [1,2,4]. Although this is likely to be an oversimplification, it again emphasizes the heterogeneity in both cognitive profile and neurochemical change in PD.

In vivo studies of brain metabolism have described reduced activity in prefrontal regions which are associated with deficits in executive and working memory. Hypometabolism in more posterior regions, including temporal, parietal and occipital lobes, have also been noted, correlated with cognitive decline, and used to distinguish PD MCI patients from cognitively intact PD patients [28–30]. Analysis of metabolic changes across the brain has identified distinct network patterns in PD [28]. In that study a rapidly developing 'motor network' with increased pallidal, thalamic and supplementary motor area metabolism and reduced pre-motor and posterior parietal metabolism was correlated with disease severity and was responsive to treatment. A separate 'cognitive network' with increased metabolism of parietal, cingulate, medial frontal and occipital lobes, and reduced metabolism of the cerebellum and brainstem, was associated with MCI in executive, language, visuospatial and mnemonic domains.

Evidence from functional neuroimaging

Functional MRI (fMRI) and positron emission tomography (PET) have been used to examine regional changes in brain activity during cognitive tasks, allowing more accurate identification of the specific brain regions involved in cognition. The TOL task requires the subject to use strategic planning and is known to reliably activate the prefrontal cortex; it is also sensitive to executive function in PD patients without dementia. Several studies have used this task during functional imaging, finding that deficits in performance on the TOL, which imply inefficient processing in the prefrontal cortex, are associated with reduced blood flow in the right caudate but no changes in prefrontal blood flow [31]. Such results have been interpreted as demonstrating that prefrontal dysfunction, indicated by poor performance on the TOL, arises from dysfunction in the caudate, which has knock-on effects on dopaminergic pathways ascending from the caudate to the prefrontal cortex. Abnormal activation in the caudate and frontal cortex has been found across a range of executive, working and attentional tasks [25,32], although other studies have found abnormal prefrontal activation and deficits in the absence of caudate dysfunction [33]. Whether prefrontal deficits are caused by dysfunction of dopaminergic corticostriatal pathways or dopaminergic mesocortical pathways is controversial, although some authors have argued a role for both and that some executive tasks require caudate activation whereas others do not [32].

Some cognitive deficits in PD appear to be ameliorated by the administration of dopaminergic therapy. Functional imaging studies have been instructive in considering how levodopa may modulate frontal lobe activity. Studies comparing performance on working memory tasks in a 'drug-off' state (following levodopa withdrawal) versus a 'drug-on' state (following levodopa administration) have shown improved performance during the drug-on state, suggesting that levodopa ameliorates deficits in working memory, and a *decrease* in prefrontal activation during the drug-on state [33,34]. This finding has been interpreted as showing that levodopa and dopamine improve performance of the working memory by increasing the signal to noise ratio within prefrontal areas, which leads to more efficient prefrontal activation. A high level of diffuse prefrontal activity would therefore indicate inefficient processing. However, it is unclear whether such beneficial effects of levodopa are limited to executive and attentional function. The issue of levodopa and cognitive performance is further complicated by evidence that high levels of medication during advanced disease may in fact increase cognitive deficits by exposing frontostriatal pathways to an 'overdose effect' [26]. The clinician may therefore face a dilemma when treating advanced disease if the motoric benefits of dopaminergic medication are outweighed by poorer cognitive performance, and it may be tricky to achieve optimal levels for both. In summary, there is clear evidence of functional, metabolic and structural prefrontal change in PD, associated with specific executive impairments, as well as more widespread metabolic change in temporal and posterior regions.

Genetic findings and cognitive phenotypes

As yet, there is little evidence for distinguishing tremor-dominant and PIGD motor profiles on a genetic basis, and little is known about whether specific familial genetic forms of PD are associated with a greater degree of cognitive decline. Mutations in the *SNCA* gene, which provides instructions for α-synuclein synthesis and is important in regulating dopamine uptake, have been implicated in the development of PD and with poorer performance on basal ganglia-mediated stimulus–reward learning in healthy volunteers [35]. It remains unclear, however, whether *SNCA* mutations in PD patients confer a higher risk of cognitive decline.

Cognitive performance in PD has an interesting interaction with functional polymorphisms in the catechol-*O*-methyltransferase (*COMT*) [36] and brain-derived neurotrophic factor (*BDNF*) [37] genes and the use of dopaminergic medication. Those individuals with alleles indicating a less active COMT (i.e. slower breakdown of dopamine) performed better on the TOL task, and this effect was magnified for those on dopaminergic therapy. Similarly, those with a polymorphism indicating slower secretion of BDNF showed better performance on the TOL, and this was only evident for those on dopaminergic medication.

There is growing genetic evidence for a role of Alzheimer-type pathology in cognitive function in PD, as functional polymorphisms indicating greater risk for Alzheimer's disease in the general population have been associated with higher rates of dementia in PD. The apolipoprotein E (*APOE*) ε4 allele is implicated in the formation of amyloid plaques, and the *MAPT* haplotype H1 is thought to increase the likelihood of neurofibrillary tangles. Both these polymorphisms have been associated with greater risk of dementia or increased rates of cognitive decline in PD [38,39]. Genotyping for common polymorphisms in PD patients may therefore help to identify those individuals with greater risk of cognitive impairment. A recent 10-year follow-up of the CamPaIGN cohort (see Cognitive impairment and dementia risk) supported the importance of *MAPT* genotype for determining dementia onset, along with 'posterior-cortical' cognitive profile [40].

Cognitive impairment and dementia risk

For those with PD, mild cognitive difficulties may sometimes seem unimportant relative to the challenges of coping with the physical symptoms of the disease. This perception may also be shared by healthcare professionals who, while aware of the risks posed by dementia, may not pay close attention to the presence and potential significance of less severe cognitive impairment. Nevertheless, such changes still have an impact on the lives of some patients, and may have important implications for delivering and planning care.

An obvious question that arises when MCI is present, is whether or not it is an early marker of dementia. Hobson and Meera [41] found baseline memory and language (including verbal fluency) function to be the best neuropsychological predictors of dementia status 4 years later in a prevalent community sample of 102 patients. Janvin et al. [42] reassessed a sample of 72 patients previously without dementia after 4 years and identified dementia in 62% of patients judged to have had MCI at baseline compared with only 20% in those without MCI [odds ratio 4.8, 95% confidence interval (CI) 1.6–14.8]. That study also assessed the prognostic significance of different subtypes of MCI. Although isolated memory impairment was not associated with a significantly increased risk of dementia, impairment of multiple domains, with or without memory impairment, or single-domain non-memory impairments (e.g. executive or visuospatial) were associated with significant increased risk. The best evidence to date comes from the prospective study of incident cohorts. Serial follow-up of the ParkWest cohort revealed that 27% of those with PD-MCI at baseline went on to develop dementia within 3 years compared with only 0.7% of those without PD-MCI (relative risk 39.2, 95% CI 5.2–296.5) [43]. A 5-year follow-up of the CamPaIGN cohort [44] found that 17% had developed dementia over that period, with initial cognitive impairment indicating parieto-temporal dysfunction (semantic fluency, drawing intersecting pentagon) predictive of dementia, but not more frontal executive impairments.

Thus, although mild cognitive difficulties do not inevitably indicate the presence of a progressive dementia, they are cause for extra clinical vigilance and monitoring of cognitive function with repeated assessments, particularly if combined with other known risk factors such as older age and the presence of hallucinations (see Chapter 10).

Cognitive impairment, disablement and daily function

Whether or not a patient becomes demented, even MCI may be a cause of significant disability and handicap and reduced quality of life [45]. Recent evidence suggests that PD-MCI can affect the ability to deal effectively and appropriately with day-to-day social problems [46].The greatest challenge will often be posed to those whose work or recreation involves cognitively challenging activity. For this reason, younger and more active patients with PD who are still in employment may suffer a greater interference from cognitive dysfunction than older patients with a narrower and less demanding daily routine. However, even 'normal' activity can suffer as a result of such impairments and be a cause of personal distress, as illustrated by the personal account in Box 8.2.

However frustrating and distressing such problems are, they become far more significant when they threaten the safety of the person with PD or others. Leaving electrical or gas appliances turned on are prime examples of when a momentary memory failure can pose a serious physical threat, while another common problem can be forgetting to lock doors and windows. Perhaps the most common cause for concern, however, is the safety of the person with PD when driving a car. While previous research has typically focused on the impact of movement control and problems with excessive daytime sleepiness, a

Box 8.2 Personal account of the impact of cognitive impairment from a 59-year-old female with a 15-year history of Parkinson's disease

I do well if I am doing things that are rote and full of habit, at least if I do them slowly. I have always been a clear thinker, with good attention to detail. I can still do that, but not if I have to think of more than one thing at a time. Today I had been helping my two grandchildren learn to play a board game. Just the teaching of things like this makes me irritable and frustrated. The 7-year-old can't sit still and spills and knocks things onto the floor all the time, while the almost 10-year-old knows everything. I was also trying to put dirty dishes into my daughter's dishwasher at the same time. By the time the game was over I was at the end of my tether. I have decided that I can only play a game with the kids one at a time, even if I have to play twice in a row.

I have become dangerously forgetful. I almost burned down my apartment two years ago. That was the time I left a pan on the cooker ALL NIGHT!! My forgetfulness is a major issue. I know this and it hurts me and frustrates me.

While doing the washing-up my daughter was trying to tell me about my forgetting to close the garage door when I park in the garage … this is a huge issue in my daughter's home. As simple as this sounds, I can't think about all these things at the same time. I get anxious, fearful, scared. By now I am almost in tears, but didn't want my daughter to see this.

growing number of recent studies have highlighted the importance of cognitive impairment in determining fitness to drive [47,48]. Simple attentional tasks are useful predictors of driving performance [49]. More specifically, some patients appear more prone to the effects of distraction during driving [50] or make driving errors when attempting to navigate unfamiliar routes [51].

Screening and assessment

While some form of periodic neuropsychological assessment should probably be standard for all patients, this is probably rarely achieved. More typically, clinical teams wait for patients or family members to report difficulties or voice concerns. However, clinically important problems may not be reported if they are thought to be signs of 'normal' ageing, while some patients, aware of the increased risk of dementia in PD, may be reluctant to mention difficulties due to stigma or fear of the diagnosis or its implications.

Instruments such as the Non-Motor Symptoms Scale (NMSS) [52] offer convenient, economical and unthreatening ways to start screening for possible cognitive problems as part of a comprehensive screen for the range of common non-motor symptoms. Patients who screen positive should receive a brief assessment of cognitive function. The standard

Mini Mental State Examination (MMSE) [53], although widely used, is not suitable for use in PD. It is not sensitive to mild cognitive decline and fails to assess executive function. Fortunately, there are a range of extended mental state examinations now available which are either designed for or are appropriate for use in PD, including the Addenbrooke's Cognitive Examination (ACE-R) [54], SCOPA-COG, the PD-Cognitive Rating Scale (PD-CRS) [55] and the increasingly used Montreal Cognitive Assessment (MoCA) [56]. Such measures can provide Level I evidence for PD-MCI or even more severe cognitive impairment (although optimum cutoffs typically remain unclear) and may indicate the need for a full neuropsychological assessment (see [8] for recommended tests).

Management of cognitive impairment

While cholinesterase inhibitors are indicated for the treatment of PD dementia, there is currently no evidence to support their use in PD-MCI. With the exception of avoiding drugs that have a significant anticholinergic action, there is no reliable evidence that conventional antiparkinsonian medication has a significant positive or negative impact on cognition, although vigilance is advised whenever medication is changed. A range of non-pharmacological approaches have been studied, including exercise and 'brain training'. Despite some positive results, a recent meta-analysis mainly highlighted the need for better quality trials [57]. Nevertheless, such strategies may provide a useful part of a multidisciplinary approach to the management of a range of non-motor symptoms alongside MCI, including depression and fatigue. Because depression, anxiety, sleep disturbance, fatigue and daytime sleepiness can all have a direct impact on cognitive performance or exacerbate existing cognitive dysfunction, these non-motor symptoms should be treated when possible and their impact on cognition monitored (see other chapters in this volume).

More broadly, management should focus on helping the patient develop strategies for coping with the cognitive difficulties that they face in particular situations, whether at work, home or during leisure activities. There is very little written specifically for PD, but the lay literature for patients and families following stroke or traumatic brain injury will often apply equally well, while occupational therapists in those services often have considerable expertise in managing cognitive dysfunction. A referral to a clinical neuropsychology service or memory clinic may provide valuable clinical input, including the appropriate use of memory aids and advice on dealing with executive problems in high-risk situations (e.g. to avoid conversations with passengers, use of hands-free mobile phones or even listening to the radio when driving). A home assessment by an occupational therapist may be indicated when there are concerns about safety, as would referral to a driving assessment centre when significant cognitive problems are identified. Where cognitive problems are a source of significant distress to the patient, referral to a clinical psychologist or counsellor also may be of value. Finally, the identification of cognitive dysfunction should trigger discussions with the patient and their family about registering lasting power of attorney before they start to experience problems managing their own affairs and their mental capacity becomes a practical and legal issue.

References

1 **Dubois B, Pillon B**. Cognitive deficits in Parkinson's disease. J Neurol 1997; **244**: 2–8.

2 **Emre M**. What causes mental dysfunction in Parkinson's disease? Mov Disord 2003;**18**(Suppl 6): S63–S71.

3 **Verleden S, Vingerhoets G, Santens P**. Heterogeneity of cognitive dysfunction in Parkinson's disease: a cohort study. Eur Neurol 2007; **58**: 34–40.

4 **Zgaljardic DJ, Borod JC, Foldi NS, et al**. An examination of executive dysfunction associated with frontostriatal circuitry in Parkinson's disease. J Clin Exp Neuropsychol 2006; **28**: 1127–44.

5 **Uc EY, Rizzo M, Anderson SW, Qian S, Rodnitzky RL, Dawson JD**. Visual dysfunction in Parkinson disease without dementia. Neurology 2005; **65**: 1907–13.

6 **Winblad B, Palmer K, Kivipelto M, et al**. Mild cognitive impairment—beyond controversies, towards a consensus: report of the International Working Group on Mild Cognitive Impairment. J Intern Med 2004; **256**: 240–6.

7 **Litvan I, Aarsland D, Adler CH, et al**. MDS Task Force on mild cognitive impairment in Parkinson's disease: critical review of PD-MCI. Mov Disord 2011; **26**: 1814–24.

8 **Litvan I, Goldman JG, Troster AI, et al**. Diagnostic criteria for mild cognitive impairment in Parkinson's disease: Movement Disorder Society Task Force guidelines. Mov Disord 2012; **27**: 349–56.

9 **Caviness JN, Driver-Dunckley E, Connor DJ, et al**. Defining mild cognitive impairment in Parkinson's disease. Mov Disord 2007; **22**: 1272–7.

10 **Aarsland D, Bronnick K, Larsen JP, Tysnes OB, Alves G**. Cognitive impairment in incident, untreated Parkinson disease: the Norwegian ParkWest study. Neurology 2009; **72**: 1121–6.

11 **Aarsland D, Bronnick K, Williams-Gray C, et al**. Mild cognitive impairment in Parkinson disease: a multicenter pooled analysis. Neurology 2010; **75**: 1062–9.

12 **Janvin C, Aarsland D, Larsen JP, Hugdahl K**. Neuropsychological profile of patients with Parkinson's disease without dementia. Dement Geriatr Cogn Disord 2003; **15**: 126–31.

13 **Goldman JG, Weis H, Stebbins G, Bernard B, Goetz CG**. Clinical differences among mild cognitive impairment subtypes in Parkinson's disease. Mov Disord 2012; **27**: 1129–36.

14 **Foltynie T, Brayne CE, Robbins TW, Barker RA**. The cognitive ability of an incident cohort of Parkinson's patients in the UK. The CamPaIGN study. Brain 2004; **127**: 550–60.

15 **Muslimovic D, Schmand B, Speelman JD, De Haan RJ**. Course of cognitive decline in Parkinson's disease: a meta-analysis. J Int Neuropsychol Soc 2007; **13**: 920–32.

16 **Lewis SJG, Foltynie T, Blackwell AD, Robbins TW, Owen AM, Barker RA**. Heterogeneity of Parkinson's disease in the early clinical stages using a data driven approach. J Neurol Neurosurg Psychiatry 2005; **76**: 343–8.

17 **Levy G, Tang MX, Cote LJ, et al**. Motor impairment in PD: relationship to incident dementia and age. Neurology 2000; **55**: 539–44.

18 **Braak H, Ghebremedhin E, Rub U, Bratzke H, Del TK**. Stages in the development of Parkinson's disease-related pathology. Cell Tissue Res 2004; **318**: 121–34.

19 **Braak H, Rub U, Del TK**. Cognitive decline correlates with neuropathological stage in Parkinson's disease. J Neurol Sci 2006; **248**: 255–8.

20 **Duncan GW, Firbank MJ, O'Brien JT, Burn DJ**. Magnetic resonance imaging: a biomarker for cognitive impairment in Parkinson's disease? Mov Disord 2013; **28**: 425–38.

21 **Hattori T, Orimo S, Aoki S, et al**. Cognitive status correlates with white matter alteration in Parkinson's disease. Hum Brain Mapp 2012 **33**: 727–39.

22 **Weintraub D, Doshi J, Koka D, et al**. Neurodegeneration across stages of cognitive decline in Parkinson disease. Arch Neurol 2011; **68**: 1562–8.

23 Kandiah N, Mak E, Ng A, et al. Cerebral white matter hyperintensity in Parkinson's disease: a major risk factor for mild cognitive impairment. Parkinsonism Relat Disord 2013; **19**: 680–3.

24 Rinne JO, Portin R, Ruottinen H, et al. Cognitive impairment and the brain dopaminergic system in Parkinson disease: [18F]fluorodopa positron emission tomographic study. Arch Neurol 2000; **57**: 470–5.

25 Lewis SJ, Dove A, Robbins TW, Barker RA, Owen AM. Cognitive impairments in early Parkinson's disease are accompanied by reductions in activity in frontostriatal neural circuitry. J Neurosci 2003; **23**: 6351–6.

26 Cools R. Dopaminergic modulation of cognitive function-implications for l-DOPA treatment in Parkinson's disease. Neurosci Biobehav Rev 2006; **30**: 1–23.

27 Brooks DJ. Imaging non-dopaminergic function in Parkinson's disease. Molec Imaging Biol 2007; **9**: 217–22.

28 Huang CR, Mattis P, Julin P. Identifying functional imaging markers of mild cognitive impairment in early Alzheimer's and Parkinson's disease using multivariate analysis. Clin Neurosci Res 2007; **6**: 367–73.

29 Wallin A, Jennersjo C, Granerus A-K. Prevalence of dementia and regional brain syndromes in long-standing Parkinson's disease. Parkinsonism Relat Disord 1999; **5**: 103–10.

30 Tachibana H, Tomino Y, Kawabata K, Sugita M, Fukuchi M. 12-month follow-up-study of regional cerebral blood-flow in Parkinson's disease. Dementia 1995; **6**: 89–93.

31 Dagher A, Owen AM, Boecker H, Brooks DJ. The role of the striatum and hippocampus in planning—a PET activation study in Parkinson's disease. Brain 2001; **124**: 1020–32.

32 Monchi O, Petrides M, Mejia-Constain B, Strafella AP. Cortical activity in Parkinson's disease during executive processing depends on striatal involvement. Brain 2007; **130**: 233–44.

33 Cools R, Stefanova E, Barker RA, Robbins TW, Owen AM. Dopaminergic modulation of high-level cognition in Parkinson's disease: the role of the prefrontal cortex revealed by PET. Brain 2002; **125**: 584–94.

34 Mattay VS, Tessitore A, Callicott JH, et al. Dopaminergic modulation of cortical function in patients with Parkinson's disease. Ann Neurol 2002; **51**: 156–64.

35 Keri S, Nagy H, Myers CE, Benedek G, Shohamy D, Gluck MA. Risk and protective haplotypes of the alpha-synuclein gene associated with Parkinson's disease differentially affect cognitive sequence learning. Genes Brain Behav 2008; **7**: 31–6.

36 Foltynie T, Goldberg TE, Lewis SG, et al. Planning ability in Parkinson's disease is influenced by the COMT val158met polymorphism. Mov Disord 2004; **19**: 885–91.

37 Foltynie T, Lewis SG, Goldberg TE, et al. The BDNF Val66Met polymorphism has a gender specific influence on planning ability in Parkinson's disease. J Neurol 2005; **252**: 833–8.

38 Goris A, Williams-Gray CH, Clark GR, et al. Tau and alpha-synuclein in susceptibility to, and dementia in, Parkinson's disease. Ann Neurol 2007; **62**: 145–53.

39 Pankratz N, Byder L, Halter C, et al. Presence of an APOE4 allele results in significantly earlier onset of Parkinson's disease and a higher risk with dementia. Mov Disord 2006; **21**: 45–9.

40 Williams-Gray CH, Mason SL, Evans JR, et al. The CamPaIGN study of Parkinson's disease: 10-year outlook in an incident population-based cohort. J Neurol Neurosurg Psychiatry 2013; **84**: 1258–64.

41 Hobson P, Meara J. Risk and incidence of dementia in a cohort of older subjects with Parkinson's disease in the United Kingdom. Mov Disord 2004; **19**: 1043–9.

42 Janvin CC, Larsen JP, Aarsland D, Hugdahl K. Subtypes of mild cognitive impairment in Parkinson's disease: progression to dementia. Mov Disord 2006; **21**: 1343–9.

43 Pedersen KF, Larsen JP, Tysnes OB, Alves G. Prognosis of mild cognitive impairment in early Parkinson disease: the Norwegian ParkWest Study. JAMA Neurol 2013; **70**: 580–6.

44 **Williams-Gray CH, Evans JR, Goris A, et al.** The distinct cognitive syndromes of Parkinson's disease: 5 year follow-up of the CamPaIGN cohort. Brain 2009; **132**: 2958–69.

45 **Reginold W, Duff-Canning S, Meaney C, et al.** Impact of mild cognitive impairment on health-related quality of life in Parkinson's disease. Dement Geriatr Cogn Disord 2013; **36**: 67–75.

46 **Anderson RJ, Simpson AC, Channon S, Samuel M, Brown RG.** Social problem solving, social cognition, and mild cognitive impairment in Parkinson's disease. Behav Neurosci 2013; **127**: 184–92.

47 **Devos H, Vandenberghe W, Nieuwboer A, Tant M, Baten G, De WW.** Predictors of fitness to drive in people with Parkinson disease. Neurology 2007; **69**: 1434–41.

48 **Stolwyk RJ, Charlton JL, Triggs TJ, Iansek R, Bradshaw JL.** Neuropsychological function and driving ability in people with Parkinson's disease. J Clin Exp Neuropsychol 2006; **28**: 898–913.

49 **Worringham CJ, Wood JM, Kerr GK, Silburn PA.** Predictors of driving assessment outcome in Parkinson's disease. Mov Disord 2006; **21**: 230–5.

50 **Uc EY, Rizzo M, Anderson SW, Sparks JD, Rodnitzky RL, Dawson JD.** Driving with distraction in Parkinson disease. Neurology 2006; **67**: 1774–80.

51 **Uc EY, Rizzo M, Anderson SW, Sparks JD, Rodnitzky RL, Dawson JD.** Impaired navigation in drivers with Parkinson's disease. Brain 2007; **130**: 2433–40.

52 **Chaudhuri KR, Martinez-Martin P, Brown RG, et al.** The metric properties of a novel non-motor symptoms scale for Parkinson's disease: results from an international pilot study. Mov Disord 2007; **22**: 1901–11.

53 **Folstein MF, Folstein SE, McHugh PR.** 'Mini—mental state'. A practical method for grading the cognitive state of patients for the clinician. J Psychiatr Res 1975; **12**: 189–98.

54 **Mioshi E, Dawson K, Mitchell J, Arnold R, Hodges JR.** The Addenbrooke's Cognitive Examination Revised (ACE-R): a brief cognitive test battery for dementia screening. Int J Geriatr Psychiatry 2006; **21**: 1078–85.

55 **Pagonabarraga J, Kulisevsky J, Llebaria G, Garcia-Sanchez C, Pascual-Sedano B, Gironell A.** Parkinson's disease-cognitive rating scale: a new cognitive scale specific for Parkinson's disease. Mov Disord 2008; **23**: 998–1005.

56 **Nasreddine ZS, Phillips NA, Bedirian V, et al.** The Montreal Cognitive Assessment, MoCA: a brief screening tool for mild cognitive impairment. J Am Geriatr Soc 2005; **53**: 695–9.

57 **Hindle JV, Petrelli A, Clare L, Kalbe E.** Nonpharmacological enhancement of cognitive function in Parkinson's disease: a systematic review. Mov Disord 2013; **28**: 1034–49.

Chapter 9

Depression, anxiety and apathy in Parkinson's disease

David A. Gallagher and Anette Schrag

Introduction

Depression, anxiety and apathy are common in Parkinson's disease (PD). Depression, in particular, has been consistently shown to be a major determinant of health-related quality of life (HR-QoL). Despite this, the application of diagnostic criteria for psychiatric or motivational difficulties in PD encounters conceptual difficulties, given the overlap between PD symptoms and the somatic features of mood disorders. Modifications to the diagnostic criteria for psychiatric disorders in PD have been proposed and are currently undergoing validation. This will be needed to determine the true prevalence of these disorders and improve diagnostic sensitivity in the clinical setting. Several pharmacotherapies are of proven efficacy in mood disorders, but depression and anxiety in PD represent a distinct neurobiological substrate and these psychotropic agents will require further well-designed double-blind placebo-controlled trials to prove their efficacy.

The prevalence and impact of depression, anxiety and apathy in Parkinson's disease

Prevalence

Disorders of mood, motivation and anxiety are common in PD, occur at higher prevalence than in the age-matched population and have a significant impact on quality of life. However, establishing the prevalence of these neuropsychiatric diagnoses in PD is challenging, for several reasons: symptomatic overlap with the underlying movement disorder and between the neuropsychiatric disorders; differences between the phenomenology of these disorders in PD and in the general population; the frequent coexistence of cognitive dysfunction; the presence of motor and non-motor fluctuations; and the difficulty of distinguishing these disorders from the psychiatric side effects of antiparkinsonian medications.

The figures for prevalence of depression in PD (dPD) vary greatly between studies (from 2.7% to more than 90% [1]), probably reflecting these difficulties and the diagnostic criteria used [e.g. Diagnostic and Statistical Manual, version IV (DSM-IV) criteria with or without structured interview, depression rating scales or clinical impression]. In a large systematic review, 104 studies on the prevalence of depression were identified [1], of which 36 met the inclusion criteria based on three elements of study quality, namely case identification, PD diagnostic criteria and depression diagnostic criteria. The weighted mean prevalence of major depression, minor depression and dysthymia were 17, 22 and 13%, respectively, with clinically significant depression in 35%. Several large cohort studies have subsequently confirmed the prevalence of clinically significant depression in PD to be approximately 30% [58].

Anxiety disorders, which are often co-morbid, are estimated to have a prevalence of 24–75% in PD [2,3], with panic disorder, general anxiety disorder (GAD) and social phobia being most common [4]. A study comparing 90 consecutive PD patients with age-matched controls [5] revealed that major depression (21.1% versus 3.3%, $P < 0.01$), dysthymia (18.8% versus 4.4%, $P < 0.05$) and panic disorder (30% versus 5.5%, $P < 0.01$) were significantly more prevalent in PD than in controls. GAD and obsessive compulsive disorder (OCD) occurred in 11.1% and 5.5%, respectively, but this did not differ from controls. Anxiety and depression combined was found in 19.3% of PD patients compared with 8.6% of controls ($P < 0.01$).

Depression and anxiety can both occur throughout the disease course and can even precede motor symptoms [6]. In a large clinico-pathological review (433 cases), 2.5% of PD patients had presented exclusively with anxiety or depression, leading to delayed diagnosis and unnecessary diagnostic and therapeutic interventions [7].

Estimates of the prevalence of apathy in PD vary depending on the clinical criteria used, but up to 60% patients have been found to have motivational difficulties in some studies [99]. Co-morbid depression and cognitive impairment, particularly fronto-temporal involvement, have a significant impact on motivation and can make a primary apathetic disorder difficult to differentiate.

Impact on health-related quality of life

Depression has consistently been shown to be one of the most debilitating non-motor features of PD, closely associated with poor HR-QoL scores, over and above motor severity and the influences of medication [9,10,62]. Several studies have also shown that anxiety has a significant correlation with HR-QoL, even when adjusted for depression or other non-motor symptoms [64–67]. Some studies have shown a significant correlation of apathy with HR-QoL [59,60], but when other variables are considered the association is less clear. In one study apathy significantly predicted poorer HR-QoL after adjustment for depression, medication and motor severity [61]. However, in other studies, despite significant bivariate correlation, apathy did not significantly contribute to HR-QoL in multivariate regression [62,63], with other non-motor features, particularly depression, showing greater association.

Diagnosis and severity rating of depression, anxiety and apathy in Parkinson's disease

Depression

Clinical diagnosis

The gold standard clinical diagnosis of depression in PD uses criteria such as DSM-IV for major, minor or subsyndromal depression or the International Statistical Classification of

Diseases and Related Health Problems, 10th revision (ICD-10) criteria for a mild, moderate or severe depressive episode. The application of such criteria in PD, however, encounters conceptual difficulties. A DSM-IV diagnosis of major depression requires at least one of the two core criteria (depressed mood and loss of interest or pleasure) and a total of five or more symptoms, including the additional criteria (significant weight change, insomnia or hypersomnia, psychomotor retardation or agitation, fatigue, expression of worthlessness or guilt, reduced concentration or decisiveness or recurrent thoughts of death), with exclusion of symptoms attributable to medication or an underlying medical condition. A National Institute of Neurological Disorders and Stroke (NINDS)/National Institute of Mental Health (NIMH) working group on depression and PD [11] suggested that application of these criteria may miss a substantial number of patients with dPD, and made the following recommendations:

1 The diagnosis of dPD should be made according to DSM-IV diagnostic criteria using an inclusive approach (as opposed to an exclusive, aetiological or substitutive approach), using all symptoms, irrespective of potential aetiological basis, as it has the greatest sensitivity and reliability and does not require clinical judgment.

2 Subsyndromal depression should be included as a diagnostic category in research studies.

3 The timing of assessment should be specified ('on' versus 'off' periods).

4 Informants should be used for cognitively impaired patients.

5 Anhedonia should only be diagnosed based on loss of pleasure rather than loss of interest (as it overlaps with apathy) for diagnosis of minor depression/subsyndromal depression.

These recommendations were upheld by studies validating the use of DSM-IV criteria in PD [12,68], which demonstrated that the components of the criteria for major depression have high internal consistency and that all DSM-IV items are significantly correlated with the core DSM-IV criterion of low mood in dPD patients. In addition, there was no difference in the influence of individual DSM-IV items (including somatic) on the overall diagnosis of depression. However, others [13] have found that somatic items (psychomotor retardation, tiredness, physical anxiety) were much poorer at discriminating between depressed and non-depressed PD patients than core symptoms (low mood or anhedonia) or other non-somatic items (guilt, suicidal ideation and psychic anxiety). In addition, masked depression (without the core symptoms of sad mood or anhedonia) is rare in dPD [12], supporting the use of low mood as a core criterion. As there is significant association between low mood and anxiety symptoms, it has also been suggested that these should be added to the DSM-IV diagnostic framework [12,68].

Clinimetric rating scales

Clinimetric rating scales are often used in large-scale epidemiological studies and other studies as they are quantifiable and do not require clinical judgment. A systematic review of depression rating scales in PD has highlighted their diverse properties and differing clinical applications [14]. A diagnosis of depression should only be made using clinical criteria, because false negatives can occur in patients with low mood and anhedonia but with relatively few somatic symptoms; conversely, false positives can occur in the absence of depression due to the large number of overlapping somatic symptoms in PD. Additionally, depressive symptoms in PD that present in atypical ways, such as in the context of motor fluctuations or dysphoria related to dopamine dysregulation syndrome (DDS), are not suitable for assessment by rating scales.

Anxiety

DSM-IV categories for anxiety include panic attacks, agoraphobia, specific phobias, social phobias, OCD, post-traumatic stress disorder, acute stress disorder and GAD. The application and clinical validity of DSM-IV anxiety criteria in PD has not undergone the same systematic analysis and critique as depression but suffers the same conceptual difficulties and problems with symptomatic overlap. For example, DSM-IV criteria for GAD include fatigability, impaired concentration, sleep disturbance and muscular tension, which are all very common in PD. As mentioned above, anxiety disorders are often co-morbid with dPD and can occur in the context of motor and non-motor fluctuations [11].

Apathy

There is no definition or diagnostic framework for apathy in DSM-IV-TR, although it has been proposed that apathy should be included in subsequent revisions. In the past diagnosis has been made using clinical judgment and clinimetric rating scales. Most commonly, the Neuropsychiatric Inventory (NPI) and the Marin Apathy Evaluation Scale have been used, and more recently the Lille Apathy Rating Scale (LARS) has been specifically designed and validated for use in PD [8]. However, diagnostic criteria for apathy, with similar content, have recently been proposed and validated in PD based on existing scales or criteria used in other neurodegenerative disorders [69,70]. Items include: (1) lack of motivation compared with the previous level of functioning, (2) diminished goal-directed behaviour, cognition or emotion, (3) symptoms severe enough to cause significant impairment of personal, social or occupational function and (4) symptoms not attributed to the effects of physical disability, impaired consciousness or the effects of medication. In one study, criteria modified from the Marin scale, showed good sensitivity and specificity compared with a neuropsychiatrist's clinical judgment [69], and in another study, consensus criteria for apathy in Alzheimer's disease and other neuropsychiatric disorders [70] were applied in PD and showed good internal consistency and concurrent and discriminant validity compared with LARS and the NPI apathy score [71]. Apathy can occur as a component of cognitive impairment or depression, although detailed psychological studies in PD have shown that apathy can exist as an independent entity [69]. A full neuropsychological assessment should be made to exclude apathy in the context of cognitive impairment or depression.

Pathophysiology of depression, anxiety and apathy in Parkinson's disease

Both endogenous (e.g. monoamine neurotransmitter depletion) and psychological (e.g. adjustment to disease) components are likely to be important in the development of neuropsychiatric illness in PD [15]. In common with depression and anxiety in patients without PD, there are numerous and varying risk factors for depression, including inheritance, environmental influences (life events, family and personal circumstances) and differences in personality and psychological adjustment to disease.

Neurobiological insights into the pathophysiology of affective disorders in PD can be gained from several sources. Experimental, neuropathological and imaging studies have demonstrated abnormal functioning of dopaminergic systems in endogenous neuropsychiatric disorders in people without PD. Secondly, the involvement of extra-striatal and non-dopaminergic neurotransmitter systems in PD (including noradrenergic, serotoninergic, glutaminergic, cholinergic and gaba-aminobutyric and neuropeptide related) has become increasingly recognized, as has their effect on the non-motor sequelae of the disease. Thirdly, the epidemiological association of PD with higher rates of mood and anxiety disorder, and the possible association of dopaminergic medication with amelioration of these symptoms and occasionally *de novo* development of neuropsychiatric complications [mania, psychosis, impulse control disorder (ICD) and DDS], have been important.

The role of dopamine

The monoamine hypothesis of depression and research into the pathogenesis of and therapeutic interventions for mood disorders has traditionally centred on noradrenergic and serotoninergic neurotransmission. However, the role of dopaminergic pathways has increasingly been shown to be important [16]. Dopaminergic neurons projecting from the ventral tegmental area (VTA) to mesolimbic areas are known to contribute to mood, motivation and reward. Polymorphisms in several genes involved in dopamine neurotransmission have been implicated in major depression and anxiety disorders [72, 19]. Chronic antidepressant use and electroconvulsive therapy (ECT) in animal models of depression have resulted in increased transcription of dopamine receptor D3 mRNA in the nucleus accumbens, an area which receives major input from the mesolimbic dopaminergic systems, and dopaminergic potentiation is a proposed mechanism for these therapies [18]. Post-mortem studies of depressed patients have demonstrated pre-synaptic dopamine transporter (DAT) downregulation and altered dopamine receptor expression in the amygdala, consistent with mesolimbic dopamine deficiency [17,73]. In PD, striatal DAT availability has been reported to correlate negatively with symptoms of depression [102] and anxiety [77, 102, 103] and functional imaging studies have demonstrated a loss of dopamine and noradrenaline innervation in the limbic system [77]. These studies suggest the involvement of dopaminergic function in mood and anxiety disorders in non-PD and PD patients that is likely to contribute to the high frequency of neuropsychiatric co-morbidities in the context of dopaminergic depletion in idiopathic PD.

Dopamine agonists (particularly the non-ergotamine derivatives with a predilection for mesolimbic D3 receptors) have been reported as a useful adjuvant in refractory depression in non-PD subjects and as a treatment with comparable efficacy to other antidepressants in major depression [20]. Conversely, in PD, the predisposition for dopamine agonists to cause ICD—disorders of the reward mechanism with inability to resist pleasurable impulses (hypersexuality, pathological gambling, excessive shopping and excessive eating [21])—is likely to be mediated by an effect on mesolimbic pathways. The influence of drugs that manipulate dopaminergic neurotransmission on mood and behaviour suggests a role for the mesolimbocortical pathways in determining mood and motivation in PD.

Non-dopaminergic involvement

Post-mortem studies of the distribution of α-synuclein containing Lewy bodies in PD [22] have demonstrated widespread involvement of the central nervous system (CNS), including the brainstem and neocortical and mesolimbic systems, and a hypothesis has been proposed by Braak et al. that these neuropathological changes follow a pattern of sequential topographical involvement [22]. Subsequent detailed pathological studies have demonstrated that this caudal–rostral progression does not apply in all cases, but confirm that involvement of serotoninergic brainstem raphe nuclei and the noradrenergic locus coeruleus (LC) can both precede basal midbrain involvement and degeneration of dopaminergic neurons of the substantia nigra. This may explain the high frequency of symptoms of depression and anxiety in PD, including during the pre-motor phase [6]. In a positron emission tomography (PET) study using serotonin transporter (SERT)-specific ligands, reduced striatal serotonin binding in the caudate and putamen in PD was shown, similar to reduced DAT density, and the changes were correlated with disease stage [23]. In another study using ^{123}I-β-CIT SPECT, striatal binding ratios (reflecting DAT density) were significantly correlated with motor disease stage in PD, whereas dorsal midbrain binding ratios (SERT receptor density) were significantly correlated with Unified Parkinson's Disease Rating Scale (UPDRS) mood, mentation and behaviour subscore, suggesting that nigral dopaminergic and dorsal raphe serotoninergic dysfunction contribute to motor and psychiatric features, respectively [24]. Other PET studies using SERT ligands have shown increased serotonin binding in the raphe nuclei and limbic structures [74] and dorsolateral and prefrontal cortices [75] in depressed PD patients, interpreted as reflecting upregulation due to lower extracellular serotonin levels in these areas. However, other studies have shown no correlation of depression with SERT binding [76]. Transcranial sonography has shown hypo-echogenicity of the dorsal raphe to be associated with the onset of depression preceding motor deficit in PD [25]. These studies support the involvement of serotoninergic transmission in depression in PD. Other neurotransmitter systems have also been implicated. For example, PET studies using ligands for cholinergic receptors [80] and examining cortical acetylcholinesterase activity [81] have demonstrated an association with symptoms of depression. Post-mortem studies in depressed PD subjects have shown particular involvement of catecholamine areas of the brain, including the LC [78,79].

Treatment of depression, anxiety and apathy in Parkinson's disease

Pharmacotherapy

Dopaminergic medication

The therapeutic potential of dopaminergic drugs is increasingly being recognized. A systematic review of dopamine agonists in non-PD psychiatric patients (24 studies) [26] revealed that pramipexole had a large effect size in both unipolar and bipolar depression, with good tolerability. In PD, two placebo-controlled studies have examined the effect of pramipexole specifically on mood in PD. The first, a large double-blind placebo-controlled trial in patients with depressive symptoms [Geriatric Depression Score (GDS) ≥ 5] showed significant benefit of pramipexole ($n = 139$) over placebo ($n = 148$) on the Beck Depression Inventory (BDI), even when adjusted for potential confounding motor benefit (UPDRS score), although the effect size was small and possibly not clinically meaningful (mean difference on BDI 1.9 units, $P = 0.01$) [82]. In the second, smaller, study ($n = 30$), comparing pramipexole, pergolide or placebo on tremor in non-depressed PD patients, there was no significant difference in the Hospital Anxiety and Depression Scale score [86]. In a meta-analysis of seven placebo-controlled trials of pramipexole that used UPDRS Part I as a secondary outcome measure, mood symptoms improved in more patients taking pramipexole than placebo [64.7% versus 43.4% for placebo; weighted odds ratio (OR) 2.41, $P < 0.001$], and motivational symptoms also improved in more patients taking pramipexole than placebo (63.2% versus 45.0% for placebo; weighted OR 2.06, $P < 0.001$) [83]. However, UPDRS Part I items are a poorer measure of mood symptoms than validated clinical scales, the studies were designed primarily to assess motor function rather mood, and in all the studies major depression was a criterion for exclusion. In the open-label extension of a double-blind study randomizing to initial treatment with pramipexole or levodopa, designed to determine the influence on motor function and particularly disease progression (the CALM-PD study [84]), there was no difference in GDS score at a mean follow-up of 6 years ($n = 222$). Another study compared dopamine agonist therapy with standard antidepressant medication. This was a 14-week open-label study of PD patients with major depression ($n = 67$) randomized to take pramipexole (1.5–4.5 mg/day) or sertraline (50 mg/day), and both groups had similar benefit on Hamilton Depression Rating Scale (HDRS) score, with a higher proportion of those taking pramipexole achieving recovery (defined as HDRS ≤ 8; $P = 0.006$) [85]. A double-blind placebo-controlled trial of an extended-release ropinirole preparation [27] reported improvement in depression using the BDI, although the effect size was small (mean difference 1.6 units). In addition, the primary outcome measures were motor function and 'on'/'off' fluctuations, and patients were not selected according to DSM-IV criteria for depression. In a small double-blind placebo-controlled study of the dopamine agonist piribedil ($n = 37$) in patients presenting with apathy following deep brain stimulation, there was no difference in the BDI ($P = 0.29$) and or Beck Anxiety Inventory ($P = 0.41$), but a trend to improvement in anhedonia measures (Snaith–Hamilton Pleasure Scale; $P = 0.08$) and the HDRS ($P = 0.05$) [88].

Other open-label studies have examined the effect of continuous apomorphine infusion and ergot dopamine agonists (which are generally less used due to potential cardiopulmonary fibrotic complications) on depression, with variable results and study design quality, but there are no double-blind or controlled trials for these agents [87].

Overall there have been four double-blind studies of dopamine agonists with depression outcome measures, of which two have shown a small but statistically significant benefit for pramipexole [82] and ropinirole [27], although it is unclear whether the effect represents a clinically significant change. In addition, as the primary role of dopaminergic medication is to ameliorate the motor symptoms of PD it may prove difficult to differentiate the improvement in depression scales due to improvement in motor symptoms from the neurotropic properties of the dopaminergic medication.

For apathy, individual case reports have suggested a benefit of ropinirole on apathy following stroke and viral encephalitis in non-PD subjects. A double-blind placebo-controlled study in patients with apathy following DBS demonstrated improvement in the Starkstein Apathy Scale score with the dopamine agonist piribedil (34.6%) versus placebo (3.2%, $P = 0.015$) although the study was small ($n = 37$) with a high number of dropouts [88]. In the post-hoc analysis of a placebo-controlled study of a transdermal rotigotine patch, assessing its impact on early morning motor function, 267 patients completed the Non-Motor Symptom Scale and there was statistically significant benefit on several items in the mood apathy domain [89].

Non-motor fluctuations, often but not always in association with motor fluctuations, are common in PD. In one questionnaire-based study [28], 60% of patients had 'off'-related non-motor features that were autonomic, sensory and neurocognitive (depression, anxiety, panic, drowsiness and confusion). Therefore, therapeutic interventions to reduce 'off' periods, including catechol-O-methyltransferase (COMT) inhibitors, oral or transdermal dopamine agonists, monoamine oxidase B (MAO-B) inhibitors, continuous subcutaneous apomorphine infusion or intra-duodenal levodopa infusions should be the first steps in attempts to ameliorate non-motor fluctuations rather than additional psychotropic medication.

Psychotropic pharmacotherapy

Pharmacological agents used for affective disorders in PD include the older tricyclic antidepressants (TCAs), the tricyclic-related drugs (trazodone), the selective serotonin reuptake inhibitors (SSRIs), the serotonin and noradrenaline reuptake inhibitor (SNRI) venlafaxine, the selective noradrenaline reuptake inhibitor reboxetine and the pre-synaptic alpha-2 adrenoreceptor antagonist mirtazapine. Consideration should be given to the potential side effects related to these medications, particularly in the elderly, their possible interaction with other drugs (particularly those metabolized via the cytochrome P450 system) resulting in variations in plasma concentration, reports of exacerbation of motor function, and their potential to exacerbate non-motor and dopaminergic drug-related complications of the disease. For example, autonomic dysfunction (constipation, genitourinary problems, orthostatic hypotension, pupillomotor impairment and hyperhidrosis) commonly occurs in PD. These symptoms are prone to exacerbation by the anticholinergic effects of TCAs, and to a lesser extent SSRIs. The anticholinergic action of these drugs can also increase confusion and worsen neuropsychiatric features of PD such as visual hallucinations and delusional thought disorder. Dopaminergic medication, levodopa and the dopamine agonists in particular, is associated with a reduction in blood pressure, and not uncommonly symptomatic orthostatic hypotension, an effect which can be exacerbated by the anticholinergic effect of antidepressant medication. The SSRIs have important pharmacological interactions with the MAO-B inhibitors selegiline and rasagiline, and thus a theoretical predilection to a serotonin syndrome. This effect is likely to be rare, given that at therapeutic doses MAO-B inhibitors produce no significant MAO-A inhibition; nonetheless, it should be considered.

A number of small studies on the efficacy of antidepressants in PD have been conducted in recent years. Systematic reviews of antidepressant use in PD [29,30] have highlighted the lack of empirical evidence for the efficacy of antidepressants, mainly due to the lack of large, well-designed randomized placebo-controlled trials. In the first meta-analysis [29] (11 studies met the inclusion criteria, of which only two were placebo-controlled), there was a very large composite reduction in depression rating scales in both active treatment and placebo groups, but no statistically significant difference between the two groups ($P = 0.44$). This was in contrast to elderly non-PD patients, in whom there was significant benefit for active treatment compared with placebo, suggesting that there is less response to standard antidepressant therapy in PD. In the second study (an evidence-based review by the Quality Standards Subcommittee of the American Academy of Neurology [30]), strict inclusion criteria and grading of evidence levels (I–IV) was employed. Only six studies met the criteria for inclusion (Level III evidence or better), three were placebo-controlled, but only one met the criteria for the Class I evidence level [31]. Of these, two underpowered placebo-controlled studies using the SSRIs citalopram [31] and sertraline [32] showed no benefit over placebo. An open-label trial comparing fluoxetine and nefazodone had benefit in both groups (BDI, $P < 0.001$) but the study was not placebo-controlled and there was no difference between the two agents ($P = 0.97$) [33]. In a study comparing nortriptyline with placebo, an improvement was reported but full statistical analysis was not given [34]. In an open-label study comparing amitriptyline with fluoxetine, there was a significant difference in favour of amitriptyline but a higher drop-out due to adverse events in that group [35]. Overall, this review concluded that there was Level C evidence (defined as possibly effective, and requiring at least one Class II or two consistent Class III studies) for the use of amitriptyline in the treatment of depression in PD, with the important caveat of potential debilitating anticholinergic side effects. In this review SSRIs had not as yet demonstrated clear efficacy compared with placebo in well-designed randomized clinical trials. In a third meta-analysis of randomized controlled trials, SSRIs were compared with placebo in six studies [combined risk ratio (RR) 1.08, 95% CI 0.77–1.55, $P = 0.67$] and TCAs in three studies (RR 0.75, 95% CI 0.39–1.42, $P = 0.37$) with no difference in treatment response, although the studies were small and false negative results could not be excluded [90]. A Movement

Disorder Society (MDS) evidence-based review of the treatment of non-motor features in PD [91] examined antidepressant medication in PD and concluded that nortriptyline and desipramine are probably efficacious (evidence suggests, but is not sufficient to show, that the intervention has a positive effect and is supported by any Level I trial without conflicting data). In a small study ($n = 52$), nortriptyline had significant benefit compared with placebo on HDRS score (effect size 1.2 units, $P < 0.002$) whereas paroxetine CR did not. There was a trend for nortriptyline over paroxetine at 8 weeks ($P < 0.079$) and response rates (>50% reduction in HDRS score) were higher for nortriptyline (53%) than paroxetine (11%) or placebo (24%) [92]. In another small study ($n = 48$), there was improvement at day 30 on the Montgomery–Åsberg Depression Rating Scale (MADRS) for both citalopram ($P = 0.03$) and desipramine ($P = 0.002$) groups compared with placebo [93]. There was insufficient evidence for SSRIs, citalopram (two studies), sertraline (three studies), fluoxetine (two studies) and paroxetine (one study) or newer antidepressants (atomoxetine and nefazodone) based on conflicting results and study methodology (small sample size, short trial duration and lack of placebo-controlled design) [91], although there were positive results in some individual studies, including recent trials. For example, in a study of 115 patients with DSM-IV defined depression there was significant benefit for paroxetine (mean difference in HDRS compared with placebo 6.2 points, 97.5% CI 2.2–10.3, $P = 0.0007$) [95] and venlafaxine (4.2 points, 97.5% CI 0.1–8.4, $P = 0.02$). A recent meta-analysis considered only placebo-controlled trials and the pooled RR for response was 1.36 (95% CI 0.98–1.87), indicating no significant benefit of antidepressants over placebo. However, the sensitivity analysis showed the RR for response was 1.41 (95% CI 1.01–1.96) after exclusion of one study with questionable results and 1.48 (95% CI 1.05–2.10) when only studies with a low risk of bias were included [94]. Atypical neuroleptics may have a role in treating depression with co-morbid psychotic features, although this may respond to antidepressants alone [36].

Without further large and comparative clinical studies, definitive recommendations for antidepressant pharmacotherapy in PD are not available and treatment should be tailored to individual patients depending on their other non-motor (particularly autonomic and cognitive) symptoms and potential for drug-related adverse events. Optimization of motor control, consideration of dopaminergic drugs and non-pharmacological interventions are likely to be important.

There has been no systematic assessment or large placebo-controlled trials for the use of anxiolytics in PD. The MDS evidence-based review of treatments for non-motor symptoms in PD failed to identify randomized controlled trials for anxiety or apathy that met inclusion criteria [91]. However, some double-blind placebo-controlled trials of antidepressant medication had anxiety measures as secondary outcomes, and in one study nortriptyline was significantly better than controlled-release paroxetine CR ($P < 0.007$) and placebo ($P < 0.0001$) in improving the HARS score and controlled-release paroxetine showed a trend over placebo ($P = 0.0740$) [92]. Neurocognitive, autonomic and sleep-related side effects are likely to be common in PD and benzodiazepines should therefore be used with caution. The SSRIs are currently favoured for the treatment of anxiety disorders in PD but their therapeutic efficacy is yet to be demonstrated.

Given the overlap of apathy and dysexecutive cognitive function, the use the cholinesterase inhibitors (donepezil, galantamine and rivastigmine) may be beneficial for apathy. A small open-label study of rivastigmine in dementia with Lewy bodies (DLB) showed a 63% reduction in the apathy domain of the NPI [37]. In one study [38], free testosterone levels were significantly correlated with apathy, suggesting a therapeutic potential for testosterone replacement in male PD patients with apathy. Methylphenidate, an amphetamine-related stimulant licensed for use in attention deficit hyperactivity disorder (ADHD), resulted in markedly increased motivation in a case study [39] but its use requires further validation.

Control of specific symptoms of PD may indirectly result in an improvement of depression in the absence of direct antidepressant effects. For example, an open-label trial of sildenafil in PD patients with erectile dysfunction resulted in improvement of depression from baseline [40].

Non-pharmacological interventions

Deep brain stimulation

Deep brain stimulation (DBS) is an intervention with proven efficacy in improving motor function and drug-related motor complications and allows a reduction in dose of dopaminergic drugs in PD. There have been conflicting reports of a beneficial or detrimental effect on neuropsychiatric symptoms of PD, in particular mood, motivation and ICD. A large meta-analysis [41] of DBS studies in PD, dystonia and essential tremor (546 articles met the inclusion criteria, 357 on PD), showed improvement in motor scales (98%), activities of daily living (96%) and HR-QoL (95%). In 37 studies where depression was prospectively assessed as a primary ($n = 3$) or secondary ($n = 34$) outcome measure, 83.3% reported an improvement. All six studies that prospectively measured anxiety reported an improvement, and there was a reported improvement in eight of nine (88.9%) studies using OCD rating scales [41]. The effect of DBS on motivation and apathy has not been clearly determined. Overall, psychiatric adverse events were reported infrequently—depression (2–4%), anxiety (0.3–0.6%) and apathy (0.3–0.6%). However, of most concern was the completed suicide rate (0.16–0.32%). This appears significantly higher than the national average. Therefore, while DBS may provide a useful treatment for both motor and non-motor (including depression and anxiety) symptoms, screening for suicidal ideation, particularly in those at most risk (young age PD onset, young age at DBS treatment, prolonged disease duration) will be important.

Repetitive transcranial magnetic stimulation

Repetitive transcranial magnetic stimulation (rTMS) has been proposed to have a beneficial effect on depression in PD, but systematic reviews of the evidence have been inconclusive [42,91] and assessment of improvement may be confounded by a potential improvement in motor and cognitive function. One study of rTMS of the motor cortex revealed no significant improvement in depression versus sham surgery [43]. However, that study was designed to assess impact on motor function and both depressed and non-depressed subjects were included at baseline. A sham controlled study of supplementary motor area stimulation on motor symptoms in PD resulted in transient benefit in UPDRS, but no change in non-motor outcomes, including HDRS scores [96]. Another small sham controlled study ($n = 18$), with rTMS stimulating the vertex, primarily aimed to assess the effect on sleep (patients were not specifically selected for depression), showed no benefit on HDRS scores [98]. A small ($n = 22$) sham controlled blinded study of left prefrontal rTMS in PD patients with DSM-IV defined depression showed significant benefit on the MADRS and BDI depression scales ($P < 0.05$) in the rTMS but not the sham group [97], although between-group statistical comparison was not given. In small double-blinded studies comparing dorsolateral prefrontal cortex (DLPFC) rTMS and fluoxetine (using placebo and sham rTMS, respectively), both agents showed comparable efficacy on depression rating scales [46–48]. Two open-label studies (PD with DSM-IV defined depression) evaluating rTMS of the left DLPFC showed significant improvement from baseline in depression indices but had no sham control [44,45]. These small pilot studies suggest that functional deficits of the DLPFC in PD depression may be amenable to reversal by rTMS, by a mechanism and at anatomical substrates distinct from those targeted by antidepressant medication.

Electroconvulsive therapy

A large meta-analysis of ECT in depressed geriatric patients (121 studies, mainly case studies with only four randomized trials) suggested that ECT was effective for acute depression in the elderly [49]. However, a Cochrane systematic review found major methodological shortcomings in these randomized trials, suggesting that no firm conclusions could be made [50]. Sub-analysis of PD (22 patients in nine case studies, none randomized controlled) patients showed substantial relapses in affective and motor symptoms [49].

Psychological treatments and education

Cognitive behavioural therapy (CBT) is well established for the treatment of depression in non-PD patients. This treatment may face particular challenges in PD because of co-existing physical disability, cognitive–psychiatric co-morbidities and the possible different pathophysiology of dPD [101]. Nevertheless, in small controlled or open-label studies in PD, CBT has been reported to reduce depressive symptoms and negative cognitions, to improve perception of social support [51] and to reduce psychological distress in caregivers [52]. In a recent controlled study of depressed PD patients (DSM IV defined) randomized to receive CBT or medical monitoring, there were significantly better depression (HDRS, $P < 0.0001$; BDI, $P = 0.001$) and anxiety scores (HARS, $P = 0.001$) and improvement in social functioning ($P = 0.02$) and positive reframing ($P = 0.05$) measures [100]. Thus, in this setting, CBT has been demonstrated to be an effective and feasible treatment for dPD. A large study of 151 patients in seven European countries has also highlighted the importance of patient education [53]. Participants completed an eight-session educational programme aimed at improving knowledge and skills related to anxiety, stress and depression in PD. This resulted in an improvement in mood and a decrease in PD-associated psychosocial problems.

Other non-pharmacological treatments

In a short controlled study with PD patients randomly assigned to have neuromuscular (massage) therapy or music relaxation, the latter group showed significant improvements in mood and anxiety [55], suggesting that application of relaxation techniques may improve anxiety and depression in PD. In a small double-blind study of electro-acupuncture in PD there was no statistical difference between the two groups but a trend towards improvement in depression and scales of activities of daily living [56]. A randomized controlled trial of the Alexander technique as add-on therapy to standard therapy resulted in improved self-assessment of disability and significantly less depression post-intervention [54]. Exercise has also been suggested to improve mood. A meta-analysis of exercise interventions in PD showed benefits in physical functioning and HR-QoL, but there was insufficient evidence for a mood benefit [57].

Conclusion

Neuropsychiatric disorders in PD have a complex pathogenesis with exogenous (psychological adjustment to disease) and endogenous (alteration of dopaminergic and non-dopaminergic neurotransmitter systems) factors likely to be important. For the diagnosis of depression in PD, PD-specific modifications have been made to the DSM diagnostic framework which will require further clinical validation. Subtypes of depression in PD, such as minor depression or subsyndromal depression, need to be examined further. Modifications to the DSM criteria for anxiety disorders in PD may also be required, as will further development of diagnostic criteria for apathetic disorders in PD. Disorders of global, and particularly frontal, cognitive impairment need to be actively sought before psychiatric diagnosis is made due to overlap of symptoms and co-morbidity. The use of psychotropic medication in PD requires special consideration given the underlying neuropathology and complex symptomatology of PD and dPD. Direct extrapolation of conclusions and evidence-based medicine for psychiatric drugs derived from studies in non-PD subjects must be conducted with extreme caution. There have been a number of recent studies providing better evidence for antidepressant medication in PD, but larger studies and more comparative studies are still needed. Special consideration needs to be given to optimization of motor function and reduction of motor fluctuations with may be associated with affective symptoms. There is also now good evidence that education and behavioural and support strategies, particularly CBT, are useful in the treatment of psychiatric complications of PD and should be considered in patients with psychiatric disorders in PD.

References

1 **Reijnders JS, Ehrt U, Weber WE, et al**. A systematic review of prevalence studies of depression in Parkinson's disease. Mov Disord 2008; **23**: 183–9.

2 **Menza M, Dobkin RD**. Anxiety. In: M Menza, L Marsh (eds) Psychiatric issues in Parkinson's disease: a practical guide, pp. 139–53. Abingdon: Taylor and Francis, 2006.

3 **Fernandez HH, Simuni T**. Anxiety. In: RF Pfeiffer, I Bodis-Wollner (eds) Parkinson's disease and nonmotor dysfunction, pp. 13–23. Totowa, NJ: Humana Press, 2005.

4 **Richard IH**. Anxiety disorders in Parkinson's disease. Adv Neurol 2005; **96**: 42–55.

5 **Nuti A, Ceravolo R, Piccinni A, et al**. Psychiatric comorbidity in a population of Parkinson's disease patients. Eur J Neurol 2004; **11**: 315–20.

6 **Shiba M, Bower JH, Maraganore DM, et al**. Anxiety disorders and depressive disorders preceding Parkinson's disease: a case-control study. Mov Disord 2000; **15**: 669–77.

7 **O'Sullivan SS, Williams DR, Gallagher DA, et al**. Nonmotor symptoms as presenting complaints in Parkinson's disease: a clinicopathological study. Mov Disord 2008; **23**: 101–6.

8 **Sockeel P, Dujardin K, Devos D, et al**. The Lille apathy rating scale (LARS): a new instrument for detecting and quantifying apathy: validation in Parkinson's disease. J Neurol Neurosurg Psychiatry 2006; **77**: 579–84.

9 **Schrag A**. Quality of life and depression in Parkinson's disease. J Neurol Sci 2006; **248**: 151–7.

10 Global Parkinson's Disease Survey Steering Committee. Factors impacting on quality of life in Parkinson's disease: results from an international survey. Mov Disord 2002; **17**: 60–7.

11 **Marsh L, McDonald WM, Cummings J, Ravina B**; NINDS/NIMH Work Group on Depression and Parkinson's Disease. Provisional diagnostic criteria for depression in Parkinson's disease. Mov Disord 2006; **21**: 148–58.

12 **Starkstein SE, Merello M, Jorge R, et al**. A validation study of depressive syndromes in Parkinson's disease. Mov Disord 2008; **23**: 538–46.

13 **Leentjens AF, Marinus J, Van Hilten JJ, et al**. The contribution of somatic symptoms to the diagnosis of depressive disorder in Parkinson's disease: a discriminant analytic approach. J Neuropsychiatry Clin Neurosci 2003; **15**: 74–7.

14 **Schrag A, Barone P, Brown RG, et al**. Depression rating scales in Parkinson's disease: critique and recommendations. Mov Disord 2007; **22**: 1077–92.

15 **Schrag A, Jahanshahi M, Quinn NP**. What contributes to depression in Parkinson's disease? Psychol Med 2001; **31**: 65–73.

16 **Dunlop BW, Nemeroff CB**. The role of dopamine in the pathophysiology of depression. Arch Gen Psychiatry 2007; **64**: 327–37.

17 **Klimek V, Schenck JE, Han H, et al**. Dopaminergic abnormalities in amygdaloid nuclei in major depression: a postmortem study. Biol Psychiatry 2002; **52**: 740–8.

18 **Lammers CH, Diaz J, Schwartz JC, Sokoloff P**. Selective increase of dopamine D3 receptor gene expression as a common effect of chronic antidepressant treatments. Mol Psychiatry 2000; **5**: 378–88.

19 **Light KJ, Joyce PR, Luty SE, et al**. Preliminary evidence for an association between a dopamine D3 receptor gene variant and obsessive-compulsive personality disorder in patients with major depression. Am J Med Genet B Neuropsychiatr Genet 2006; **141**: 409–13.

20 **Corrigan MH, Denahan AQ, Wright CE, et al**. Comparison of pramipexole, fluoxetine, and placebo in patients with major depression. Depress Anxiety 2000; **11**: 58–65.

21 **Voon V, Fox SH**. Medication-related impulse control and repetitive behaviors in Parkinson disease. Arch Neurol 2007; **64**: 1089–96.

22 **Braak H, Bohl JR, Müller CM, et al**. Stanley Fahn Lecture 2005: the staging procedure for the inclusion body pathology associated with sporadic Parkinson's disease reconsidered. Mov Disord 2006; **21**: 2042–51.

23 **Kerenyi L, Ricaurte GA, Schretlen DJ, et al**. Positron emission tomography of striatal serotonin transporters in Parkinson disease. Arch Neurol 2003; **60**: 1223–9.

24 **Murai T, Müller U, Werheid K, et al**. In vivo evidence for differential association of striatal dopamine and midbrain serotonin systems with neuropsychiatric symptoms in Parkinson's disease. J Neuropsychiatry Clin Neurosci 2001; **13**: 222–8.

25 Walter U, Hoeppner J, Prudente-Morrissey L, et al. Parkinson's disease-like midbrain sonography abnormalities are frequent in depressive disorders. Brain 2007; **130**: 1799–807.

26 Aiken CB. Pramipexole in psychiatry: a systematic review of the literature. J Clin Psychiatry 2007; **68**: 1230–6.

27 Pahwa R, Stacy MA, Factor SA, et al.; EASE-PD Adjunct Study Investigators. Ropinirole 24-hour prolonged release: randomized, controlled study in advanced Parkinson disease. Neurology 2007; **68**: 1108–15.

28 Raudino F. Non motor off in Parkinson's disease. Acta Neurol Scand 2001; **104**: 312–15.

29 Weintraub D, Morales KH, Moberg PJ, et al. Antidepressant studies in Parkinson's disease: a review and meta-analysis. Mov Disord 2005; **20**: 1161–9.

30 Miyasaki JM, Shannon K, Voon V, et al. for the Quality Standards Subcommittee of the American Academy of Neurology. Practice parameter: evaluation and treatment of depression, psychosis, and dementia in Parkinson disease (an evidence-based review): report of the Quality Standards Subcommittee of the American Academy of Neurology. Neurology 2006; **66**: 996–1002.

31 Wermuth L, Sorensen P, Timm S, et al. Depression in idiopathic Parkinson's disease treated with citalopram: a placebo-controlled trial. Nord J Psychiatry 1998; **52**: 163–9.

32 Leentjens AF, Vreeling FW, Luijckx GJ, Verhey FR. SSRIs in the treatment of depression in Parkinson's disease. Int J Geriatr Psychiatry 2003; **18**: 552–4.

33 Avila A, Cardona X, Martin-Baranera M, et al. Does nefazodone improve both depression and Parkinson disease? A pilot randomized trial. J Clin Psychopharmacol 2003; **23**: 509–13.

34 Andersen J, Aabro E, Gulmann N, et al. Anti-depressive treatment in Parkinson's disease. A controlled trial of the effect of nortriptyline in patients with Parkinson's disease treated with L-DOPA. Acta Neurol Scand 1980; **62**: 210–19.

35 Serrano-Dueñas M. Dosis bajas de amitriptilina frente a dosis bajas de fluoxetine en el tratamiento de la depression de enfermos con Parkinson [A comparison between low doses of amitriptyline and low doses of fluoxetine used in the control of depression in patients suffering from Parkinson's disease]. Rev Neurol 2002; **35**: 1010–14.

36 Voon V, Fox S, Butler TR, Lang AE. Antidepressants and psychosis in Parkinson disease: a case series. Int J Geriatr Psychiatry 2007; **22**: 601–4.

37 McKeith IG, Grace JB, Walker Z, et al. Rivastigmine in the treatment of dementia with Lewy bodies: preliminary findings from an open trial. Int J Geriatr Psychiatry 2000; **15**: 387–92.

38 Ready RE, Friedman J, Grace J, Fernandez H. Testosterone deficiency and apathy in Parkinson's disease: a pilot study. J Neurol Neurosurg Psychiatry 2004; **75**: 1323–6.

39 Chatterjee A, Fahn S. Methylphenidate treats apathy in Parkinson's disease. J Neuropsychiatry Clin Neurosci 2002; **14**: 461–2.

40 Raffaele R, Vecchio I, Giammusso B, et al. Efficacy and safety of fixed-dose oral sildenafil in the treatment of sexual dysfunction in depressed patients with idiopathic Parkinson's disease. Eur Urol 2002; **41**: 382–6.

41 Appleby BS, Duggan PS, Regenberg A, Rabins PV. Psychiatric and neuropsychiatric adverse events associated with deep brain stimulation: a meta-analysis of ten years' experience. Mov Disord 2007; **22**: 1722–8.

42 Helmich RC, Siebner HR, Bakker M, et al. Repetitive transcranial magnetic stimulation to improve mood and motor function in Parkinson's disease. J Neurol Sci 2006; **248**: 84–96.

43 Okabe S, Ugawa Y, Kanazawa I. 0.2-Hz repetitive transcranial magnetic stimulation has no add-on effects as compared to a realistic sham stimulation in Parkinson's disease. Mov Disord 2003; **18**: 382–8.

44 **Dragasevic N, Potrebić A, Damjanović A, et al**. Therapeutic efficacy of bilateral prefrontal slow repetitive transcranial magnetic stimulation in depressed patients with Parkinson's disease: an open study. Mov Disord 2002; **17**: 528–32.

45 **Epstein CM, Evatt ML, Funk A, et al**. An open study of repetitive transcranial magnetic stimulation in treatment-resistant depression with Parkinson's disease. Clin Neurophysiol 2007; **118**: 2189–94.

46 **Fregni F, Santos CM, Myczkowski ML, et al**. Repetitive transcranial magnetic stimulation is as effective as fluoxetine in the treatment of depression in patients with Parkinson's disease. J Neurol Neurosurg Psychiatry 2004; **75**: 1171–4.

47 **Cardoso EF, Fregni F, Martins Maia F, et al**. rTMS treatment for depression in Parkinson's disease increases BOLD responses in the left prefrontal cortex. Int J Neuropsychopharmacol 2008; **11**: 173–83.

48 **Boggio PS, Fregni F, Bermpohl F, et al**. Effect of repetitive TMS and fluoxetine on cognitive function in patients with Parkinson's disease and concurrent depression. Mov Disord 2005; **20**: 1178–84.

49 **Van der Wurff FB, Stek ML, Hoogendijk WJ, Beekman AT**. The efficacy and safety of ECT in depressed older adults: a literature review. Int J Geriatr Psychiatry 2003; **18**: 894–904.

50 **Van der Wurff FB, Stek ML, Hoogendijk WL, Beekman AT**. Electroconvulsive therapy for the depressed elderly. Cochrane Database Syst Rev 2003: CD003593.

51 **Dobkin RD, Allen LA, Menza M**. Cognitive-behavioral therapy for depression in Parkinson's disease: a pilot study. Mov Disord 2007; **22**: 946–52.

52 **Secker DL, Brown RG**. Cognitive behavioural therapy (CBT) for carers of patients with Parkinson's disease: a preliminary randomised controlled trial. J Neurol Neurosurg Psychiatry 2005; **76**: 491–7.

53 **Macht M, Gerlich C, Ellgring H, et al**. Patient education in Parkinson's disease: formative evaluation of a standardized programme in seven European countries. Patient Educ Counsel 2007; **65**: 245–52.

54 **Stallibrass C, Sissons P, Chalmers C**. Randomized controlled trial of the Alexander technique for idiopathic Parkinson's disease. Clin Rehabil 2002; **16**: 695–708.

55 **Craig LH, Svircev A, Haber M, Juncos JL**. Controlled pilot study of the effects of neuromuscular therapy in patients with Parkinson's disease. Mov Disord 2006; **21**: 2127–33.

56 **Cristian A, Katz M, Cutrone E, Walker RH**. Evaluation of acupuncture in the treatment of Parkinson's disease: a double-blind pilot study. Mov Disord 2005; **20**: 1185–8.

57 **Goodwin VA, Richards SH, Taylor RS, et al**. The effectiveness of exercise interventions for people with Parkinson's disease: a systematic review and meta-analysis. Mov Disord 2008; **23**: 631–40.

58 **Aarsland D, Påhlhagen S, Ballard CG, Ehrt U, Svenningsson P**. Depression in Parkinson disease—epidemiology, mechanisms and management. Nat Rev Neurol 2011; **8**: 35–47.

59 **Gómez-Esteban JC, Tijero B, Somme J, et al**. Impact of psychiatric symptoms and sleep disorders on the quality of life of patients with Parkinson's disease. J Neurol. 2011; **258**: 494–9.

60 **Barone P, Antonini A, Colosimo C, et al**. PRIAMO study group. The PRIAMO study: A multicenter assessment of nonmotor symptoms and their impact on quality of life in Parkinson's disease. Mov Disord. 2009; **24**: 1641–9.

61 **Benito-León J, Cubo E, Coronell C; ANIMO Study Group**. Impact of apathy on health-related quality of life in recently diagnosed Parkinson's disease: the ANIMO study. Mov Disord. 2012; **27**: 211–18.

62 **Gallagher DA, Lees AJ, Schrag A**. What are the most important nonmotor symptoms in patients with Parkinson's disease and are we missing them? Mov Disord. 2010; **25**: 2493–500.

63 **Leroi I, Ahearn DJ, Andrews M, McDonald KR, Byrne EJ, Burns A**. Behavioural disorders, disability and quality of life in Parkinson's disease. Age Ageing 2011; **40**: 614–21.

64 Hinnell C, Hurt CS, Landau S, Brown RG, Samuel M; PROMS-PD Study Group. Nonmotor versus motor symptoms: how much do they matter to health status in Parkinson's disease? Mov Disord 2012; **27**: 236–41.

65 Havlikova E, van Dijk JP, Nagyova I, et al. The impact of sleep and mood disorders on quality of life in Parkinson's disease patients. J Neurol 2011; **258**: 2222–9.

66 Quelhas R, Costa M. Anxiety, depression, and quality of life in Parkinson's disease. J Neuropsychiatry Clin Neurosci. 2009; **21**: 413–19.

67 Carod-Artal FJ, Ziomkowski S, Mourão Mesquita H, Martínez-Martin P. Anxiety and depression: main determinants of health-related quality of life in Brazilian patients with Parkinson's disease. Parkinsonism Relat Disord. 2008; **14**: 102–8.

68 Starkstein S, Dragovic M, Jorge R, et al. Diagnostic criteria for depression in Parkinson's disease: a study of symptom patterns using latent class analysis. Mov Disord 2011; **26**: 2239–45.

69 Starkstein SE, Merello M, Jorge R, Brockman S, Bruce D, Power B. The syndromal validity and nosological position of apathy in Parkinson's disease. Mov Disord 2009; **24**: 1211–16.

70 Robert P, Onyike CU, Leentjens AF, et al. Proposed diagnostic criteria for apathy in Alzheimer's disease and other neuropsychiatric disorders. Eur Psychiatry 2009; **24**: 98–104.

71 Drijgers RL, Dujardin K, Reijnders JS, Defebvre L, Leentjens AF. Validation of diagnostic criteria for apathy in Parkinson's disease. Parkinsonism Relat Disord 2010; **16**: 656–60.

72 Opmeer EM, Kortekaas R, Aleman A. Depression and the role of genes involved in dopamine metabolism and signalling. Prog Neurobiol 2010; **92**: 112–33.

73 Xiang L, Szebeni K, Szebeni A, et al. Dopamine receptor gene expression in human amygdaloid nuclei: elevated D4 receptor mRNA in major depression. Brain Res 2008; **1207**: 214–24.

74 Politis M, Wu K, Loane C, et al. Depressive symptoms in PD correlate with higher 5-HTT binding in raphe and limbic structures. Neurology 2010; **75**: 1920–7.

75 Boileau I, Warsh JJ, Guttman M, et al. Elevated serotonin transporter binding in depressed patients with Parkinson's disease: a preliminary PET study with [11C]DASB. Mov Disord 2008; **23**: 1776–80.

76 Strecker K, Wegner F, Hesse S, et al. Preserved serotonin transporter binding in de novo Parkinson's disease: negative correlation with the dopamine transporter. J Neurol 2011; **258**: 19–26.

77 Remy P, Doder M, Lees A, Turjanski N, Brooks D. Depression in Parkinson's disease: loss of dopamine and noradrenaline innervation in the limbic system. Brain 2005; **128**: 1314–22.

78 Frisina PG, Haroutunian V, Libow LS. The neuropathological basis for depression in Parkinson's disease. Parkinsonism Relat Disord 2009; **15**: 144–8.

79 Chan-Palay V, Asan E. Alterations in catecholamine neurons of the locus coeruleus in senile dementia of the Alzheimer type and in Parkinson's disease with and without dementia and depression. J Comp Neurol 1989; **287**: 373–92.

80 Meyer PM, Strecker K, Kendziorra K, et al. Reduced alpha4beta2*-nicotinic acetylcholine receptor binding and its relationship to mild cognitive and depressive symptoms in Parkinson disease. Arch Gen Psychiatry 2009; **66**: 866–77.

81 Bohnen NI, Kaufer DI, Hendrickson R, Constantine GM, Mathis CA, Moore RY. Cortical cholinergic denervation is associated with depressive symptoms in Parkinson's disease and parkinsonian dementia. J Neurol Neurosurg Psychiatry 2007; **78**: 641–3.

82 Barone P, Poewe W, Albrecht S, et al. Pramipexole for the treatment of depressive symptoms in patients with Parkinson's disease: a randomised, double-blind, placebo-controlled trial. Lancet Neurol 2010; **9**: 573–80.

83 Leentjens AF, Koester J, Fruh B, Shephard DT, Barone P, Houben JJ. The effect of pramipexole on mood and motivational symptoms in Parkinson's disease: a meta-analysis of placebo-controlled studies. Clin Ther 2009; **31**: 89–98.

84 **Parkinson Study Group CALM Cohort Investigators**. Long-term effect of initiating pramipexole vs levodopa in early Parkinson disease. Arch Neurol 2009; **66**: 563–70.

85 **Barone P, Scarzella L, Marconi R, et al**.; Depression/Parkinson Italian Study Group. Pramipexole versus sertraline in the treatment of depression in Parkinson's disease: a national multicenter parallel-group randomized study. J Neurol 2006; **253**: 601–7.

86 **Navan P, Findley LJ, Jeffs JA, Pearce RK, Bain PG**. Randomized, double-blind, 3-month parallel study of the effects of pramipexole, pergolide, and placebo on Parkinsonian tremor. Mov Disord 2003; **18**: 1324–31.

87 **Leentjens AF**. The role of dopamine agonists in the treatment of depression in patients with Parkinson's disease: a systematic review. Drugs 2011; **71**: 273–86.

88 **Thobois S, Lhommée E, Klinger H, et al**. Parkinsonian apathy responds to dopaminergic stimulation of D2/D3 receptors with piribedil. Brain 2013; **136**: 1568–77.

89 **Ray Chaudhuri K, Martinez-Martin P, Antonini A, et al**. Rotigotine and specific non-motor symptoms of Parkinson's disease: Post hoc analysis of RECOVER. Parkinsonism Relat Disord. 2013; **19**: 660–5.

90 **Skapinakis P, Bakola E, Salanti G, Lewis G, Kyritsis AP, Mavreas V**. Efficacy and acceptability of selective serotonin reuptake inhibitors for the treatment of depression in Parkinson's disease: a systematic review and meta-analysis of randomized controlled trials. BMC Neurol 2010; **10**: 49.

91 **Seppi K, Weintraub D, Coelho M, et al**. The Movement Disorder Society evidence-based medicine review update: treatments for the non-motor symptoms of Parkinson's disease. Mov Disord 2011; **26**(Suppl 3): S42–S80.

92 **Menza M, Dobkin RD, Marin H, et al**. A controlled trial of antidepressants in patients with Parkinson disease and depression. Neurology 2009; **72**: 886–92.

93 **Devos D, Dujardin K, Poirot I, et al**. Comparison of desipramine and citalopram treatments for depression in Parkinson's disease: a double-blind, randomized, placebo-controlled study. Mov Disord 2008; **23**: 850–7.

94 **Rocha FL, Murad MG, Stumpf BP, Hara C, Fuzikawa C**. Antidepressants for depression in Parkinson's disease: systematic review and meta-analysis. J Psychopharmacol 2013; **27**: 417–23.

95 **Richard IH, McDermott MP, Kurlan R, et al**. A randomized, double-blind, placebo-controlled trial of antidepressants in Parkinson disease. Neurology 2012; **78**: 1229–36.

96 **Shirota Y, Ohtsu H, Hamada M, Enomoto H, Ugawa Y; Research Committee on rTMS Treatment of Parkinson's Disease**. Supplementary motor area stimulation for Parkinson disease: a randomized controlled study. Neurology 2013; **80**: 1400–5.

97 **Pal E, Nagy F, Aschermann Z, Balazs E, Kovacs N**. The impact of left prefrontal repetitive transcranial magnetic stimulation on depression in Parkinson's disease: a randomized, double-blind, placebo-controlled study. Mov Disord 2010; **25**: 2311–17.

98 **Arias P, Vivas J, Grieve KL, Cudeiro J**. Double-blind, randomized, placebo controlled trial on the effect of 10 days low-frequency rTMS over the vertex on sleep in Parkinson's disease. Sleep Med 2010; **11**: 759–65.

99 **Oguru M, Tachibana H, Toda K, Okuda B, Oka N**. Apathy and depression in Parkinson disease. J Geriatr Psychiatry Neurol 2010; **23**: 35–41.

100 **Dobkin RD, Menza M, Allen LA, et al**. Cognitive-behavioral therapy for depression in Parkinson's disease: a randomized, controlled trial. Am J Psychiatry 2011; **168**: 1066–74.

101 **Charidimou A, Seamons J, Selai C, Schrag A**. The role of cognitive-behavioural therapy for patients with depression in Parkinson's disease. Parkinsons Dis 2011; **2011**: 737523.

102 **Weintraub, D, Newberg, AB, Cary, MS**. Striatal dopamine transporter imaging correlates with anxiety and depression symptoms in Parkinson's disease. J Nucl Med 2005; **46**: 227–32.

103 **Erro R, Pappatà S, Amboni M, et al**., Anxiety is associated with striatal dopamine transporter availability in newly diagnosed untreated Parkinson's disease patients Parkinsonism Relat Disord 2012; **18**: 1034–8.

Chapter 10

Dementia in Parkinson's disease

David J. Burn and Alison J. Yarnall

Background

Amongst the many non-motor symptoms that may occur in Parkinson's disease (PD), dementia is pre-eminent in terms of its impact upon patients and their families. Dementia in PD (PDD) is associated with increased mortality and a greater likelihood of hospitalization and nursing home placement, and constrains effective management of the motor features of the disorder. Nearly 90% of people with PDD also experience troublesome neuropsychiatric symptoms, with depression, apathy, anxiety and hallucinations being most frequent [1]. Visual hallucinations are strongly predictive of nursing home placement for PD [2], while the carers of PD patients with dementia are more likely to experience higher levels of stress and depression compared with carers of PD patients without dementia [3].

PDD shares a close, and at times confusing, relationship with dementia with Lewy bodies (DLB). Both PDD and DLB are termed 'Lewy body dementias'. They are separated by the so-called one-year rule which states that if extra-pyramidal motor features have been present for 12 months or more before the onset of dementia, the diagnosis should be PDD, while if dementia occurs within 12 months of the motor features, or even precedes the motor features, the diagnosis should be DLB. Both PDD and DLB are now widely regarded as part of a Lewy body disease spectrum, underpinned by abnormalities of α-synuclein metabolism. Indeed, other than age of onset (generally older in DLB), temporal course and possibly levodopa responsiveness, no major differences between PDD and DLB have been determined, including cognitive profile, neuropsychiatric features, type and severity of parkinsonism, sleep disorder, autonomic dysfunction, neuroleptic sensitivity and responsiveness to cholinesterase inhibitors [4].

Epidemiology

Descriptive observations

In a UK community-based incidence study, 36% of people with PD had evidence of cognitive impairment at presentation [5]. At a mean of 3.5 years from diagnosis 10% of these patients had developed dementia, corresponding to an annual dementia incidence of 30.0 (95% confidence interval 16.4–52.9) per 1000 person-years [6]. Someone with PD is five to six times more likely than an age-matched control to develop dementia. A systematic review suggested that 24–31% of people with PD have dementia (i.e. PDD), and that 3–4% of dementia in the general population is due to PDD [7]. The estimated prevalence of PDD in the general population aged 65 years and over is thus 0.2–0.5%, while from community-based longitudinal studies the cumulative incidence of dementia in PD is over 80% [8]. Dementia associated with PD is therefore a common complication and an integral part of the neurodegenerative process.

Analytical observations

Increasing age, and not age at disease onset per se, is the most important risk factor for incident dementia in PD [9]. Increasing motor disability, symmetric motor presentation and axial motor impairment with reduced tremor, longer disease duration and male gender have been associated with increased risk of PDD. Furthermore, older age and more severe motor impairment are synergistic for dementia risk. Other risk factors may include low educational attainment, previous and current smoking habit, depression, excessive daytime somnolence, rapid eye movement (REM) sleep behaviour disorder (RBD) and orthostatic hypotension. Anticholinergic drug use may be a risk factor for PDD, and prolonged use of these agents has been associated with an increased frequency of cortical plaques and tangles in PD patients without dementia. Poor response to levodopa and hallucinations on dopaminergic treatment may predict dementia. Levodopa-induced hyperhomocysteinaemia could contribute towards cognitive failure, while amantadine and simvastatin may delay or attenuate dementia, although these observations require further evaluation [10,11]. Visual hallucinations in PD appear to predict more rapid cognitive deterioration. Psychosis requiring antipsychotic therapy has been associated with the development and progression of dementia, while the use of atypical antipsychotics may have adverse disease-modifying effects. Posterior cortical cognitive deficits, as measured by impaired pentagon copying and semantic fluency, have been associated with increased risk of cognitive failure in PD, as has mild cognitive impairment at baseline assessment. Recent studies suggest that apathy may herald cognitive decline and dementia.

Unlike Alzheimer's disease (AD), PDD is not associated with *APOE* polymorphisms [12]. Inherited genetic variation in the tau gene (*MAPT*) may influence the rate of cognitive decline in PD and the development of dementia [13]. The *MAPT* H1/H1 genotype has been associated with a greater rate of cognitive decline in 109 incident PD patients prospectively followed up over a 3.5-year period. For 15% of H1/H1 homozygotes, but none of the H2 carriers, the rate of cognitive decline was sufficient for them to develop dementia within the follow-up period [13].

Clinical features

Cognitive impairment

The onset of cognitive decline in PD is insidious. In one prospective study, the mean annual decline on the Mini Mental State Examination (MMSE) during 4 years was 1 point in the non-dementia group and 2.3 points in the PDD group, the latter figure being similar to the decline observed in patients with AD [14]. A similar rate of decline was reported in another study where the mean decline in MMSE over 2 years was 4.5 points, comparable to that seen in DLB [15]. There is heterogeneity of cognitive impairment in mild cognitive impairment associated with PD and also in full-blown PDD [5,16]. Some patients may have a 'DLB-like' phenotype, with prominent dysexecutive and visuospatial deficits, while others display greater amnestic deficit (more in common with AD). Dysexecutive problems are particularly common in PDD, however, and comprise difficulties in the realization of complex cognitive tasks requiring the selection of information to be processed, finding a rule, shifting mental set, solving multiple-step problems, resisting cognitive interference, sharing attentional resources and actively retrieving information.

Comparing the profiles of cognitive impairment in 488 AD patients with a similar number of PDD patients using the MMSE and the Alzheimer's Disease Assessment Scale-cognitive subscale (ADAS-cog) the diagnosis was predicted with an overall accuracy of 74.7% [17]. Poor performance of the AD patients on the orientation test in ADAS-cog best discriminated between the groups, followed by poor performance of the PDD patients on the attentional task in the MMSE. This is significant, as attentional deficit is an important determinant of the inability to perform instrumental and physical activities of daily living [18]. Despite the heterogeneous cognitive deficits found in PDD, therefore, the cognitive profile generally differs from that found in AD. These differences are more apparent in the early to middle stages of the dementia process. Table 10.1 summarises the cognitive deficits associated with PDD.

Neuropsychiatric symptoms

Neuropsychiatric symptoms are very common in PDD and not infrequently pre-date the onset of dementia. In a study of 537 PDD patients, 89% presented at least one symptom

Table 10.1 Cognitive profile typical of dementia associated with Parkinson's disease

Domain	Characterization of deficit
Executive function	Severely impaired verbal fluency, concept formation; may influence deficits in other domains (e.g. memory)
Attention	Impairments may be marked and also variable, with 'fluctuations' demonstrable on computerized testing
Visuospatial function	Globally impaired visual perception (as measured by tests of visual discrimination, space-motion and object-form perception without needing manual responses)
Construction and praxis	Markedly impaired clock-drawing test—performance may be influenced by executive and motor deficits
Memory	Impaired verbal and visual memory (but less than that seen in AD); recognition memory may be less affected than recall in mild to moderate PDD
Language	Few studies performed but core language functions less impaired than in AD

PD, Parkinson's disease dementia; AD, Alzheimer's disease.

when assessed using the Neuropsychiatric Inventory (NPI), while 77% had two or more symptoms [1]. Hallucinations occur in 45–65% of PDD patients, whereas in AD typically fewer than 10% of patients are affected. Visual hallucinations in PDD are twice as frequent as auditory ones, the majority being complex, formed hallucinations. Tactile hallucinations are uncommon. Initially, visual hallucinations may be simple and ill-defined—a feeling that someone is behind the patient ('presence'), or that something, or someone, has passed across their visual field ('passage'). Subsequently, the hallucinations become more formed and detailed, often in colour, static and centrally located. Anonymous people and family members (living or dead) are common contents, as are animals. Delusional misinterpretation of the hallucinations may occur as insight is lost. Overall, delusions have a frequency in PDD of 25–30%. Paranoid ideation, such as spousal infidelity and 'phantom boarder' (believing strangers are living in the house) are common themes.

When applying formal diagnostic criteria to a community-based sample, the rate of major depression in PDD was 13%, compared with 9% for PD patients without dementia [19]. Anxiety is also common in PDD (30–50%) and tends to cluster with depressed mood. Irritability and aggression are not prominent features in PDD. Apathy affects over 50% of people with PDD and in 70% this may be severe [1].

Other clinical features

A 'postural instability and gait disorder' (PIGD) phenotype is over-represented in PDD compared with PD [20], while more severe cognitive failure is associated with significantly more impairment in motor and autonomic domains [21]. Falls are more common in PDD than in PD patients without dementia, and are multifactorial in nature. Using the Epworth Sleepiness Scale, 57% of PDD, 50% of DLB and 41% of PD subjects were classified as having excessive daytime somnolence, compared with 18% of AD and 10% of controls [22]. Furthermore, sleep quality was poorer in PDD, PD and DLB patients compared with AD and normal controls. A higher frequency of symptomatic orthostasis has been reported in association with cognitive impairment in PD [23]. PDD patients show consistent impairment of both parasympathetic and sympathetic function tests in comparison with controls and AD [24], while higher autonomic symptom scores in PDD are associated with poorer outcomes in all measures of physical activity, activities of daily living, depression and quality of life [25]. Although some reports have suggested reduced responsiveness to levodopa in PDD patients, this has not been formally established. There are insufficient data to infer differences in the occurrence and phenomenology of levodopa-induced motor complications in PDD compared with PD.

Diagnosis of PDD

When dementia develops in the context of well-established PD there is usually no doubt about the diagnosis. Routine structural imaging adds little to the clinical picture in these circumstances. In certain situations, for example a new referral where the temporal sequence of events is unclear, with significant co-morbid illness or when the clinical course is atypical (e.g. a rapid onset of confusion), the differential may include vascular parkinsonism, AD with or without drug-induced parkinsonism, delirium, depressive pseudo-dementia and DLB. Many of these conditions may be excluded by a careful collateral history, blood tests and structural (e.g. computed tomography or magnetic resonance imaging) and functional (e.g. dopamine transporter) imaging. Mild depression or dysthymia has little, if any, impact on cognition in PD while severe depressive symptoms may impair executive function and memory [26].

Although widely used as measure of global cognitive function, over-reliance upon a single MMSE score less than the traditional value of 24 out of 30 is insensitive because this instrument does not include robust measures of executive function and is heavily biased towards memory deficits. Thus, patients with scores above this cutoff may still have dementia. Furthermore, cognition in PD may vary considerably, probably because of fluctuating attention, such that at the time of one assessment a 'spuriously' high score may be obtained that is not representative of day-to-day impairment.

Diagnostic criteria for PDD from the Movement Disorder Society Task Force [27] (Tables 10.2 and 10.3) were developed through a comprehensive literature review in which the characteristic cognitive, behavioural, motor and other features of PDD were defined. On the basis of this review, four groups of features were derived (Table 10.2). Two levels of certainty for the diagnosis of PDD (probable or possible) are suggested, based upon the presence and/or absence of these features (Table 10.3). The defining feature of PDD is that the dementia develops in the context of established PD. The diagnosis of dementia must be based on the presence of deficits in two or more of the four core cognitive domains (attention, memory, executive and visuospatial functions) and be severe enough to affect normal functioning. Neuropsychiatric and behavioural symptoms are frequent in PDD, but are not invariable, and this is reflected in the criteria.

The operationalization of these criteria was described by the Movement Disorder Society Task Force [28]. Those guidelines are based on a two-level process, depending upon the clinical scenario and the expertise of the evaluator. Level I assessment is aimed primarily at the clinician with no particular expertise in neuropsychological methods (Table 10.4) and requires, in addition to clinical history and care-giver account, the MMSE, a clock drawing test and the four-item NPI. Fluctuating attention, which, as described above, is a dominant factor in determining disability in PDD, is examined by asking the patient to give the months of the year backwards, starting from December, or by repeatedly subtracting 7, starting at 100. It remains to be established whether these tests are sufficiently sensitive to detect this problem.

The Level I assessment can be used alone or in combination with Level II. The latter is more suitable when there is a need to specify the pattern and severity of dementia associated with PD [28]. The Level II assessment requires neuropsychological expertise and is more time-consuming. It is suitable for detailed clinical monitoring, research studies or pharmacological trials.

Table 10.2 Features of dementia associated with Parkinson's disease (modified from [27])

I: Core features

(1) Diagnosis of Parkinson's disease according to Queen Square Brain Bank criteria

(2) A dementia syndrome with insidious onset and slow progression, developing within the context of established Parkinson's disease and diagnosed by history, clinical and mental examination, defined as:
  ◆ Impairment in more than one cognitive domain
  ◆ Representing a decline from pre-morbid level
  ◆ Deficits severe enough to impair daily life (social, occupational or personal care), independent of the impairment ascribable to motor or autonomic symptoms

II: Associated clinical features

(1) Cognitive features
  ◆ Attention: impairment in spontaneous and focused attention, poor performance in attentional tasks; performance may fluctuate during the day and from day to day
  ◆ Executive functions: impairment in tasks requiring initiation, planning, concept formation, rule finding, set shifting or set maintenance; impaired mental speed (bradyphrenia)
  ◆ Visuospatial functions: impairment in tasks requiring visual–spatial orientation, perception or construction
  ◆ Memory: impairment in free recall of recent events or in tasks requiring learning new material, memory usually improves with cueing, recognition is usually better than free recall
  ◆ Language: core functions largely preserved, although may be word-finding difficulties and impaired comprehension of complex sentences

(2) Behavioural features
  ◆ Apathy: decreased spontaneity; loss of motivation, interest and effortful behaviour
  ◆ Changes in personality and mood including depressive features and anxiety
  ◆ Hallucinations: mostly visual, usually complex, formed visions of people, animals or objects
  ◆ Delusions: usually paranoid, such as infidelity, or phantom boarder (unwelcome guests living in the home) delusions
  ◆ Excessive daytime sleepiness

III: Features which do not exclude PDD, but make the diagnosis uncertain

  ◆ Coexistence of any other abnormality, which may by itself cause cognitive impairment, but is judged not to be the cause of dementia, e.g. presence of relevant vascular disease in imaging
  ◆ Time interval between the development of motor and cognitive symptoms not known

IV: Features suggesting other diseases as cause of mental impairment, which when present make it impossible to reliably diagnose PDD

  ◆ Cognitive and behavioural symptoms appearing solely in the context of other conditions such as:
    – acute confusion due to systemic diseases or abnormalities or drug intoxication
    – major depression according to DSM-IV
  ◆ Features compatible with 'probable vascular dementia' criteria according to NINDS-AIREN (dementia in the context of cerebrovascular disease as indicated by focal signs in a neurological exam such as hemiparesis, sensory deficits and evidence of relevant cerebrovascular disease by brain imaging AND a relationship between the two as indicated by the presence of one or more of the following: onset of dementia within 3 months after a recognized stroke, abrupt deterioration in cognitive functions, and fluctuating, stepwise progression of cognitive deficits)

Table 10.3 Criteria for the diagnosis of probable and possible Parkinson's disease dementia (PDD) (modified from [27])

Probable PDD
(A) Core features[1]: both must be present
(B) Associated clinical features: • Typical profile of cognitive deficits including impairment in at least two of the four core cognitive domains (impaired attention which may fluctuate, impaired executive functions, impairment in visuospatial functions and impaired free recall memory which usually improves with cueing) • The presence of at least one behavioural symptom (apathy, depressed or anxious mood, hallucinations, delusions, excessive daytime sleepiness) supports the diagnosis of Probable PDD; the lack of behavioural symptoms, however, does not exclude the diagnosis
(C) None of the Group III criteria present
(D) None of the Group IV criteria present
Possible PDD
(A) Core features[1]: both must be present
(B) Associated clinical features: • Atypical profile of cognitive impairment in one or more domains, such as prominent or receptive-type (fluent) aphasia, or pure storage-failure type amnesia (memory does not improve with cueing or in recognition tasks) with preserved attention • Behavioural symptoms may or may not be present
OR
(C) One or more of the Group III criteria present
(D) None of the Group IV criteria present

[1] See Table 10.2 for core features and Group II and IV criteria.

Pathology

As described above, the clinical phenotype of PDD is variable, suggesting heterogeneity of the underlying pathological processes. Biological candidates include Lewy bodies and sy-nuclein pathology, Alzheimer-type pathology, vascular changes, neuronal loss and neuro-chemical deficits. More recent studies emphasize the importance of amyloid-β deposition in the development of PDD [29]. The observation that amyloid-β plaque burden, specif-ically diffuse plaque load, correlates with overall cortical Lewy body burden strengthens the concept of a synergistic effect between these major pathological proteins. Age at dis-ease onset and disease duration also contribute to pathological findings associated with PDD [30]. Furthermore, parallel to a massive accumulation of pre-synaptic α-synuclein, morphological changes in the form of loss of post-synaptic dendritic spines have also been reported in DLB, implying that synaptic dysfunction may be fundamental to the patholog-ical process in the Lewy body dementias [31].

The relative amounts and topographical distribution of abnormal proteins are likely to be determined by a number of factors, including genetic factors. Such factors may rep-resent a balance of 'resistance' and 'susceptibility' to the dementia process, with the end

Table 10.4 Guidelines for diagnosis of Parkinson's disease (PD) dementia (PDD) at Level I (modified from [28])

1. A diagnosis of PD based on the Queen's Square Brain Bank criteria
2. PD developed prior to the onset of dementia
3. Mini Mental State Examination (MMSE) score below 26
4. Cognitive deficits severe enough to impact upon daily living (elicited via caregiver interview or 'pill questionnaire'[1])

5. Impairment in at least two of the following cognitive domains:
    ◆ months reversed or seven backwards
    ◆ lexical fluency or clock drawing
    ◆ MMSE pentagons
    ◆ MMSE three-word recall

The presence of one of the following behavioural symptoms: apathy or depressed mood or delusions or excessive daytime sleepiness supports the diagnosis of probable PDD[2]
The presence of major depression or delirium or any other abnormality which may by itself cause significant cognitive impairment makes the diagnosis uncertain[3]

[1] This item, described in an appendix in [28], requires validation. In brief, the patient is asked to describe verbally their treatment and its time schedule. Even if the patient does not manage their own treatment, it is suggested that they have lost at least a part of their autonomy if they can no longer describe their treatment. The criterion of impairment is met if the patient is no longer able to explain their daily PD medication, or if errors are made that are considered clinically significant.

[2] These can be assessed with the four-item Neuropsychiatric Inventory which includes hallucinations, depression, delusions and apathy. A cutoff score of ≥ 3 for each item is proposed. Excessive daytime sleepiness may be assessed by specific questions.

[3] Should be absent to permit diagnosis of 'probable' PDD.

result being how soon the person develops dementia during the course their PD. Some support for this comes from a study which suggested that people developing dementia after a relatively short duration of PD had a greater burden of cortical α-synuclein and amyloid compared with those with longer duration of PD before the onset of dementia [32].

The variability in certain clinical features in PDD, not least fluctuating cognition, suggests a functional rather than structural substrate. In this context, loss of ascending cholinergic afferents from basal forebrain and brainstem nuclei (e.g. the nucleus basalis of Meynert and pedunculopontine nucleus, respectively) with relatively preserved postsynaptic cholinergic muscarinic receptors may be relevant. This is corroborated by evidence from post-mortem and *in vivo* imaging studies in AD and PDD demonstrating a greater cholinergic deficit in PDD compared with AD.

Management

General approach

A clear and unambiguous diagnosis of PDD followed by careful and sensitive explanation to the patient and carer is an essential first step in the management process. Non-pharmacological treatments should always be considered and may, for example, benefit depression, visual hallucinations and apathy [33]. Attention to nutrition can reduce the risk of infection and mortality [34].

To avoid exacerbating neuropsychiatric problems without leading to unacceptable immobility, a gradual and systematic simplification of the antiparkinsonian drug regimen is necessary, withdrawing anticholinergic drugs, selegiline, dopamine agonists and catechol-O-methyltransferase inhibitors, one at a time. The aim is to maintain the patient on the lowest possible dose of levodopa monotherapy in order to preserve function. Anticholinergic drugs prescribed to control urinary urgency and frequency should be stopped if they cross the blood–brain barrier and other medications to treat co-morbid medical problems should also be reviewed and rationalized.

There should be a low threshold to treat if depression is suspected, although there are no randomized controlled trial (RCT) data to inform on the choice of antidepressant in PDD. The usual choice is a selective serotonin reuptake inhibitor, although mixed reuptake inhibitors (i.e. serotonin and noradrenaline reuptake inhibitors) could, in theory, benefit apathy and inattention. If excessive daytime drowsiness and inattention are problematic, the reasons for nocturnal sleep fragmentation should be considered and treated, if possible. RBD may respond to a small dose of clonazepam at a starting dose 0.25 mg and increasing very gradually to avoid increasing the risk of falls. Melatonin may also be useful in the treatment of RBD and avoids the morbidity and mortality associated with benzodiazepine treatment. Preliminary data suggest that a cholinesterase inhibitor such as rivastigmine may reduce the frequency of RBD in refractory cases, but this needs further confirmation [35].

Antipsychotic treatment

The choice of atypical antipsychotics in PDD is limited by extrapyramidal side effects and concerns over an increased risk of stroke with several of these agents in elderly demented patients. In practice, the choice usually lies between quetiapine or clozapine, although trial data are far stronger for clozapine. Management guidelines from the UK and the United States and a meta-analysis have summarized the evidence to support the use of clozapine in this indication [36] and explicitly stated that olanzepine should not be used to manage psychosis in PD (both Level B evidence) [37–39]. If clozapine is used, then registration with a mandatory monitoring scheme is required. Quetiapine may have useful hypnotic benefits when prescribed at night in gradually increasing doses (starting with 25–50 mg), although PDD patients may be more susceptible to worsening of motor symptoms with quetiapine compared with PD patients with psychosis.

Regarding newer atypical antipsychotic agents, eight of 14 PD subjects with drug-induced psychosis had to be withdrawn in an open-label study of the partial dopamine receptor agonist aripiprazole [40]. Ziprasidone, an antagonist at $5\text{-}HT_{2A}$ and dopamine D2 receptors improved refractory drug-induced psychosis in three of four PD patients with psychosis but resulted in worsening of extrapyramidal features in one subject and, curiously, 'pathological laughter' in two [41]. A more recent open-label study found ziprasidone to be as effective as clozapine in treating psychosis in PD [42]. Pimavanserin

(ACP-103) is a 5-HT$_{2A}$ inverse agonist/antagonist that did not worsen motor function and which showed antipsychotic potential in a Phase II RCT of 60 PD patients [43]. Most recently, pimavanserin met the primary endpoint in a Phase III trial by demonstrating significant antipsychotic efficacy as measured using the nine-item Schedule for Assessment of Positive Symptoms (SAPS)-PD scale. Pimavanserin also met the key secondary endpoint for motoric tolerability as measured using Parts II and III of the UPDRS. In addition, clinical benefits were observed in all exploratory efficacy measures with significant improvements in night-time sleep, daytime wakefulness and caregiver burden (see <http://www.businesswire.com/news/home/20121127005529/en>).

Cholinesterase inhibitors

Just two adequately sized RCTs have been performed for the use of cholinesterase inhibitors (ChEIs) in PDD: the EXPRESS study of rivastigmine ($n = 541$) [44] and the EDON study of donepezil ($n = 549$) [45]. The other trials have been very small, recruiting a *total* of 52 patients between them [46–48]. Both the EXPRESS and the EDON studies recruited PD patients with mild to moderate dementia, with treatment durations of 24 weeks. EXPRESS study participants were also offered the chance to enter an active treatment extension phase over an additional 24 weeks. Using ADAS-cog (range 0–70 points maximum), modest but statistically significant benefits were noted at 24 weeks in the EXPRESS study (a 2.8-point improvement in active versus placebo groups). For the EDON study, mean ADAS-cog changes from baseline to week 24 were not significant for donepezil in the intent-to-treat population by the predefined statistical model but subsequent analysis, removing the treatment-by-country interaction term from the model, revealed a significant dose-dependent benefit with donepezil (difference from placebo –2.08 for 5 mg and –3.31 for 10 mg). Significant improvements were also noted in the EXPRESS study in several secondary outcome measures, including activities of daily living and burden of neuropsychiatric symptoms. For EDON, both doses of donepezil were associated with significant benefit in a number of secondary endpoints, including the MMSE, the Delis–Kaplan Executive Function System and Brief Test of Attention. Interestingly, neuropsychiatric symptom burden was not significantly improved by donepezil, although this may have represented a 'floor' effect since baseline NPI scores were relatively modest in all groups. Both ChEIs were relatively well tolerated with 73% of those assigned to rivastigmine and over 75% of those assigned to donepezil completing treatment; the main reason for premature withdrawal in both studies was adverse events.

A recent Cochrane review, pooling 1236 subjects with DLB, concluded that current evidence supports the use of ChEI in patients with PDD, with positive impacts on global assessment, cognitive function, behavioural disturbance and activities of daily living rating scales [49]. The use of ChEIs in managing PDD therefore represents a therapeutic advance, but heterogeneity of drug response (i.e. some patients respond dramatically and others derive no benefit at all), balancing benefits against side effects and uncertainties over 'real life' benefit to the patient and their carers remain areas where further research is needed.

The transdermal mode of administering rivastigmine may reduce side effects without loss of efficacy. In the IDEAL (investigation of transdermal exelon in Alzheimer's disease) study, 1195 patients with AD were randomized to placebo or one of three active treatment target dose groups [50]. All rivastigmine treatment groups showed significant improvement relative to placebo with the 10-cm^2 patch showing similar efficacy to capsules. A recent study in 583 PDD subjects evaluated the long-term safety of rivastigmine capsules and patches over 76 weeks [51]. Adverse events relating to increased tremor, nausea and vomiting were all lower in the patch group.

Small case series gave conflicting results as to whether the N-methyl-D-aspartate (NMDA) antagonist memantine may be beneficial in PDD. But two recent controlled studies that included both PDD and DLB patients showed that memantine did not improve cognition in PDD [52,53].

Future developments

Given the high cumulative incidence of dementia in PD, there is a tremendous opportunity to develop interventional treatments that may modify, delay or attenuate the onset of cognitive impairment in a pre-defined 'high-risk' group. Although increasing age is the main determinant of PDD, not everyone with PD will develop dementia and the underlying pathophysiology is likely to differ between patients. It is therefore vital to develop clinical and biomarker predictors of PDD. Plasma or cerebrospinal fluid markers and neuroimaging may help in this regard. Fluorodeoxyglucose positron emission tomography (PET) can highlight cortical hypometabolism in PD patients without dementia, for example, while amyloid-binding PET ligands may give insight into the relative accumulation of abnormal protein and even guide the type of disease-modifying treatment to use [54]. Ideally, such studies should be combined with pathological analysis.

Regarding symptomatic treatments, the use of available drugs, notably ChEIs, should be better evaluated. Identification of responsive subgroups, determination of change in 'real-life' endpoints and measurement of cost-effectiveness should all be addressed. The on-going UK multicentre MUSTARDD-PD study (<http://clinicaltrials.gov/show/NCT01014858>) aims to address these issues. The development of receptor-specific cholinergic agonists may represent a more potent means of influencing the cholinergic system than ChEIs per se.

The ultimate aim must be to develop disease-modifying treatments for PDD. These may be based upon generic anti-PD approaches, perhaps by inhibiting the accumulation of oligomeric α-synuclein in susceptible cells. Alternatively, therapeutic strategies adopted from the field of AD research to prevent or diminish accumulation of insoluble β-amyloid may prove to be useful in PDD. Such approaches could include secretase inhibitors or modulators, active or passive vaccines [55], tau kinase inhibitors, cholesterol-lowering statins, anti-inflammatory drugs (e.g. minocycline) and omega-3 fatty acids. Finally, as for AD, the use of non-pharmacological interventions such as physical exercise, cognitive training and nutrition should also be explored in PDD.

References

1 **Aarsland D, Brønnick K, Ehrt U, et al**. Neuropsychiatric symptoms in patients with Parkinson's disease and dementia: frequency, profile and associated care giver stress. J Neurol Neurosurg Psychiatry 2007; **78**: 36–42.

2 **Goetz CG, Stebbins GT**. Risk factors for nursing home placement in advanced Parkinson's disease. Neurology 1993; **43**: 2227–9.

3 **Schrag A, Hovris A, Morley D, Quinn N, Jahanshahi M**. Caregiver-burden in Parkinson's disease is closely associated with psychiatric symptoms, falls, and disability. Parkinsonism Relat Disord 2006; **2006**: 35–41.

4 **Lippa CF, Duda JE, Grossman M, et al**. DLB and PDD boundary issues: diagnosis, treatment, molecular pathology and biomarkers. Neurology 2007; **68**: 812–19.

5 **Foltynie T, Brayne CEG, Robbins TW, Barker RA**. The cognitive ability of an incident cohort of Parkinson's disease patients in the UK. The CamPaIGN study. Brain 2004; **127**: 550–60.

6 **Williams-Gray CH, Foltynie T, Brayne CEG, Robbins TW, Barker RA**. Evolution of cognitive dysfunction in an incident Parkinson's disease cohort. Brain 2007; **130**: 1787–98.

7 **Aarsland D, Zaccai J, Brayne C**. A systematic review of prevalence studies of dementia in Parkinson's disease. Mov Disord 2005; **10**: 1255–63.

8 **Hely MA, Reid WG, Adena MA, Halliday GM, Morris JG**. The Sydney multicenter study of Parkinson's disease: the inevitability of dementia at 20 years. Mov Disord 2008; **23**: 837–44.

9 **Aarsland D, Kvaløy JT, Andersen K, et al**. The effect of age of onset of PD on risk of dementia. J Neurol 2007; **254**: 38–45.

10 **Inzelberg R, Bonuccelli U, Schechtman E, et al**. Association between amantadine and the onset of dementia in Parkinson's disease. Mov Disord 2006; **21**: 1375–9.

11 **Wolozin B, Wang SW, Li NC, Lee A, Lee TA, Kazis LE**. Simvastatin is associated with a reduced incidence of dementia and Parkinson's disease. BMC Med 2007; **5**: 20.

12 **Jasinska-Myga B, Opala G, Goetz CG, et al**. Apolipoprotein E gene polymorphism, total plasma cholesterol level, and Parkinson disease dementia. Arch Neurol 2007; **64**: 261–5.

13 **Goris A, Williams-Gray CH, Clark GR, et al**. Common variation in tau and alpha synuclein genes influences risk of developing idiopathic Parkinson disease and related cognitive impairment. Ann Neurol 2007; **62**: 145–53.

14 **Aarsland D, Andersen K, Larsen JP, et al**. The rate of cognitive decline in Parkinson's disease. Arch Neurol 2004; **61**: 1906–11.

15 **Burn D, Rowan E, Allan L, Molloy S, O'Brien J, McKeith I**. Motor subtype and cognitive decline in Parkinson's disease, Parkinson's disease with dementia, and dementia with Lewy bodies. J Neurol Neurosurg Psychiatry 2006; **77**: 585–9.

16 **Verleden S, Vingerhoets G, Santens P**. Heterogeneity of cognitive dysfunction in Parkinson's disease: a cohort study. Eur Neurol 2007; **58**: 34–40.

17 **Bronnick K, Emre M, Lane R, Tekin S, Aarsland D**. Profile of cognitive impairment in dementia associated with Parkinson's disease compared with Alzheimer's disease. J Neurol Neurosurg Psychiatry 2007; **78**: 1064–8.

18 **Bronnick K, Ehrt U, Emre M, et al**. Attentional deficits affect activities of daily living in dementia-associated with Parkinson's disease. J Neurol Neurosurg Psychiatry 2006; **77**: 1136–42.

19 **Aarsland D, Ballard CG, Larsen JP, McKeith IG**. A comparative study of psychiatric symptoms in dementia with Lewy bodies and Parkinson's disease with and without dementia. Int J Geriatr Psychiatry 2001; **16**: 528–36.

20 **Burn DJ, Rowan EN, Minnett T, et al**. Extrapyramidal features in Parkinson's disease with and without dementia and dementia with Lewy bodies: a cross-sectional comparative study. Mov Disord 2003; **18**: 884–9.

21 Verbaan D, Marinus J, Visser M, et al. Cognitive impairment in Parkinson's disease. J Neurol Neurosurg Psychiatry 2007; **78**: 1182–7.

22 Boddy F, Rowan EN, Lett D, O'Brien JT, McKeith IG, Burn DJ. Sleep quality and excessive daytime somnolence in Parkinson's disease with and without dementia, dementia with Lewy bodies and Alzheimer's disease: a comparative, cross-sectional study. Int J Geriatr Psychiatry 2007; **22**: 529–35.

23 Graham JM, Sagar HJ. A data-driven approach to the study of heterogeneity in idiopathic Parkinson's disease: identification of three distinct subtypes. Mov Disord 1999; **14**: 10–20.

24 Allan LM, Ballard CG, Allen J, et al. Autonomic dysfunction in dementia. J Neurol Neurosurg Psychiatry 2007; **78**: 671–7.

25 Allan L, McKeith I, Ballard C, Kenny RA. The prevalence of autonomic symptoms in dementia and their association with physical activity, activities of daily living and quality of life. Dement Geriatr Cogn Disord 2006; **22**: 230–7.

26 Tröster AI, Stalp LD, Paolo AM, Fields JA, Koller WC. Neuropsychological impairment in Parkinson's disease with and without depression. Arch Neurol 1995; **52**: 1164–9.

27 Emre M, Aarsland D, Brown R, et al. Clinical diagnostic criteria for dementia associated with Parkinson disease. Mov Disord 2007; **22**: 1689–707.

28 Dubois B, Burn D, Goetz C, et al. Diagnostic procedures for Parkinson's disease dementia. Mov Disord 2007; **22**: 2314–24.

29 Compta Y, Parkkinen L, O'Sullivan SS, et al. Lewy- and Alzheimer-type pathologies in Parkinson's disease dementia: which is more important? Brain 2011; **134**: 1493–505.

30 Kempster PA, O'Sullivan SS, Holton JL, Revesz T, Lees AJ. Relationships between age and late progression of Parkinson's disease: a clinico-pathological study. Brain 2010; **133**: 1755–62.

31 Kramer ML, Schulz-Schaeffer WJ. Presynaptic alpha-synuclein aggregates, not Lewy bodies, cause neurodegeneration in dementia with Lewy bodies. J Neurosci 2007; **27**: 1405–10.

32 Ballard C, Ziabreva I, Perry R, et al. Differences in neuropathologic characteristics across the Lewy body dementia spectrum. Neurology 2006; **67**: 1931–4.

33 Cohen-Mansfield J, Mintzer JE. Time for change: the role of non-pharmacological interventions in treating behavior problems in nursing home residents with dementia. Alzheimer Dis Assoc Disord 2005; **19**: 37–40.

34 Gil Gregorio P, Ramirez Diaz SP, Ribera Casado JM, on behalf of the DEMENU group. Dementia and nutrition: intervention study in institutionalized patients with Alzheimer disease. J Nutr Health Aging 2003; **7**: 304–8.

35 Di Giacopo R, Fasano A, Quaranta D, Della Marca G, Bove F, Bentivoglio AR. Rivastigmine as alternative treatment for refractory REM behavior disorder in Parkinson's disease. Mov Disord 2012; **27**: 559–61.

36 Seppi K, Weintraub D, Coelho M, et al. The Movement Disorder Society evidence-based medicine review update: treatments for the non-motor symptoms of Parkinson's disease. Mov Disord 2011; **26**: S42–S80.

37 National Institute for Health and Clinical Excellence. Parkinson's disease: diagnosis and management in primary and secondary care. NICE Clinical Guidelines 35. London: National Institute for Health and Care Excellence, 2006. Available at: <http://guidance.nice.org.uk/CG35>.

38 Miyasaki J, Shannon K, Voon V, et al. Practice parameter: evaluation and treatment of depression, psychosis, and dementia in Parkinson disease (an evidence-based review). Report of the Quality Standards Subcommittee of the American Academy of Neurology. Neurology 2006; **66**: 996–1002.

39 Frieling H, Hillemacher T, Ziegenbein M, Neundörfer B, Bleich S. Treating dopamimetic psychosis in Parkinson's disease: structured review and meta-analysis. Eur Neuropsychopharmacol 2007; **17**: 165–71.

40 Friedman J, Berman RM, Goetz CG, et al. Open-label flexible-dose pilot study to evaluate the safety and tolerability of aripiprazole in patients with psychosis associated with Parkinson's disease. Mov Disord 2006; **21**: 2078–81.

41 **Schindehütte J, Trenkwalder C.** Treatment of drug-induced psychosis in Parkinson's disease with ziprasidone can induce severe dose-dependent off-periods and pathological laughing. Clin Neurol Neurosurg 2007; **109**: 188–91.

42 **Pintor L, Valldeoriola F, Baillés E, Martí MJ, Muñiz A, Tolosa E.** Ziprasidone versus clozapine in the treatment of psychotic symptoms in Parkinson disease: a randomized open clinical trial. Clin Neuropharmacol 2012; **35**: 61–6.

43 **Friedman J, Vanover KE, Taylor EM, Weiner D, Davis RE, van Kammen DP.** ACP-103 reduces psychosis without impairing motor function in Parkinson's disease. Mov Disord 2006; **21**: 1546.

44 **Emre M, Aarsland D, Albanese A, et al.** Rivastigmine for dementia associated with Parkinson's disease. N Engl J Med 2004; **351**: 2509–18.

45 **Dubois B, Tolosa E, Katzenschlager R, et al.** Donepezil in Parkinson's disease dementia: a randomized, double-blind efficacy and safety study. Mov Disord 2012; **27**: 1230–8.

46 **Aarsland D, Laake K, Larsen JP, Janvin C.** Donepezil for cognitive impairment in Parkinson's disease: a randomised controlled study. J Neurol Neurosurg Psychiatry 2002; **72**: 708–12.

47 **Leroi I, Brandt J, Reich SG, et al.** Randomized placebo-controlled trial of donepezil in cognitive impairment in Parkinson's disease. Int J Geriatr Psychiatry 2004; **19**: 1–8.

48 **Ravina B, Putt M, Siderowf A, et al.** Donepezil for dementia in Parkinson's disease: a randomised, double blind, placebo controlled, crossover study. J Neurol Neurosurg Psychiatry 2005; **76**: 934–9.

49 **Rolinski M, Fox C, Maidment I, McShane R.** Cholinesterase inhibitors for dementia with Lewy bodies, Parkinson's disease dementia and cognitive impairment in Parkinson's disease. Cochrane Database Syst Rev 2012; CD006504.

50 **Winblad B, Grossberg G, Frölich L, et al.** IDEAL: a 6-month, double-blind, placebo-controlled study of the first skin patch for Alzheimer disease. Neurology 2007; **69**: S14–S22.

51 **Emre M, Poewe W, De Deyn PP, et al.** A 76-week study on the long-term safety of rivastigmine capsules and patch in patients with dementia associated with Parkinson's disease. Mov Disord 2011; **26**: S125.

52 **Aarsland D, Ballard C, Walker Z, et al.** Memantine in patients with Parkinson's disease dementia or dementia with Lewy bodies: a double-blind, placebo-controlled, multicentre trial. Lancet Neurol 2009; **8**: 613–18.

53 **Emre M, Tsolaki M, Bonuccelli U, et al.** Memantine for patients with Parkinson's disease dementia or dementia with Lewy bodies: a randomised, double-blind, placebo-controlled trial. Lancet Neurol 2010; **9**: 969–77.

54 **Gomperts SN, Locascio JJ, Rentz D, et al.** Amyloid is linked to cognitive decline in patients with Parkinson disease without dementia. Neurology 2013; **80**: 85–91.

55 **Bombois S, Maurage CA, Gompel M, et al.** Absence of beta-amyloid deposits after immunization in Alzheimer disease with Lewy body dementia. Arch Neurol 2007; **64**: 583–7.

Chapter 11

Fatigue in Parkinson's disease

Benzi M. Kluger and Joseph H. Friedman

Background

Fatigue is one of the most common symptoms seen in medicine, and particularly in neurological illnesses including Parkinson's disease (PD) [1]. Unfortunately, our understanding of the pathophysiology of fatigue in PD is quite limited and we currently have no specific treatments. While fatigue was noted by James Parkinson in his original description of the disorder in 1817, it was not until 1993 that studies began describing its prevalence, progression and impact [2,3].

In healthy adults, fatigue is a transient phenomenon brought about by prolonged exertion which diminishes with rest and does not interfere with daily functioning. This contrasts with pathological fatigue, which is chronic, brought on by no or minimal exertion, does not fully improve with rest and causes disability [4]. While pathological fatigue may arise in otherwise healthy individuals, it is most frequently associated with disease states either as a primary or secondary manifestation of the illness [5]. For example, fatigue in cancer patients is frequently secondary to anaemia and responds to treatment of the anaemia [6]. Alternatively, the classical motor decrements seen with prolonged exertion in myasthenia gravis are due to pathological changes at the neuromuscular junction and respond to treatment of the primary disease process [7]. Muscle fatigue, as occurs with repeated contractions, is a different and unrelated condition from the fatigue described by PD patients.

Possible secondary causes of fatigue in individuals with PD include sleep disorders, medications and depression [8]. However, population-based studies in PD demonstrate that sleep disorders [9] and excessive daytime sleepiness (EDS) [10] do not account for fatigue in the majority of PD subjects, and patients are often able to distinguish between EDS and fatigue. Similarly, studies of the most common medications used in PD show no effect or even slight improvements in fatigue, despite the EDS associated with these same medications [11]. While several studies demonstrate a correlation between measures of depression and fatigue [12], this may in part be due to methodological issues related to the overlap of symptoms that are assessed by fatigue and depression inventories. Even in studies demonstrating this correlation, half of PD patients without depression still report fatigue [13]. Fatigue often appears to be present at the time of diagnosis, and is independent of motor symptoms and disease severity [3,9]. Longitudinal studies suggest that PD patients with fatigue continue to have fatigue, while those without fatigue generally do not develop it [12]. Taken as a whole, these studies suggest that, in the majority of PD patients, fatigue is intrinsic to the disease.

Components of fatigue

Ryan [14] defined two distinct fatigue components:

1 feelings of tiredness, weariness or exhaustion (perceptions of fatigue);

2 a reductions in the capacity to perform a task as a result of continuous performance on the same task (objective fatigability).

Objective fatigability, by definition, always affects performance on the task that induced the fatigue and may affect performance on other tasks, particularly if the task-related stress shares common physiological substrates. Like many complex constructs, advances in our understanding of the phenomenology and physiology of fatigue will depend on appropriately identifying distinct components. Figure 11.1 shows a separation of fatigue into potential causal factors based on current behavioural and neurophysiological evidence [15]. These factors are not meant to be mutually exclusive but may serve to focus research efforts on the predominant source(s) of fatigue in particular populations.

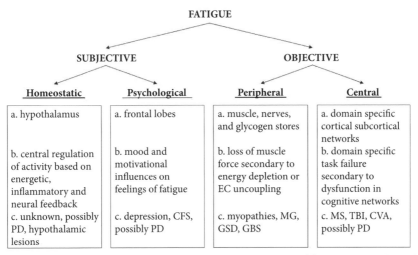

Fig. 11.1 Diagram of major factors contributing to the two domains of fatigue: perceptions of fatigue and fatigability. While separated in this diagram, it should be noted that perceptions of fatigue and performance fatigability have the potential to influence each other. Letters in boxes refer to: (a) known neuroanatomical sites mediating this factor; (b) normal function of this factor; (c) pathological states involving this factor. Abbreviations: CFS, chronic fatigue syndrome; EC, excitation/contraction; MG, myasthenia gravis; GSD, glycogen storage diseases; GBS, Guillain–Barré syndrome; TBI, traumatic brain injury; CVA, cerebrovascular accident.

Homeostatic factors serve a regulatory function in protecting the organism from the physical stress and energetic loss of prolonged activity. Several lines of research suggest that structures within the central nervous system (CNS) act as a 'central governor' to prevent total energy depletion [16]. While the signalling mechanisms and CNS targets are incompletely known, potential pathways include inflammatory (interleukin-6), metabolic (cerebral glycogen depletion) and neuronal (increases of serotonin and decreases of dopamine) ones [17]. Animal models demonstrate that the hypothalamus is at least one of the CNS structures responsible for energy regulation [18]. While fatigue has been noted with lesions of the hypothalamus, it is difficult to attribute fatigue directly to those lesions as these patients frequently have additional CNS lesions, abnormalities of circadian rhythm and endocrine disturbances [1]. While PD may affect the hypothalamus [19], it is unknown if these lesions are associated with fatigue.

Psychological factors may affect both perceptions of fatigue and objective performance, and include expectations, motivation and mood. The strong association of depression and fatigue in PD supports the role of mood as a contributor to fatigue complaints [12]. Experiments in healthy subjects have shown that objective performance and subjective fatigue may be altered by giving false temporal or force feedback during their performance [20]. Disturbances of temporal perception in PD subjects may similarly cause a heightened sense of effort on a given task [21].

Peripheral factors refer to performance decrements on the basis of dysfunction at the level of muscles or peripheral nerves that is typically brought on by physically demanding motor tasks involving repetitive or prolonged muscle contractions. Peripheral factors are predominant in many diseases of the peripheral nervous system and muscles [1]. Many physiological and cellular mechanisms have been proposed on the basis of direct electrical stimulations of nerves and muscles [22]. However, distinguishing between peripheral and central factors can be quite challenging in a living organism under physiological conditions. Although decrements in cognitive tasks are almost always due to central factors, decrements in motor tasks are rarely due to isolated peripheral dysfunction as there is typically a concurrent decrement in central drive [15]. Objective motor fatigability in PD is presumed to arise from central causes [23,24].

Central factors refer to decrements in task performance due to changes within the CNS. Studies of fatigability of cognitive performance in multiple sclerosis (MS) have suggested that central fatigue in clinical populations may disproportionately affect specific neuropsychological domains [25]. Preliminary studies in PD have also demonstrated heightened cognitive fatigability versus age-matched controls, but it is unknown whether specific domains are particularly affected [26]. Unlike peripheral factors, the mechanisms underlying central factors are unknown but may generally be divided into neurophysiological and energetic explanations [27]. These explanations are not mutually exclusive, and may in fact be complementary, as energetic deficits can affect neuronal function. Central factors in PD may conceivably be caused by alterations in global energy expenditure or mitochondrial dysfunction [28,29] or dysfunction within the circuitry of the basal ganglia [30].

Measurement of fatigue

Although standardized batteries have not been developed, fatigability may be objectively measured using the definitions given in the section Components of fatigue by looking for decrements in cognitive [25] or physical performance [24] on a specific task over time. Regarding perceptions of fatigue, there are a number of rating instruments which have been developed, with the Fatigue Severity Scale (FSS) being the most commonly used [31]. This scale has been used in many disorders, particularly MS, due to its ease of scoring. However, it has not been validated in PD. The Multidimensional Fatigue Inventory (MFI) is another rating instrument for fatigue which has the advantage of assessing five dimensions of fatigue but is more difficult to score and also has not been validated in PD [32]. The only PD-specific rating scale is the Parkinson Fatigue Scale, developed by Brown et al. [33]. It has the advantage of being PD-specific, and having been validated both in the UK and the United States [34].

Epidemiology

Fatigue is common to all people and is a normal concomitant of any mental or physical activity. Clinically significant or pathological fatigue, no matter how defined, is common in virtually all somatic and mental disorders. In a random sample of primary-care patients, 25% considered fatigue to be a 'major problem' [35]. Five to ten per cent of all visits to primary-care surgeries are for the assessment of fatigue, and this figure has been fairly constant for decades [36,37]. It is a major problem in MS, affecting about 75% [38] but is common in anaemia, congestive heart failure, systemic lupus erythematosus and cancer patients receiving chemotherapy, and is a cardinal sign in the DSM-IV diagnosis of major depression and anxiety [39,40]. As both depression and anxiety are markedly increased in PD it is difficult to distinguish fatigue that is primary to PD from that which is secondary to these problems.

The first epidemiological report of fatigue in PD was made in 1967 by Hoehn and Yahr [41] who reported that 2% of their PD patients presented with fatigue. While this is still an uncommon presenting symptom to a neurologist it needs to be better recognized. For instance, the famous British soccer player, Ray Kennedy, who was still playing professionally after his PD developed, reported that fatigue was his first symptom. While he first noted that he took much longer to recover from his matches, it took an estimated 10 years for the development of other signs and 14 years before a diagnosis of PD was finally made [42].

Fatigue was not recognized as an important clinical entity until 1993, with near simultaneous reports [3,43]. These and subsequent publications consistently describe fatigue as affecting between 33 and 58% of the population surveyed, varying with definitions and study populations [44]. In the first published report, a Dutch study found that fatigue was considerably more common in PD patients than in controls, affecting nearly 50% of their sample [43]. In the US study of 100 consecutive PD patients, one-half considered fatigue to be one of their three most disabling symptoms and one-third listed fatigue as their single most disabling symptom [3]. The majority described their fatigue with PD as different from their experience of fatigue prior to developing PD. In that study, there was a statistically significant association between fatigue and depression. A Dutch study of non-depressed PD patients found that 43% of PD patients suffered from fatigue and that half of them noted that the fatigue had pre-dated the onset of motor symptoms [10]. Only 15% rated it as their single worst symptom, but 54% considered it as severe as their other symptoms. Of 233 PD patients from Norway, 44% were fatigued versus 18% of the controls [45]. As in the US study already mentioned, the fatigue correlated with depression, but not disease severity. Controls without depression, dementia or sleepiness also suffered from increased fatigue. The PD group from the University of Maryland found that fatigue affected 40% of a selected group. Fatigue was not associated with gender or disease severity but, unlike other reports, this study found no association with depression [46]. Perhaps most significantly, this study also looked at physician awareness of non-motor symptoms and reported that over 80% of PD patients complaining of significant fatigue did not have their fatigue recognized by their PD specialist neurologists.

PD patients have to contend with their disease and co-morbidities. They also have to deal with the side effects of their medications, which frequently include sedation. The results of the multicentre ELLDOPA trial are particularly important [47]. In this study, designed to determine whether levodopa altered disease progression, the FSS was included. Participants were untreated, non-depressed volunteers without dementia, with early PD but not yet requiring dopaminergic therapy. Even in this sample of motivated patients, the point prevalence of fatigue was greater than 33%, with 127 of 349 subjects endorsing fatigue prior to any treatment. Although this study did find an association between fatigue and motor impairment, measured with both the Unified Parkinson's Disease Rating Scale (UPDRS) motor and the activities of daily life measures, the cohort was highly selected with a very narrow range of impairments.

The natural history of fatigue has been less well studied. The first report was a follow-up to the first US study and found that, after 9 years, the patients who were initially fatigued remained fatigued, but were more so [12]. On the other hand, few patients who were not initially fatigued developed fatigue, implying that fatigue is an early feature of PD which remains a stable problem. A much larger Norwegian cohort followed for 8 years using the Nottingham Health Profile found that only 56% of those initially fatigued were fatigued at follow-up measurements at 4 and 6 years [13]. They found that on their initial assessment 36% were fatigued, and the follow-up numbers were 43%, then 56%, suggesting an increasing prevalence.

These data indicate that fatigue, no matter how measured, is a common problem in PD, affecting, in a significant manner, about half the PD population. Fatigue occurs early, often pre-dating the onset or recognition of the motor symptoms of the disease, and is not correlated, in general, with disease severity as measured by motor function. It probably correlates with depression but not with gender or age. While the presence or absence of fatigue may fluctuate in many patients, it appears to be persistent in the majority.

Pathophysiology of fatigue

Little is known about the pathophysiology of contributions of the CNS to fatigue, although significant data exist concerning fatigue at the level of the muscles and peripheral nerves [22]. The observation that fatigue follows stereotypic courses when associated with certain chemotherapy regimes, infections and radiation therapy indicates that there must be organic mediators of this syndrome in some circumstances [48]. The fact that fatigue is such a prominent feature in psychiatric diagnoses supports the importance of psychological and emotional components as well. In short, it is likely that the complaint of fatigue may result from any process that disrupts normal human performance or the perception of effort. From this it follows that fatigue in different patient populations may have very distinctive features and pathophysiological causes. The fact that fatigue is not associated with the severity of PD and that it often pre-dates recognition of the disorder indicates that fatigue is often a primary problem and not directly related to motor deficits.

Studies of PD patients have shown that they are less efficient than age-matched controls in performing identical motor activities and have a greater percentage decrement in their performance over time (objective fatigability) [49,50]. However, these studies have been unable to demonstrate any correlation between motor fatigability and subjective ratings of fatigue, including subjective ratings of 'physical fatigue' and 'activities' from the MFI [50]. PD patients require more energy, as measured by oxygen utilization, for breathing [51], which in part explains why their resting energy requirements are higher [52]. While this energy inefficiency improves with drug treatment, fatigue complaints generally do not [53]. However, levodopa-induced dyskinesias further increase energy use. Garber and Friedman [28] used a series of exercises to compare PD patients with and without fatigue to determine whether fatigue correlated with motor inefficiency. This study found no difference in energy utilization, but did find that self-reported activity levels between the groups were different, with fatigued patients being less likely to have engaged in very effortful activities and, in general, considerably more sedentary. The authors could not determine whether fatigue induced the inactivity or vice versa.

Hypothesized physiological mechanisms of fatigue in PD include altered activation of the hypothalamic–pituitary–adrenal axis, alterations in neurotransmitters and neurotransmission within the CNS and disruption of the non-motor functions in the basal ganglia and dysfunction of frontal striato-thalamo-cortical loops [1,30]. One study found reduced frontal lobe blood perfusion in fatigued PD patients, but only 26 subjects were involved and the work has not been subsequently replicated [54]. However, studies of fatigue in MS similarly found hypometabolism in the frontal lobes and basal ganglia [55]. Chaudhuri and Behan have reviewed other evidence, including both imaging and pathological studies, from a wide range of neurological and psychiatric diseases, adding support for a basal ganglia hypothesis of fatigue [30].

Transcranial magnetic stimulation (TMS) and pharmacological studies offer a means of assessing the influence of cortical excitability and neurotransmitters on fatigue. A single study has used both TMS and double-blinded levodopa administration to study PD fatigue [50]. This study examined the relationship of several TMS measures and levo-dopa administration to both subjective fatigue ratings and objective motor fatigability. As discussed, objective motor fatigability did not correlate with subjective ratings. As a secondary outcome, the study found that lower baseline motor thresholds (reflecting a net balance towards hyperexcitability versus inhibition) correlated with increased subjective fatigue complaints but not objective performance. In contrast, these measures of cortical excitability improved with levodopa treatment, as did objective fatigability, but subjective ratings were unchanged [50]. This study is consistent with the ELLDOPA trial in which only a small percentage of treated patients had improvements in their fatigue with levodopa treatment [47]. In fact, most fatigued patients with PD are taking levodopa and do not report lessened fatigue with treatment of motor symptoms.

Shulman et al. [9] first noted the clustering of fatigue and other non-motor symptoms in PD. This tendency toward the aggregation of multiple non-motor symptoms in individual patients was recently confirmed in a study on autonomic dysfunction in which autonomic dysfunction correlated with depression and cognitive dysfunction [56]. Fatigue was unfortunately not measured in that study. This clustering suggests that there may be overlapping causes or at least significant interactions among these various symptoms. One theory posits that this interaction works through a positive-feedback loop in which symptoms such as pain, fatigue, depression, inactivity and deconditioning mutually augment one another and lead to global disability [57]. Such a feedback loop would imply that any effective approach to treatment will need to take each of these non-motor symptoms into account.

Treatment of fatigue

As fatigue in PD is probably multifactorial, it is unlikely that a single approach will be helpful for all patients. In addition, without an understanding of the pathophysiology of fatigue, our treatments will be limited to an empirical approach based on plausible hypotheses rather than specifically targeted treatments based on sound theoretical and physiological evidence. Thus, the average patient may require several treatment trials and/or more than one therapeutic approach.

We believe that the first, and possibly most important, step in treating fatigue in PD is to establish in the mind of the patient and the family the notion that this is a bona fide symptom of PD, affecting about half of all PD patients. Too many people, both those with PD and those in the network around the patient, are prone to consider fatigue a moral weakness, indicative of laziness. Putting fatigue in the same category as the other symptoms of PD, including the motor symptoms, will help establish the trust that is necessary to enhance the likelihood that the patient will invest the effort required for an exercise programme, research protocol or drug treatment.

The next most important step in treating fatigue is to try to determine whether the fatigue is primary or secondary. Secondary fatigue, due to depression, anxiety, apathy, sleep disorder, medications, pain or another concomitant medical condition, obviously needs to be treated first. It must be noted, however, that the successful treatment of depression in people who do not suffer from PD frequently does not improve their complaint of fatigue even when the same treatment relieves their other symptoms of depression such as sadness [58]. Although current guidelines on the treatment of depression in PD do not have enough evidence to endorse any particular treatment strategy, it is likely that fatigue will remain in a significant proportion of patients, including those who attribute their fatigue to depression [59]. However, a small controlled study of nortriptyline in depression reported an improvement in fatigue as a secondary outcome [60].

The only positive published report on the treatment of fatigue in PD tested methylphenidate, 10 mg three times a day, in a double-blind placebo-controlled trial lasting 6 weeks [61]. Seventeen subjects received active drug and 19 placebo. Clinically and statistically significant improvements were measured in the FSS and the MFI (General Fatigue) on active drug, with fewer side effects from methylphenidate than placebo, including insomnia. There was no change in UPDRS motor scores, suggesting that the benefit was not simply an indirect measure of improved motor efficiency. Mood was not assessed, meaning that a secondary effect via mood benefit cannot be excluded. While the ELLDOPA trial reported that levodopa improved fatigue to a small degree as measured on the FSS [44], the majority of trials, including trials of dopamine agonists [62], testosterone supplements in men with low hormone levels [63], and modafinil at doses of 200–400 mg daily in patients with EDS [64], were not beneficial.

Reports that exercise improves fatigue in other fatigue disorders [65], and the observation that PD patients with fatigue often report that fatigue improves after exercise [33], support a non-medicinal approach with a graduated exercise programme. Exercise has also been shown to be an effective treatment for patients with major depression [66]. Finally, forced exercise in animal models of PD has demonstrated neuroprotective effects, providing a physiological rationale for exercise programmes even in those in PD patients without fatigue.

This approach is often met with scepticism by the patient who describes inertia so great that the idea of exercising for even a few minutes is inconceivable: 'If I could I would'.

Future directions

The past 15 years of research on fatigue in PD has clearly demonstrated the prevalence and impact of fatigue on patients with PD. It has also demonstrated the significant amount of research still needed. Although there is an increasing amount of interest in and support for this research, we are still several steps from achieving the goal of being able to offer an effective treatment for PD patients with fatigue.

As discussed, the challenges of defining fatigue and its phenomenology are quite significant. However, this is a critical step in developing a long-term strategy for understanding fatigue in PD. Although it appears that the fatigue is not due to secondary causes in the majority of PD patients we still do not have positive proof that it is a primary symptom of PD. It is conceivable that PD fatigue may be secondary to a factor which has not been discovered or that on an epidemiological level fatigue may be due to multiple different causes distributed over individual patients, such that only the minority of patients remain with a primary or unexplained cause.

Studies are currently planned to investigate whether objective cognitive fatigability is associated with subjective complaints. Alternatively, it may be that fatigue is a subjective symptom, more akin to depression, apathy and motivation, or it could be performance-based, the latter being the traditional view. To fully address this issue, better standardized measures or batteries will be needed to provide objective fatigue measurements of various physical and cognitive domains.

Once these phenomenological and measurement issues are addressed, the next major step will be to determine the physiological bases for some fatigue subtypes in PD. There are many complementary paths this research may take, such as studies using functional imaging and TMS. Pharmacological intervention studies combined with these modalities, as was done by Lou et al. [24], are also needed to improve our understanding of the role of neurotransmitters and potential treatment modalities.

Ultimately, the goal of all clinical researchers is the prevention or effective treatment of fatigue. Given the probable heterogeneity of fatigue, even within PD patients, this may involve a complex approach in which specific causes or types of fatigue are paired with specific treatments. While trials are now under way to empirically test medications currently approved for other indications, true advances in our ability to treat fatigue is likely to await improvements in our understanding of its pathophysiology.

References

1 **Chaudhuri A, Behan P**. Fatigue in neurological disorders. Lancet 2004; 363: 978–88.

2 **Parkinson J**. An essay on the shaking palsy. London: Sherwood, Neely and Jones, 1817.

3 **Freidman JH, Friedman H**. Fatigue in Parkinson's disease. Neurology 1993; 43: 2016–18.

4 **Fukuda K, Strauss SE, Hickie I, et al.**, for the International Chronic Fatigue Syndrome Study Group. The chronic fatigue syndrome: a comprehensive approach to its definition and study. Ann Intern Med 1994; 15: 953–9.

5 **Krupp LB, Pollina DA**. Mechanisms and management of fatigue in progressive neurological disorders. Curr Opin Neurol 1996; 9: 456–60.

6 **Harper P, Littlewood T**. Anaemia of cancer: impact on patient fatigue and long-term outcome. Oncology 2005; 69(Suppl 2): 2–7.

7 **Keesey JC**. Clinical evaluation and management of myasthenia gravis. Muscle Nerve 2004; 29: 484–505.

8 **Yoshii F, Takahashi H, Kumazawa R, Kobori S**. Parkinson's disease and fatigue. J Neurol 2006; 253(Suppl 7): 48–53.

9 **Shulman LM, Taback RL, Bean J, Weiner WJ**. Comorbidity of the nonmotor symptoms of Parkinson's disease. Mov Disord 2001; 16: 507–10.

10 **Van Hilten JJ, Weggeman M, van der Velde EA, et al**. Sleep, excessive daytime sleepiness and fatigue in Parkinson's disease. J Neural Trans Park Dis Dement Sect 1993; 5: 235–44.

11 **Abe K, Takanashi M, Yanagihara T, Sakoda S**. Pergolide mesilate may improve fatigue in patients with Parkinson's disease. Behav Neurol 2001; 13: 117–21.

12 **Freidman JH, Friedman H**. Fatigue in Parkinson's disease: a nine-year follow-up. Mov Disord 2001; 16: 1120–2.

13 **Alves G, Wentzel-Larsen T, Larsen JP**. Is fatigue an independent and persistent symptom in patients with Parkinson disease? Neurology 2004; 63: 1908–11.

14 **Ryan TA**. Work and effort: the psychology of production. New York: The Ronald Press Company, 1947.

15 **Kluger B, Krupp L, Enoka R**. Fatigue and fatigability in neurologic illnesses: proposal for a unified taxanomy. Neurology 2013; 80: 409–16.

16 **Noakes TD, St Clair Gibson A, Lambert EV**. From catastrophe to complexity: a novel model of integrative central neural regulation of effort and fatigue during exercise in humans. Br J Sports Med 2004; 38: 511–14.

17 **Davis JM, Bailey SP**. Possible mechanisms of central nervous system fatigue during exercise. Med Sci Sports Exer 1997; 29: 45–57.

18 **Soares DD, Coimbra CC, Marubayashi U**. Tryptophan-induced central fatigue in exercising rats is related to serotonin content in preoptic area. Neurosci Lett 2007; 415: 274–8.

19 **Braak H, Braak E**. Pathoanatomy of Parkinson's disease. J Neurology 2000; 247(Suppl 2): 3–10.

20 **Wells CM, Collins D, Hale BD**. The self-efficacy–performance link in maximum strength performance. J Sports Sci 1993; 11: 167–75.

21 **Pastor MA, Artieda J, Jahanshahi M, Obeso JA**. Time estimation and reproduction is abnormal in Parkinson's disease. Brain 1992; 115: 211–25.

22 **Enoka R, Duchateau J**. Muscle fatigue: what, why, and how it influences muscle function. J Physiol 2007; 586: 11–23.

23 **Stevens-Lapsley J, Kluger BM, Schenkman M**. Quadriceps muscle weakness, activation deficits, and fatigue with Parkinson disease. Neurorehabil Neural Repair 2012; 26: 533–41.

24 **Lou JS, Kearns G, Benice T, et al**. Levodopa improves physical fatigue in Parkinson's disease: a double-blind, placebo-controlled crossover study. Mov Disord 2003; 18: 1108–14.

25 **Krupp LB, Elkins E**. Fatigue and declines in cognitive functioning in multiple sclerosis. Neurology 2000; 55: 934–9.

26 **Lou JS**. Physical and mental fatigue in Parkinson's disease: epidemiology, pathophysiology and treatment. Drugs Aging 2009; 26: 195–208.

27 **Dalsgaard MK, Secher NH**. The brain at work: a cerebral metabolic manifestation of central fatigue? J Neurosci Res 2007; 85: 3334–9.

28 **Garber CE, Freidman JH**. Effects of fatigue on physical activity and function in patients with Parkinson's disease. Neurology 2003; 60: 1119–24.

29 **Martin LJ**. Mitochondriopathy in Parkinson disease and amyotrophic lateral sclerosis. J Neuropathol Exp Neurol 2006; 65: 1103–10.

30 **Chaudhuri A, Behan P**. Fatigue and basal ganglia. J Neurol Sci 2000; 179(Suppl 1–2): 34–42.

31 **Krupp LB, LaRocca NG, Muir-Nash J, Steinberg AD**. The Fatigue Severity Scale. Application to patients with multiple sclerosis and systemic lupus erythematosus. Arch Neurol 1989; 46: 1121–3.

32 **Smets EM, Garssen B, Bonke B, De Haes JC**. The Multidimensional Fatigue Inventory (MFI) psychometric qualities of an instrument to assess fatigue. J Psychosom Res 1995; 39: 315–25.

33 **Brown RG, Dittner A, Findley L, Wessely SC**. The Parkinson Fatigue Scale. Parkinsonism Relat Disord 2005; 11: 49–55.

34 **Grace J, Mendelsohn A, Friedman JH**. A comparison of fatigue measures in Parkinson disease. Park Rel Disord 2007; 13: 443–5.

35 **Kroenke K, Wood DR, Mangelsdorff AD, et al**. Chronic fatigue in primary care. Prevalence, patient characteristics, and outcome. J Am Med Assoc 1988; 260: 929–34.

36 **Cathebras PJ, Robbins JM, Kirmayer LJ, Hayton BC**. Fatigue in primary care: prevalence, psychiatric comorbidity, illness behavior and outcome. J Gen Intern Med 1992; 7: 276–86.

37 French G. The clinical significance of tiredness. Can Med Assoc J 1960; 82: 665–71.

38 Schwid SR, Covington M, Segal BM, Goodman AD. Fatigue in multiple sclerosis: current understanding and future directions. J Rehabil Res Dev 2002; 39: 211–24.

39 Sharpe M, Wilks D. Fatigue. Br Med J 2002; 325: 480–3.

40 American Psychiatric Association. Diagnostic and statistical manual of mental disorders, 4th edition, text revision (DSM-IV-TR). Washington DC: American Psychiatric Association, 2000.

41 Hoehn MM, Yahr MD. Parkinsonism: onset, progression and mortality. Neurology 1967; 17: 427–42.

42 Lees AJ. When did Ray Kennedy's Parkinson's disease begin? Mov Disord 1992; 7: 110–16.

43 Van Hilten JJ, Hoogland G, van der Velde EA, et al. Diurnal effects of motor activity and fatigue in Parkinson's disease. J Neurol Neurosurg Psychiatry 1993; 56: 874–7.

44 Friedman JH, Brown RG, Comella C. Fatigue in Parkinson's disease: a review. Mov Disord 2007; 22: 297–308.

45 Karlsen K, Larsen JP, Tandberg E, Jorgensen K. Fatigue in patients with Parkinson's disease. Mov Disord 1999; 14: 237–41.

46 Shulman LM, Taback R, Rabinstein AA, Weiner WJ. Non-recognition of depression and other non-motor symptoms in Parkinson's disease. Parkinsonism Relat Disord 2002; 8: 193–7.

47 Shiffito G, Friedman JH, Oakes D. Fatigue in ELLDOPA. Paper presented at the World Congress on Parkinson's Disease, Washington DC, 22–26 February 2006.

48 Irvine D, Vincent L, Graydon JE, et al. The prevalence and correlates of fatigue in patients receiving treatment with chemotherapy and radiotherapy. A comparison with the fatigue experienced by healthy individuals. Cancer Nurs 1994; 17: 367–78.

49 Ziv I, Avraham M, Michaelov Y. Enhanced fatigue during motor performance in patients with Parkinson's disease. Neurology 1998; 51: 1583–6.

50 Lou JS, Benice T, Kearns G, et al. Levodopa normalizes exercise related cortico-motoneuron excitability abnormalities in Parkinson's disease. Clin Neurophysiol 2003; 114: 930–7.

51 Tzelepis GE, McCool FD, Friedman JH, Hoppin FG Jr. Respiratory muscle dysfunction in Parkinson's disease. Am Rev Respir Dis 1988; 138: 266–71.

52 Levi S, Coz M, Lugon M, et al. Increased energy expenditure in PD. Br Med J 1990; 301: 1256–7.

53 Markus HS, Cox M, Tomkins AM. Raised resting energy expenditure in PD and its relationship to muscle rigidity. Clin Sci 1992; 83: 199–204.

54 Abe K, Takanashi M, Yanagihara T. Fatigue in patients with Parkinson's disease. Behav Neurol 2000; 12: 103–6.

55 Filippi M, Rocca MA, Colombo B. Functional magnetic resonance imaging correlates of fatigue in multiple sclerosis. NeuroImage 2002; 15: 559–67.

56 Verbaan D, Marinus J, Visser M, et al. Patient-reported autonomic symptoms in Parkinson's disease. Neurology 2007; 69: 333–41.

57 Covington EC. Depression and chronic fatigue in the patient with chronic pain. Prim Care 1991; 18: 341–58.

58 Nirenberg AA, Keefe BR, Leslie VC. Residual symptoms in depressed patients who respond acutely to fluoxetine. J Clin Psychiatry 1999; 60: 221–5.

59 Weintraub D, Morales KH, Moberg PJ. Antidepressant studies in patients with Parkinson's disease: a review and meta-analysis. Mov Disord 2005; 20: 1161–9.

60 Andersen J, Aabro E, Gulmann N, et al. Anti-depressive treatment in Parkinson's disease. A controlled trial of the effect of nortryptiline in patients with Parkinson's disease treated with L-DOPA. Acta Neurol Scand 1980; 62: 210–19.

61 Mendonca DA, Menezes K, Jog MS. Methylphenidate improves fatigue scores in Parkinson disease: a randomized controlled trial. Mov Disord 2007; 22: 2070–6.

62 **Oved D, Ziv I, Treves TA**. Effect of dopamine agonists on fatigue and somnolence in Parkinson disease. Mov Disord 2006; 21: 1257–61.

63 **Okun MS, Fernandez HH, Rodriguez RL**. Testosterone therapy in men with Parkinson disease: results of the TEST-PD study. Mov Disord 2006; 63: 729–35.

64 **Ondo WG, Fayle R, Atassi R, Jankovic J**. Modafinil for daytime somnolence in Parkinson disease: double blind, placebo controlled parallel trial. Mov Disord 2005; 76: 1636–9.

65 **Nail LM**. Fatigue in patients with cancer [abstract]. Oncol Nurs Forum 2002; 29: 537.

66 **Cohen AD, Tillerson JL, Smith AD, et al**. Neuroprotective effects of prior limb use in 6-hydroxydopamine-treated rats: possible role of GDNF. J Neurochem 2003; 85: 299–305.

Chapter 12

Psychosis in Parkinson's disease

Christopher G. Goetz, Nico J. Diederich
and Gilles Fénelon

Introduction

Hallucinations are spontaneous aberrant perceptions and illusions are misinterpretations of real perceptual stimuli [1]. Secondary delusional interpretation can lead to psychosis. In Parkinson's disease (PD) these phenomena are generally considered together, although psychiatric semiology draws distinctions between them. Visual hallucinations are the most frequent psychiatric signs in PD, although the frequency of hallucinations in other modalities may be underestimated [2]. In cross-sectional studies, visual hallucinations occur in approximately one-third of chronically treated PD subjects [3,4]. Visual hallucinations are the primary risk factor for nursing home placement [5]. The present chapter summarizes our knowledge on prevalence and incidence, the broad phenomenological spectrum and the present treatment strategies. The pathophysiology of psychotic phenomena in PD remains an incomplete framework; only the most relevant research data in this domain are referred to.

Historical background

In the pre-dopaminergic era, psychotic signs were rarely described in PD patients. Ball [6] probably referred to the signs of rapid eye movement (REM) sleep behaviour disorder (RBD) in post-encephalitic parkinsonism when describing a 53-year-old man who saw and heard enemies invading his room. The subject tried to escape the visions by shaking violently. These episodes occurred only at nighttime, with no persecutory visions during the day. In a study of 326 parkinsonian patients, Mjönes [7] described two patients with haptic hallucinations; one of them experienced auditory and visual hallucinations. The author estimated the frequency of psychoses in PD as being between 3.2 and 6.4%. In untreated patients with post-encephalitic parkinsonism, visual hallucinations were occasionally embedded in 'crises' with the simultaneous occurrence of various motor symptoms. Sacks et al. [8] described a patient with post-encephalitic parkinsonism, who ordered an 'old painting of the shanty-town … for the sole and express purpose of hallucinating with it'. The impact of anticholinergic delirium confounds clear estimates of visual hallucinations in the pre-dopaminergic era. Further, the distinction between PD and dementia with

Lewy bodies (DLB) was not appreciated. Nevertheless, these historical descriptions suggest that hallucinations may be an inherent, though rare, part of the disease itself [9].

Reports on the frequent occurrence and morbidity of visual hallucinations in PD patients date from the era after the discovery of levodopa treatment. Thus, Klawans and colleagues [10–12] presented a wide spectrum of levodopa-associated psychiatric signs in PD, ranging from vivid dreams, nightmares, night terrors, hypnagogic hallucinations and hallucinations with retained insight or loss of insight to delusional psychosis.

Prevalence

Cross-sectional studies

Prevalence studies on visual hallucinations in PD have yielded varying results depending on the setting, for example field studies, cross-sectional studies and observational studies on selected ambulant or hospitalized patients. PD patients may not report having experienced visual hallucinations when completing self-report screening questionnaires. In one study, only 23% reported visual hallucinations in a self-report questionnaire, but the percentage rose to 44% when the same patients were specifically interviewed about visual hallucinations [13]. The percentage of patients who hallucinate is also reported as lower in interviews with family members or caregivers [14]. Overall, cross-sectional figures estimate that one-third of PD patients hallucinate, as found by Tanner et al. in a very large retrospective study with 775 patients in 1983 [3] and subsequently confirmed by others (Table 12.1) [15]. However, percentages may substantially increase if the assessment also includes isolated minor visual hallucinations. The overall lifetime prevalence of hallucinations in PD patients is estimated to be around 50% [15,16].

Longitudinal studies

The proportion of PD patients suffering hallucinations also increases with time, as established in a prospective longitudinal assessment over 4 years [17]. In this study, 33% of the patients had visual hallucinations at baseline, 44% at 18 months and 63% at 48 months. Having hallucinations at baseline or at any given assessment was a strong predictor at all follow-up evaluations of continued hallucinations, thus showing the chronicity of the hallucinatory syndrome. In a population-based study, over 200 PD patients were followed up prospectively over 12 years. By the study's end, 60% had developed psychotic features (hallucinations or delusions) [18]. The evolution of so-called benign hallucinations, defined as hallucinations with retained insight, has been investigated. Surprisingly, after 3 years, 81% of the patients had hallucinations with *loss* of insight, if no specific treatment was initiated [19].

Genetic forms of parkinsonism

Knowledge on the prevalence of psychotic symptoms in genetic forms of parkinsonism is limited and relies mostly on case series. Consequently, proper prevalence numbers are missing. However, it is clear that hallucinations occur in these genetic forms of

Table 12.1 Prevalence of hallucinations in PD in cross-sectional prospective studies

	n	Total prevalence	Complex visual hallucinations	Minor hallucinations/ illusions	Auditory hallucinations	Delusions	Study period
Sanchez-Ramos et al. 1996 [61]	214[a]	26	26	–	0	–	ND
Graham et al. 1997 [36]	129[a]	25	23	–	12	7	Past and present
Inzelberg et al. 1998 [43]	121[a]	37	37	–	8	–	Past and present
Fénelon et al. 2000 [15]	216[a]	40	22	25	10	–	Past 3 months
Holroyd et al. 2001 [39]	98[a]	–	27	–	2	1	Past week
Bailbé et al. 2002 [165]	152[b]	23	21	–	6	7	Past 15 days
Aarsland et al. 1999 [14]	235[c]	16	–	–	–	–	Past week
Schrag et al. 2002 [166]	124[c]	23	–	–	–	–	Past and present
Paleacu et al. 2005 [4]	276[a]	32	–	–	3	–	Past and present
Pacchetti et al. 2005 [112]	289[a]	30	30	17	8	7	Past 6 months
Williams et al. 2007 [167]	115[a]	75	38	72	22	–	Past 3 months

ND, not disclosed. All the authors used a questionnaire on hallucinations, with the exception of Aarsland et al. [14] who used Section I of the Unified Parkinson's Disease Rating Scale. Values are expressed as percentages.

[a] Patients from movement disorder clinics.

[b] Patients from hospitals or private clinics.

[c] Population-based study.

parkinsonism. Kasten and co-workers [20] have estimated frequencies of between 3 and 29% based on their own data and literature review; *LRRK2* G2019S carriers similarly displayed a high frequency of hallucinations in another study [21]. The most solid data have been reported for glucocerebrosidase (*GBA*) mutations: in a cohort of 33 patients with *GBA* mutations and parkinsonism (most of them also with a pathological post-mortem analysis), hallucinations were reported in 45% [22].

Impact on Parkinson's disease prognosis and mortality

Goetz and Stebbins [23] used a case–control methodology to compare PD patients about to enter nursing homes with PD patients remaining in the community. Each nursing home subject was matched with two control patients for age, gender and disease duration. The authors examined motor disability, dementia and hallucinations as putative risks for nursing home placement. Visual hallucinations were the only differentiating factor: 82% of the patients placed in nursing homes had regular hallucinations in comparison with only 5% of the patients staying at home. These results were confirmed by Aarsland et al. [24] who found that the presence of visual hallucinations was a stronger predictor for institutionalization than functional impairment and old age. Goetz and Stebbins [5] followed the two patient groups for 5 years and showed that all patients who entered a nursing home died within 2 years. In contrast, only 32% died within the same period in the original community dwellers. However, it remains uncertain whether the high mortality in these end-stage PD patients is more closely associated with nursing home placement than with visual hallucinations [17]. Meanwhile it appears that prognosis has improved with atypical antipsychotic therapy, as only 28% of the hallucinating patients placed in a nursing home died within 2 years in a more recent study [25].

Signs and symptoms

Clear versus clouded sensorium

The clinical context of the hallucinatory syndrome under consideration is essential because PD patients may develop hallucinations for other, non-disease-related, reasons. As part of a toxic delirium, hallucinations occur in the context of a clouded sensorium. In this syndrome, patients usually show signs of distractibility, agitation and myoclonus. Such a diffuse encephalopathy occurs with fever, infections, renal failure and with anticholinergic treatment [26]. Subjects with mild renal failure who receive amantadine can experience acute delirium with hallucinations as well. In the perioperative state, especially when PD patients receive pain medications, they have a significantly increased risk of a confusional state with hallucinations [27]. In general, all these situations are short-lived, and the hallucinations clear when the underlying medical condition is treated.

Early versus late appearance

Early hallucinations are one of the three clinical features that most accurately distinguish DLB from PD [28,29]. However, the cutoff between these conditions, although

Box 12.1 Diagnostic criteria for PD-associated psychosis

Presence of at least one of the following symptoms:

- Illusions
- False sense of presence
- Hallucinations
- Delusions
- Symptoms occur *after* the onset of PD
- They are recurrent or continuous for at least 1 month
- No triggering psychiatric or general medical condition (fever, infection, phase after surgery)
- Associated with/without: insight, dementia, specific PD treatment

Modified from: Ravina et al. [31].

theoretically well defined, may be more difficult to establish in clinical practice, and the phenomenology of visual hallucinations linked to PD and DLB is similar [30].

Prototypical hallucinations

A group of experts sponsored by the National Institutes of Health (NIH) has recently formulated very detailed diagnostic criteria [31] (Box 12.1). Furthermore, Duvoisin's classical description [32] perfectly illustrates the panoply of psychotic phenomena in PD patients (Box 12.2).

Box 12.2 Duvoisin's protypical description of psychotic phenomena in PD [32]

. . . Visual illusions are especially frequent. Familiar objects may be mistaken for something else. The patient may mention seeing worms on the floor, whereas actually there is a design in the flooring which is misinterpreted because the pattern seems to move. Spectral illusions generally of a benign if not pleasant character are experienced. There may be hallucinations of people or animals roaming around the house. . . . Complex scenes with a group of people wandering around, having a party . . . seem to go about their business without disturbing the patient. Patients may experience these visions for long periods of time but are afraid to mention them to anyone for fear of being thought 'crazy'.

Finally, however, the patient reacts, angrily ordering the strangers out of the house, accusing them of stealing. . . .

Establishing the time of the first true visual hallucinations may be difficult as they may begin insidiously, out of seemingly normal heightened perceptions, misperceptions (illusions) and very fleeting impressions with preserved insight that cause no concern to the patient. Even after patients recognize the hallucinations as a false perception, many remain hesitant to admit them to family members [13]. The feeling of presence of another person (FP) (*sensation de presence* or *Anwesenheit*) was first described in PD in 1982 [33]. About half of the PD patients with FP claim to recognize the 'identity' of the presence. FP are mostly short-lasting and non-distressing and insight is preserved [34]. The sensation of movement in the peripheral visual field (*sensation de passage*) seems to be more frequent in PD patients with dementia than those without [35]. Fénelon et al. [15] also systematically investigated these phenomena as presumably pre-hallucinatory symptoms. Isolated occurrence was noted in 14% and combined occurrence with formed hallucinations in another 9% of the patients. PD patients also frequently misinterpret non-living objects, especially moving ones, as living beings (see Fig. 12.1 and Plate 3). These illusions may be facilitated by dim light and/or reduced vigilance and attentiveness during drowsiness. Their frequency has rarely been investigated separately, because in systematic interviews it is often difficult for the PD patient to differentiate illusions from visual hallucinations. [36,37]. However, taken together, FP, passage hallucinations and visual illusions occurred in 45% of 116 consecutive PD patients [38].

The content and contextual framework of the prototypic or core hallucinatory syndrome has been investigated by different research groups, and similar descriptive core features have been reported [37–40]. The hallucinators unanimously reported visual hallucinations that represent human beings, animals or both and were often mobile, appearing in

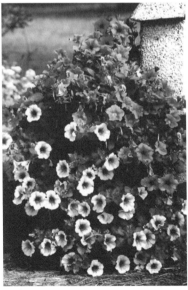

Fig. 12.1 A cognitively impaired Parkinson's disease patient took these petunias for numerous little faces staring at him. (See also Plate 3)

scenes of short duration, often lasting only for seconds. They were usually moving, doing otherwise appropriate activities without disturbing the patient. By their repetitive and stereotyped character, the figures in the visual hallucinations became familiar to the patient, who, as a bystander, observed them with amused interest (the 'marketplace effect'). The patients never involved themselves in the activities of the hallucinations. Favoured by dim light or reduced vigilance, visual hallucinations appeared suddenly, without any known trigger or voluntary effort. They also vanished suddenly, sometimes when the patient tried to check their reality by approaching or touching them. It is notable that simple visual hallucinations, consisting of elementary geometrical patterns, are uncommon in PD [30]. Visual hallucinations were not regularly bound to the same motoric state ('on' or 'off') and had no direct temporal relation to ingestion of antiparkinsonian medication. Often a given visual hallucination occurred when the PD patient was in a specific environmental setting. Real objects might contribute to the scene by being mistaken in an illusory way. Visual hallucinations often had blurred borders, but had neither colour predominance nor a specific localization to a field of vision (lateral versus central) (Table 12.2). Affectively, patients usually expressed little concern about the visual hallucinations, although some patients found themselves anxious or depressed and a few felt terrified [15,41]. Comparative prevalence and phenomenology during the day or at night was not extensively studied, although one report found that diurnal visual hallucinations were more common than nocturnal visual hallucinations, with 46% of patients indicating only diurnal visual hallucinations,

Table 12.2 Prototypic psychotic phenomena in PD

Phenomenon	Comments, examples
Minor hallucinations:	
Sensation de passage, sensation de présence	Syn: extracampine hallucinations
	Sense of moving figure out of the corner of one's vision
Illusional misinterpretations	Favoured by dim light
	Patient mistakes a standing lamp for a person
Core syndrome:	
Scenic, complex, repetitive visual hallucinations, mostly of normal size; micropsia and metaphormopsia are rare	Not frightening, patient often an amused bystander, efficient coping
Accompanying hallucinations of other modalities	Auditory hallucinations as 'soundtrack' of visual scenes
Full-blown psychosis:	
Secondary delusional interpretations	Frightening, rather rare, more frequent in patients with dementia; poor prognosis [20]
	Patient now actively involved in the hallucinatory events (for instance chasing after hallucinations of robbers who are trying to steal objects from the house)

13% only nocturnal visual hallucinations and 41% both types [37]. Another study with continuous polysomnographic recording found that in 20 hallucinating patients, 14 experienced visual hallucinations during the day, eight during a 'wakeful state', five during a twilight state and one on awaking from napping in the afternoon. In contrast, four patients developed visual hallucinations upon awakening at night [42].

Hallucinations in other sensory modalities

Auditory hallucinations were registered in 8% of PD patients [43] (see Table 12.2). They may be elementary (ringing, knocks, etc.) or, more often, complex. The vocal content is neutral or incomprehensible and differs from the pejorative or threatening auditory hallucinations of schizophrenia. Auditory hallucinations may constitute the 'soundtrack' of visual hallucinations, with the patient hearing the conversation of unreal persons. Tactile hallucinations [44] involve contact with small animals, although they do not generate the belief of infestation. They may also manifest as the feeling of being touched by someone. Originally described only in series or case reports [39,45,46], olfactory and gustatory hallucinations may have been underestimated, and in one study they occurred in 10% of patients in a cohort of 87 [47]. Both, olfactory and tactile hallucinations can be experienced as very unpleasant, but are rarely long-lasting [44,48–50]. Remarkably, pleasant olfactory hallucinations or phantosmias have been described as a pre-motor syndrome in PD [51,52].

Multimodal hallucinations

Most patients experiencing visual hallucinations may also experience non-visual hallucinations, although not report them. A combination of often visual with non-visual hallucinations even predominates in late PD [53]. When focusing on new-onset hallucinations, it has been shown that elderly patients were more likely to have multimodal hallucinations than pure visual hallucinations, suggesting that age and ageing processes may influence the phenomenology of hallucinations [46].

Delusional psychosis

Full-blown psychotic decompensation with frightening paranoid delusions and loss of insight has been a rare phenomenon in most studies. However, underestimation is possible, as a prospective study that specifically focused on delusional misidentification syndromes documented this problem in 17% of PD patients with dementia. Most of these subjects also exhibited severe hallucinations as well as marked memory and language deficits [54]. PD patients with Capgras syndrome (named after a French psychiatrist, and also called *illusions des sosies*) mistake familiar persons, mostly their spouses, for impostors or doubles. They still correctly identify the physiognomy of the family members, but have lost the sense of familiarity (hypoidentification) [55]. Subjects with the Othello syndrome develop marked delusional jealousy and accuse their spouse of infidelity [56,57]. Most of the patients with one or the other of these syndromes are male.

Assessment by questionnaire

While most clinicians may gather information on psychotic symptoms through an open interview method, standardized and internationally recognized measurement tools are desired for prevalence and interventional studies. In a review and critique of available rating scales for PD psychosis none of 12 available scales for assessing psychosis in PD could be recommended without restriction [58]. The review highlighted that none covered the broad phenomenological spectrum, and only three had been validated in a PD population, all of them without sufficient clinimetric properties. For the 12 scales reviewed, the Movement Disorder Society (MDS) Task Force on Rating Scales in PD favoured four scales as potential primary outcome scales, although all were noted to have limitations: the Neuropsychiatric Inventory (NPI), the Brief Psychiatric Rating Scale (BPRS), the Positive and Negative Syndrome Scale (PANSS) and the Schedule Assessment Positive Symptoms (SAPS).

A definitive rating tool is for psychosis in PD is a still unmet scientific need, and the MDS has officially endorsed the development of such a scale [59]. One of the major challenges in developing such a scale is the common reluctance of patients to endorse symptoms that they fear may be interpreted as 'crazy', as evidenced in one study where standard interview techniques yielded a non-declaration rate of 42% for hallucinations and 62% for delusions. [60]. Details on the progress of a MDS-sponsored rating scale for psychosis in PD can be accessed at the society's website (<http://www.movementdisorders.org>).

Pathophysiology

Recent work has extended the classical aetiological concepts of pharmacotoxicity ('levodopa psychosis') by showing that peripheral and central visual perception disorders and dysfunction of sleep (regulating centres) are associated factors, in addition to dysexecutive signs and dementia.

Biochemistry

Psychotic signs were first thought to represent a medication-induced toxic syndrome due to overstimulation of mesolimbic D3 and D4 dopaminergic receptors. Moskowitz et al. [10] postulated a pharmacological kindling model to suggest enhanced sensitivity of dopaminergic receptors after chronic treatment. Thus, excess dopamine from medications could overflow onto supersensitive receptors, inducing psychotic signs. However, several observations have challenged this hypothesis. The daily dose of levodopa is no different between patients who hallucinate and those who don't [44,61], and in predisposed patients high-dose intravenous levodopa cannot provoke visual hallucinations in a predefined clinical setting [62]. Especially in patients with cognitive impairment, visual hallucinations can easily be triggered by anticholinergic treatment, possibly because there is profound neocortical loss of cholinergic neurons and choline acetyltransferase (ChAT) in patients with PD dementia and DLB. Additional losses are seen in the temporal cortex involved with visual recognition [63,64]. New neurophysiological tools permitting researchers to probe neocortical cholinergic function more directly by using the short latency afferent inhibition (SAI) technique confirm marked reduction of SAI in PD patients with hallucinations [65]. It has been hypothesized that with reduced cortical levels of acetylcholine, irrelevant intrinsic and sensory information, normally processed in parallel at a subconscious level, enters conscious awareness in the form of visual hallucinations [66]. Finally, enhanced serotonergic neurotransmission has been postulated as well. Thus, increased serotonin 2A ($5\text{-}HT_{2A}$) receptor binding has been demonstrated *in vivo* in the ventral visual pathway of PD patients with visual hallucinations [67], echoed by increased levels of $5\text{-}HT_{2A}$ in the temporal cortex of such patients in post-mortem studies [68]. In contrast $5\text{-}HT_{1A}$ levels cannot discriminate between PD patients with or without hallucinations [69].

Taken together, these studies suggest that dopaminergic stimulation by itself [70], secondary imbalance with the cholinergic system [71] and enhanced serotonergic transmission are part of the pathophysiological framework, probably more as a triggering factors than as the primary causal factors.

Visual impairment

Quite different investigational tools have been used to explore the impact of visual deficits on hallucinations in PD. Besides traditional autopsy studies, there are morphometric *in vivo* studies focused specifically on the comparative grey matter volume of different cortical areas associated with hallucinations. Network involvement can be evaluated by psychophysiological studies and by activation studies using functional magnetic resonance imaging (fMRI). We shall review step by step the results obtained with each of these techniques, keeping in mind that all tools have specific limitations and that an integrated final synthesis has yet to be unveiled.

In PD there is a reduction in dopaminergic innervation around the fovea and retinal dopamine concentration [72,73], and there is secondary thinning of the retinal nerve fibre layer [74]. Furthermore there are numerous *in vivo* electrophysiological and psychophysical arguments for the disruption of retinal function in PD patients [75]. At the supraretinal level, selective reductions in grey matter volume have been reported in hallucinating PD patients for the lingual gyrus, the right or left orbitofrontal lobe and the superior parietal, and more surprisingly for the pedunculopontine nucleus and for the head of the hippocampus [76–80]. It should be mentioned that differing reductions in grey matter volume have been seen in patients with DLB and visual hallucinations [77]. Although autopsy studies have not yet focused on PD, DLB patients with hallucinations have increased muscarinic binding in Brodman area 36, which includes the posterior hippocampal formation, the parahippocampal gyrus and the lingual and fusiform gyri [63], and high densities of Lewy bodies (LBs) in the parahippocampus and the amygdala [81].

At the clinical level, visual acuity in the best eye is significantly reduced in PD patients with visual hallucinations in comparison with PD patients without such hallucinations [39,82]. PD patients with visual hallucinations show substantially reduced performances on colour discrimination or contrast sensitivity tests [83]. It is remarkable that these colour discrimination deficits are already present at a potential pre-motor phase, namely 'idiopathic' RBD [84]. More complex visual deficits concern 'reality monitoring' and involve visual silhouette agnosia [85]. PD patients with visual hallucinations also perform less well in image recognition, especially with black and white or monochrome images [79,86]. Recognition speed is slower and delayed visual as well as spatial memory is impaired [87,88]. When using a facial discrimination paradigm in order to elicit event-related visual potentials, PD dementia patients with visual hallucinations produce longer latencies of the visual P_2 and P_3 potentials, suggesting impairment in the early stage of facial information processing [89]. Even in a virtual reality environment, PD patients are also at risk of experiencing visual hallucinations [90].

Neuroimaging of visual hallucinations, by directly tracking the responsible cerebral pathways, has not yet been successful. However, a surrogate visual paradigm has been used in order to test the functional cerebral activation pattern in response to visual stimuli: fMRI has been performed during stroboscopic or kinematic visual excitation in PD patients with or without a history of visual hallucinations [91]. The PD patients with visual hallucinations showed decreased cerebral activation in occipital, parietal and temporoparietal regions, and in parallel increased frontal activation in the region of the frontal eye fields. Another fMRI study similarly reported reduced activation of occipital–temporal areas before image recognition in PD patients with visual hallucinations [92]. However, increased top-down frontal activation was not seen. It must be pointed out here that, due to differing paradigm choices, differing areas of interest or calculation methods, the interpretation of fMRI studies remains difficult and even more conflicting results have to be reported. Thus, in another fMRI study, visualization of facial stimuli produced reduced activation of several right-sided prefrontal areas in hallucinating PD patients [93], whereas in a third study increased activation in the fusiform gyrus was reported during a facial perception paradigm [94]. Despite these restrictions, these findings seem to suggest a dysfunctional interplay between primary visual and associative visual areas on one side and selective visual attention pathways on the other [95]. Impairment in bottom-up visual signalling and secondary or adaptive hyperfunction of attention areas has also been confirmed by positron emission tomography (PET) studies, showing frontal hypermetabolism in PD patients with visual hallucinations [96], orypoperfusion in the right fusiform gyrus, hyperperfusion in the right superior and middle temporal gyri [97] and, finally, reduced metabolism in occipitotemporoparietal regions, sparing the occipital pole [98]. Thus, while the visual data processing in V1 seems to remain intact, there is probably pressing dysfunction of visual object recognition [85].

Taken together, the numerous studies on low- and high-level visual impairment in PD suggest that higher visual processing deficits occur in the selective visual attention pathways, and most reproducibly in the extra-striatal visual cortices. The functional neuroanatomy of visual hallucinations in PD may also be variable, and functional parallelism has been proposed with both Charles Bonnet syndrome, where hyperperfusion of the temporal cortex as well as increased cerebral activation in the ventral extra-striatal region [99,100] have been reported, and DLB, where patients with visual hallucinations show hypoperfusion or decreased glucose utilization in the occipital cortex [101].

Sleep dysregulation

Sleep problems are very common in PD and commonly coexist with hallucinations, but no sleep problem is specifically predictive of future hallucinations [102]. The relationship between sleep aberrations and hallucinations has been actively debated for several years. First, sleep disruption and vivid dreams have been proposed as elements of a long-lasting, hidden, subclinical phase of the hallucinatory syndrome [10,12], but in a prospective longitudinal study [17] the presence of vivid dreams/nightmares did not predict future visual hallucinations. Furthermore, sleep fragmentation does not predict the later occurrence of hallucinations in PD. However, numerous nocturnal sleep abnormalities as well as dysfunctional wake–sleep cycles have been reported in patients with hallucinations, including frequent nocturnal awakenings, increased motor activity during the night with secondary nocturnal sleep fragmentation, vivid dreams and nightmares, unpredictable circadian rest–activity rhythms and increased daytime sleepiness. [103–105]. As such, the odds of experiencing any psychotic symptoms are five times higher in PD patients with co-morbid disorders of sleep–wakefulness and depression [106]. Recent research has focused more on REM sleep pathology. RBD has been recognized as the harbinger of a more diffuse neurodegenerative process, most importantly PD and DLB [107,108]. This neurodegenerative process includes a predilection for complex visuospatial, visuoconstructional or visuoperceptual functions [109,110], attention deficits or poor fluency performances [111]. The presence of RBD and reduced REM sleep atonia at PD onset, before or after PD diagnosis, has been advocated as a harbinger of increased risk for hallucinations in the long term, although this assumption has been contested as it is not a consistent finding [112–114]. Visual hallucinations may represent intrusions of REM into wakefulness [115,116], although phenomenological comparison between dreams and visual hallucinations in PD attests to a poor parallelism between the two. However, cognitive 'bizarreness' in daytime dreams and 'heightened aggressiveness' in nighttime dreams have been reported in PD patients [117,118]. In addition, RBD in PD patients may resolve with antiparkinsonian medications given at bedtime, while visual hallucinations in PD are easily triggered by such treatment. Perturbation of the physiological sleep–wake cycle has been the latest research avenue in this domain. PD patients have early degeneration of the brainstem sleep centres, such as the locus coeruleus and pedunculopontine nucleus [78], and have low numbers of the hypothalamic cells producing hypocretin, an essential regulator of the sleep–wake cycle [119]. Polysomnography-based studies in PD patients with visual hallucinations demonstrate greater levels of daytime sleep, and one-third of the registered hallucinatory episodes were related to daytime non-REM sleep or nocturnal REM sleep [42].

Cognitive impairment

Cognitive impairment and/or dementia is an independent risk factor for hallucinations [15,120,122], and the prevalence of hallucinations is higher in PD patients with dementia. In patients with early PD, a lower Mini Mental State Examination at baseline was associated with a higher risk of developing hallucinations under treatment [122].

Box 12.3 Factors contributing to hallucinations in PD

- Faulty or incomplete visual input
- Reduced cortical activation of visual cortex
- Aberrant activation of associative visual cortex
- Impaired processing of facial recognition
- Defective visual memory
- Lack of suppression or spontaneous reappearance of internally generated imagery
- Impaired bottom-up visual activation
- Increased adaptive activation of top-down attentional networks
- Intrusion of REM dreaming imagery ('REM fragments') into wakefulness
- Erratic changes of the filtering capacities through fluctuating vigilance or perturbation of the physiological sleep–wake cycle
- Medication-related overactivation of mesolimbic systems
- Medication-induced imbalance or blockade of the cholinergic transmission of the associative visual cortex

Various neuropsychological tests have established specific dysfunctions in visuoperceptive [30,76,85], visuoexecutive [123], executive [124], language [123] and memory tasks [76]. Widespread cognitive dysfunction is also echoed by similarly widespread atrophy, including limbic, paralimbic and neocortical grey-matter loss [125].

The numerous disparate findings derived from several investigative domains have precluded a unitary pathophysiological model of visual hallucinations in PD. We have adapted Hobson's work on the states of consciousness [1] and propose that visual hallucinations should be considered as a dysregulation of the gating/filtering of both external and internal perception mechanisms. In this model it is easy to integrate numerous contributory factors (Box 12.3).

Modelling hallucinations in Parkinson's disease

It seems to be a Sisyphean endeavour to compact the panoply of predisposing or causative factors of hallucinations in one causal model. All attempts must exclude or minimize some factors. Also, phenomenologically different hallucinations may have different causes. Nevertheless, such efforts are helpful in order to 'get an overview' and open new avenues for therapeutic research. While detailed exploration of this topic is beyond the scope of the present chapter, most notable models should be mentioned. In the *perception and attention deficit model* proto-objects are an essential concept, as these unconscious object templates are proposed during the process of perception, by top-down mechanisms for further processing [126]. Finally one of them is chosen and also actually seen. Bottom-up factors strongly influence the selection process. PD patients with visual hallucinations erroneously take an incorrect proto-object as a real object. This defective processing is due to 'a combination of impaired attentional binding and poor sensory activation of the correct proto-objects in conjunction with a relatively intact scene representation that biases perception towards an incorrect image' [126]. Hobson's activation–input–modulation (AIM) model of consciousness has also been proposed as a multidimensional model [127]. Hallucinations in PD 'should be considered as a dysregulation of the gating and filtering of external perception and internal image production' [127]. Meanwhile this aetiological multimodal model has been confirmed in clinics by demonstration in a large cohort that impaired visual processing, sleep–wake dysfunction, brainstem abnormalities and impairment of dysexecutive frontal all independently predispose to visual hallucinations in PD [128]. More focused models have addressed the defective interplay of higher-order visual performances and attentional networks [79,129]. Finally, it should be mentioned that, based on fMRI studies of the resting state network, alterations in this default mode network have been proposed as causing auditory hallucinations in schizophrenic patients, and applicability to visual hallucinations in Parkinson's disease has to be investigated [130,131].

Treatment (evidence-based and practical recommendations)

As a first-line strategy, patients with new onset or a sudden exacerbation of hallucinations need to be checked for metabolic disturbances and infections. In cases of subacute onset or exacerbation of hallucinations an ophthalmological evaluation can help detect primary visual disturbances that can play a role in misinterpretation of visual perceptions. Next, decreases in medication or elimination of one or more antiparkinsonian agents should be considered. Agents with the lowest antiparkinsonian efficacy or a high anticholinergic potential (anticholinergics, amantadine, selegiline) should be eliminated first. This intervention may still allow the use of adequate doses of levodopa and dopaminergic agonists to alleviate any worsening of the parkinsonian symptoms. Whereas a drug holiday was once used in the treatment of psychosis in PD, its major potential complications (lengthy hospitalizations, aspiration, pulmonary emboli, neuroleptic-like malignant syndrome) actually limit its utility [132]. However, substantial reduction of dopaminergic treatment is also feasible by use of subthalamic nucleus deep brain stimulation (STN DBS) and a small case series has reported drastic reduction of psychotic features in PD patients treated by STN DBS [133].

Neuroleptics

So far it is unresolved when to start treatment of hallucinations in PD. In a small cohort study it could be demonstrated that the PD patients with very early treatment mostly maintained insight, whereas those without treatment (reduction of dopaminergic medication or antipsychotic drugs) tended to deteriorate with lost insight within 12 months [134]. However, larger randomized treatment trials are needed to confirm the usefulness of this strategy.

Typical low-potency neuroleptics frequently cause intolerable worsening of motor function and should therefore be avoided. New 'atypical' antipsychotics, including clozapine [135,136], risperidone [137], remoxipride [138], zotepine [139], olanzapine [140] and ondansetron [141], appear in some cases to have a better profile concerning potential side effects and have been used in open-label studies with mixed success. Clozapine, olanzapine and quetiapine are the only agents that have been compared with placebo in randomized, double-blind controlled trials. Clozapine is a drug that belongs to the dibenzodiazepine class of chemicals and has a regional selectivity for action at dopamine receptors in the mesolimbic behavioural system. It has also marked affinity for the 5-HT$_{2A}$ receptor. In general, over 80% of PD patients respond to clozapine with complete or partial resolution of psychosis. The recommended initial daily dose of clozapine is 6.25–12.5 mg every other day with an incremental increase of 12.5 mg every 4–7 days until symptoms are adequately controlled or adverse effects occur. A more rapid increase can be achieved during a hospitalization. Typically, most PD patients can be maintained on 12.5–37.5 mg four times a day. Despite the efficacy of clozapine at very low doses, side effects like sedation, orthostatic hypotension and agranulocytosis can occur. The latter potential complication underlies governmental regulations on frequent blood testing in patients treated with clozapine. Long-term efficacy of clozapine has been demonstrated for up to 3 years. It is unclear, however, whether PD patients who respond to clozapine require chronic maintenance therapy and for what duration. In one study, however, a high relapse rate occurred after withdrawal of clozapine [136].

Olanzapine was shown to significantly aggravate the motor signs of parkinsonism [142] and should not be considered as a first-choice drug. Quetiapine has been examined in two double-blind studies, but both trials found that it was not efficacious in treating hallucinations [143,144]. A double-blind comparator study between clozapine and quetiapine found that both agents were effective in treating hallucinations [145]. The results of the placebo-controlled trial contrast with wide utilization of quetiapine in clinical settings, positive open-label results [146] and overall favourable experience with the drug in the present authors' personal experience. One potential explanation for this dichotomy between clinical experience and evidence-based data lies in the possibility that quetiapine has more sleep-promoting effects than pure antihallucinatory impact and that clinical perception of improvement relates to this effect. However, sleep normalization has not been confirmed in a polysomnography-based study [147]. The US Food and Drug Administration has determined that the use of atypical antipsychotic agents in elderly patients with dementia is associated with increased mortality risk, based on an analysis of 17 placebo-controlled trials [148]. In this analysis, the mean mortality among subjects on antipsychotic agents was 4.5% versus 2.6% in subjects receiving placebo. Given that the PD population is often elderly and may have cognitive impairment, these warnings need to be incorporated into best medical management decisions.

Cholinesterase inhibitors

Based on observations that cholinesterase inhibitors can abate hallucinations in patients with DLB, small series of PD patients, with or without significant cognitive impairment, have been tested with these agents [149,150]. Positive outcomes have been reported, but no large randomized placebo or comparator controlled trial has been conducted specifically on hallucinations. A large study of rivastigmine in PD patients with dementia showed that global improvement occurred in those with and without hallucinations, but the hallucinations in the hallucinating group did not significantly improve [151]. The presence of hallucinations in PD patients with dementia, however, has been reported to predict a better overall response to rivastigmine in comparison with PD subjects without hallucinations [152, 153]. Donepezil provides general improvement of cognition and behaviour in PD patients with dementia with or without hallucinations [154,155]. No direct antipsychotic role of cholinesterase inhibitors can be affirmed from these studies.

Selective serotonin 2A antagonist

More recently, research interest has especially focused on development of 5-HT_{2A} antagonists or also 5-HT_{2A} inverse agonists, fuelled by the knowledge that both effective atypical neuroleptics, clozapine and quetiapine, develop action at the 5-HT_{2A} receptor and that enhanced serotonergic transmission has been shown in PD patients with hallucinations [67–69,156]. Furthermore the hallucinogenic $5\text{-HT}_{2A/1A}$ agonist psilocybin substantially disturbs visual object completion, while causing visual hallucinations [157]. Psychotic-like behaviours can indeed be disrupted in a rodent model of PD by the use of pimavanserin, a 5-HT_{2A} inverse agonist [158]. In a clinical pilot study pimavanserin significantly reduced psychotic features and did not produce noticeable side effects [159]. It should be noted that the serotonin receptor antagonist ondansetron has also been reported to be useful for PD-associated hallucination. While these approaches may well represent a novel 'targeted' treatment for hallucinations in PD, carefully designed and executed double-blind studies are essential before conclusions can be made.

Other treatment options

The encouragement of good sleep habits and keeping lights on at night so that dark shadows do not foster visual misinterpretations are easily applied recommendations [1]. Some patients can learn coping strategies (rubbing their eyes or focusing intently on the hallucination to make it disappear, or consciously reminding themselves of the false nature of the experience) [41]. Corrective measures to improve best eyesight are another reasonable, though untested, approach [82]. Light therapy had no clear benefit for visual hallucinations in one small study [160]. Antidepressants have been used in hallucinating and depressed PD patients with some success [161,162].

Future developments

As alluded to above, multiple brain areas, ranging from the eye itself to brainstem nuclei to the associative visual cortex, may be involved in the generation of psychotic symptoms in PD. Neuropathological research has identified progressive degeneration of most of these regions in PD, but contrasting findings as well as various methodological issues have so far precluded specificity of the findings. At present fMRI and other neuroimaging techniques, including the use of transmitter-specific markers, are most promising, as they are applicable *in vivo* and hopefully, in the near future, while the patient is actually hallucinating. While therapeutic research has understandably focused on the transmitter systems known to be involved in hallucinations, a deeper look at fundamental cellular mechanisms potentially involved in hallucinations could be fruitful as well. In this context increased oxidative stress, reflected by increased urinary excretion of 8-hydroxydeoxyguanosine, has been linked with hallucinations but not with motor symptoms in PD [163]. Finally, alterations in lipid pathways within the primary visual cortex of PD patients offer another glimpse at fundamental, possibly adaptive, changes, again with the potential to open up novel routes for treatment [164].

We propose that future research should examine, using fMRI, other neuroimaging techniques and autopsy studies, three domains of interest for visual hallucinations in PD:

Visual pathways: the retinal dopaminergic layers as visualized by optical coherence tomography; the associative (extra-striatal) visual cortex involving visual attention and motion detection; the white matter tracts of the visual system; fundamental changes within these pathways including deregulation of gene expression, alteration of lipid metabolism and oxidative stress status.

Sleep–wake and REM sleep regulation systems: the pedunculopontine nucleus and its thalamic target areas; the locus coeruleus and its involvement in cognitive dysfunction; the dopaminergic tegmental area of the mesencephalus; the amygdala.

Specific frontal/temporal lobe areas: underlying specific or non-specific visual attention; underlying verbal (categorical) fluency; underlying 'source monitoring'; underlying facial recognition; underlying spatial object recognition.

References

1 **Diederich NJ, Goetz CG, Stebbins GT**. Repeated visual hallucinations in Parkinson's disease as disturbed external/internal perceptions: focused review and a new integrative model. Mov Disord 2005; **20**: 130–40.

2 **Chou K, Messing S, Oakes D, et al**. Drug-induced psychosis in Parkinson disease: phenomenology and correlations among psychosis rating instruments. Clin Neuropharmacol 2005; **28**: 215–19.

3 **Tanner CM, Vogel C, Goetz CG, Klawans H**. Hallucinations in Parkinson's disease: a population study [abstract]. Ann Neurol 1983; **14**: 13.

4 **Paleacu D, Schechtman E, Inzelberg R**. Association between family history of dementia and hallucinations in Parkinson disease. Neurology 2005; **64**: 1712–15.

5 **Goetz CG, Stebbins GT**. Mortality and hallucinations in nursing home patients with advanced Parkinson's disease. Neurology 1995; **45**: 669–71.

6 **Ball B**. De l'insanité dans la paralysie agitante. L'Encéphale 1882; **2**: 22–32.

7 **Mjönes H**. Paralysis agitans. A clinical and genetic study. Copenhagen: Ejnar Munksgaard, 1949.

8 **Sacks OW, Kol MS, Messeloff CR, Schwartz WF**. Effects of levodopa in parkinsonian patients with dementia. Neurology 1972; **22**: 516–19.

9 **Fénelon G, Goetz CG, Karenberg A**. Hallucinations in Parkinson's disease in the prelevodopa era. Neurology 2006; **66**: 93–8.

10 Moskovitz C, Moses H, Klawans HL. Levodopa induced psychosis: a kindling phenomenon. Am J Psych 1978; **135**: 669–75.

11 Sharf B, Moskowitz C, Lupton MD, Klawans HL. Dream phenomena induced by chronic levodopa therapy. J Neural Transm 1978; **43**: 143–51.

12 Nausieda PA, Weiner W, Kaplan L, et al. Sleep disruption and psychosis in chronic levodopa therapy. Clin Neuropharm 1982; **5**: 183–94.

13 Haeske-Dewick HC. Hallucinations in Parkinson's disease: characteristics and associated features. Int J Geriatr Psych 1995; **10**: 487–95.

14 Aarsland D, Larsen JP, Cummins JL, Laake K. Prevalence and clinical correlates of psychotic symptoms in Parkinson's disease: a community-based study. Arch Neurol 1999; **56**: 595–601.

15 Fénelon G, Mahieux F, Huon R, Ziegler M. Hallucinations in Parkinson's disease. Prevalence, phenomenology and risk factors. Brain 2000; **123**: 733–45.

16 Fénelon G, Alves G. Epidemiology of psychosis in Parkinson's disease. J Neurol Sci 2010; **289**: 12–17.

17 Goetz CG, Leurgans S, Pappert EJ, et al. Prospective longitudinal assessment of hallucinations in Parkinson's disease. Neurology 2001; **57**: 2078–82.

18 Forsaa EB, Larsen JP, Wentzel-Larsen T, et al. A 12-year population-based study of psychosis in Parkinson disease. Arch Neurol 2010; **67**: 996–1001.

19 Goetz CG, Wuu J, Curgian L, Leurgans S. Age-related influences on the clinical characteristics of new-onset hallucinations in Parkinson's disease patients. Mov Disord 2006; **21**: 267–70.

20 Kasten M, Kertelge L, Brüggemann N, et al. Nonmotor symptoms in genetic Parkinson's disease. Arch Neurol 2010; **67**: 670–6.

21 Belarbi S, Hecham N, Lesage S, et al. LRRK2 G2019S mutation in Parkinson's disease: a neuropsychological and neuropsychiatric study in a large Algerian cohort. Parkinsonism Relat Disord 2010; **16**: 676–9.

22 Neumann J, Bras J, Deas E, et al. Glucocerebrosidase mutations in clinical and pathologically proven Parkinson's disease. Brain 2009; **132**: 1783–94.

23 Goetz CG, Stebbins GT. Risk factors for nursing home placement in advanced Parkinson's disease. Neurology 1993; **43**: 2227–9.

24 Aarsland D, Larsen JP, Tandberg E, Laake K. Predictors of nursing home placement in Parkinson's disease: a population-based, prospective study. J Am Geriatr Soc 2000; **48**: 938–42.

25 Factor SA, Feustel PJ, Friedman JH, et al. Longitudinal outcome of Parkinson's disease patients with psychosis. Neurology 2003; **60**: 1756–61.

26 De Smet Y, Ruberg M, Serdaru M, et al. Confusion, dementia and anticholinergics in Parkinson's disease. J Neuro Neurosurg Psychiatry 1982; **45**: 1161–4.

27 Golden WE, Lavender RC, Metzer WS. Acute postoperative confusion and hallucinations in Parkinson's disease. Ann Intern Med 1989; **111**: 218–22.

28 Lippa CF, Duda JE, Grossman M, et al. DLB and PDD boundary issues: diagnosis, treatment, molecular pathology, and biomarkers. Neurology 2007; **68**: 812–19.

29 Litvan I, MacIntyre A, Goetz CG, et al. Accuracy of the clinical diagnoses of Lewy body disease, Parkinson's disease and dementia with Lewy bodies: a clinicopathologic study. Arch Neurol 1998; **55**: 969–78.

30 Mosimann UP, Rowan EN, Partington CE, et al. Characteristics of visual hallucinations in Parkinson disease dementia and dementia with Lewy bodies. Am J Geriatr Psychiatry 2006; **14**: 153–60.

31 Ravina B, Marder K, Fernandez HH, et al. Diagnostic criteria for psychosis in Parkinson's disease: report of an NINDS, NIMH work group. Mov Disord 2007; **22**: 1061–8.

32 Duvoisin RC. Parkinson's disease. A guide for patient and family. New York: Raven, 1991.

33 Thompson C. Anwesenheit: psychopathology and clinical associations. Br J Psychiatry 1982; **141**: 628–30.

34 Fénelon G, Soulas T, Cleret de Langavant L, Trinkler I, Bachoud-Lévi AC. Feeling of presence in Parkinson's disease. J Neurol Neurosurg Psychiatry 2011; **2**: 1219–24.

35 Archibald NK, Clarke MP, Mosimann UP, Burn DJ. Visual symptoms in Parkinson's disease and Parkinson's disease dementia. Mov Disord 2011; **26**: 2387–95.

36 Graham JM, Gruenewald RA, Sagar HJ. Hallucinosis in idiopathic Parkinson's disease. J Neurol Neurosurg Psychiatry 1997; **63**: 434–40.

37 Diederich NJ, Pieri V, Goetz CG. Die visuellen Halluzinationen des Parkinson-Patienten und das Charles Bonnet Syndrom. Eine phänomenologische und pathogenetische Gegenüberstellung. Fortschr Neurol Psychiat 2000; **68**: 129–36.

38 Fénelon G, Soulas T, Zenasni F, Cleret de Langavant L. The changing face of Parkinson's disease-associated psychosis: a cross-sectional study based on the new NINDS-NIMH criteria. Mov Disord 2010; **25**: 763–6.

39 Holroyd S, Currie L, Wooten GF. Prospective study of hallucinations and delusions in Parkinson's disease. J Neurol Neurosurg Psychiatry 2001; **70**: 734–8.

40 Barnes J, David AS. Visual hallucinations in Parkinson's disease: a review and phenomenological survey. J Neurol Neurosurg Psychiatry 2001; **70**: 727–33.

41 Diederich NH, Pieri V, Goetz CG. Coping strategies for visual hallucinations in Parkinson's disease. Mov Disord 2003; **18**: 831–8.

42 Manni R, Pacchetti C, Terzaghi M, et al. Hallucinations and sleep-wake cycle in PD: a 24-hour continuous polysomnographic study. Neurology 2002; **59**: 1979–81.

43 Inzelberg R, Kipervasser S, Korczyn AD. Auditory hallucinations in Parkinson's disease. J Neurol Neurosurg Psychiatry 1998; **64**: 533–5.

44 Fénelon G, Thobois S, Bonnet AM, et al. Tactile hallucinations in Parkinson's disease. J Neurol 2002; **12**: 1699–703.

45 Tousi B, Frankel M. Olfactory and visual hallucinations in Parkinson's disease. Parkinsonism Relat Dis 2004; **10**: 253–4.

46 Goetz CG, Wuu J, Curgian LM, Leurgans S. Hallucinations and sleep disorders in PD: six-year prospective longitudinal study. Neurology 2005; **64**: 81–6.

47 Bannier S, Berdagué JL, Rieu I, et al. Prevalence and phenomenology of olfactory hallucinations in Parkinson's disease. J Neurol Neurosurg Psychiatry 2012; **83**: 1019–21.

48 Sandyk R. Olfactory hallucinations in Parkinson's disease [letter]. S Afr Med J 1981; **60**: 950.

49 Jimenez-Jimenez FJ, Orti-Pareja M, Gasalla T, et al. Cenesthetic hallucinations in a patient with Parkinson's disease [letter]. J Neurol Neurosurg Psychiatry 1997; **63**: 120.

50 Clark J. Case history of a patient with musical hallucinations and Parkinson's disease [letter]. Int J Geriatr Psychiatry 1998; **13**: 886–7.

51 Landis BN, Burkhard PR. Phantosmias and Parkinson disease. Arch Neurol 2008; 65: 1237–9.

52 Hirsch AR. Parkinsonism: the hyposmia and phantosmia connection. Arch Neurol 2009; **66**: 538–9 [author reply 539].

53 Goetz CG, Stebbins GT, Ouyang B. Visual plus nonvisual hallucinations in Parkinson's disease: development and evolution over 10 years. Mov Disord 2011; **26**: 2196–200.

54 Pagonabarraga J, Llebaria G, García-Sánchez C, Pascual-Sedano B, Gironell A, Kulisevsky J. A prospective study of delusional misidentification syndromes in Parkinson's disease with dementia. Mov Disord 2008; **23**: 443–8.

55 Josephs KA. Capgras syndrome and its relationship to neurodegenerative disease. Capgras syndrome and its relationship to neurodegenerative disease. Arch Neurol 2007; **64**: 1762–6.

56 Cannas A, Solla P, Floris G, et al. Othello syndrome in Parkinson disease patients without dementia. Neurologist 2009; **15**: 34–6.

57 Georgiev D, Danieli A, Ocepek L, et al. Othello syndrome in patients with Parkinson's disease. Psychiatr Danub 2010; **22**: 94–8.

58 Fernandez HH, Aarsland D, Fénelon G, et al. Scales to assess psychosis in Parkinson's disease: Critique and recommendations. Mov Disord 2008; **23**: 484–500.

59 Goetz CG. Scales to evaluate psychosis in Parkinson's disease. Parkinsonism Relat Disord 2009; 15(Suppl 3): S38–S41.

60 Chaudhuri KR, Prieto-Jurcynska C, Naidu Y, et al. The nondeclaration of nonmotor symptoms of Parkinson's disease to health care professionals: an international study using the nonmotor symptoms questionnaire. Mov Disord 2010; **25**: 704–9.

61 Sanchez-Ramos JR, Ortoll R, Paulsen GW. Visual hallucinations associated with Parkinson's disease. Arch Neurol 1996; **53**: 1265–8.

62 Goetz CG, Pappert EJ, Blasucci LM, et al. Intravenous levodopa in hallucinating Parkinson's disease patients: high-dose challenge does not precipitate hallucinations. Neurology 1998; **50**: 515–17.

63 Ballard C, Piggott M, Johnson M, et al. Delusions associated with elevated muscarinic binding in dementia with Lewy bodies. Ann Neurol 2000; **48**: 868–76.

64 Francis PT, Perry EK. Cholinergic and other neurotransmitter mechanisms in Parkinson's disease, Parkinson's disease dementia, and dementia with Lewy bodies. Mov Disord 2007; 22(Suppl 17): S351–S357.

65 Manganelli F, Vitale C, Santangelo G, Pisciotta C, et al. Functional involvement of central cholinergic circuits and visual hallucinations in Parkinson's disease. Brain 2009; **132**: 2350–5.

66 Perry EK, Perry RH. Acetylcholine and hallucinations: disease-related compared to drug-induced alterations in human consciousness. Brain Cognition 1995; **28**: 240–58.

67 Ballanger B, Strafella AP, van Eimeren T, et al. Serotonin$_{2A}$ receptors and visual hallucinations in Parkinson disease. Arch Neurol 2010; **67**: 416–21.

68 Huot P, Johnston TH, Darr T, et al. Increased 5-HT$_{2A}$ receptors in the temporal cortex of parkinsonian patients with visual hallucinations. Mov Disord 2010; **25**: 1399–408.

69 Huot P, Johnston TH, Visanji NP, et al. Increased levels of 5-HT$_{1A}$ receptor binding in ventral visual pathways in Parkinson's disease. Mov Disord 2012; **27**: 735–42.

70 Goetz CG, Tanner CM, Klawans HL. Pharmacology of hallucinations induced by long-term drug therapy. Am J Psych 1982; **139**: 494–7.

71 Perry EK, Marshall E, Kerwin J, et al. Evidence of a monoaminergic-cholinergic imbalance related to visual hallucinations in Lewy body dementia. J Neurochem 1990; **55**: 1454–6.

72 Nguyen-Legros J. Functional neuroarchitecture of the retina: Hypothesis on the dysfunction of retinal dopaminergic circuitry in Parkinson's disease. Surg Radiol Anat 1988; **10**: 137–44.

73 Harnois C, Di Paolo T. Decreased dopamine in the retinas of patients with Parkinson's disease. Invest Ophthalmol Visual Sci 1990; **31**: 2473–5.

74 Inzelberg R, Ramirez JA, Nisipeanu P, Ophir A. Retinal nerve fiber layer thinning in Parkinson disease. Vision Res 2004; **44**: 2793–7.

75 Archibald NK, Clarke MP, Mosimann UP, Burn DJ. The retina in Parkinson's disease. Brain 2009; **132**: 1128–45.

76 Ramírez-Ruiz B, Martí MJ, Tolosa E, et al. Cerebral atrophy in Parkinson's disease patients with visual hallucinations. Eur J Neurol 2007; **14**: 750–6.

77 Sanchez-Castaneda C, Rene R, Ramirez-Ruiz B, Campdelacreu J, et al. Frontal and associative visual areas related to visual hallucinations in dementia with Lewy bodies and Parkinson's disease with dementia. Mov Disord 2010; **25**: 615–22.

78 Janzen J, van't Ent D, Lemstra AW, et al. The pedunculopontine nucleus is related to visual hallucinations in Parkinson's disease: preliminary results of a voxel-based morphometry study. J Neurol 2012; **259**: 147–54.

79 Shine JM, Halliday GH, Carlos M, Naismith SL, Lewis SJ. Investigating visual misperceptions in Parkinson's disease: a novel behavioral paradigm. Mov Disord 2012; **27**: 500–5.

80 Ibarretxe-Bilbao N, Ramírez-Ruiz B, Tolosa E, et al. Hippocampal head atrophy predominance in Parkinson's disease with hallucinations and with dementia. J Neurol 2008; **255**: 1324–31.

81 Harding AJ, Broe GA, Halliday GM. Visual hallucinations in Lewy body disease relate to Lewy bodies in the temporal lobe. Brain 2002; **125**: 391–403.

82 Matsui H, Udaka F, Tamura A, et al. Impaired visual acuity as a risk factor for visual hallucinations in Parkinson's disease. J Geriatr Psychiatry Neurol 2006; **19**: 36.

83 Diederich NJ, Goetz CG, Raman R, et al. Poor visual discrimination and visual hallucinations in Parkinson's disease. Clin Neuropharm 1998; **21**: 289–95.

84 Postuma RB, Lang AE, Massicotte-Marquez J, Montplaisir J. Potential early markers of Parkinson disease in idiopathic REM sleep behavior disorder. Neurology 2006; **66**: 845–51.

85 Barnes J, Boubert L, Harris J, et al. Reality monitoring and visual hallucinations in Parkinson's disease. Neuropsychologia 2003; **41**: 565–74.

86 Barnes J, Boubert L. Visual memory errors in Parkinson's disease patient with visual hallucinations. Int J Neurosci 2011; **121**: 159–64.

87 Meppelink AM, Koerts J, Borg M, Leenders KL, van Laar T. Visual object recognition and attention in Parkinson's disease patients with visual hallucinations. Mov Disord 2008; **23**: 1906–12.

88 Shin S, Lee JE, Hong JY, et al. Neuroanatomical substrates of visual hallucinations in patients with non-demented Parkinson's disease. J Neurol Neurosurg Psychiatry 2012; **83**: 1156–61.

89 Kurita A, Murakami M, Takagi S, Matsushima M, Suzuki M.Visual hallucinations and altered visual information processing in Parkinson disease and dementia with Lewy bodies. Mov Disord 2010; **25**: 167–71.

90 Onofrj M, Bonanni L, Albani G, et al. Visual hallucinations in Parkinson's disease: clues to separate origins. J Neurol Sci 2006; **248**: 143–50.

91 Stebbins GT, Goetz CG, Carrillo MC, et al. Altered cortical visual processing in PD with hallucinations: an fMRI study. Neurology 2004; **63**: 1409–16.

92 Meppelink AM, de Jong BM, Renken R, et al. Impaired visual processing preceding image recognition in Parkinson's disease patients with visual hallucinations. Brain 2009; **132**: 2980–93.

93 Ramírez-Ruiz B, Martí MJ, Tolosa E, et al. Brain response to complex visual stimuli in Parkinson's patients with hallucinations: a functional magnetic resonance imaging study. Mov Disord 2008; **23**: 2335–43.

94 Cardoso EF, Fregni F, Maia FM, et al. Abnormal visual activation in Parkinson's disease patients. Mov Disord 2010; **25**: 1590–6.

95 Ibarretxe-Bilbao N, Junque C, Marti MJ, Tolosa E. Cerebral basis of visual hallucinations in Parkinson's disease: structural and functional MRI studies. J Neurol Sci 2011; **310**: 79–81.

96 Nagano-Saito A, Washimi Y, Arahata Y, et al. Visual hallucination in Parkinson's disease with FDG PET. Mov Disord 2004; **19**: 801–6.

97 Oishi N, Udaka F, Kameyama M, et al. Regional cerebral blood flow in Parkinson disease with nonpsychotic visual hallucinations. Neurology 2005; **65**: 1708–15.

98 Boecker H, Ceballos-Baumann AO, Volk D, et al. Metabolic alterations in patients with Parkinson disease and visual hallucinations. Arch Neurol 2007; **64**: 984–8.

99 Ffytche DH, Howard RJ, Brammer MJ, et al. The anatomy of conscious vision: an fMRI study of visual hallucinations. Nat Neurosci 1998; **1**: 738–42.

100 **Adachi N, Watanabe T, Matsuda H, Onuma T.** Hyperperfusion in the lateral temporal cortex, the striatum and the thalamus during complex visual hallucinations: single photon emission computed tomography findings in patients with Charles Bonnet syndrome. Psychiat Clin Neurosci 2000; **54**: 157–62.

101 **Imamura T, Ishii K, Hirono N, et al.** Visual hallucinations and regional cerebral metabolism in dementia with Lewy bodies (DLB). NeuroReport 1999; **10**: 1903–7.

102 **Goetz CG, Ouyang B, Negron A, Stebbins GT.** Hallucinations and sleep disorders in PD: ten-year prospective longitudinal study. Neurology 2010; **75**: 1773–9.

103 **Pappert EJ, Goetz CG, Niederman FG, et al.** Hallucinations, sleep fragmentation, and altered dream phenomena in Parkinson's disease. Mov Disord 1999; **14**: 117–21.

104 **Whitehead DL, Davies AD, Playfer JR, Turnbull CJ.** Circadian rest–activity rhythm is altered in Parkinson's disease patients with hallucinations. Mov Disord 2008; **23**: 1137–45.

105 **Barnes J, Connelly V, Wiggs L, Boubert L, Maravic K.** Sleep patterns in Parkinson's disease patients with visual hallucinations. Int J Neurosci 2010; **120**: 564–9.

106 **Lee AH, Weintraub D.** Psychosis in Parkinson's disease without dementia: common and comorbid with other non-motor symptoms. Mov Disord 2012; **27**: 858–63.

107 **Schenck CH, Mahowald MW.** Delayed emergence of a parkinsonian disorder in 38% of 29 older males initially diagnosed with idiopathic REM sleep behavior disorder. Neurology 1996; **46**: 388–93.

108 **Iranzo A, Molinuevo JL, Santamaría J, et al.** Rapid-eye-movement sleep behavior disorder as an early marker for a neurodegenerative disorder: a descriptive study. Lancet Neurol 2006; **5**: 572–7.

109 **Vendette M, Gagnon JF, Décary A, et al.** REM sleep behavior disorder predicts cognitive impairment in Parkinson disease without dementia. Neurology 2007; **69**: 1843–9.

110 **Ferman TJ, Boeve BF, Smith GE, et al.** REM sleep behavior disorder and dementia: cognitive differences when compared with AD. Neurology 1999; **52**: 951–7.

111 **Terzaghi M, Sinforiani E, Zucchella C, et al.** Cognitive performance in REM sleep behaviour disorder: a possible early marker of neurodegenerative disease? Sleep Med 2007; **9**: 343–51.

112 **Pacchetti C, Manni R, Zangaglia R, et al.** Relationship between hallucinations, delusions, and rapid eye movement sleep behavior disorder in Parkinson's disease. Mov Disord 2005; **20**: 1439–48.

113 **Postuma RB, Bertrand JA, Montplaisir J, et al.** Rapid eye movement sleep behavior disorder and risk of dementia in Parkinson's disease: a prospective study Mov Disord 2012; **27**: 720–6.

114 **Lavault S, Leu-Semenescu S, Tezenas du Montcel S, et al.** Does clinical rapid eye movement behavior disorder predict worse outcomes in Parkinson's disease? J Neurol 2010; **257**: 1154–9.

115 **Comella CL, Tanner CM, Ristanovic RK.** Polysomnographic sleep measures in Parkinson's disease patients with treatment- induced hallucinations. Ann Neurol 1993; **34**: 710–14.

116 **Manni R, Terzaghi M, Ratti PL, et al.** Hallucinations and REM sleep behaviour disorder in Parkinson's disease: dream imagery intrusions and other hypotheses. Conscious Cogn 2011; **20**: 1021–6.

117 **D'Agostino A, De Gaspari D, Antonini A, et al.** Cognitive bizarreness in the dream and waking mentation of nonpsychotic patients with Parkinson's disease. J Neuropsychiatry Clin Neurosci 2010; **22**: 395–400.

118 **Bugalho P, Paiva T.** Dream features in the early stages of Parkinson's disease. J Neural Transm 2011; **118**: 1613–19.

119 **Fronczek R, Overeem S, Lee SY, et al.** Hypocretin (orexin) loss in Parkinson's disease. Brain 2007; **130**: 1577–85.

120 **Williams DR, Lees AJ.** Visual hallucinations in the diagnosis of idiopathic Parkinson's disease: a retrospective autopsy study. Lancet Neurol 2005; **4**: 605–10.

121 Uc EY, McDermott MP, Marder KS, et al. Incidence of and risk factors for cognitive impairment in an early Parkinson disease clinical trial cohort. Neurology 2009; **73**: 1469–77.

122 Biglan KM, Holloway RG, McDermott MP, Richard IH, Parkinson Study Group CALM-PD Investigators. Risk factors for somnolence, edema, and hallucinations in early Parkinson disease. Neurology 2007; **69**: 187–95.

123 Llebaria G, Pagonabarraga J, Martínez-Corral M, et al. Neuropsychological correlates of mild to severe hallucinations in Parkinson's disease. Mov Disord 2010; **25**: 2785–91.

124 Grossi D, Trojano L, Pellecchia MT, et al. Frontal dysfunction contributes to the genesis of hallucinations in non-demented parkinsonian patients. Int J Geriatr Psychiatry 2005; **20**: 1–6.

125 Ibarretxe-Bilbao N, Ramirez-Ruiz B, Junque C, et al. Differential progression of brain atrophy in Parkinson's disease with and without visual hallucinations. J Neurol Neurosurg Psychiatry 2010; **81**: 650–7.

126 Collerton D, Perry E, McKeith I. Why people see things that are not there: a novel perception and attention deficit model for recurrent visual hallucinations. Behav Brain Sci 2005; **28**: 737–57.

127 Diederich NJ, Goetz CG, Stebbins GT. Repeated visual hallucinations in Parkinson's disease as disturbed external/internal perceptions: focused review and a new integrative model. Mov Disord 2005; **20**: 130–40.

128 Gallagher DA, Parkkinen L, O'Sullivan SS, et al. Testing an aetiological model of visual hallucinations in Parkinson's disease. Brain 2011; **134**: 3299–309.

129 Shine JM, Halliday GM, Naismith SL, Lewis SJ. Visual misperceptions and hallucinations in Parkinson's disease: dysfunction of attentional control networks? Mov Disord 2011; **26**: 2154–9.

130 Northoff G, Qin P. How can the brain's resting state activity generate hallucinations? A 'resting state hypothesis' of auditory verbal hallucinations. Schizophr Res 2011; **127**: 202–14.

131 Onofrj M, Taylor JP, Monaco D, et al. Visual hallucinations in PD and Lewy body dementias: old and new hypotheses. Behav Neurol 2013; **27**: 479–93.

132 Goetz CG. Hallucinations in Parkinson's disease: the clinical syndrome. Adv Neurol 1999; **80**: 419–23.

133 Umemura A, Oka Y, Okita K, Matsukawa N, Yamada K. Subthalamic nucleus stimulation for Parkinson disease with severe medication-induced hallucinations or delusions. J Neurosurg 2011; **114**: 1701–5.

134 Goetz CG, Fan W, Leurgans S. Antipsychotic medication treatment for mild hallucinations in Parkinson's disease: positive impact on long-term worsening. Mov Disord 2008; **23**: 1541–5.

135 The Parkinson Study Group. Low-dose clozapine for the treatment of drug-induced psychosis in Parkinson's disease. N Engl J Med 1999; **340**: 757–63.

136 Pollak P, Tison F, Rascol O, et al. Clozapine in drug-induced psychosis in PD: a randomized placebo-controlled study with open follow-up. J Neurol Neurosurg Psychiatry 2004; **75**: 689–95.

137 Meco G, Bernardi S. Antidepressant use in treatment of psychosis with comorbid depression in Parkinson's disease. Prog Neuropsycholpharmacol Biol Psychiatry 2007; **31**: 311–13.

138 Lang AE, Sandor P, Duff J. Remoxipride in Parkinson's disease: differential response in patients with dyskinesias fluctuations versus psychosis. Clin Neuropharmacol 1995; **18**: 39–45.

139 Spieker S, Stetter F, Klockgether T. Zotepine in levodopa-induced psychosis. Mov Disord 1995; **10**: 795–6.

140 Wolters EC, Jansen ENH, Tuynman-Qua HG, Bergmans PLM. Olanzapine in the treatment of dopaminomimetic psychosis in patients with Parkinson's disease. Neurology 1996; **47**: 1085–7.

141 Zoldan J, Friedberg G, Weizman A, Melamed E. Ondansetron, a 5HT3 antagonist for visual hallucinations and paranoid delusional disorder associated with chronic L-dopa therapy in advanced Parkinson's disease. Adv Neurol 1996; **69**: 541–4.

142 Goetz CG, Blasucci LM, Leurgans S, Pappert EJ. Olanzapine and clozapine: comparative effects on motor function in hallucinating PD patients. Neurology 2000; **55**: 789–94.

143 Ondo WG, Levy HJ, Vuong K, Jankovic J. Olanzapine for the treatment of dopaminergic induced hallucinations. Mov Disord 2005; **20**: 958–63.

144 Rabey JM, Prokhorov T, Miniovitz A, et al. Effect of quetiapine in psychotic PD patients: a double blind labeled study of 3 months duration. Mov Disord 2007; **22**: 313–18.

145 Merims D, Balas M, Peretz C, et al. Rater-blinded, prospective comparison: quetiapine vs. clozapine for PD psychosis. Clin Neuropharmacol 2006; **29**: 331–7.

146 Juncos JL, Roberts VJ, Evatt ML, et al. Quetiapine improves psychotic symptoms and cognition in Parkinson's disease. Mov Disord 2004; **19**: 29–35.

147 Fernandez HH, Okun MS, Rodriguez RL, et al. Quetiapine improves visual hallucinations in Parkinson disease but not through normalization of sleep architecture: results from a double-blind clinical-polysomnography study. Int J Neurosci 2009; **119**: 2196–205.

148 Singh S, Wooltorton E. Increased mortality among elderly patients with dementia using atypical antipsychotics [abstract]. Can Med Assoc J 2005; **173**: 252.

149 Kurita A, Ochyiai Y, Kono Y, et al. The beneficial effect of donepezil on visual hallucinations in patients with Parkinson's disease. J Geriatr Psychiatry Neurol 2003; **16**: 184–8.

150 Sobow T. Parkinson's disease-related visual hallucinations unresponsive to atypical antipsychotics treated with cholinesterase inhibitors. Neurol Neurochir Pol 2007; **41**: 276–9.

151 Burn D, Emre M, McKeith I, et al. Effects of rivastigmine in patients with and without visual hallucinations in dementia associated with PD. Mov Disord 2006; **21**: 1899–907.

152 Emre M, Cummings JL, Lane RM. Rivastigmine in dementia associated with Parkinson's disease and Alzheimer's disease: similarities and differences. J Alzheimer's Dis 2007; **11**: 509–14.

153 Williams-Gray CH, Barker RA. Visual hallucinations predict increased benefits from rivastigmine in Parkinson's disease dementia. Nature Clin Pract Neurol 2007; **3**: 250–1.

154 Thomas AJ, Burn DJ, Rowan EN, et al. A comparison of the efficacy of donepezil in Parkinson's disease with dementia and dementia with Lewy bodies. Int J Geriatr Psychiatry 2005; **20**: 938–44.

155 Dubois B, Tolosa E, Katzenschlager R, et al. Donepezil in Parkinson's disease dementia: a randomized, double-blind efficacy and safety study. Mov Disord 2012; **27**: 1230–8.

156 Rabey JM. Hallucinations and psychosis in Parkinson's disease. Parkinsonism Relat Disord 2009; 15(Suppl 4): S105–S110.

157 Kometer M, Cahn BR, Andel D, Carter OL, Vollenweider FX. The 5-HT2A/1A agonist psilocybin disrupts modal object completion associated with visual hallucinations. Biol Psychiatry 2011; **69**: 399–406.

158 McFarland K, Price DL, Bonhaus DW. Pimavanserin, a 5-HT2A inverse agonist, reverses psychosis-like behaviors in a rodent model of Parkinson's disease. Behav Pharmacol 2011; **22**: 681–92.

159 Meltzer HY, Mills R, Revell S, et al. Pimavanserin, a serotonin(2A) receptor inverse agonist, for the treatment of Parkinson's disease psychosis. Neuropsychopharmacology 2010; **35**: 881–92.

160 Willis GL, Turner EJD. Primary and secondary features of Parkinson's disease improve with strategic exposure to bright light. Chronbiol Int 2007; **24**: 521–37.

161 Voon V, Lang AE. Antidepressants in the treatment of psychosis with comorbid depression in PD. Clin Neuropharmacol 2004; **27**: 90–2.

162 Meco G, Alessandri A, Guistini P, Vonifati V. Risperidone in levodopa-induced psychosis in advanced Parkinson's disease: an open-label, long-term study. Mov Disord 1997; **12**: 610–12.

163 Hirayama M, Nakamura T, Watanabe H, et al. Urinary 8-hydroxydeoxyguanosine correlate with hallucinations rather than motor symptoms in Parkinson's disease. Parkinsonism Relat Disord 2011; **17**: 46–9.

164 **Cheng D, Jenner AM, Shui G, et al**. Lipid pathway alterations in Parkinson's disease primary visual cortex. PLoS One 2011; **6**: e17299.

165 **Bailbé M, Korolewicz S, Neau JP**. Hallucinations, delusions, and nocturnal events in 152 Parkinson's patients. Rev Neurol 2002; **158**: 203–10.

166 **Schrag A, Ben-Shlomo Y, Quinn N**. How common are complications of Parkinson's disease? J Neurol 2002; **249**: 419–23.

167 **Williams DR, Warren JD, Lees AJ**. Using the presence of visual hallucinations to differentiate Parkinson's disease from atypical parkinsonism. J Neurol Neurosurg Psychiatry 2008; **79**: 652–5.

Chapter 13

Neurobiology of sleep: the role of dopamine in Parkinson's disease-related sleep disorders

Lynn Marie Trotti and David B. Rye

Introduction

Sleep problems are common and troubling for people with Parkinson's disease (PD). One survey found that 98% of respondents had some PD-related problems during the night or upon awakening, although not all subjects rated their overall sleep quality as poor [1]. Sleep problems in PD are not uniform, and not everything that patients may experience or report as sleepiness is truly an increased propensity to sleep. For example, a number of patients report fatigue that seems more related to their motor disability than to sleepiness per se [2]. However, genuine sleepiness is undeniably common in PD. Self-reported sleepiness or unintended sleep severe enough to interfere with activities of daily living occurs in 10–75% of PD patients [3]. The most common sleep complaints in PD are fragmented sleep, reduced sleep time, dream enactment, nocturia and nocturnal motor manifestations of PD, including stiffness, decreased ability to move and dystonia [4,5] (Table 13.1). Objective detailing of sleep in PD via polysomnography shows sleep fragmentation, poor sleep efficiency, rapid eye movement (REM) sleep behaviour disorder (RBD) or REM sleep without atonia (RWA) and periodic limb movements of sleep (PLMS) [5].

While specific sleep disorders and symptoms such as RBD, restless legs syndrome (RLS)/PLMS, sleep apnoea and excessive sleepiness are discussed in Chapters 14–16, this chapter will divide the sleep disorders of PD into those of excessive sleepiness and those of excessive nocturnal movement, and discuss the potential role of dopamine in their pathophysiology. There are five subtypes of seven transmembrane G-protein coupled dopamine receptors, named D1 to D5 [6]. These are traditionally divided into two classes, the D1-like receptors (consisting of the D1 and D5 molecularly defined receptors) and the D2-like receptors (i.e. the D2, D3 and D4 receptors). Activation of the D1-like receptors results in increased activity of glutamate receptors, calcium channels and cyclic adenosine monophosphate (cAMP) response element-binding proteins, with decreased activity of *gamma-aminobutyric acid* (GABA)-A receptors, sodium channels and the sodium–potassium ATPase [6]. Activation of D2-like receptors stimulates the G1 transduction pathway to decrease adenylylcylase and increases intracellular calcium [6]. In addition to post-synaptic

Table 13.1 Subjective and objective sleep disturbances in Parkinson's disease

Subjective patient reports:
- ◆ Sleepiness
- ◆ Fragmented sleep
- ◆ Short sleep time
- ◆ Dream enactment
- ◆ Stiffness/decreased ability to move/dystonia
- ◆ Nocturia

Objective findings:
- ◆ Sleep fragmentation/poor sleep efficiency
- ◆ Disorders of impaired thalamocortical arousal
  - – short sleep latency
  - – loss of sleep spindles
  - – loss of slow wave sleep
  - – intrusion of REM sleep into daytime naps (SOREMS)
- ◆ Disorders of excessive nocturnal movement:
  - – periodic limb movements of sleep (PLMS)
  - – REM sleep behaviour disorder (RBD)

effects, D2-like receptors are also found pre-synaptically on dopaminergic neurons, and are a critical source of autoinhibition of dopamine neurons [6].

There are several key dopaminergic pathways within the central nervous system. The nigrostriatal pathway is implicated in the primary motor manifestations of PD. The mesocorticolimbic dopamine system, which originates in the midbrain in the ventral tegmental area (VTA) and targets the nucleus accumbens, limbic system, hippocampus, prefrontal cortex and midline thalamic nuclei, is classically implicated in reward, abuse of illicit drugs and working memory, but may also prove important with respect to the sleepiness observed in PD [7]. The diencephalospinal pathway, originating in the A11 cell group of the hypothalamus and projecting to the spinal cord, may have particular relevance to nocturnal movement in PD, in the form of PLMS [7].

Excessive daytime sleepiness in Parkinson's disease

Excessive daytime sleepiness is reported by many patients with PD or their caregivers. While self-reported sleepiness is common, relying solely on self-reports may be problematic, as some patients with PD fail to appreciate the severity of their own objectively measured sleepiness [8]. Objective assessments of sleepiness are commonly captured using the Multiple Sleep Latency Test (MSLT), a standardized testing paradigm where subjects are given four or five 20-minute daytime opportunities to nap. A mean sleep latency of less than 5 minutes is considered strong evidence of excessive daytime sleepiness; sleep latencies of less than 8 minutes are required for the diagnosis of narcolepsy and idiopathic hypersomnia [9,10]. When measured by MSLT testing, 19–37% of PD patients who are not pre-selected for a complaint of sleepiness have mean sleep latencies of less than or equal to 5 minutes [2,8]. When considering only those parkinsonian patients who report sleepiness, the rates increase to 42–71% [11–13]. Daytime sleepiness can also be assessed using the Maintenance of Wakefulness Test (MWT). In this testing paradigm, patients are asked to remain awake in a dark and soporific environment for four 40-minute periods [9]. As in the MSLT, a substantial portion of PD patients show objective evidence of sleepiness when measured by the MWT, although the percentage identified by the MWT may be lower than that measured by the MSLT (26% versus 47%) [14]. Continuous electroencephalographic monitoring of PD patients also supports the presence of excessive sleep and daytime sleepiness, as manifested by frequent microsleeps, sleep attacks and intentional daytime naps [15].

Dissecting the pathophysiological basis of excessive daytime sleepiness in PD is difficult given the complicated effects of dopamine *in vivo*. There is an apparent paradox, in that the loss of endogenous dopamine in PD appears to contribute to sleepiness yet sleepiness has also been associated with administration of either dopamine agonists or dopamine antagonists (e.g. antipsychotics) [16]. It is becoming increasingly clear that in PD sleepiness is impacted by the effects of both drugs and the disease.

Sleepiness in Parkinson's disease: drug effects

Animal studies of dopaminergic medications have shown that both dose and receptor type modulate the effects of exogenous dopamine. Agonists of the D1-like receptors increase wakefulness and decrease REM sleep in rats [17,18]. The effects of D2-like receptor agonists are more complicated due to their ability to autoregulate via pre-synaptic autoreceptors; low doses of D2-like receptor agonists increase sleep (presumably by binding to the pre-synaptic receptors, which have a 10-fold higher affinity than post-synaptic receptors), while higher doses result in wakefulness [19–21]. However, this pattern of low doses promoting sleep and high doses promoting wakefulness observed in animal studies is not entirely consistent with clinical experience in PD patients.

In healthy human controls levodopa can be sedating. In one study, both levodopa and the benzodiazepine triazolam were more sedating than placebo, although the sleepiness emerging with daily doses of levodopa wore off over 11 days, while the effects of triazolam remained constant [22]. Ropinirole, a D2/D3 receptor agonist, was shown to decrease MSLT-measured sleep latency (i.e. it increased sleepiness) in 18 healthy volunteers, more so than did placebo [23]. An open-label study of the dopamine agonist apomorphine in healthy controls also showed a sedative effect [24].

Multiple studies have assessed the effects of prescribed dopaminergics on sleepiness in PD patients, although the heterogeneity of PD complicates such analyses. In a meta-analysis of clinical trials of dopamine agonists for the treatment of early PD, Stowe et al. [25] reported an odds ratio (OR) of 2.71 [95% confidence interval (CI) 2.09–3.50] for somnolence with non-ergot derived dopamine agonists. Considering individual dopamine agonists, the OR for somnolence from pramipexole was 2.16 (CI 1.53–3.03) and for ropinirole it was 3.75 (CI 2.52–5.59); the effect was larger in studies comparing dopamine agonists with placebo than in those comparing dopamine agonists with levodopa. Yet a very mixed picture regarding the association between sleepiness and levodopa equivalent dosage emerges from studies of sleepiness in clinic samples of PD. Some studies demonstrate an association and other studies show no effect [8,26–28]. Part of the discrepancy across studies may be explained by the use of a levodopa-equivalent score that assumes a similar effect of dopamine agonists and levodopa on sleepiness. Recently, a divergent effect of these two classes of medication on sleepiness has been described, such that higher doses of dopamine agonists worsened MWT-derived sleepiness metrics in PD patients, whereas higher doses of levodopa were associated with less sleepiness [26].

Sleepiness in Parkinson's disease: disease effects

Separate from the effects of dopaminergics on daytime alertness, it is also clear that sleepiness is intrinsic to PD in the untreated state. Three different population-based studies have demonstrated an association between measures of excessive sleepiness and the subsequent development of PD [29–31]. The consistent association in these three studies establishes that sleepiness precedes motor dysfunction in many patients with PD, and thus implicates the disease as the cause of sleepiness, rather than the subsequent treatment. Clinical studies of PD patients provide modest support for this hypothesis, with some, but not all, studies demonstrating worsening of sleepiness with longer disease duration [4,26–28]. More compelling support comes from animal models of parkinsonism that demonstrate sleepiness in the absence of dopaminergic medications. In particular, non-human primates given MPTP lesions (1-methyl-4-phenyl-1,2,3,6-tetrahydropyridine, a dopamine toxin) become parkinsonian and also develop excessive daytime sleepiness [32].

The role of dopamine in wake/sleep state control

Historically, the role of dopamine in alertness has been controversial. Early investigations into midbrain dopaminergic neurons revealed that they had stable group mean firing rates in both sleep and wake states, leading to the conclusion that dopamine was not important in state control [16]. However, further investigation has shown that burst firing is more important than mean firing rates in the release of synaptic dopamine, and that there are changes in the temporal pattern of firing of these neurons that vary with state [16]. Additionally, dopamine is known to modulate a variety of behaviours that only occur during the wake state, including movements, motivation, reward, cognition and feeding [6]. Anatomically, dopamine is ideally situated to affect state control. The midbrain dopaminergic neurons have inputs from multiple regions that receive important information about the external and internal environment that would be useful in regulating state. Specifically, the extended amygdala receives second-order chemoreceptor, baroreceptor and other visceral information from the nucleus of the solitary tract, and hypocretin-producing neurons receive information about levels of circulating glucose and insulin [7]. The pedunculopontine nucleus also provides input into the midbrain dopaminergic neurons and is known to promote the wake state and REM sleep [7]. Additionally, the axons of these dopaminergic neurons branch extensively and innervate multiple brain regions, a configuration that would allow them to coordinate behaviours of different brain regions and potentially state;

this pattern of branching looks similar to that of the output from the reticular activating system, which is also involved in state control [6].

Further evidence for the role of dopamine in contributing to wakefulness comes from studies of wake-promoting medications. Amphetamines increase wakefulness but have multiple sites of action, blocking plasma membrane transporters for dopamine, norepinephrine, serotonin and vesicular monoamines [33]. However, their ability to increase wakefulness is dependent on their affinity for the dopamine transporter (DAT), and DAT knockout mice do not have increased wakefulness in response to amphetamines [6,33]. In contrast, despite the effects of amphetamine on plasma norepinephrine transporters, cats with lesions of the locus coeruleus still show increased wakefulness when given amphetamines [33]. Similarly, dopamine uptake inhibitors increase wakefulness in normal and narcoleptic dogs, while selective norepinephrine uptake inhibitors do not [34]. Modafinil is a newer stimulant, thought perhaps to have its effect through norepinephrine, hypocretin or GABA [33]. However, DAT knockout mice do not have increased wakefulness in response to modafinil, suggesting a dopaminergic mode of action for this medication in maintaining wakefulness [33].

Dopamine and the two-process model of sleep/wake regulation

Sleep/wake regulation is thought to reflect the interaction of two processes: a circadian timing system and a homeostatic drive to sleep that increases as wake time increases [35]. Dysfunction of either component might contribute to the sleepiness experienced in PD. In animals, there is diurnal variation in expression of tyrosine hydroxylase (the rate-limiting step in dopamine synthesis), dopamine receptors and DAT [36]. Plasma dopamine levels in healthy men similarly show a circadian pattern, with lower levels during sleep [37]. At the molecular level, there are bidirectional relationships between dopamine and the clock genes that regulate circadian rhythmicity. In particular, expression of *PER1* and *PER2* may be affected by stimulation of striatal dopamine receptors, and *PER2* regulates striatal dopamine metabolism [38]. Rats given intracerebroventricular *6-hydroxydopamine* (6-OHDA; in combination with desipramine to prevent noradrenergic cell loss) show alterations in activity patterns, consistent with a disruption in circadian rhythms [39]. MPTP treatment in mice changes the rhythm of expression of several of the circadian clock genes [40]. Mice engineered to overexpress α-synuclein also show disruption of their circadian rhythms [39].

It might be expected, then, that PD patients would demonstrate alterations in circadian rhythmicity. This manifests as decreased diurnal variation of several markers of circadian rhythm, including melatonin and cortisol [38], as well as measured rest–activity cycles (i.e. with actigraphy) [41]. *BMAL1*, one of the genes regulating the circadian system, shows reduced expression in lymphocytes of PD patients [40]. In addition to these intrinsic effects, exogenous dopaminergic medications may also alter the rhythmicity of the circadian system, with a tendency to phase advance melatonin levels (i.e. to make sleep occur earlier) [38,41]. This might contribute to the sleepiness in PD, in that a phase advance would be expected to result in the major sleep period advancing into what was previously considered 'daytime' [4]. Although still preliminary, evidence suggests that light therapy might provide symptomatic benefit to some PD patients [38,41], but the optimal timing, dosage and duration of such therapy remains to be determined.

Clinical evidence suggests that the homeostatic sleep drive is also altered in patients with PD. In subjects with a normally functioning homeostatic sleep drive, poorer nocturnal sleep is associated with more daytime sleepiness, and better nocturnal sleep prevents daytime sleepiness. In contrast, while fragmented nocturnal sleep is a common problem in PD patients, multiple studies have shown that sleepiness and measured nocturnal sleep time or sleep efficiency are positively correlated (such that patients with the most nocturnal sleep also demonstrate the highest levels of daytime sleepiness) or unrelated [2,8,11,26,27]. These findings are contrary to what would be predicted if the homeostatic sleep drive were functioning in PD, although the molecular basis underlying this alteration remains to be fully defined.

Localization of the effect of dopamine on sleepiness

Some data indicate that sleepiness in PD is related to loss of nigrostratal dopamine function. In particular, subjective sleepiness in PD patients is inversely correlated to DAT binding within this pathway (striatum, caudate, putamen) during single-photon emission computed tomography (SPECT) scanning, at least in patients with Hoehn and Yahr Stage 2 disease [42]. Despite this, clinical experience with sleepy PD patients suggests that dopamine-mediated arousal may not be solely a function of this pathway. Excessive daytime sleepiness and motor disability are frequently, although not always, unrelated [2,8,26–28,42–45], suggesting a different progression of motor dysfunction and sleepiness. Further, injection of D2/D3 agonists, which typically cause sleepiness when given systemically, directly into the substantia nigra in a group of narcoleptic dogs did not increase sleepiness [46], as would be expected if this pathway mediated arousal.

Alternatively, it is possible that dopaminergic cell loss in the VTA or its targets (the prefrontal cortex, cholinergic magnocellular basal forebrain and midline thalamus) may mediate sleepiness in PD [5]. Administration of apomorphine into the VTA in rats increases sleep, whereas injection into the substantia nigra or caudate does not [47]. Injection of D2/D3 agonists into the VTA in narcoleptic dogs also increases drowsiness and sleep [46]. Injection of D2 receptor antagonists into the VTA blocks the sedative effects of administration of a systemic dopamine agonist in rats [47]. Injection of amphetamines into the medial basal forebrain, a target of the VTA, results in wakefulness in rats [48]. Thus, animal data suggest that this region may be relevant to PD-related sleepiness (see Fig. 13.1).

Because the generation of wakefulness is a process that is regulated by multiple neurotransmitters, non-dopaminergic cell loss might also contribute to sleepiness in PD. The hypocretin-containing neurons of the lateral hypothalamus are a particularly intriguing possibility as a site of impaired arousal in PD, because their loss gives rise to narcolepsy, the prototypical disorder of excessive daytime sleepiness. Analyses of hypocretin in the cerebrospinal fluid (CSF) of PD patients have been mixed in this regard, with several studies showing normal levels but others demonstrating low values in a subset of PD patients

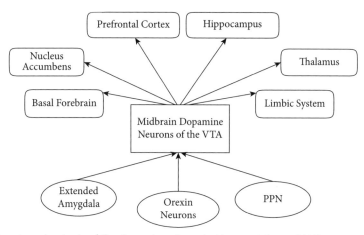

Fig. 13.1 Inputs and outputs of the dopaminergic ventral tegmental area (VTA) neurons. PPN, pedunculopontine nucleus.

[49–51]. More recently, Wienecke et al. [27] demonstrated normal hypocretin levels in patients with both early and advanced PD, but also noted a significant inverse relationship between objectively measured sleepiness and hypocretin levels ($r = 0.60$, $P = 0.02$) as well as a decrease in hypocretin levels over time in the two PD patients in whom it was measured serially. This suggests that hypocretin cell loss, while not as severe as that seen in narcolepsy, might contribute to sleepiness in PD.

Disorders of nocturnal movement in Parkinson's disease

Both subjective reports and polysomnographic monitoring have revealed that excess nocturnal movements are common in PD, raising the question of whether dopamine loss may underlie these movements. In general, the excessive nocturnal movements of PD appear clinically to be best controlled when daytime motor symptoms are also controlled [5]. In animal models, depletion of striatal dopamine in rats results in increased nocturnal movement [52] and in a non-human primate resulted in increased electromyogram (EMG) activity during REM sleep [53]. To fully assess the role of dopamine loss in nocturnal movement in PD, the two major causes of nocturnal movement will be considered separately.

Nocturnal movement in PD: periodic limb movements of sleep

PLMS are repetitive, periodic movements of the limbs, most commonly the legs, occurring during sleep. They may be seen in association with RLS, RBD or sleep-disordered breathing, but are also more common in PD patients than in age-matched controls or patients with other neurodegenerative diseases such as Alzheimer's [54]. Dopamine dysfunction has been implicated as a cause of PLMS in patients who have RLS rather than PD, in part because of the consistent clinical response of RLS/PLMS to treatment with dopaminergic medications [55]. The clinical response of RLS to dopaminergics is pronounced enough that a positive response is included as a supportive criterion for the diagnosis itself [56]. Further, dopamine antagonists (e.g. metoclopramide, prochlorperazine, antipsychotics) can unveil or exacerbate RLS symptoms [57]. In patients with PD, dopaminergic dysfunction as a cause of PLMS is suggested by the fact that the number of PLMS is correlated with PD disease severity and disease duration [58,59], and dopamine agonist therapy reduces the severity of PLMS in PD patients [58,60].

However, the dopaminergic pathway or pathways responsible for PLMS in PD patients have yet to be clearly defined. Happe et al. [61] found that the number of PLMS in PD patients was inversely correlated with striatal pre-synaptic DATs (as measured by SPECT). Despite this, deep brain stimulation of the subthalamic nucleus does not decrease PLMS counts [62,63]. Furthermore, functional imaging studies of the nigrostriatal pathway in idiopathic RLS/PLMS have not demonstrated consistent abnormalities [64], and it has been hypothesized that the smaller diencephalospinal dopamine pathway may underlie idiopathic RLS/PLMS, and possibly PLMS occurring in PD [7].

Nocturnal movement in Parkinson's disease: REM sleep behaviour disorder

In the case of RBD there are relatively robust associations between idiopathic RBD (i.e. RBD occurring without co-morbid neurodegenerative disease) and dopaminergic markers of disease progression. In PET studies of patients with idiopathic RBD, both striatal dopamine terminal and DAT binding are reduced, and serial imaging of the DAT shows a progressive decline in striatal tracer uptake over 3 years in patients more than in controls [65–67]. However, it is possible that this is a marker of the impending development of PD rather than a marker specific to idiopathic RBD. In PD patients, the amount of striatal dopamine denervation does not distinguish those with and without RBD, but rather those patients with RBD demonstrate greater cholinergic denervation (neocortical, limbic and thalamic) [68].

First-line treatments for RBD are non-dopaminergic (i.e. clonazepam and melatonin), and studies of dopaminergic treatments have shown inconsistent effects on RBD [69]. Three open-label studies or case series of RBD patients (who were predominantly idiopathic RBD patients, with only two of 33 total subjects having coexisting PD) demonstrated fewer nocturnal behaviours either by subjective report or polysomnography when treated with pramipexole [70–72]. In both polysomnographic studies, REM without atonia was unchanged, despite an improvement from pramipexole on RBD [71,72]. In contrast to this experience, levodopa administered to treatment-naïve PD patients increased phasic EMG activity, and levodopa dose may correlate with more RBD [58,73]. In PD patients with RBD on chronic levodopa therapy, the addition of pramipexole did not improve either subjective symptom report or polysomnographic measures of RBD severity [74]. As with PLMS, deep brain stimulation of the subthalamic nucleus does not reduce RBD or phasic EMG activity during REM [62,63]. PD patients with RBD do not typically appear parkinsonian during dream enactment behaviours, which has led Arnulf [75] to speculate that the generation of movements during RBD episodes, unlike waking movements, may bypass the basal ganglia entirely. Emerging models of the pathophysiology of RBD emphasize the critical importance of non-dopaminergic brainstem structures [75,76].

In summary, PD patients frequently exhibit disorders of excessive daytime somnolence and nocturnal movement. The sleepiness of PD is likely to be multifactorial, with contributions from both dopamine loss and exogenous dopaminergic medications, as well as other non-dopaminergic dysfunctions. Dopamine loss may also contribute to some forms of excessive nocturnal movement.

References

1 **Lees AJ, Blackburn NA, Campbell VL**. The nighttime problems of Parkinson's disease. Clin Neuropharmacol 1988; **11**: 512–19.

2 **Rye DB, Bliwise DL, Dihenia B, Gurecki P**. FAST TRACK: daytime sleepiness in Parkinson's disease. J Sleep Res 2000; **9**: 63–9.

3 **Rye DB**. Excessive daytime sleepiness and unintended sleep in Parkinson's disease. Curr Neurol Neurosci Rep 2006; **6**: 169–76.

4 **Ondo WG, Dat Vuong K, Khan H, Atassi F, Kwak C, Jankovic J**. Daytime sleepiness and other sleep disorders in Parkinson's disease. Neurology 2001; **57**: 1392–6.

5 **Rye DB, Iranzo A**. The nocturnal manifestations of waking movement disorders—focus on Parkinson's disease. In: C Guilleminault (ed.) Clinical neurophysiology of sleep disorders, pp. 263–72 New York: Elsevier, 2005.

6 **Freeman A, Rye D**. Dopamine in behavioral state control. In: C Sinton, P Perumal, J Monti (eds) The neurochemistry of sleep and wakefulness, pp. 179–223. Cambridge: Cambridge University Press, 2008.

7 **Rye DB**. The two faces of Eve: dopamine's modulation of wakefulness and sleep. Neurology 2004; **63**(Suppl 3): S2–S7.

8 **Razmy A, Lang AE, Shapiro CM**. Predictors of impaired daytime sleep and wakefulness in patients with Parkinson disease treated with older (ergot) vs newer (nonergot) dopamine agonists. Arch Neurol 2004; **61**: 97–102.

9 **Littner MR, Kushida C, Wise M, et al**. Practice parameters for clinical use of the multiple sleep latency test and the maintenance of wakefulness test. Sleep 2005; **28**: 113–21.

10 **American Academy of Sleep Medicine**. International classification of sleep disorders: diagnostic and coding manual (ICSD-2), 2nd edn. Westchester, IL: AASM, 2005.

11 **Roth T, Rye DB, Borchert LD, et al**. Assessment of sleepiness and unintended sleep in Parkinson's disease patients taking dopamine agonists. Sleep Med 2003; **4**: 275–80.

12 **Baumann C, Ferini-Strambi L, Waldvogel D, Werth E, Bassetti CL**. Parkinsonism with excessive daytime sleepiness—a narcolepsy-like disorder? J Neurol 2005; **252**: 139–45.

13 **Arnulf I, Konofal E, Merino-Andreu M, et al**. Parkinson's disease a sleepiness: an integral part of PD. Neurology 2002; **58**: 1019–24.

14 **Stevens S, Cormella CL, Stepanski EJ**. Daytime sleepiness and alertness in patients with Parkinson disease. Sleep 2004; **27**: 967–72.

15 **Pacchetti C, Martignoni E, Terzaghi M, et al**. Sleep attacks in Parkinson's disease: a clinical and polysomnographic study. Neurol Sci 2003; **24**: 195–6.

16 **Rye DB, Jankovic J**. Emerging views of dopamine in modulating sleep/wake state from an unlikely source: PD. Neurology 2002; **58**: 341–6.

17 **Trampus M, Ferri N, Monopoli A, Ongini E**. The dopamine D1 receptor is involved in the regulation of REM sleep in the rat. Eur J Pharmacol 1991; **194**: 189–94.

18 Monti JM, Fernandez M, Jantos H. Sleep during acute dopamine D1 agonist SKF 38393 or D1 antagonist SCH 23390 administration in rats. Neuropsychopharmacology 1990; **3**: 153–62.

19 Monti JM, Jantos H, Fernandez M. Effects of the selective dopamine D-2 receptor agonist, quinpirole on sleep and wakefulness in the rat. Eur J Pharmacol 1989; **169**: 61–6.

20 Monti JM, Hawkins M, Jantos H, D'Angelo L, Fernandez M. Biphasic effects of dopamine D-2 receptor agonists on sleep and wakefulness in the rat. Psychopharmacology 1988; **95**: 395–400.

21 Lagos P, Scorza C, Monti JM, et al. Effects of the D3 preferring dopamine agonist pramipexole on sleep and waking, locomotor activity and striatal dopamine release in rats. Eur Neuropsychopharmacol 1998; **8**: 113–20.

22 Andreu N, Chale JJ, Senard JM, Thalamas C, Montastruc JL, Rascol O. L-Dopa-induced sedation: a double-blind cross-over controlled study versus triazolam and placebo in healthy volunteers. Clin Neuropharmacol 1999; **22**: 15–23.

23 Ferreira JJ, Galitzky M, Thalamas C, et al. Effect of ropinirole on sleep onset: a randomized, placebo-controlled study in healthy volunteers. Neurology 2002; **58**: 460–2.

24 Bassi S, Albizzati MG, Frattola L, Passerini D, Trabucchi M. Dopamine receptors and sleep induction in man. J Neurol Neurosurg Psychiatry 1979; **42**: 458–60.

25 Stowe RL, Ives NJ, Clarke C, et al. Dopamine agonist therapy in early Parkinson's disease. Cochrane Database Syst Rev 2008; CD006564.

26 Bliwise DL, Trotti LM, Wilson AG, et al. Daytime alertness in Parkinson's disease: potentially dose-dependent, divergent effects by drug class. Mov Disord 2012; **27**: 1118–24.

27 Wienecke M, Werth E, Poryazova R, et al. Progressive dopamine and hypocretin deficiencies in Parkinson's disease: is there an impact on sleep and wakefulness? J Sleep Res 2012; **21**: 710–17.

28 Tan EK, Lum SY, Fook-Chong SM, et al. Evaluation of somnolence in Parkinson's disease: comparison with age- and sex-matched controls. Neurology 2002; **58**: 465–8.

29 Chen H, Schernhammer E, Schwarzschild MA, Ascherio A. A prospective study of night shift work, sleep duration, and risk of Parkinson's disease. Am J Epidemiol 2006; **163**: 726–30.

30 Gao J, Huang X, Park Y, et al. Daytime napping, nighttime sleeping, and Parkinson disease. Am J Epidemiol 2011; **173**: 1032–8.

31 Abbott RD, Ross GW, White LR, et al. Excessive daytime sleepiness and subsequent development of Parkinson disease. Neurology 2005; **65**: 1442–6.

32 Barraud Q, Lambrecq V, Forni C, et al. Sleep disorders in Parkinson's disease: the contribution of the MPTP non-human primate model. Exp Neurol 2009; **219**: 574–82.

33 Wisor JP, Nishino S, Sora I, Uhl GH, Mignot E, Edgar DM. Dopaminergic role in stimulant-induced wakefulness. J Neurosci 2001; **21**: 1787–94.

34 Nishino S, Mao J, Sampathkumaran R, Shelton J. Increased dopaminergic transmission mediates the wake-promoting effects of CNS stimulants. Sleep Res Online 1998; **1**: 49–61.

35 Borbely AA. A two process model of sleep regulation. Hum Neurobiol 1982; **1**: 195–204.

36 McClung CA. Circadian rhythms, the mesolimbic dopaminergic circuit, and drug addiction. Sci World J 2007; **7**: 194–202.

37 Sowers JR, Vlachakis N. Circadian variation in plasma dopamine levels in man. J Endocrinol Invest 1984; **7**: 341–5.

38 Rutten S, Vriend C, van den Heuvel OA, Smit JH, Berendse HW, van der Werf YD. Bright light therapy in Parkinson's disease: an overview of the background and evidence. Parkinson's Dis 2012; **2012**: 767105.

39 McDowell K, Chesselet MF. Animal models of the non-motor features of Parkinson's disease. Neurobiol Dis 2012; **46**: 597–606.

40 Hayashi A, Matsunaga N, Okazaki H, et al. A disruption mechanism of the molecular clock in a MPTP mouse model of Parkinson's disease. Neuromol Med 2013; **15**: 238–51.

41 Videnovic A, Golombek D. Circadian and sleep disorders in Parkinson's disease. Exp Neurol 2013; **243**: 45–56.

42 Happe S, Baier PC, Helmschmied K, Meller J, Tatsch K, Paulus W. Association of daytime sleepiness with nigrostriatal dopaminergic degeneration in early Parkinson's disease. J Neurol 2007; **254**: 1037–43.

43 Brodsky MA, Godbold J, Roth T, Olanow CW. Sleepiness in Parkinson's disease: a controlled study. Mov Disord 2003; **18**: 668–72.

44 Hobson DE, Lang AE, Martin WR, Razmy A, Rivest J, Fleming J. Excessive daytime sleepiness and sudden-onset sleep in Parkinson disease: a survey by the Canadian Movement Disorders Group. J Am Med Assoc 2002; **287**: 455–63.

45 Pal S, Bhattacharya KF, Agapito C, Chaudhuri KR. A study of excessive daytime sleepiness and its clinical significance in three groups of Parkinson's disease patients taking pramipexole, cabergoline and levodopa mono and combination therapy. J Neural Transm 2001; **108**: 71–7.

46 Honda K, Riehl J, Mignot E, Nishino S. Dopamine D3 agonists into the substantia nigra aggravate cataplexy but do not modify sleep. NeuroReport 1999; **10**: 3717–24.

47 Bagetta G, De Sarro G, Priolo E, Nistico G. Ventral tegmental area: site through which dopamine D2-receptor agonists evoke behavioural and electrocortical sleep in rats. Br J Pharmacol 1988; **95**: 860–6.

48 Berridge CW, O'Neil J, Wifler K. Amphetamine acts within the medial basal forebrain to initiate and maintain alert waking. Neuroscience 1999; **93**: 885–96.

49 Drouot X, Moutereau S, Nguyen J, et al. Low levels of ventricular CSF orexin/hypocretin in advanced PD. Neurology 2003; **61**: 540–3.

50 Overeem S, van Hilten JJ, Ripley B, Mignot E, Nishino S, Lammers GJ. Normal hypocretin-1 levels in Parkinson's disease patients with excessive daytime sleepiness. Neurology 2002; **58**: 498–9.

51 Baumann C, Dauvilliers Y, Mignot E, Bassetti C. Normal CSF hypocretin-1 (orexin A) levels in dementia with Lewy bodies associated with excessive daytime sleepiness. Eur Neurol 2004; **52**: 73–6.

52 Decker MJ, Keating GL, Freeman AA, Rye DB. Parkinsonian-like sleep-wake architecture in rats with bilateral striatal 6-OHDA lesions. Soc Neurosci Abstr 2000; **26**: 1514.

53 Daley JT, Turner RS, Bliwise DL, Rye DB. Nocturnal sleep in daytime alertness in the MPTP-treated primate. Sleep 1999; 22(Suppl): S218–S219.

54 Bliwise DL, Trotti LM, Yesavage JA, Rye DB. Periodic leg movements in sleep in elderly patients with Parkinsonism and Alzheimer's disease. Eur J Neurol 2012; **19**: 918–23.

55 Scholz H, Trenkwalder C, Kohnen R, Riemann D, Kriston L, Hornyak M. Dopamine agonists for restless legs syndrome. Cochrane Database Syst Rev 2011; CD006009.

56 Allen RP, Picchietti D, Hening WA, Trenkwalder C, Walters AS, Montplaisi J. Restless legs syndrome: diagnostic criteria, special considerations, and epidemiology. A report from the restless legs syndrome diagnosis and epidemiology workshop at the National Institutes of Health. Sleep Med 2003; **4**: 101–19.

57 Earley CJ, Allen RP, Beard JL, Connor JR. Insight into the pathophysiology of restless legs syndrome. J Neurosci Res 2000; **62**: 623–8.

58 Sixel-Doring F, Trautmann E, Mollenhauer B, Trenkwalder C. Age, drugs, or disease: what alters the macrostructure of sleep in Parkinson's disease? Sleep Med 2012; **13**: 1178–83.

59 Poewe W, Hogl B. Akathisia, restless legs, and periodic limb movements in sleep in Parkinson's disease Neurology 2004; 63(Suppl 3): S12–S16.

60 Hogl B, Rothdach A, Wetter TC, Trenkwalder C. The effect of cabergoline on sleep, periodic leg movements in sleep, and early morning motor function in patients with Parkinson's disease. Neuropsychopharmacology 2003; **28**: 1866–70.

61 **Happe S, Pirker W, Klosch G, Sauter C, Zeitlhofer J**. Periodic leg movements in patients with Parkinson's disease are associated with reduced striatal dopamine transporter binding. J Neurol 2003; **250**: 83–6.

62 **Iranzo A, Valldeoriola F, Santamaria J, Tolosa E, Rumia J**. Sleep symptoms and polysomnographic architecture in advanced Parkinson's disease after chronic bilateral subthalamic stimulation. J Neurol Neurosurg Psychiatry 2002; **72**: 661–4.

63 **Arnulf I, Bejjani BP, Garma L, et al**. Improvement of sleep architecture in PD with subthalamic nucleus stimulation. Neurology 2000; **55**: 1732–4.

64 **Trotti LM, Rye DB**. Restless legs syndrome. Handb Clin Neurol 2011; **100**: 661–73.

65 **Albin RL, Koeppe RA, Chervin RD, et al**. Decreased striatal dopaminergic innervation in REM sleep behavior disorder. Neurology 2000; **55**: 1410–12.

66 **Eisensehr I, Linke R, Noachtar S, Schwarz J, Gildehaus FJ, Tatsch K**. Reduced striatal dopamine transporters in idiopathic rapid eye movement sleep behaviour disorder. Comparison with Parkinson's disease and controls. Brain 2000; **123**: 1155–60.

67 **Iranzo A, Valldeoriola F, Lomena F, et al**. Serial dopamine transporter imaging of nigrostriatal function in patients with idiopathic rapid-eye-movement sleep behaviour disorder: a prospective study. Lancet Neurol 2011; **10**: 797–805.

68 **Kotagal V, Albin RL, Muller ML, et al**. Symptoms of rapid eye movement sleep behavior disorder are associated with cholinergic denervation in Parkinson disease. Ann Neurol 2012; **71**: 560–8.

69 **Trotti LM**. REM sleep behaviour disorder in older individuals: epidemiology, pathophysiology and management. Drugs Aging 2010; **27**: 457–70.

70 **Schmidt MH, Koshal VB, Schmidt HS**. Use of pramipexole in REM sleep behavior disorder: results from a case series. Sleep Med 2006; **7**: 418–23.

71 **Fantini ML, Gagnon JF, Filipini D, Montplaisir J**. The effects of pramipexole in REM sleep behavior disorder. Neurology 2003; **61**: 1418–20.

72 **Sasai T, Inoue Y, Matsuura M**. Effectiveness of pramipexole, a dopamine agonist, on rapid eye movement sleep behavior disorder. Tohoku J Exp Med 2012; **226**: 177–81.

73 **Garcia-Borreguero D, Caminero AB, De La Llave Y, et al**. Decreased phasic EMG activity during rapid eye movement sleep in treatment-naive Parkinson's disease: effects of treatment with levodopa and progression of illness. Mov Disord 2002; **17**: 934–41.

74 **Kumru H, Iranzo A, Carrasco E, et al**. Lack of effects of pramipexole on REM sleep behavior disorder in Parkinson disease. Sleep 2008; **31**: 1418–21.

75 **Arnulf I**. REM sleep behavior disorder: motor manifestations and pathophysiology. Mov Disord 2012; **27**: 677–89.

76 **Boeve BF, Silber MH, Saper CB, et al**. Pathophysiology of REM sleep behaviour disorder and relevance to neurodegenerative disease. Brain 2007; **130**: 2770–88.

Chapter 14

Rapid eye movement sleep behaviour disorder in Parkinson's disease

Alex Iranzo and Eduard Tolosa

Introduction: definition and importance of rapid eye movement sleep behaviour disorder

Rapid eye movement (REM) sleep behaviour disorder (RBD) is characterized by dream-enacting behaviours (e.g. punching, shouting, jumping out of bed, etc.) linked to unpleasant dreams (e.g. being attacked or robbed) and excessive electromyographic activity during REM sleep [1–3]. Accurate diagnosis of RBD requires a history of abnormal sleep behaviours and nocturnal video-polysomnographic (VPSG) demonstration of prominent tonic and/or phasic electromyographic activity associated with abnormal vocal and motor manifestations in REM sleep [1]. VPSG is required because dream-enacting behaviours resembling those typically seen in RBD may occur in people affected by obstructive sleep apnoea, periodic limb movement disorder, visual hallucinations, isolated nightmares, confusional awakenings in demented subjects and more rarely by somnambulism and nocturnal epilepsy. One study showed that patients with Parkinson's disease (PD), particularly when associated with dementia, had non-RBD episodes of sleep-enactment behaviours occurring upon arousals from either REM or non-REM sleep [4].

The pathophysiology of RBD is thought to be related to dysfunction of the brainstem REM sleep centres (e.g. the locus subcoeruleus nucleus in the pons and the magnocellularis nucleus in the medulla) and their anatomical connections (e.g. amygdala, pallidum, neocortex) [5]. Available data indicate that there is no strong evidence indicating that RBD is caused by dopaminergic deficiency alone, and that it is probably the result of a complex neurotransmitter dysfunction involving GABA-ergic, glutamatergic and monoaminergic systems and networks in the brainstem nuclei that inhibit muscle activation during REM sleep. RBD may be idiopathic (IRBD) or secondary to neurological diseases, particularly the synucleinopathies of PD, dementia with Lewy bodies (DLB) and multiple system atrophy (MSA). Most subjects with IRBD will develop the classic motor and cognitive symptoms of one of these three neurodegenerative diseases after several years of follow-up [6–10], particularly those individuals with hyposmia and subclinical damage of the substantia nigra demonstrated by dopamine transporter imaging and transcranial sonography. RBD occurs in 25–58% of PD patients, pre-dating the onset of parkinsonism by several years in about 20% [11–20]. Less frequently RBD may be present in subjects with focal brainstem lesions, narcolepsy, Machado–Joseph disease, Guadeloupean parkinsonism, progressive supranuclear palsy and Alzheimer's disease [1,2]. RBD in PD is associated with the rigid–akinetic motor subtype, older age, male predominance, autonomic dysfunction and an increased risk of developing dementia over time. This suggests that the presence of RBD in PD predicts the development of widespread neuropathological changes in the brain. In this chapter we review the clinical and pathophysiological relevance of RBD in PD.

RBD as a predictor of PD

Idiopathic RBD occurs when patients with confirmed RBD have no known neurological diseases, no cognitive complaints and RBD is not explained by the introduction or withdrawal of any medication or substance. The following data, however, indicate that iRBD is not an isolated parasomnia and that in the majority of cases it represents the prelude of a neurodegenerative disease such as PD. First, the only two IRBD subjects examined neuropathologically to date (April 2014) had the pathological hallmarks of PD, namely brainstem neuronal cell loss and Lewy bodies involving the substantia nigra [21,22]. Second, the following abnormalities have been identified in subjects with iRBD: olfactory deficits [23,24], impairment of colour vision [24], subclinical cognitive abnormalities on neuropsychological testing, subtle cortical electroencephalographic slowing, dysautonomic abnormalities, reduced cardiac ^{123}I-labelled metaiodobenzyguanidine (MIBG) scintigraphy, decreased dopamine transporters in the striatum and increased echogenicity of the substantia nigra [25,26] (Table 14.1). All these disturbances are characteristic features of sporadic PD.

Table 14.1 Clinical and subclinical abnormalities in idiopathic REM sleep behaviour disorder

- Reduced arm swinging
- Facial akinesia
- Depression
- Impaired olfaction
- Colour vision impairment
- Asymptomatic cognitive abnormalities on cognitive tests, especially in the executive, memory and visuospatial domains
- Cortical electroencephalographic slowing
- Orthostatic hypotension
- Systolic blood pressure drop
- Decreased beat-to-beat variability in the cardiac rhythm
- Constipation
- Reduced post-prandial ghrelin response
- Urinary symptoms
- Erectile symptoms
- Episodes of acute psychosis after minor or major surgery
- Reduced cardiac scintigraphy ^{123}I-MIBG
- Decreased dopamine transporter in the striatum, particularly in the left putamen
- Substantia nigra hyper-echogenicity
- Brainstem changes in diffusion tensor imaging
- Decreased cortical and increased pontine perfusion

Third, longitudinal studies from three different groups have shown that subjects with iRBD eventually develop a synucleinopathy. In the study by Schenck et al. [6], parkinsonism developed in 11 of 29 (38%) subjects with IRBD nearly 4 years after their diagnosis and at a mean interval of nearly 13 years after the onset of RBD symptoms. After 16 additional years of follow-up, 21 IRBD patients from the original cohort developed PD, DLB or MSA [7]. In the series reported by Postuma et al. [8], 26 of 93 (28%) IRBD patients developed a neurological disorder over a mean follow-up period of 5 years. Fourteen developed PD, seven DLB, one MSA and four isolated dementia. In a study conducted in our institution, 20 of 44 (45%) IRBD patients [3] developed a defined neurodegenerative syndrome after a mean follow-up of 5 years [9]. Emerging disorders were PD, DLB and less frequently MSA and mild cognitive impairment (MCI). We found that patients who developed a motor or cognitive disorder were those with a longer clinical follow-up. This suggested that the conversion rate toward these disorders would be increased with extended follow-up. To test this hypothesis, in a subsequent study we aimed to determine the frequency and nature of the neurodegenerative syndromes that emerged in our original cohort after 7 years of additional follow-up. Of the 44 subjects from the original cohort diagnosed with VPSG between 1991 and 2003, 36 (82%) developed a defined neurodegenerative syndrome [10]. Sixteen patients were diagnosed with PD, 14 with DLB, one with MSA and five with MCI. The rates of neurological disease-free survival from IRBD diagnosis at our centre were 65.2% at 5 years, 26.6% at 10 years and 7.5% at 14 years. Of the four remaining disease-free individuals who underwent neuroimaging and olfactory tests, all four had decreased striatal dopamine transporter uptake, one had hyper-echogenicity of the substantia nigra on transcranial sonography and two had impaired olfaction on smell tests. In three patients, the ante-mortem diagnoses of PD and DLB were confirmed by neuropathological examination showing widespread Lewy bodies in the brain and α-synuclein aggregates in the peripheral autonomic nervous system in one of them. In these three cases, neuronal loss and Lewy body pathology were found in the substantia nigra and in brainstem nuclei that regulate REM sleep atonia. Thus, the majority of individuals with IRBD from our cohort developed a synucleinopathy disorder with time. Subjects who remained disease-free at follow-up showed markers of increased short-term risk for developing PD and DLB in IRBD, such as decreased striatal dopamine transporter binding and hyposmia. To confirm these results, we estimated the risk of developing a neurodegenerative syndrome in all the 174 IRBD subjects diagnosed in our centre with VPSG between November 1991 and July 2013 after a median follow-up of 4 years. We found that the risk of a defined neurodegenerative syndrome from the time of IRBD diagnosis was 33.1% at 5 years, 75.7% at 10 years and 90.9% at 14 years. The median conversion time was 7.5 years. There were emerging diagnoses (37.4%) of DLB in 29 subjects, PD in 22, MSA in 2 and MCI in 12. In six cases, in whom post mortem was performed, neuropathological examination disclosed neuronal loss and widespread Lewy-type pathology in the brain in each case [27].

These data challenge the current diagnostic criteria of PD based exclusively on the clinical presence of parkinsonism. Of note, a patient from our institution presented with IRBD and during a 10-year follow-up he developed constipation, hyposmia, depression, MCI and abnormal dopamine transporter imaging but neither parkinsonism nor dementia. Post-mortem examination demonstrated neuronal loss and Lewy body pathology in the peripheral autonomic nervous system (e.g. the cardiac and myenteric plexus), olfactory bulb, medulla, pons, substantia nigra pars compacta (estimated cell loss of 20–30%), nucleus basalis of Meynert and amygdala, sparing the neocortex [28].

Several longitudinal studies have determined which factors are linked to short development of PD and other neurodegenerative disorders in subjects diagnosed with iRBD. These studies have shown that IRBD individuals with hyposmia [24] and subclinical damage of the substantia nigra demonstrated by dopamine transporter imaging and transcranial sonography [25] have an increased short-term risk of developing a synucleinopathy. This may be of great interest for the design of future clinical trials before the onset of parkinsonism. Longitudinal ^{123}I-FP-CIT single-photon emission computed tomography (SPECT) could be used to monitor the progression of nigrostriatal deficits in patients with iRBD, and could be useful in studies of potential disease-modifying compounds in these patients. In contrast, serial olfactory evaluation [24,29] and transcranial sonography of the substantia nigra shows no worsening with time.

Taken together, available data indicate that IRBD represents the prodromal phase of the synucleinopathies and that it is an optimal target for testing disease-modyfing agents before the development of parkinsonism and dementia.

RBD in PD

RBD occurs in 25–58% of patients with sporadic PD, pre-dating the onset of parkinsonism by several years in about 20% of them [11–20]. RBD may precede parkinsonism or may develop concomitantly with or after the onset of parkinsonism [19,20]. In one study involving 27 PD patients affected with RBD, parkinsonism preceded RBD in six. PD patients in whom RBD developed with or after parkinsonism showed more severe parkinsonism, longer disease duration and higher dopaminergic therapy [18]. RBD is seen in 25–30% of drug naïve newly diagnosed PD patients. RBD occurs in sporadic PD patients whether treated or untreated with dopaminergic agents [11–20] (Table 14.2–14.4). RBD confirmed by polysomnography (PSG) may also occur in patients with PD linked to *PARK2* mutations, but in this condition RBD-related clinical manifestations are usually mild. RBD was not detected in one *PARK6* family, an autosomal recessive disorder that manifests as early-onset PD with a particularly mild progression.

Characteristics of RBD in subjects with PD

RBD-related motor and vocal behaviours in PD are generally identical to those described in IRBD, and include gesturing, elaborated pseudo-purposeful behaviours, punching, kicking, biting, knocking over the bedside table, jumping out of bed, sitting on the bed, whispering, talking, shouting, swearing, crying, laughing and singing [1–3,14]. As a consequence, patients and bed partners may be injured. One study showed that in subjects with PD a report of sleep-related falling out of bed was clinically suggestive of RBD [30].

Table 14.2 Demographic and clinical findings in 231 RBD patients with MSA, DLB, PD and the idiopathic form seen at our sleep centre. RBD was confirmed by VPSG in all subjects

	MSA (*n* = 67)	DLB (*n* = 17)	PD (*n* = 65)	IRBD (*n* = 102)
Male (%)	56.7	94.1	70.8	86.3
Age at diagnosis of RBD (years)	61.5 ± 7.9	74.2 ± 6.5	65.8 ± 7.5	68.4 ± 6.7
Age at RBD onset (years)	54.7 ± 10.2	65.3 ± 11.8	61.0 ± 7.7	61.0 ± 8.8
RBD duration (years)	7.3 ± 6.9	8.9 ± 10.4	4.6 ± 4.0	7.2 ± 7.2
Age at disease onset (years)	57.1 ± 8.2	71.7 ± 8.4	56.2 ± 9.7	NA
Duration of disease (years)	4.4 ± 2.7	3.2 ± 4.4	9.6 ± 6.0	NA
RBD preceding disease onset (%)	52.2	100.0	18.5	NA

n, number of subjects; RBD, rapid eye movement sleep behaviour disorder; MSA, multiple system atrophy; DLB, dementia with Lewy bodies; PD, Parkinson's disease; iRBD, idiopathic RBD; VPSG, video-polysomnography; NA, not applicable.

In a study involving PD patients without dementia with RBD, VPSG analysis and bed partners' reports demonstrated alleviation of parkinsonism during elaborated and complex RBD episodes. Movements during RBD episodes were faster, stronger and smoother than those seen when the PD patient was awake. In the same manner, speech during RBD was more intelligible, better articulated and louder than during wakefulness [12].

Recalled dreams commonly have a negative emotional content, including being attacked, robbed or chased by unfamiliar people for unknown reasons. Other common nightmares are being frightened or attacked by animals (snakes, insects, dogs, lions, donkeys) and falling from a cliff. A few patients recall funny dreams that are associated with smiling and laughing during sleep. However, about 14% of RBD patients do not recall fearful dreams [14].

When the diagnosis of RBD is based on clinical history alone or on questionnaires, the prevalence of RBD in PD varies from 15 to 55% [31–40]. This is somewhat lower than the 25–58% figure [11–20] which is reported when diagnosis of RBD is performed using clinical and VPSG diagnostic criteria.

Several studies using VPSG criteria have evaluated the frequency and characteristics of RBD in consecutive PD patients. It has been shown that some PD patients undergoing PSG exhibit increased muscle tone during REM sleep without motor and vocal manifestations. This subclinical situation has been termed REM sleep without atonia, and its clinical significance is still unknown. One study involving 45 patients without dementia found that 18 (40%) showed either RBD (in six men and one woman; 16%) or subclinical REM sleep without atonia (in six men and five women; 24%). Patients with REM sleep disturbances had longer disease duration, more severe stage of the disease and were treated with a higher dose of dopaminergic agents [11]. In another study, 33 non-depressed patients without dementia or hallucinations with a mild to moderate stage of PD were evaluated. Nineteen (58%) had REM sleep without submental atonia. Of these, 11 (33%, ten men and one woman, nine treated with dopaminergic agents and two untreated) were symptomatic.

Table 14.3 Findings of reported dream content and witnessed abnormal behaviours in 231 RBD patients with MSA, DLB, PD and the idiopathic form seen at our sleep centre. RBD was confirmed by PSG in all subjects

	MSA (*n* = 67)	DLB (*n* = 17)	PD (*n* = 65)	iRBD (*n* = 102)
Self-awareness of behaviours (%)	23.9	29.4	35.4	53.9
Unpleasant dream recall (%)	65.7	82.4	86.2	92.1
Most frequent unpleasant dreams				
Attacked by someone (%)	38.8	64.7	67.7	84.3
Arguing with someone (%)	35.8	41.2	53.1	58.8
Chased by someone (%)	35.8	47.1	53.8	52.9
Falling from a cliff (%)	29.9	11.8	44.6	48.0
Attacked by animals (%)	26.9	29.4	32.3	42.2
Most frequent abnormal behaviours				
Talking (%)	89.6	94.1	95.4	96.1
Shouting (%)	79.1	82.4	89.2	89.2
Swearing (%)	26.9	23.5	29.2	33.3
Crying (%)	52.2	41.2	49.2	42.2
Laughing (%)	61.2	52.9	47.7	54.9
Singing (%)	13.4	0	13.8	17.6
Punching (%)	73.1	64.7	69.2	83.3
Kicking (%)	56.7	41.2	66.2	78.4
Falling out of bed (%)	46.3	82.4	38.5	77.5
Patient injured (%)	13.4	41.2	15.4	55.9
Bed partners injured (%)	6.0	5.9	10.8	23.5
Treatment?				
Treatment with clonazepam (%)	29.9	35.3	46.2	65.7
Dose of clonazepam (mg/day)	0.58 ± 0.20	0.90 ± 0.65	0.66 ± 0.35	0.94 ± 0.93

n, number of subjects; RBD, rapid eye movement sleep behaviour disorder; MSA, multiple system atrophy; DLB, dementia with Lewy bodies; PD, Parkinson's disease; iRBD, idiopathic RBD; PSG, polysomnography.

The remaining eight were either unaware of their abnormal nocturnal behaviours or REM sleep without atonia was not associated with abnormal clinical manifestations on VPSG. RBD and REM sleep without atonia was more frequent in males than in females. Differences between patients with and without RBD were not reported in this study [17]. In another study, 41 of 51 consecutive patients without dementia undergoing VPSG had RBD. RBD occurred before (22%), at the same time as (23%) or after (55%) the onset of parkinsonism. VPSG demonstrated somnambulism in one patient reporting typical symptoms of RBD. VPSG demonstrated RBD in six asymptomatic patients. A longer duration of parkinsonism was the only variable that distinguished these 41 PD patients with RBD from

Table 14.4 Polysomnographic findings in 231 RBD patients with MSA, DLB, PD and the idiopathic form seen at our sleep centre. RBD was confirmed by VPSG in all subjects

	MSA (*n* = 67)	DLB (*n* = 17)	PD (*n* = 45)	iRBD (*n* = 102)
Sleep efficiency (%)	64.2 ± 16.0	74.9 ± 10.8	65.9 ± 17.0	73.9 ± 12.8
Total sleep time (min)	285.4 ± 74.0	346.5 ± 52.5	309 ± 91.8	340.5 ± 68.4
Sleep onset latency (min)	34.3 ± 33.4	36.6 ± 40.0	21.7 ± 21.4	25.5 ± 21.5
Arousal index	22.1 ± 13.3	27.7 ± 20.5	25.4 ± 17.6	23.3 ± 13.9
N1 sleep stage (%)	17.2 ± 11.4	24.2 ± 18.2	19.0 ± 14.1	22.2 ± 12.6
N2 sleep stage (%)	44.8 ± 12.6	46.6 ± 14.9	47.2 ± 14.6	46.3 ± 11.4
N3 stage (%)	21.8 ± 14.7	17.3 ± 13.4	16.3 ± 9.8	14.2 ± 9.1
REM (%)	16.0 ± 9.3	11.8 ± 7.5	17.5 ± 8.0	17.6 ± 7.3
REM sleep latency (min)	140.0 ± 85.9	195.5 ± 109.3	134.0 ± 86.2	131.2 ± 86.3
REM sleep stages (*n*)	2.4 ± 1.3	1.9 ± 0.8	2.6 ± 1.4	2.8 ± 1.1
PLMS index	27.9 ± 36.8	21.5 ± 34.6	10.4 ± 17.9	12.8 ± 22.3
Apnoea–hypopnoea index	10.5 ± 11.4	14.1 ± 17.3	13.9 ± 19.3	13.4 ± 16.4

n, number of subjects; RBD, rapid eye movement sleep behaviour disorder; MSA, multiple system atrophy; DLB, dementia with Lewy bodies; PD, Parkinson's disease; IRBD, idiopathic RBD; PLMS, periodic leg movements in sleep VPSG, video-polysomnography.

a group of PD patients without RBD [12]. In an unselected cohort of 457 PD subjects undergoing PSG, the overall frequency of RBD was 46%. RBD was associated with older age, longer disease duration, more severe parkinsonism, more falls, more fluctuations, more psychiatric morbidity and a higher dose of levodopa [15]. In contrast, one study found that 17 RBD and 40 non-RBD patients did not differ in age, gender, disease duration, motor symptom and severity, cognitive performance or sleep architecture [19]. In one study involving 41 PD patients without dementia and 29 with dementia, RBD was seen in 37% of those without dementia and in 79% of those with dementia [14]. In one study conducted in Japan with 82 subjects, 33% had RBD, 28% had subclinical REM sleep without atonia and the remaining 39% PD patients had normal REM sleep muscle atonia. Some of the subjects with subclinical REM sleep without atonia developed dream-enacting symptoms after a few years of follow-up [16].

The natural history of RBD in PD has been examined in a few studies [36,41,42]. In one study involving 231 PD patients at baseline, 15% reported symptoms suggestive of RBD, 27% did so after 4 years and 15% after 8 years. One-third of those with possible RBD at baseline were without RBD symptoms 4 years later. Only three patients reported symptoms suggestive of RBD at all three study time points [36]. In another longitudinal study with 61 PD patients, 39 had a history suggestive of RBD and did 22 not. After 2 years of follow-up, 11 patients reported the disappearance of RBD symptoms and 4 reported the new onset of RBD symptoms [41]. In one study, in a cohort of 61 PD patients, 25 had a clinical history suggestive of RBD at baseline and 35 patients 2 years later. Three subjects with possible

RBD changed to non-RBD at follow-up, while 10 non-RBD subjects developed symptoms suggestive of RBD at follow-up (annual incidence of 12.5%) [42]. These data should be interpreted with caution, since a limitation of these studies is the lack of PSG assessment to confirm the presence or absence of RBD at baseline and during follow-up assessments. It is certainly our experience that there is a group of PD patients and bed partners who report that the frequency and intensity of their RBD symptoms (nightmares and vigorous behaviours) decrease with time and can even disappear (personal observations). This may be explained by reduction of REM sleep time due to either destruction by the degenerative process of the nuclei that originate REM sleep or by the use of antidepressants in advanced stages of the disease (these medications are known to reduce the amount of REM sleep).

Characteristics of PD in subjects with RBD

In patients with iRBD who developed parkinsonism with time, vocal and facial akinesia appeared earliest (estimated prodromal interval of nearly 10 years) followed by rigidity (4.4 years), gait abnormalities (4.4 years) and limb bradykinesia (4.2 years) [43]. In one prospective study following 44 IRBD patients clinically, 16 (13 men and 3 women) were diagnosed with PD [10]. The mean age at PD diagnosis was 75 years, the duration of RBD at the time of the diagnosis of PD was 13 years, and the interval between diagnosis of RBD and diagnosis of PD was 5.5 years. Five PD patients developed dementia. In these five patients, the median interval between diagnosis of PD and development of dementia was 6 years.

Most studies using PSG have shown that in sporadic PD patients without dementia or hallucinations the presence of RBD in PD is not associated with age [11,12], hypersomnia [12], sleep benefit [12], disruption of sleep architecture [11,12], olfactory dysfunction [44] or lower daily levodopa equivalent dose [11,12]. In contrast, RBD in PD has been associated with male gender [45], longer duration of parkinsonism [11,12], akinetic–rigid subtype [46], presence of freezing [45], falls [15,45], fluctuations [15], depression [45], a higher dose of levodopa [15,16], cognitive deficits in neuropsychological tests [47], orthostatic hypotension [15,16] and other dysautonomic variables such as abnormalities in measures of beat-to-beat heart variability and reduced ^{123}I-labelled MIBG in myocardial scintigrams. When sporadic PD patients exhibit RBD, this parasomnia precedes the onset of parkinsonism in 18–22% of cases [12,14]. In one study, RBD preceded parkinsonism only when parkinsonian signs developed after the age of 50 years [46]. In subjects with *PARK2* mutations, RBD develops after the onset of parkinsonism and the intensity of the RBD symptomatology is not usually severe.

Available data suggest that RBD in the setting of PD is linked to cognitive impairment. Established risks for dementia in PD such as duration of parkinsonism, severity of parkinsonism and akinetic–rigid subtype are more frequent in PD patients with RBD than in those without. Studies in patients without dementia suggest that RBD in PD is linked to asymptomatic abnormalities in neuropsychological testing, MCI, impaired cortical activation during wakefulness and the future development of dementia. In one study involving PD patients without dementia those with associated RBD showed poorer performance in executive function, verbal memory and visuospatial abilities than those without RBD and controls [47]. One study showed that the proportion of PD patients with RBD having MCI (73%) was higher than in PD patients without RBD (8%) [48]. Another study showed that after 4 years of follow-up 48% of PD patients with RBD developed dementia compared with 0% of those PD subjects without RBD. Of note, 19 of 27 patients with RBD at base-line had MCI compared with only 4 of 15 patients without RBD [49]. In one study with 65 PD subjects, 24 had symptoms suggestive of RBD and 41 did not. Of the 24 patients with probable RBD, 10 had dementia (42%) and the remaining 14 did not (58%). The frequency of RBD was higher in the group of subjects with dementia (77%) than those without de-mentia (14%) [50]. In another study, PD patients with RBD but without dementia showed widespread cortical electroencephalographic slowing during wakefulness [51]. It has been speculated that in RBD these observations are the result of primary damage to the brain-stem structures that regulate REM sleep, leading to cortical dysfunction and subsequent cognitive deficits. However, this does not explain the fact than in MSA cognitive function is generally preserved and RBD is universal [14].

Between 65 and 75% of the PD patients with RBD are male [11,14], a figure similar to the frequency of men in sporadic PD. The origin of the male preponderance in RBD is un-known. It has been hypothesized that sex hormone abnormalities might account for this male predominance and the violent nature of the RBD-associated behaviours. However, in male patients with IRBD and RBD linked to PD there are no differences in circulating sex hormone levels between patients and controls.

Pathophysiology of RBD in PD

It is thought that RBD is the result of dysfunction of brain structures that modulate REM sleep (e.g. the locus subcoeruleus, pedunculopontine nucleus, nucleus magnocellularis) and their anatomical connections (e.g. the amygdala, pallidum, neocortex). These areas modulate REM sleep atonia and the emotional content of dreams. In animals, experimen-tal lesions in the dorsolateral pontine tegmentum (involving the subcoeruleus nucleus) or in the ventromedial medulla (including the magnocellularis nucleus) eliminate muscle atonia and induce abnormal behaviours during REM sleep. Dysfunction of the amygdala probably explains the negative emotional content of dreams occurring in RBD (e.g. being threatened or attacked by people and animals). Cats with unilateral damage to the central nucleus of the amygdala preceded by bilateral pontine lesions exhibit attack behaviours associated with REM sleep without atonia. Furthermore, RBD may occur in patients with limbic encephalitis impairing the amygdala and sparing the brainstem. Cortical (motor and language) areas may also be involved in the pathogenesis of RBD as patients display purposeful behaviours, sing and give long speeches [3]. In PD, pathological changes are common and severe in the structures that modulate REM sleep, such as the brainstem and amygdala. In contrast, full-blown expression of RBD is not common in diseases associated with widespread cell loss in the brainstem but little in the limbic system, such as progres-sive supranuclear palsy, and in diseases with no marked cell loss in the brainstem, such as Alzheimer's disease.

Braak et al. [52] reported that in sporadic PD, Lewy pathology (Lewy bodies and neu-rites) begins in the dorsal motor nucleus of the vagus nerve in the medulla (Stage 1) and advances upwards through the magnocellularis nucleus, the subcoeruleus–coeruleus complex (Stage 2), the substantia nigra, the pedunculopontine nucleus, the amygdala (Stage 3), the temporal mesocortex (Stage 4), finally reaching the neocortex (Stages 5 and 6). This temporal sequence of Lewy pathology may account for the finding that in some PD patients, RBD (Stage 2) precedes the onset of parkinsonism (Stage 3). This temporal sequence, however, does not explain the more common observations that RBD never de-velops in some PD patients or that parkinsonism precedes the onset of RBD. One possible explanation is that, in these situations, the severity of neuronal dysfunction in the brain-stem structures that modulate REM sleep does not reach a critical threshold for the clinical expression of RBD [53].

Available data indicate that RBD is not mediated by dopaminergic deficiency alone [1]. Recent studies suggest that dysfunction of the GABA-ergic, glutamatergic and glycinergic systems located in the lower brainstem may be directly involved in the pathogenesis of RBD [54,55]. The pathophysiology of RBD in PD is probably explained by the regional distribution and severity of neuronal dysfunction in the brainstem structures that regulate REM sleep and their anatomical connections. PD subjects without RBD are probably those in whom neuronal dysfunction does not occur in these regions or in whom the threshold for clinical symptomatology is not exceeded.

Treatment of RBD in PD

The severity of RBD symptoms in PD ranges from mild to severe. Overall, RBD has little impact on the patient's quality of life and daily performance. In most patients, REM sleep fragmentation caused by abnormal behaviours is not sufficient to cause either a feeling of non-restorative sleep upon awakening or excessive daytime sleepiness. An important proportion of patients consider RBD a minor problem compared with the impact of their disabling waking motor condition. Treatment of RBD may be required to prevent injuries in patients with violent dream-enacting behaviour, to decrease the intensity of unpleasant dreams in those subjects who consider them an uncomfortable experience and when RBD significantly disturbs the bed partner's quality of sleep.

There is no strong evidence that dopaminergic agents have a marked influence on the development, evolution or severity of RBD. In PD, pramipexole [56] and subthalamic deep brain stimulation [57,58] do not improve RBD-related symptoms and PSG measures. For unknown reasons, RBD in PD (and also RBD associated with any other condition) re-sponds to small doses of clonazepam (0.25–4 mg) at bedtime. Effective treatment with clonazepam, however, does not prevent the development of parkinsonism in subjects with IRBD. In refractory cases or when clonazepam is associated with side effects (e.g. dizziness, somnolence, impotence) melatonin can be tried. A double-blind crossover pilot trial in 12 PD subjects with RBD symptoms refractory to both clonazepam and melatonin showed significant reduction of the frequency of RBD episodes for 3 weeks using a patch of the cho-linesterase inhibitor rivastigmine at a dose of 4.6 mg daily [59]. Methods of self-protection from injury, such as placing a mattress on the floor or removal of furniture from the room, may be needed to minimize the risk of self-injuries. It should be noted that antidepressants and lipophilic beta-blockers such as bisoprolol may induce or aggravate RBD.

Key features of RBD in PD

- RBD is characterized by vigorous movements associated with unpleasant dreams and increased electromyographic activity during REM sleep.
- The majority of patients diagnosed with idiopathic RBD will develop PD and other synucleinopathies with time.
- RBD in PD occurs in 20–58% of patients. In about 20% of cases it develops before the onset of classic waking motor symptoms.
- Some 65% of PD patients with RBD are unaware of their dream-enacting behaviours.
- About 20% of patients with RBD do not recall fearful dreams.
- PD patients with RBD tend to have the rigid–akinetic motor subtype, are of older age and predominantly male, have autonomic dysfunction and an increased risk of developing dementia over time. This suggests that the presence of RBD in PD is indicative of the development of widespread neuropathological changes in the brain.
- Polysomnography with audiovisual recording is needed to confirm the diagnosis of RBD and exclude other conditions that can mimic its symptoms, including severe sleep apnoea, nocturnal hallucinations and confusional awakenings.
- In PD, RBD is thought to result from involvement in the pathological process of those brain structures that regulate REM sleep atonia and the emotional content of dreams.
- RBD is probably the result of a complex neurotransmitter dysfunction mainly involving GABA-ergic, glutamatergic and monoaminergic systems.
- There is no strong evidence to indicate that RBD is caused by dopaminergic deficiency alone.
- The severity of RBD symptoms range from mild to severe, occasionally leading to injuries. When clinically required, small doses of clonazepam and melatonin at bedtime are the treatments of choice.

References

1 **Iranzo A, Santamaria J, Tolosa E.** The clinical and pathophysiological relevance of REM sleep behavior disorder in neurodegenerative diseases. Sleep Med Rev 2009; **13**: 385–401.

2 **Boeve B.** REM sleep behavior disorder. Ann NY Acad Sci 2010; **1184**: 15–54.

3 **Arnulf I.** REM sleep behavior disorder: motor manifestations and pathophysiology. Mov Disord 2012; **27**: 677–89.

4 **Ratti PL, Terzaghi M, Minafra B, et al.** REM and NREM sleep enactment behaviors in Parkinson's disease, Parkinson disease dementia and dementia with Lewy bodies. Sleep Med 2012; **13**: 926–32.

5 **Boeve BF, Silber MH, Saper CB, et al.** Pathophysiology of REM sleep behaviour disorder and relevance to neurodegenerative disease. Brain 2007; **130**: 2770–88.

6 Schenck CH, Bundlie SR, Mahowald MW. Delayed emergence of a parkinsonian disorder in 38% of 29 older men initially diagnosed with idiopathic rapid eye movement sleep behavior disorder: Neurology 1996; **46**: 388–93.

7 Schenck CH, Boeve BF, Mahowald MW. Delayed emergence of a parkinsonian disorder or dementia in 81% of older males initially diagnosed with idiopathic REM sleep behavior disorder (IBD): 16 year update on a previously reported series. Sleep Med 2013; **14**: 744–8.

8 Postuma RB, Gagnon JF, Vendette M, Fantini ML, Massicotte-Marquez J, Montplaisir J. Quantifying the risk of neurodegenerative disease in idiopathic REM sleep behavior disorder. Neurology 2009; **72**: 1296–300.

9 Iranzo A, Molinuevo JL, Santamaria J, et al. Rapid-eye-movement sleep behaviour disorder as an early marker for a neurodegenerative disease: a descriptive study. Lancet Neurol 2006; **5**: 572–7.

10 Iranzo A, Tolosa E, Gelpi E, et al. Neurodegenerative status and post-mortem pathology in idiopathic rapid-eye-movement disorder: an observational cohort study. Lancet Neurol 2013: **12**: 443–53.

11 Wetter TC, Trenkwalder C, Gershanik O, Högl B. Polysomnographic measures in Parkinson's disease: a comparison between patients with and without REM sleep disturbances. Wien Klin Wochenschr 2001; **113**: 249–53.

12 De Cock VC, Vidailhet M, Leu S, et al. Restoration of normal muscle control in Parkinson's disease during REM sleep. Brain 2007; **130**: 450–6.

13 Diederich NJ, Vaillant V, Mancuso G, et al. Progressive sleep destructuring in Parkinson's disease. A polysomnographic study in 46 patients. Sleep Med 2005; **6**: 313–18.

14 Iranzo A, Rye DB, Santamaria J et al. Characteristics of idiopathic REM sleep behavior disorder and that associated with MSA and PD. Neurology 2005; **65**: 247–52.

15 Sixel-Doring F, Trautmann E, Mollenhauer B, Trenkwalder C. Associated factors for REM sleep behaviour disorder in Parkinson disease. Neurology 2011; **77**: 1048–54.

16 Nomura T, Inoue Y, Kagimura T, Nakashima K. Clinical significance of REM sleep behaviour disorder in Parkinson's disease. Sleep Med 2013; **14**: 131–5.

17 Gagnon JF, Bédard MA, Fantini ML, et al. REM sleep behavior disorder and REM sleep without atonia in Parkinson's disease. Neurology 2002; **59**: 585–9.

18 Ferri R, Consentino FII, Pizza F, Arico D, Plazzi G. The timing between REM sleep behavior disorder and Parkinson's disease. Sleep Breath 2013; doi: 10.1007/s11325-013-0887-3.

19 Mollenhauer B, Trautman E, Sixel-Doring F, et al. Nonmotor and diagnostic findings in subjects with de novo Parkinson disease of the DeNoPa cohort. Neurology 2013; **81**: 1–9.

20 Plomhause L, Dujardin K, Duhamel A, et al. Rapid eye movement sleep behavior in treatment-naïve Parkinson disease patients. Sleep Med 2013; **14**: 1035–7.

21 Uchiyama M, Isse K, Tanaka K, et al. Incidental Lewy body disease in a patient with REM sleep behavior disorder. Neurology 1995; **45**: 709–12.

22 Boeve BF, Dickson DW, Olson EJ, et al. Insights into REM sleep behavior disorder pathophysiology in brainstem-predominant Lewy body disease. Sleep Med 2007; **8**: 60–4.

23 Fantini ML, Postuma RB, Montplaisir J, Ferini-Strambi L. Olfactory deficit in idiopathic rapid eye movements sleep behavior disorder. Brain Res Bull 2006; **70**: 386–90.

24 Postuma RB, Gagnon JF, Vendette M, Desjardins C, Montplaisir JY. Olfaction and color vision identify impending neurodegeneration in rapid eye movement sleep behavior disorder. Ann Neurol 2011; **69**: 811–18.

25 Iranzo A, Lomeña F, Stockner H, et al., for the Sleep Innsbruck Barcelona (SINBAR) group. Decreased striatal dopamine transporter uptake and substantia nigra hyperechogenicity as risk markers of synucleinopathy in patients with idiopathic rapid-eye-movement sleep behaviour disorder: a prospective study. Lancet Neurol 2010; **9**: 1070–7.

26 Iranzo A, Valldeoriola F, Lomeña F, et al. Serial dopamine transporter imaging of nigrostriatal function in patients with idiopathic rapid-eye-movement sleep behaviour disorder: a prospective study. Lancet Neurol 2011; **10**: 797–805.

27 Iranzo A, Fernández-Arcos A, Tolosa E, et al. Neurodegenerative disorder risk in idiopathic REM sleep behavior disorder: study in 174 patients. PLoS ONE 9(2): e89741.

28 Iranzo A, Gelpi E, Tolosa E, et al. Neuropathology of prodromal Lewy body disease. Mov Disord 29(Suppl 3): 410–15.

29 Iranzo A, Serradell M, Vilaseca I, et al. Longitudinal assessment of olfactory function in idiopathic REM sleep behavior disorder. Parkinsonism Relat Disord 2013; **19**: 600–4.

30 Wallace DM, Shafazand S, Carvalho DZ, et al. Sleep-related falling out of bed in Parkinson's disease. J Clin Neurol 2012; **8**: 51–7.

31 Borek LL, Kohn R, Friedman JH. Phenomenology of dreams in Parkinson's disease. Mov Disord 2007; **22**: 198–202.

32 Comella C, Nardine TM, Diederich NJ, Stebbins GT. Sleep-related violence, injury, and REM sleep behavior disorder in Parkinson's disease. Neurology 1998; **51**: 526–9.

33 Antonini A, Pezzoli G, Castronovo V, et al. REM sleep behavior disorder and Parkinson's disease (PD): relationship to PD onset and treatment. Sleep 2002; **25**: A494.

34 Scaglione C, Vignatelli L, Plazzi G, et al. REM sleep behaviour disorder in Parkinson's disease: a questionnaire-based study. Neurol Sci 2005; **25**: 316–21.

35 Meral H, Aydemir, Ozer F, et al. Relationship between visual hallucinations and REM sleep behavior disorder in patients with Parkinson's disease. Clin Neurol Neurosurg 2007; **109**: 862–7.

36 Gjerstad MD, Boeve B, Wentzel-Larsen T, et al. Occurrence and clinical correlates of REM sleep behaviour disorder in patients with Parkinson's disease over time. J Neurol Neurosurg Psychiatry 2007; **79**: 387–91.

37 Yoritaka A, Ohizumi H, Tanaka S, Hattori N. Parkinson's disease with and without REM sleep behavior disorder: are there any clinical differences? Eur Neurol 2009; **61**: 164–70.

38 Bugalho P, Alves da Silva J, Neto B. Clinical features associated with REM sleep behaviour disorder symptoms in the early stages of Parkinson's disease. J Neurol 2011; **258**: 50–5.

39 Vibha D, Shulka G, Goyal S, Singh S, Srivastava AK, Behari M. RBD in Parkinson's disease: a clinical case control from North India. Clin Neurol Neurosurg 2011; **113**; 472–6.

40 Nihei Y, Takahashi K, Koto A, et al. REM sleep behaviour disorder in Japanese patients with Parkinson's disease: a multicentre study using the REM sleep behaviour disorder screening questionnaire. J Neurol 2012; **259**: 1606–12.

41 Levault S, Leu-Semenescu S, Tezenas du Monteel S, Cochen de Cock V, Vidailhet M, Arnulf I. Does clinical rapid eye movement behaviour disorder predict worse outcomes in Parkinson's disease? J Neurol 2010; **257**: 1154–9.

42 Bugalho P, Viana-Baptista M. REM sleep behavior disorder and motor dysfunction in Parkinson's disease–a longitudinal study. Parkinsonism Relat Disord 2013; **19**: 1084–7.

43 Postuma RN, Lang AE, Gagnon JF, Pelletier A, Montplaisir JY. How does parkinsonism start? Prodromal parkinsonism motor changes in idiopathic REM sleep behaviour disorder. Brain 2012; **27**: 617–26.

44 Postuma RB, Gagnon JF, Vendette M, et al. REM sleep behavior disorder in Parkinson's disease is associated with specific motor features. J Neurol Neurosurg Psychiatry 2008; **79**: 1117–21.

45 Romenets SR, Ggnon JF, Latreille V, et al. Rapid eye movement sleep behaviour disorder and subtypes of Parkinsons's disease. Mov Disord 2012; **27**: 996–1003.

46 Kumru H, Santamaria J, Tolosa E, Iranzo A. Relation between subtype of Parkinson's disease and REM sleep behavior disorder. Sleep Med 2007; **8**: 779–83.

47 **Vendette M, Gagnon JF, Décary A, et al**. REM sleep behavior disorder predicts cognitive impairment in Parkinson disease without dementia. Neurology 2007: **69**: 1843–9.

48 **Gagnon JF, Vendette M, Postuma R, et al**. Mild cognitive impairment in rapid eye movement sleep behaviour disorder and Parkinson disease. Ann Neurol 2009; **66**: 39–47.

49 **Postuma RB, Bertrand JA, Montplaisir J, et al**. Rapid eye movement sleep behaviour disorder and risk of dementia in Parkinson's disease: a prospective study. Mov Disord 2012; **27**: 720–6.

50 **Marion HM, Qurasgi M, Marshall G, Foster O**. Is REM sleep behaviour disorder (RBD) a risk factor for Parkinson's disease. J Neurol 2008; **255**: 192–6.

51 **Gagnon JF, Fantini ML, Bédard MA, et al**. Association between waking EEG slowing and REM sleep behavior disorder in PD without dementia. Neurology 2004; **62**: 401–6.

52 **Braak H, Del Tredici K, Rub U, et al**. Staging of brain pathology related to sporadic Parkinson's disease. Neurobiol Aging 2003; **24**: 197–211.

53 **Boeve BF**. Idiopathic REM sleep behaviour disorder in the development of Parkinson's disease. Lancet Neurol 2013; **12**: 469–82.

54 **Boissard R, Fort P, Gervasoni D, et al**. Localization of the GABAergic and non-GABAergic neurons projecting to the sublaterodorsal nucleus and potentially gating paradoxical sleep onset. Eur J Neurosci 2003; **18**: 1627–39.

55 **Lu J, Sherman D, Devor M, Saper CB**. A putative flip-flop switch for control of REM sleep. Nature 2006; **441**: 589–94.

56 **Kumru H, Iranzo A, Carrasco E, et al**. Lack of effect of pramipexole on REM sleep behavior disorder in subjects with Parkinson's disease. Sleep 2008; **31**: 1418–21.

57 **Iranzo A, Valldeoriola F, Santamaria J, et al**. Sleep symptoms and polysomnographic architecture in advanced Parkinson's disease after chronic bilateral subthalamic stimulation. J Neurol Neurosurg Psychiatry 2002; **72**: 661–4.

58 **Arnulf I, Bejjani BP, Garma L, et al**. Improvement of sleep architecture in PD with subthalamic stimulation. Neurology 2000; **55**: 1732–4.

59 **Giacopo R, Fasano A, Quaranta D, et al**. Rivastigmine as alternative treatment for refractory REM behaviour disorder in Parkinson's disease. Mov Disord 2012; **27**: 559–61.

Chapter 15

Parkinson's disease and restless legs syndrome

William G. Ondo

Introduction

Parkinson's disease (PD) is a complex neurodegenerative disorder. Although clinically defined by rigidity, bradykinesia and tremor, numerous sensory, sleep symptoms and other non-motor symptoms are commonly reported. Some of these symptoms probably result from dopamine cell loss while others do not.

Restless legs syndrome (RLS) and PD both respond to dopaminergic treatments, both show some dopaminergic abnormalities on functional imaging and both are variably associated with periodic limb movements in sleep [1]. Therefore, a relationship between the two conditions has long been sought. Earlier results, however, were mixed. Prior to the development of current RLS criteria, some studies [2,3], but not others [4,5], reported a higher prevalence of RLS in patients with PD. Diagnostic inconsistency makes these reports difficult to interpret. Most reports employing current criteria do suggest that PD patients have higher rates of RLS than the general population, but clear pathophysiological connections are lacking.

Restless legs syndrome

A 2003 National Institutes of Health consensus summit defined RLS by the simultaneous presence of: (1) desire to move the extremities, often associated with paraesthesia/dysaesthesia; (2) worsening of symptoms at rest; (3) transient improvement with movement; and (4) worsening of symptoms in the evening or at night [6]. No widely available biomarker or test corroborates the diagnosis, which is made exclusively via interview. However, patients often have difficulty describing the sensory component of their RLS. The descriptions are quite varied and tend to be suggestive and education-dependent. The limb sensation is always unpleasant but not necessarily painful. It is usually deep within the legs. In one study of RLS patients, the most common terms used, in descending order of frequency, included: 'need to move', 'crawling', 'tingling', 'restless', 'cramping', 'creeping', 'pulling', 'painful', 'electric', 'tension', 'discomfort' and 'itching' [7]. Patients usually deny any 'burning' or 'pins and needles' sensations, commonly experienced in neuropathies or nerve entrapments, although neuropathic pain and RLS can coexist. RLS differs from akathisia, also reported in PD, in that the urge to move is isolated to the limbs, rather than the entire body, there is more dramatic relief with ambulation and there is a more robust worsening at night, with near complete cessation of symptoms in the early morning.

RLS is extremely common, affecting about 10% of Caucasian populations [8], although it appears to be less common in Asian and African populations [9]. In roughly 60% of cases a family history of RLS can be found, although this is often not initially reported by the patient, and multiple genes and additional loci have been published [10–14].

Pathophysiology of RLS and PD

The pathology of idiopathic RLS involves homeostatic dysregulation of central nervous system (CNS) iron. Cerebrospinal fluid (CSF) ferritin and other measures of iron are lower in people with RLS [15]. Specially sequenced magnetic resonance imaging (MRI) studies and transcranial ultrasound show reduced iron stores in the striatum and substantia nigra [16,17]. Most importantly, pathological data in autopsied brains of RLS patients show reduced ferritin staining, reduced iron staining, increased transferrin stains and reduced iron regulatory protein-1 activity, but also reduced transferrin receptors [18,19]. The transferrin receptor downregulation is particularly telling as a simple reduction in iron availability to the area would upregulate these receptors. It therefore appears that primary RLS involves reduced intracellular iron indices secondary to a perturbation of homeostatic mechanisms that regulate iron influx and/or efflux from the cell. In contrast, PD is associated with increased iron in dopaminergic areas [16].

CNS dopaminergic systems are implicated in RLS, but a pathophysiological understanding of this is lacking. Dopaminergic medications, especially dopamine agonists, robustly improve RLS, even at low doses. Normal circadian dopaminergic variation is also augmented in patients with RLS [20]. Dopamine imaging studies in RLS, however, have been inconsistent and difficult to interpret. Positron emission tomography (PET) studies measuring levodopa/dopamine have shown normal levels [21] or slight reductions [22,23]. Imaging of dopamine transporter protein is normal [24–26] or shows modest reductions (Allen R, personal communication). Imaging of dopamine receptors showed normal [26] or a modestly reduced availability of receptors [23,24], suggesting either decreased receptors or increased endogenous dopamine occupancy. Possible explanations for these disparities include: different severities of RLS in the subjects, the variable use of dopaminergic medications as treatments, different times of data acquisition (day versus night), different ligands and other technical considerations. The imaging studies are difficult to reconcile, but may be limited by only assessing nigral–striatal dopamine. Some models and theories of RLS suggest that spinal dopaminergic areas are culpable [27]. These areas, however, are too small to image.

Pathological data do not suggest reduced dopamine in RLS. CSF studies and human brain studies of the nigrostriatal system generally suggest normal or even increased dopaminergic turnover [28,29]. Specifically, dopaminergic cells in the substantia nigra are not reduced in number, nor are there markers associated with neurodegenerative diseases, such as τ or α-synuclein abnormalities [19,30]. PD, of course, exhibits reduced numbers of dopamine cells and multiple neurodegenerative markers.

In RLS, the relationship between reduced iron pathology and effective treatment with dopaminergics is not clearly understood, and is beyond the scope of this chapter. However, some evidence suggests that the bridge is Thy-1. This cell adhesion molecule, which is robustly expressed on dopaminergic neurons, is reduced in brain homogenates in iron-deprived mice [31] and in brains of patients with RLS [32]. Thy-1 regulates the vesicular release of monoamines, including dopamine [33]. A leading hypothesis suggests that reduced iron stores decrease Thy-1, which is necessary for the transmission of dopamine across the synapse. Thy-1 status in PD has not been explored.

Both PD and, especially, RLS have a genetic contribution. One large family with PD caused by *PARK2* mutations included a large number of members with RLS, both with and without concurrent PD [34]. The pattern of RLS inheritance was consistent with an autosomal dominant pattern; however, the authors did not find an association between RLS and *PARK2* mutations within the family.

In summary, there are no clear pathological similarities between PD and idiopathic RLS. Brain iron is decreased in RLS but increased in PD. Dopamine and dopamine cells are overtly reduced in PD, but not in RLS, where the dopaminergic dysfunction is not clear. Nevertheless, most studies suggest that RLS is more common in subjects with PD than in controls.

Clinical RLS in patients with PD

Multiple surveys have queried the prevalence of RLS symptoms in PD populations (Table 15.1). Most were performed at tertiary centres but there is little reason to suspect ascertainment bias. Some reports seek associations and/or include a control group. In general, most studies suggest a higher rate of RLS in PD than control populations or historic controls.

In a prospective survey of 303 consecutive PD patients, we found that 20.8% of all patients with PD met the diagnostic criteria for RLS [35]. Despite this high number of cases, several caveats tend to lessen its clinical significance. The RLS symptoms in PD patients are often ephemeral, are usually not severe and might be confused with other PD symptoms such as wearing off dystonia, akathisia or internal tremor. We specifically attempted to differentiate between these conditions. Most patients in our group were not previously diagnosed with RLS and few recognized that this was separate from other PD symptoms. Finally, the presence of RLS did not affect Epworth scores of daytime sleepiness.

After determining the prevalence of RLS in PD, we next evaluated for factors that could predict RLS in this population, and determined that only lower serum ferritin levels predicted RLS symptoms in the PD population. RLS did not correlate with duration of PD, age, Hoehn and Yahr stage, gender, dementia, use of levodopa, use of dopamine agonists, history of pallidotomy or history of deep brain stimulation (DBS). PD symptoms preceded RLS symptoms in 35/41 cases (85.4%; $\chi^2 = 20.5$, $P < 0.0001$) in which patients confidently

Table 15.1 Summary of restless legs syndrome (RLS) in Parkinson's disease (PD) studies

Study	Population	RLS in PD	Risk factors	Onset of RLS and PD	Comment
Ondo, 2002 [35]	US	63/303 (20.8%)	Reduced serum ferritin	PD first in 85%	Older age of onset and less family history than idiopathic RLS
Driver-Dunckly, 2006 [37]	US undergoing STN DBS	6/25 (24%)	NR	NR	Improved with STN DBS
Peralta, 2005 [36]	Austria	28/113 (24%)	Younger age. Lower 'on' Hoehn and Yahr	PD first in 83%	RLS symptoms during 'wearing off' episodes
Simuni, 2000 [38]	US	42/200 (21%)	Tendency for 'fluctuators' ($P = 0.14$)	PD first in 93%	RLS undiagnosed in 59%
Braga-Neto, 2004 [62]	Brazil	45/86 (49.9%)	Longer duration of PD, but not age	NR	RLS not associated with daytime sleepiness
Chaudhuri, 2006 [63]	US and Europe	46/123[a] (37.4), controls (28.1)		NR	Part of a non-motor survey
Kumar, 2002 [40]	India	21/149 (14.1%), controls (0.9%)	NR	NR	RLS diagnosis based on a single question
Krishman, 2003 [39]	India	10/126 (7.9%), controls (1.3%)	Older age Depression	NR	
Nomora, 2005 [41]	Japan	20/165 (12%), controls (2.3%)	Younger age	PD first in 95%	RLS worsened PSQI
Tan, 2002 [42]	Singapore	1/135 (0.6%), controls (0.1%)			Motor restlessness in 15.2%
Verbaan, 2010 [64]	Holland	269 (11%)	Female	NR	
Loo, 2008 [54]	Singapore	400 (3.0%), controls (0.5%)	Correlated with Hoehn and Yahr stage and poor sleep	Mean RLS onset 62	RLS severity correlated with PD severity

STN DBS, subthalamic nucleus deep brain stimulation; NR, not relevant; PSQI, Pittsburgh Sleep Quality Index.
[a]A single written question, not full RLS criteria.

remembered the initial onset of both symptoms. We compared the PD/RLS group with patients with RLS not associated with PD (idiopathic RLS). Only 20.2% of all PD/RLS patients reported a positive family history of RLS, compared with more than 60% of our non-PD RLS population. Serum ferritin was also lower in the PD/RLS group compared with the idiopathic RLS group. In the cases with PD who did have a family history of RLS, the RLS symptoms usually preceded PD and generally resembled typical RLS. In short,

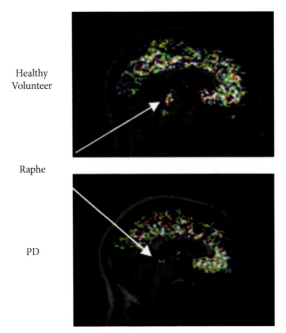

Healthy
Volunteer

Raphe

PD

Plate 1 ^{11}C-WAY 100635 PET images of serotonin HT$_{1A}$ binding in the brain of a control subject and a patient with Parkinson's disease (PD). Decreased ^{11}C-WAY 100635 binding in the median raphe is visible in the PD patient. (See Fig. 6.2)

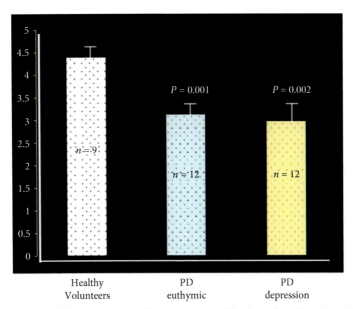

Plate 2 Mean values of ^{11}C-WAY 100635 binding in the midbrain raphe of healthy volunteers, patients with Parkinson's disease without depression, and patients with Parkinson's disease and depression. The two PDD groups show similar reductions in HT$_{1A}$ binding. (See Fig. 6.3)

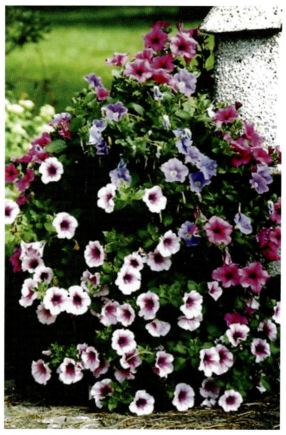

Plate 3 A cognitively impaired Parkinson's disease patient mistook these petunias for numerous little faces staring at him. (See Fig. 12.1)

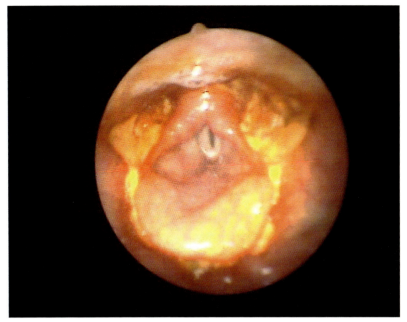

Plate 4 Retention of a melted tablet in the low back part of the mouth. The tablet was taken 90 minutes before the fluoroscopy. (See Fig. 19.1)

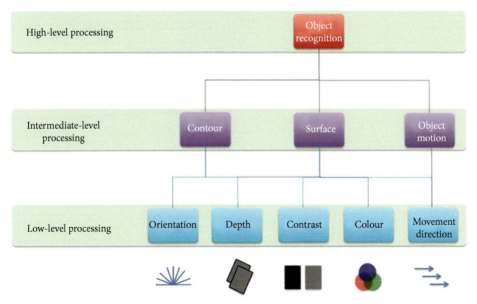

Plate 5 The visual system is organized in both a hierarchical and a parallel manner. Low-level visual information is integrated at the intermediate-level processing stage. (See Fig. 24.2)

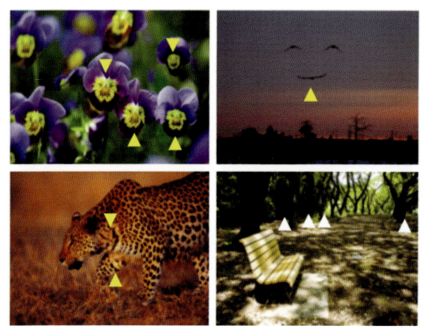

Plate 6 Examples of the pareidolia test. Patients with dementia with Lewy bodies often misidentify objects or patterns in a picture as human faces (yellow triangles) or as people and animals (white triangles). (See Fig. 24.4)

our results did not suggest that RLS is a *forme fruste* or a risk factor for the subsequent development of PD, but rather that PD is a risk factor for RLS, which probably constitutes a non-motor feature of PD.

In an abstract, Peralta et al. [36] reported that 28/113 (24%) of Austrian PD patients met criteria for RLS. PD/RLS subjects were younger and had lower (less severe) 'on' medicine PD severity. PD preceded RLS in 83%. Two other US studies reported that 24% and 21% of PD patients had RLS [37,38].

Krishnan et al. [39] evaluated the prevalence of RLS in patients with PD compared with normal controls in a population from India. Interestingly, they found that 10 of 126 cases of PD (7.9%) versus only one of 128 controls (0.8%) ($P = 0.01$) reported RLS. PD patients with RLS were older and reported more depression. Another report from India similarly found RLS in 14.1% of PD patients versus only 0.9% in controls [40]. Although both prevalences are lower than US reports, the difference in RLS prevalence between PD and controls is similar. This probably reflects baseline epidemiology that suggests RLS is less common in non-Caucasian populations.

A Japanese survey reported similar results. RLS was seen in 12% of PD subjects compared with 2.3% of controls [41]. They associated RLS with a younger age of PD and with poor sleep. PD almost always preceded RLS. The only study that did not find any increased risk of RLS in PD was reported from Singapore. Tan and colleagues [42], in a mostly Chinese population, found only a single case of RLS out of 125 patients presenting with PD. They also reported a very low prevalence of RLS in the general population [9].

In summary, studies done since modern RLS criteria were established, aside from one Singapore study, report the absolute differences in the rates of RLS in PD to be about 10% greater (range 6.6–14%) than in historic controls or actual controls. All reports that queried symptom onset show that PD preceded RLS in the majority.

Prevalence of PD in patients with RLS

Evaluating the prevalence of PD in populations presenting with RLS is problematic, as PD symptoms would usually be more overt and precipitate an evaluation. Banno et al. [3], however, reported that 'extrapyramidal disease or movement disorders' were previously diagnosed in 17.5% of male RLS patients versus 0.2% of male controls and in 23.5% of female patients versus 0.2% of female controls ($P < 0.05$). They did not clarify whether they felt that these prior diagnoses were correct or truly represented a different disease. In an abstract, Fazzini et al. [43] reported that 19/29 RLS patients had symptoms of PD. In contrast, Walters et al. [44] did not report any patients presenting with RLS who had PD. In the author's experience, RLS does not predispose to the development of PD; however, definitive longitudinal epidemiology does not exist for this scenario.

Over 15 years we collected 36 cases in which subjects developed RLS long before PD, and/or had a family history of RLS in a first-degree relative and had well-documented RLS before the onset of their PD. In this RLS/PD group, 13 were female, 18 had a positive family history of RLS and six had a family history of PD. We compared these with a 'control' group of idiopathic PD without RLS (n = 36, 10 females, 1 with family history of RLS, 9 with family history of PD). The age at motor onset of RLS/PD was older (64.25 ± 6.4 versus 56.8 ± 10.7 years) than for patients with idiopathic PD ($P \leq 0.001$). Patients with idiopathic PD developed dyskinesia more (21/36) than RLS/PD (4/32) at last follow-up ($P = 0.0001$). PD phenotype and levodopa dose were similar. We concluded that idiopathic RLS may actually delay the onset of PD, reduce the occurrence of dyskinesia and possibly reduce progression of PD. This is potentially supported by the aforementioned pathological studies that show increased dopamine turnover in RLS and reduced iron, as opposed to increased iron seen in PD. Assessments of brain iron in this unique group (idiopathic RLS followed by PD) have not been done.

Periodic limb movements in sleep in RLS and PD

Periodic limb movements in sleep (PLMS) are strongly associated with RLS. PLMS are defined by the Association of Sleep Disorders as 'periodic episodes of repetitive and highly stereotyped limb movements that occur during sleep'. The incidence in the general population increases with age and is reported to occur in as many as 57% of elderly people [45–47]. One large study reported that 81% of RLS patients showed pathological PLMS [48]. The prevalence increased to 87% if recordings were done over two nights. Although PLMS accompany most cases of RLS, data evaluating the prevalence of RLS in the setting of polysomnographically documented PLMS found that only 9 of 53 (17.0%) PLMS patients complained of RLS symptoms [49]. Therefore, most people with RLS have PLMS but many patients with isolated PLMS do not have RLS. Although the exact relationship between the two phenotypes is unclear, recent genetic research suggests a strong biological association [11].

PD is also associated with higher rates of PLMS in some [1,50], but not all [51], reports. The assessment of PLMS in PD is clearly confounded by dopaminergic treatment, which improves PLMS [52]. There is more compelling evidence that, when present, PLMS correlate with the severity of PD, both clinically and in imaging studies [53]. Most evidence suggests that PLMS do not seem to contribute to excessive daytime sleepiness in PD.

One study that performed polysomnography in PD subjects with and without RLS did find that PLMS were more common in the PD/RLS group [54]. In contrast, another study segregating PD based on the presence of PLMS did not find higher rates of RLS in the PLMS + PD group [55].

The assessment of PLMS in PD is clearly confounded by dopaminergic treatment, which improves PLMS in general and did improve PLMS specifically in PD in one prospective trial [56].

Treatment of RLS in PD

No formal study has ever prospectively assessed the treatment of RLS in the setting of PD. Anticholinergic and antihistaminergic drugs, including amitriptyline, mirtazapine, quetiapine and many others used in PD, can exacerbate RLS in general and should be discontinued if possible. One may consider checking serum ferritin and supplementing this if it is low; however, it is not known whether this could affect the course of PD. Dopamine agonists and levodopa improve RLS as well as PD, so adjustment of these medications may improve RLS. One case report stated that pergolide treated RLS in a PD patient who was already being treated with levodopa [57]. Another polysomnographic study found that PD patients already treated with clonazepam had fewer periodic leg movements and less daytime sleepiness than those not treated with clonazepam [58].

Interestingly, several reports suggest that CNS surgery for PD may affect RLS in the PD/RLS population. Rye and DeLong [59] first reported a single case of RLS symptoms improving in a PD patient following pallidotomy. Driver-Dunkley et al. [37] found RLS in 6/25 PD subjects prior to them undergoing bilateral deep brain stimulation (DBS) of the subthalamic nucleus (STN). All six had some improvement in RLS at 3–24 months after DBS. Three had complete resolution and the mean International RLS Rating Scale improved by 84%. PD medications were lowered by 56% and the Unified Parkinson's Disease Rating Scale 'off' motor scores improved by 63%, suggesting an excellent clinical response to the DBS. In contrast, Kedia et al. [60] reported the emergence of RLS post-operatively after STN DBS in 11 of 195 patients. The mean reduction in antiparkinsonian medication was 74%, which they felt may have unmasked the RLS symptoms. Parra et al. [61] also reported a case of emergence of RLS after DBS.

Conclusions

The majority of studies suggest that RLS is more common in PD than in the general population. All studies of predominantly Caucasian populations demonstrate a rate of RLS in PD at least twice as high as that in non-PD subjects. PD/RLS rates in Asian surveys are lower, as are the baseline rates of RLS. Reported risk factors for RLS in the PD population include reduced serum iron stores, older age, younger age and depression. RLS symptom severity is less than in those seeking treatment for idiopathic RLS but may be similar to the idiopathic RLS population as a whole. Although the data are mixed, the overall effect of RLS on daytime sleepiness and quality of life in PD is probably modest. Importantly, there is no good evidence to suggest that RLS is a *forme fruste* of PD, and in fact the pathophysiologies are markedly different, despite similar responses to dopaminergic medications. Therefore, it appears that RLS is one of many non-motor features intrinsic to PD, presumably secondary to dopaminergic loss, although this is not actually known.

References

1 Wetter TC, Collado-Seidel V, Pollmacher T, et al. Sleep and periodic leg movement patterns in drug-free patients with Parkinson's disease and multiple system atrophy. Sleep 2000; **23**: 361–7.
2 Horiguchi J, Inami Y, Nishimatsu O, et al. Sleep–wake complaints in Parkinson's disease [in Japanese]. Rinsho Shinkeigaku 1990; **30**: 214–16.
3 Banno K, Delaive K, Walld R, Kryger MH. Restless legs syndrome in 218 patients: associated disorders. Sleep Med 2000; **1**: 221–9.

4 Lang AE. Restless legs syndrome and Parkinson's disease: insights into pathophysiology. Clin Neuropharmacol 1987; **10**: 476–8.

5 Paulson G. Is restless legs a prodrome to Parkinson's disease. J Am Geriatr Soc 1997; **12**(Suppl 1): 68.

6 Allen RP, Picchietti D, Hening WA, et al. Restless legs syndrome: diagnostic criteria, special considerations, and epidemiology. A report from the restless legs syndrome diagnosis and epidemiology workshop at the National Institutes of Health. Sleep Med 2003; **4**: 101–19.

7 Ondo W, Jankovic J. Restless legs syndrome: clinicoetiologic correlates. Neurology 1996; **47**: 1435–41.

8 Hening W, Walters AS, Allen RP, et al. Impact, diagnosis and treatment of restless legs syndrome (RLS) in a primary care population: the REST (RLS epidemiology, symptoms, and treatment) primary care study. Sleep Med 2004; **5**: 237–46.

9 Tan EK, Seah A, See SJ, et al. Restless legs syndrome in an Asian population: a study in Singapore. J Am Geriatr Soc 2001; **16**: 577–9.

10 Winkelmann J, Schormair B, Lichtner P, et al. Genome-wide association study of restless legs syndrome identifies common variants in three genomic regions. Nat Genet 2007; **39**: 1000–6.

11 Stefansson H, Rye DB, Hicks A, et al. A genetic risk factor for periodic limb movements in sleep. N Engl J Med 2007; **357**: 639–47.

12 Chen S, Ondo WG, Rao S, et al. Genomewide linkage scan identifies a novel susceptibility locus for restless legs syndrome on chromosome 9p. Am J Hum Genet 2004; **74**: 876–85.

13 Desautels A, Turecki G, Montplaisir J, et al. Identification of a major susceptibility locus for restless legs syndrome on chromosome 12q [see comment]. Am J Hum Genet 2001; **69**: 1266–70.

14 Bonati MT, Ferini-Strambi L, Aridon P, et al. Autosomal dominant restless legs syndrome maps on chromosome 14q. Brain 2003; **126**: 1485–92.

15 Earley CJ, Connor JR, Beard JL, et al. Abnormalities in CSF concentrations of ferritin and transferrin in restless legs syndrome. Neurology 2000; **54**: 1698–700.

16 Schmidauer C, Sojer M, Stocckner H, et al. Brain parenchyma sonography differentiates RLS patients from normal controls and patients with Parkinson's disease. J Am Geriatr Soc 2005; **20**(Suppl 10): S43.

17 Allen RP, Barker PB, Wehrl F, et al. MRI measurement of brain iron in patients with restless legs syndrome. Neurology 2001; **56**: 263–5.

18 Connor JR, Wang XS, Patton SM, et al. Decreased transferrin receptor expression by neuromelanin cells in restless legs syndrome. Neurology 2004; **62**: 1563–7.

19 Connor JR, Boyer PJ, Menzies SL, et al. Neuropathological examination suggests impaired brain iron acquisition in restless legs syndrome. Neurology 2003; **61**: 304–9.

20 Garcia-Borreguero D, Larrosa O, Granizo JJ, et al. Circadian variation in neuroendocrine response to L-dopa in patients with restless legs syndrome. Sleep 2004; **27**: 669–73.

21 Trenkwalder C, Walters AS, Hening WA, et al. Positron emission tomographic studies in restless legs syndrome. J Am Geriatr Soc 1999; **14**: 141–5.

22 Ruottinen HM, Partinen M, Hublin C, et al. An FDOPA PET study in patients with periodic limb movement disorder and restless legs syndrome. Neurology 2000; **54**: 502–4.

23 Turjanski N, Lees AJ, Brooks DJ. Striatal dopaminergic function in restless legs syndrome: ^{18}F-dopa and ^{11}C-raclopride PET studies. Neurology 1999; **52**: 932–7.

24 Michaud M, Soucy JP, Chabli A, et al. SPECT imaging of striatal pre- and postsynaptic dopaminergic status in restless legs syndrome with periodic leg movements in sleep. J Neurol 2002; **249**: 164–70.

25 Linke R, Eisensehr I, Wetter TC, et al. Presynaptic dopaminergic function in patients with restless legs syndrome: are there common features with early Parkinson's disease? Mov Disord 2004; **19**: 1158–62.

26 Eisensehr I, Wetter TC, Linke R, et al. Normal IPT and IBZM SPECT in drug-naive and levodopa-treated idiopathic restless legs syndrome. Neurology 2001; **57**: 1307–9.

27 Qu S, Le W, Zhang X, Xie W, et al. Locomotion is increased in a11-lesioned mice with iron deprivation: a possible animal model for restless legs syndrome. J Neuropathol Exp Neurol 2007; **66**: 383–8.

28 Stiasny-Kolster K, Moller JC, Zschocke J, et al. Normal dopaminergic and serotonergic metabolites in cerebrospinal fluid and blood of restless legs syndrome patients. J Am Geriatr Soc 2004; **19**: 192–6.

29 Earley CJ, Hyland K, Allen RP. CSF dopamine, serotonin, and biopterin metabolites in patients with restless legs syndrome. J Am Geriatr Soc 2001; **16**: 144–9.

30 Pittock SJ, Parrett T, Adler CH, et al. Neuropathology of primary restless leg syndrome: absence of specific tau- and alpha-synuclein pathology. Mov Disord 2004; **19**: 695–9.

31 Ye Z, Connor JR. Identification of iron responsive genes by screening cDNA libraries from suppression subtractive hybridization with antisense probes from three iron conditions. Nucleic Acids Res 2000; **28**: 1802–7.

32 Wang X, Wiesinger J, Beard J, et al. Thy1 expression in the brain is affected by iron and is decreased in restless legs syndrome. J Neurol Sci 2004; **220**: 59–66.

33 Jeng CJ, McCarroll SA, Martin TF, et al. Thy-1 is a component common to multiple populations of synaptic vesicles. J Cell Biol 1998; **140**: 685–98.

34 Adel S, Djarmati A, Kabakci K, et al. Co-occurrence of restless legs syndrome and Parkin mutations in two families. Mov Disord 2006; **21**: 258–63.

35 Ondo WG, Vuong KD, Jankovic J. Exploring the relationship between Parkinson disease and restless legs syndrome. Arch Neurol 2002; **59**: 421–4.

36 Peralta CM, Wolf E, Seppi K, et al. Restless legs in idiopathic Parkinson' disease. J Am Geriatr Soc 2005; **20**(Suppl 10): S108.

37 Driver-Dunckley E, Evidente VG, Adler CH, et al. Restless legs syndrome in Parkinson's disease patients may improve with subthalamic stimulation. Mov Disord 2006; **21**: 1287–9.

38 Simuni T, Wilson R, Stern MB. Prevalence of restless legs syndrome in Parkinson's disease. J Am Geriatr Soc 2000; **15**(Suppl 5): 1043.

39 Krishnan PR, Bhatia M, Behari M. Restless legs syndrome in Parkinson's disease: a case-controlled study. Mov Disord 2003; **18**: 181–5.

40 Kumar S, Bhatia M, Behari M. Sleep disorders in Parkinson's disease. Mov Disord 2002; **17**: 775–81.

41 Nomura T, Inoue Y, Miyake M, et al. Prevalence and clinical characteristics of restless legs syndrome in Japanese patients with Parkinson's disease. Mov Disord 2006; **21**: 380–4.

42 Tan EK, Lum SY, Wong MC. Restless legs syndrome in Parkinson's disease. J Neurol Sci 2002; **196**: 33–6.

43 Fazzini E, Diaz R, Fahn S. Restless legs in Parkinson's disease-clinical evidence for underactivity of catecholamine neurotransmission [abstract]. Ann Neurol 1989; **26**: 142.

44 Walters AS, LeBrocq C, Passi V, et al. A preliminary look at the percentage of patients with restless legs syndrome who also have Parkinson disease, essential tremor or Tourette syndrome in a single practice. J Sleep Res 2003; **12**: 343–5.

45 Ancoli-Israel S, Kripke DF, Klauber MR, et al. Periodic limb movements in sleep in community-dwelling elderly. Sleep 1991; **14**: 496–500.

46 Mosko SS, Dickel MJ, Paul T, et al. Sleep apnea and sleep-related periodic leg movements in community resident seniors. J Am Geriatr Soc 1988; **36**: 502–8.

47 Roehrs T, Zorick F, Sicklesteel J, et al. Age-related sleep–wake disorders at a sleep disorder center. J Am Geriatr Soc 1983; **31**: 364–70.

48 Montplaisir J, Boucher S, Poirier G, et al. Clinical, polysomnographic, and genetic characteristics of restless legs syndrome: a study of 133 patients diagnosed with new standard criteria. J Am Geriatr Soc 1997; **12**: 61–5.

49 Coleman RM, Miles LE, Guilleminault CC, et al. Sleep–wake disorders in the elderly: polysomnographic analysis. J Am Geriatr Soc 1981; **29**: 289–96.

50 Trenkwalder C. Sleep dysfunction in Parkinson's disease. Clin Neurosci 1998; **5**: 107–14.

51 Wetter TC, Trenkwalder C, Gershanik O, Hogl B. Polysomnographic measures in Parkinson's disease: a comparison between patients with and without REM sleep disturbances. Wien Klin Wochenschr 2001; **113**: 249–53.

52 Hogl B, Rothdach A, Wetter TC, Trenkwalder C. The effect of cabergoline on sleep, periodic leg movements in sleep, and early morning motor function in patients with Parkinson's disease. Neuropsychopharmacology 2003; **28**: 1866–70.

53 Happe S, Pirker W, Klosch G, et al. Periodic leg movements in patients with Parkinson's disease are associated with reduced striatal dopamine transporter binding. J Neurol 2003; **250**: 83–6.

54 Loo HV, Tan EK. Case-control study of restless legs syndrome and quality of sleep in Parkinson's disease. J Neurol Sci 2008; **266**: 145–9.

55 Covassin N, Neikrug AB, Liu L, et al. Clinical correlates of periodic limb movements in sleep in Parkinson's disease. J Neurol Sci 2012; **316**: 131–6.

56 Hogl B, Rothdach A, Wetter TC, Trenkwalder C. The effect of cabergoline on sleep, periodic leg movements in sleep, and early morning motor function in patients with Parkinson's disease. Neuropsychopharmacology 2003; **28**: 1866–70.

57 Imamura A, Tsuboi Y, Tanaka M, et al. Effect of high dose pergolide mesilate on restless legs syndrome associated with Parkinson disease [in Japanese]. Rinsho Shinkeigaku 2007; **47**: 156–9.

58 Shpirer I, Miniovitz A, Klein C, et al. Excessive daytime sleepiness in patients with Parkinson's disease: a polysomnography study. Mov Disord 2006; **21**: 1432–8.

59 Rye DB, DeLong MR. Amelioration of sensory limb discomfort of restless legs syndrome by pallidotomy. Ann Neurol 1999; **46**: 800–1.

60 Kedia S, Moro E, Tagliati M, et al. Emergence of restless legs syndrome during subthalamic stimulation for Parkinson disease. Neurology 2004; **63**: 2410–12.

61 Parra J, Brocalero-Camacho A, Sancho J, et al. [Severe restless legs syndrome following bilateral subthalamic stimulation to treat a patient with Parkinson's disease]. Rev Neurol 2006; **42**: 766–7.

62 Braga-Neto P, da Silva FP, Jr, Sueli Monte F, et al. Snoring and excessive daytime sleepiness in Parkinson's disease. J Neurol Sci 2004; 217: 41–5 [erratum in J Neurol Sci **2004**; **219**: 171].

63 Chaudhuri KR, Martinez-Martin P, Schapira AH, et al. International multicenter pilot study of the first comprehensive self-completed nonmotor symptoms questionnaire for Parkinson's disease: the NMSQuest study. Mov Disord 2006; **21**: 916–23.

64 Verbaan D, van Rooden SM, van Hilten JJ, Rijsman RM. Prevalence and clinical profile of restless legs syndrome in Parkinson's disease. Mov Disord 2010; **25**: 2142–7.

Chapter 16

Excessive daytime sleepiness in Parkinson's disease

Birgit Frauscher and Werner Poewe

At the last, constant sleepiness, with slight delirium, and other marks of extreme exhaustion, announce the wished-for release.
J. Parkinson, 1817

Introduction

While in his 'Essay on the shaking palsy' Parkinson referred to excessive sleepiness as an end-stage feature of the disease now bearing his name [1], different manifestations of dysregulation of the sleep–wake cycle have meanwhile become recognized as common non-motor problems across all stages of Parkinson's disease (PD), and rapid eye movement (REM) sleep behaviour disorder (RBD) may even occur as a 'pre-clinical' sign prior to the development of the cardinal motor symptoms. Depending on definitions and types of assessment, excessive daytime sleepiness (EDS) has been found in up to 50% of patients [2,3] and episodes of sudden-onset sleep (SOS) have now been identified as an important adverse reaction to dopaminergic therapy—in particular with dopamine agonists [4]. This chapter will review the current definitions, prevalence and underlying mechanisms as well as treatment of EDS in PD.

Definition and clinical assessment of EDS

EDS is inappropriate and undesirable sleepiness during waking hours even after adequate nighttime sleep. Sudden involuntary sleep onset and microsleeps are common complications. SOS has been defined as abrupt episodes of unplanned sleep during activities of daily living when they are not expected to occur (e.g. while speaking, eating or driving). These episodes may be preceded by somnolence and last from a few minutes to several hours [5].

In clinical practice, assessment of EDS and SOS usually has to rely on subjective information provided by the patient with possible involvement of third parties such as spouses or caregivers. Several sleepiness scales are available to formalize and quantify this information. Perhaps the most frequently used are the Stanford Sleepiness Scale (SSS) [6] and the Epworth Sleepiness Scale (ESS) [7]. In the SSS, patients are required to rate their current state, choosing from different levels of sleepiness (from fully alert to fully asleep), whereas the ESS measures sleepiness in recent times. The ESS is an eight-item questionnaire with four response options regarding the probability of falling asleep in eight different everyday situations. A cutoff value of >10 is used in most studies to define EDS. To assess the risk of falling asleep, the inappropriate sleep composite score was developed by Hobson and co-workers [8]. This score includes items 6 and 8 of the ESS and four additional questions regarding pathological aspects of sleepiness, such as falling asleep while conversing (question 6 of the ESS), stopping in traffic while driving (question 8 of the ESS), driving, eating, working and during household activities. Each question is rated from 0 to 3. Recently, a specific daytime sleepiness scale for PD has been developed (SCOPA-DL) [9]. It has similarities to the ESS and consists of six items with four response options. One disadvantage of all subjective scales is that they are entirely dependent on patients' perceptions of their problems. In PD in particular misperception of sleepiness is common. In a recent study, 38% of 47 sleepy PD patients were unaware of at least one nap during the multiple sleep latency test [10]. The involvement of spouses or caregivers in completing questionnaires like the ESS may increase the reliability of this subjective type of information.

In contrast, objective measures of sleepiness are independent of the patient's perception but require sleep laboratory facilities and are much more time-consuming. Two broadly accepted standardized electrophysiological measures in this context are the Multiple Sleep Latency Test (MSLT) [11] and the Maintenance of Wakefulness Test (MWT) [12]. The MSLT measures the ability of an individual to fall asleep. It is assessed during five 20-minute examinations with an inter-nap interval of 2 hours after a night of polysomnographic registration. A mean sleep latency of less than 8 minutes is considered to be pathological. Sleep-onset rapid eye movement (REM) episodes (SOREMs) are defined as a REM sleep latency of less than 15 minutes in the MSLT. REM sleep is characterized by rapid eye movements, muscle atonia (or rather hypotonia) and a mixed-frequency, low-voltage electroencephalogram (EEG) pattern [13]. SOREMs are a typical hallmark of narcolepsy with cataplexy, but have been observed in PD patients exhibiting EDS [14]. The MWT measures the ability to stay awake and is therefore better suited to assessing the risk of SOS. During the MWT, subjects remain inactive in a seated position for periods of 20–40 minutes and are instructed to stay awake for as long as possible. In the 20-minute variant, a latency shorter than 11 minutes is abnormal [12]. Despite their potential limitations, the ESS and the MSLT have been used repeatedly in PD, and together with the MWT currently appear to be the best available methods for measuring EDS in this condition.

Prevalence and risk factors

Depending on the definitions and assessments used, EDS has been found in 16–51% of all PD patients [8,9,15–28] (see Table 16.1). It is also common in PD patients without dementia who are otherwise functionally fully independent [8]. Episodes of SOS were reported by 4–6% of subjects in two large questionnaire-based surveys [8,21]. The risk of SOS was found to be 2.9% with levodopa monotherapy, 5.3% with dopamine agonist

Table 16.1 Prevalence of excessive daytime sleepiness (EDS) in Parkinson's disease (PD)

Author	Number of patients (controls)	Method	EDS PD (%)	EDS controls (%)
Van Hilten et al., 1993 [15]	90 (71)	EDS score ≥ 3	44	31 (n = 71)
Tandberg et al., 1999 [16]	245 (100)	Questionnaire[a]	16	1 (n = 100)
Ondo et al., 2001 [17]	303	ESS > 10	50	–
Hobson et al., 2002 [8]	638	ESS > 7	51	–
Tan et al., 2002 [18]	201/214	ESS ≥ 10	20	10 (n = 214)
Brodsky et al., 2003 [19]	101/100	ESS ≥ 10	41	19 (n = 100)
Högl et al., 2003 [20]	99/44	ESS ≥ 10	33	11 (n = 44)
Paus et al., 2003 [21]	177[b]	ESS > 10	75	–
Marinus et al., 2003 [9]	143 (104)	ESS > 10	27	3 (n = 104)
Kumar et al., 2003 [22]	149 (115)	ESS > 8	21	3 (n = 115)
Monaca et al., 2006 [23]	222	ESS > 10	43	–
Ferreira et al., 2006 [24]	176 (174)	ESS ≥ 15	34	16 (n = 174)
Ghorayeb et al., 2007 [26]	1625	ESS ≥ 10	29	–
Verbaan et al., 2008 [25]	419 (150)	SCOPA-DS ≥ 5	43	10 (n = 150)
Suzuki et al., 2008 [27]	188	ESS ≥ 10	21%	–
Breen et al., 2013 [28]	118	ESS > 10	49%-	–

Note that only studies with n ≥ 90 participants are included.

EDS, excessive daytime sleepiness; ESS, Epworth sleepiness score; SCOPA-DS, scales for outcomes in Parkinson's disease–daytime sleepiness.

[a] Falling asleep three or more times or total sleep time during the day >2 hours.

[b] PD patients with episodes of sudden onset of sleep.

monotherapy and 7.3% with a combined levodopa and dopamine agonist therapy [21]. The type of dopamine agonist used, however, does not differentially affect the risk of EDS or SOS [8,19,21,29], indicating that the induction of sleepiness represents a class effect common to all currently used agonists. Total dopaminergic drug dose [19,21,29], ESS score [8,19,21], disease duration [8,21], disease severity [30], male sex [17], benzodiazepine use [31], co-morbid dementia or psychosis [32], autonomic failure [33] as well as heavy snoring [20,34] have all been identified as risk factors for EDS or SOS in various studies. An ESS score >7 predicted a 75% chance of SOS while driving. Its specificity, however, was low at 52% [8]. Using the MSLT in 54 sleepy PD patients, a narcolepsy-like phenotype (a sleep latency of less than 8 minutes plus two or more periods of REM sleep onset) was detected in 39% of cases [14].

Pathophysiological mechanisms

A number of different mechanisms have been implicated in the pathophysiology of EDS in PD. They include a dysfunctional sleep–wakefulness control intrinsic to PD, secondary effects of the motor and non-motor symptoms of PD on sleep (e.g. nocturnal akinesia, tremor, rigidity, nocturnal off-period dystonia and pain as well as nocturia), side effects of medication, co-morbid conditions and genetic factors.

Intrinsic dysfunction of sleep–wakefulness control in PD

The pathology of PD is now known to affect a number of key brainstem areas critical for regulation of the sleep–wake cycle, including the hypothalamus and lower brainstem [35]. Although the exact clinico-pathological correlations are far from established, it appears likely that abnormalities of sleep–wakefulness control observed in PD are at least partially explained by such pathologies.

A recent hypothesis suggests that EDS and SOS are based on a disturbed corticothalamic arousal system [36]. While the nigrostriatal dopamine system is involved in motor control, dopaminergic neurons in the mesocorticolimbic circuits seem to play an important role in sleep–wakefulness control [37]. Arnulf and co-workers [14] found that the severity of sleepiness was not dependent on nocturnal sleep abnormalities, motor and cognitive impairment or antiparkinsonian medication in patients with PD pre-selected for sleepiness, but it seemed to be an integral part of the disease itself. The same was shown for non-selected PD patients in a MSLT study. The authors showed that EDS was in fact inversely related to the integrity of nighttime sleep [31]. EDS can rarely be a prominent feature at disease onset, as reported for a previously untreated woman with juvenile PD who was found to have deficits in remaining awake—probably as a consequence of central dopaminergic depletion or other early neuropathological changes characteristic of PD [38]. In addition, healthy subjects with evidence for EDS were found to have an increased risk of developing PD, suggesting that EDS could even be an early pre-motor sign of the disease [39].

In contrast to narcolepsy, however, spinal cerebrospinal fluid (CSF) hypocretin-1 (hcrt-1) in PD revealed normal findings, even in PD patients with EDS [40–48]. The only study which found decreased CSF hcrt-1 values in PD assessed ventricular hcrt-1 [49], but found no association between reduced CSF hcrt-1 and measures of objective sleepiness [50].

Effects of medication

The induction of sleepiness via dopaminergic drugs is not unique to PD and was described in healthy volunteers decades ago [51]. One study even found similar degrees of drug-induced sleepiness in healthy volunteers who were challenged with either levodopa or a benzodiazepine [52]. Drug-induced somnolence has also been documented for the newer non-ergot dopamine agonists [53,54]. In addition to dopaminergic therapies, sedating antidepressants, anxiolytics and atypical neuroleptics, which are commonly used to treat the neuropsychiatric co-morbidities of PD, are important contributors to consider in patients with EDS.

While SOS in PD was initially described in patients treated with the non-ergot D2/D3-receptor agonists pramipexole and ropinirole [4], this was soon followed by reports of SOS in PD patients treated with all other non-ergot and ergot dopamine agonists as well as with levodopa [55–57]. However, available evidence suggests that the prevalence of drug-induced EDS is higher with dopamine agonists than with levodopa alone, as exemplified by a prospective 6-year follow-up study investigating the long-term effect of initial pramipexole versus levodopa monotherapy in early PD where EDS occurred in 57% of the pramipexole group compared with 35% of the levodopa group [58]. No significant differences could be detected between ergot and non-ergot dopamine agonists in relation to ESS scores or EDS [8,19,21,29], but the risk of EDS seemed to increase with combination therapies using levodopa plus dopamine agonists [21].

Co-morbid conditions

Sleep-related breathing disorders

Polysomnographic studies in PD patients investigating the presence of sleep-related breathing disorders found rates of relevant obstructive sleep apnoea (apnoea–hypopnoea index >15/hour) between 15 and 34% [14,59–61]. A recent study found no difference in the frequency of sleep apnoea between PD patients and age-matched healthy controls [62], which is in line with studies in the general population that have shown a prevalence of relevant obstructive sleep apnoea of up to 18% [63].

Restless legs syndrome/periodic limb movements in sleep

Whereas several studies have reported rates of restless legs syndrome (RLS) affecting around 20% of PD patients [64,65] compared with only 10% in the general elderly population [66], more recent studies in both treated and untreated PD patients failed to confirm differences in prevalence of RLS between PD patients and controls [67,68]. This discrepancy might in part be explained by confounding motor and non-motor fluctuations in earlier studies, which have the potential to mimic RLS via bedtime wearing-off symptoms producing unpleasant sensations and an urge to move. Periodic limb movements in sleep (PLMS) were found in 15% of sleepy PD patients [14]. While RLS and PLMS are associated with sleep disturbance, their exact contribution to sleep fragmentation and EDS in PD has not yet been clarified.

Genetics

Genetic risk factors for EDS in PD have not been extensively investigated [30,69–72] and the data available so far have remained inconclusive. Significant associations of EDS with the low-activity allele of the *COMT* polymorphism were found in one pilot study [69], but not confirmed in a replication sample of 240 patients [30]. Other genetic studies found an association of EDS and the *DRD4* *2 allele [70], the *DRD2* A2 allele [71] and pre-prohypocretin polymorphisms [72]. All these await replication.

Management

Management of EDS has to target underlying mechanisms. Therefore, a careful evaluation of causative factors including drug history, co-morbid conditions affecting sleep–wake regulation and PD-related contributors to reduced wakefulness is required. EDS or SOS following the introduction or dose increase of a dopamine agonist requires down-titration or discontinuation, depending on the severity of the EDS, the occurrence of SOS and the availability of alternatives to treat parkinsonism. PD patients on dopamine agonists must be warned not to drive or handle machinery if they experience symptoms of increased daytime sleepiness. While down-titration of a given agonist often helps, switching from one agonist to another is unlikely to solve the problem, given that agonist-induced EDS is a class effect common to all agents of this type. Levodopa rarely causes EDS compared with dopamine agonists, but similar actions such as down-titration need to be considered when a given patient on levodopa complains of daytime somnolence. New-onset EDS in patients on combined regimens of levodopa with or without catechol-O-methyltransferase (COMT) inhibitors, dopamine agonists and monoamine oxidase B (MAO-B) inhibitors should usually have their dopamine agonist dose reviewed before changes of other agents are considered. MAO-B inhibitors are unlikely culprits in these situations since EDS with SOS has not been reported with MAO-B inhibitor monotherapy. Sedatives, anxiolytics, sedating antidepressants and hypnotic medications should also be reviewed and—depending on the context in which EDS symptoms first appeared—should possibly be eliminated before changes of dopaminergics are implemented (see Table 16.2).

The specific treatment of sleep-related co-morbidities such as sleep-related breathing disorders or RLS/PLMS may improve EDS in some patients, although systematic controlled trials are lacking. In PD patients, nasal continuous positive airway pressure treatment resulted in less improvement of sleep architecture than found in patients with obstructive sleep apnoea syndrome alone [73]. If a dose reduction of dopaminergic or other contributing drugs is not feasible or treatment of underlying co-morbid conditions does not significantly improve EDS scores, symptomatic treatment of daytime sleepiness may sometimes be achieved with wake-enhancing or stimulant drugs (see Table 16.2).

Most of the evidence on efficacy of drugs to treat EDS in PD is related to modafinil. Modafinil appears to promote wakefulness by improving dopaminergic transmission, although its precise mechanism of action is unknown [74]. It has been approved by the US Food and Drug Administration (FDA) for the treatment of narcolepsy, persisting EDS despite sufficiently treated obstructive sleep apnoea/hypopnoea syndrome and shift-work sleep disorder. In 2010, the European Medical Agency restricted the use of modafinil for narcolepsy only after reviewing the safety profile of this drug (serious skin reactions, psychiatric adverse reactions as well as hypertension and cardiac arrhythmias). There is one open-label study in ten PD patients [75] and three randomized placebo-controlled studies in 15, 21 and 40 patients [76–78]. At modafinil doses of approximately 200 mg/day, significant positive effects on the ESS but not on the MWT were reported in two cross-over trials [76,77], while the larger parallel group study failed to show significant differences compared with placebo in the ESS or the MSLT [78]. A recent evidence-based review of treatments targeting the non-motor symptoms of PD therefore concluded that there is insufficient evidence for efficacy of modafinil to treat EDS in PD [79]. Stimulants such as methylphenidate or amphetamines have also been proposed as second-line therapy for

Table 16.2 Practical management of excessive daytime sleepiness

Symptom	Management
Primary sleep-wake dysregulation	
Sleep fragmentation	Zolpidem 10 mg, melatonin 3–6 mg at bedtime
Rapid eye movement sleep behaviour disorder	Clonazepam 0.25–2 mg at bedtime, melatonin 3–6 mg at bedtime
'Narcoleptic phenotype'	First line: modafinil 100–400 mg. Second line: stimulants, buproprion after careful evaluation
Secondary effects of PD symptoms	
Nocturnal akinesia, tremor and rigidity	Optimized PD treatment regimen
Nocturnal off-period dystonia and pain	Optimized PD treatment regimen
Effects of medications	
Levodopa/dopamine agonists	Dose reduction, dose splitting or switch to another drug
Non-dopaminergic agents	
Benzodiazepines	Eliminate if possible
Atypical neuroleptics	Careful risk/benefit evaluation
Sedative antidepressants	Careful risk/benefit evaluation
Antihistaminergic drugs	Eliminate if possible
Effects of co-morbid conditions	
Sleep-related breathing disorders	Nasal continuous positive airway pressure treatment
RLS/PLMS	Dopamine agonists, opiods or antiepileptics (e.g. pregabalin)

PD, Parkinson's disease; PLMS, periodic limb movements in sleep; RLS, restless legs syndrome.

EDS in PD, but there is no evidence from randomized, controlled trials to support their use in this indication. The same is true for buproprion, an antidepressant which is thought to be an indirect dopaminergic agonist. Recent clinical Phase II and III studies in the United States and Europe have investigated the effects of the selective inverse histamine H3 receptor agonist pitolisant, as well as of caffeine and sodium oxybate on EDS in PD. While the results of pitolisant for EDS in PD have not yet been published, an open-label polysomnographic study with sodium oxybate showed promising results [80]. A randomized controlled trial of caffeine for treatment of PD failed to demonstrate an effect on EDS in patients with PD [81].

Conclusion

Daytime sleepiness is a common and potentially disabling non-motor symptom of PD with complex underlying mechanisms. They include dysfunctional sleep–wake regulation resulting from PD pathology affecting the brainstem–cortical networks subserving wakefulness as well as a multitude of interacting factors comprising side effects of medication, disturbed and fragmented sleep via the effects of nocturnal motor and non-motor symptoms as well as the effects of co-morbidities like sleep-disordered breathing. Careful history taking is essential to dissect out the different components contributing to EDS in a given patient and will often require information from bed partners or carers. Similarly complex are the resulting management issues, which often call for combinations of therapeutic approaches focusing on reviews of the current drug regimen with the aim of eliminating drug-induced EDS and the control of PD symptoms and co-morbidities impacting on sleep quality. These measures are particularly important since, to date, no agent has been identified as being unequivocally efficacious in improving EDS in PD.

References

1 **Parkinson J**. An essay on the shaking palsy. London: Sherwood, Neely, and Jones, 1817.

2 **Factor SA, McAlarney T, Sanchez-Ramos JR, Weiner WJ**. Sleep disorders and sleep effect in Parkinson's disease. Mov Disord 1990; **5**: 280–5.

3 **Poewe W, Högl B**. Parkinson's disease and sleep. Curr Opin Neurol 2000; **13**: 423–6.

4 **Frucht S, Rogers JD, Greene PE, et al**. Falling asleep at the wheel: motor vehicle mishaps in persons taking pramipexole and ropinirole. Neurology 1999; **52**: 1908–10.

5 European Agency for the Evaluation of Medical Products. CPMP position statement. Dopaminergic substances and sudden sleep onset. London: EMEA, 2002.

6 **Hoddes E, Zarcone V, Smythe H, et al**. Quantification of sleepiness: a new approach. Psychophysiology 1973; **10**: 431–6.

7 **Johns MW**. A new method for measuring daytime sleepiness: the Epworth sleepiness scale. Sleep 1991; **14**: 540–5.

8 **Hobson DE, Lang AE, Martin WR**. Excessive daytime sleepiness and sudden-onset sleep in Parkinson disease: a survey by the Canadian Movement Disorders Group. J Am Med Assoc 2002; **287**: 455–63.

9 **Marinus J, Visser M, van Hilten JJ, et al**. Assessment of sleep and sleepiness in Parkinson's disease. Sleep 2003; **26**: 1049–54.

10 **Merino-Andreu M, Arnulf I, Konofal E, et al**. Unawareness of naps in Parkinson's disease and in disorders with excessive daytime sleepiness. Neurology 2003; **60**: 1553–4.

11 **Carskadon MA, Dement WC, Mitler MM, et al**. Guidelines for the multiple sleep latency test (MSLT): a standard measure of sleepiness. Sleep 1986; **9**: 519–24.

12 **Doghramji K, Mitler MM, Sangal RB, et al**. A normative study of the maintenance of wakefulness test (MWT). Electroencephalogr Clin Neurophysiol 1997; **103**: 554–62.

13 **Berry RB, Brooks R, Gamaldo CE, Harding SM, Marcus CL, Vaughn BF**; for the American Academy of Sleep Medicine. The AASM manual for the scoring of sleep and associated events: rules, terminology and technical specifications, Version 2.0. Westchester, IL: AASM, 2012.

14 **Arnulf I, Konofal E, Merino-Andreu M, et al**. Parkinson's disease and sleepiness. An integral part of PD. Neurology 2002; **58**: 1019–24.

15 **Van Hilten JJ, Weggeman M, Van der Velde EA, et al**. Sleep, excessive daytime sleepiness and fatigue in Parkinson's disease. J Neural Transm Park Dis Dement Sect 1993; **5**: 235–44.

16 **Tandberg E, Larsen JP, Karlsen K**. Excessive daytime sleepiness and sleep benefit in Parkinson's disease: a community-based study. Mov Disord 1999; **14**: 922–7.

17 **Ondo W, Dat Vuong K, Khan H, et al**. Daytime sleepiness and other sleep disorders in Parkinson's disease. Neurology 2001; **57**: 1392–6.

18 **Tan EK, Lum SY, Fook-Chong SM, et al**. Evaluation of somnolence in Parkinson's disease: comparison with age- and sex-matched controls. Neurology 2002; **58**: 465–8.

19 Brodsky MA, Godbold J, Roth T, Olanow CW. Sleepiness in Parkinson's disease: a controlled study. Mov Disord 2003; **18**: 668–72.

20 Högl B, Seppi K, Brandauer E, et al. Increased daytime sleepiness in Parkinson's disease: a questionnaire survey. Mov Disord 2003; **18**: 319–23.

21 Paus S, Brecht HM, Köster J, et al. Sleep attacks, daytime sleepiness, and dopamine agonists in Parkinson's disease. Mov Disord 2003; **18**: 659–67.

22 Kumar S, Bhatia M, Behari M. Excessive daytime sleepiness in Parkinson's disease as assessed by Epworth sleepiness scale (ESS). Sleep Med 2003; **4**: 339–42.

23 Monaca C, Duhamel A, Jacquesson JM, et al. Vigilance troubles in Parkinson's disease: a subjective and objective polysomnographic study. Sleep Med 2006; **7**: 448–53.

24 Ferreira JJ, Desboeuf K, Galitzky M, et al. Sleep disruption, daytime somnolence and 'sleep attacks' in Parkinson's disease: a clinical survey in PD patients and age-matched healthy volunteers. Eur J Neurol 2006; **13**: 209–14.

25 Verbaan D, van Rooden SM, Visser M, et al. Nighttime sleep problems and daytime sleepiness in Parkinson's disease. Mov Disord 2008; **23**: 35–41.

26 Ghorayeb I, Loundou A, Auquier P, et al. A nationwide survey of excessive daytime sleepiness in Parkinson's disease in France. Mov Disord 2007; **22**: 1567–72.

27 Suzuki K, Miyamoto T, Miyamoto M, et al. Excessive daytime sleepiness and sleep episodes in Japanese patients with Parkinson's disease. J Neurol Sci 2008; **271**: 47–52.

28 Breen DP, Williams-Gray CH, Mason SL, Foltynie T, Barker RA. Excessive daytime sleepiness and its risk factors in incident Parkinson's disease. J Neurol Neurosurg Psychiatry 2013; **84**: 233–4.

29 Razmy A, Lang AE, Shapiro CM. Predictors of impaired daytime sleep and wakefulness in patients with Parkinson disease treated with older (ergot) vs. newer (nonergot) dopamine agonists. Arch Neurol 2004; **61**: 97–102.

30 Rissling I, Frauscher B, Kronenberg F, et al. Daytime sleepiness and the COMT va1158met polymorphism in patients with Parkinson disease. Sleep 2006; **29**: 108–11.

31 Rye DB, Bliwise DL, Dihenia B, Gurecki P. Daytime sleepiness in Parkinson's disease. J Sleep Res 2000; **9**: 63–9.

32 Gjerstad MD, Aarsland D, Larsen JP. Development of daytime somnolence over time in Parkinson's disease. Neurology 2002; **58**: 1544–6.

33 Montastruc JL, Brefel-Courbon C, Senard JM, et al. Sleep attacks and antiparkinsonian drugs: a pilot prospective pharmacoepidemiologic study. Clin Neuropharmacol 2001; **24**: 181–3.

34 Braga-Neto P, da Silva-Junior FP, Sueli Monte F, et al. Snoring and excessive daytime sleepiness in Parkinson's disease. J Neurol Sci 2004; **217**: 41–5.

35 Braak H, Del Tredici K, Rüb U, et al. Staging of brain pathology related to sporadic Parkinson's disease. Neurobiol Aging 2003; **24**: 197–211.

36 Rye DB. Excessive daytime sleepiness and unintended sleep in Parkinson's disease. Curr Neurol Neurosci Rep 2006; **6**: 169–76.

37 Rye DB. The two faces of Eve. Dopamine's modulation of wakefulness and sleep. Neurology 2004; 63(Suppl 3): S2–S7.

38 Rye D, Johnston LH, Watts RL, Bliwise DL. Juvenile Parkinson's disease with REM sleep behavior disorder, sleepiness and daytime REM-onsets. Neurology 1999; **53**: 1868–70.

39 Abbott RD, Ross GW, White LR, et al. Excessive daytime sleepiness and subsequent development of Parkinson disease. Neurology 2005; **65**: 1442–6.

40 Ripley B, Overeem S, Fujiki N, et al. CSF hypocretin/orexin levels in narcolepsy and other neurological conditions. Neurology 2001; **57**: 2253–8.

41 Mignot E, Lammers GJ, Ripley B, et al. The role of cerebrospinal fluid hypocretin measurement in the diagnosis of narcolepsy and other hypersomnias. Arch Neurol 2002; **59**: 1553–62.

42 Overeem S, van Hilen JJ, Ripley B, et al. Normal hypocretin-1 levels in Parkinson's disease patients with excessive daytime sleepiness. Neurology 2002; **58**: 49–9.

43 Yasui K, Inoue Y, Kanbayashi T, Nomura T, Kusumi M, Nakashima K. CSF orexin levels of Parkinson's disease, dementia with Lewy bodies, progressive supranuclear palsy and corticobasal degeneration. J Neurol Sci 2006; **250**: 120–3.

44 Baumann CR, Scammel TE, Bassetti CL. Parkinson's disease, sleepiness and hypocretin/orexin. Brain 2008; **131**: e91.

45 Compta Y, Santamaria J, Ratti L, et al. Cerebrospinal hypocretin, daytime sleepiness and sleep architecture in Parkinson's disease dementia. Brain 2009; **132**: 3308–17.

46 Poceta JS, Parsons L, Engelland S, Kripke DF. Circadian rhythm of CSF monoamines and hypocretin-1 in restless legs syndrome and Parkinson's disease. Sleep Med 2009; **10**: 129–33.

47 Asai H, Hirano M, Furiya Y, et al. Cerebrospinal fluid-orexin levels and sleep attacks in four patients with Parkinson's disease. Clin Neurol Neurosurg 2009; **111**: 341–4.

48 Wienecke M, Werth E, Poryazova R, et al. Progressive dopamine and hypocretin deficiencies in Parkinson's disease: is there an impact on sleep and wakefulness? J Sleep Res 2012; **21**: 710–17.

49 Drouot X, Moutereau S, Lefaucheur JP, et al. Low level of ventricular CSF orexin-A is not associated with objective sleepiness in PD. Sleep Med 2011; **12**: 936–7.

50 Drouot X, Moutereau S, Nguyen JP, et al. Low levels of ventricular CSF orexin/hypocretin in advanced PD. Neurology 2003; **61**: 540–3.

51 Bassi S, Albizzati MG, Fratolla L, et al. Dopamine receptors and sleep induction in man. J Neurol Neurosurg Psychiatry 1979; **42**: 458–60.

52 Andreu N, Chalé JJ, Senard JM, et al. L-Dopa induced sedation: a double-blind cross-over controlled study versus triazolam and placebo in healthy volunteers. Clin Neuropharmacol 1999; **22**: 15–23.

53 Ferreira JJ, Galitzky M, Thalamas C, et al. Effect of ropinirole on sleep onset: a randomized, placebo-controlled study in healthy volunteers. Neurology 2002; **58**: 460–2.

54 Micallef J, Rey M, Eusebio A, et al. Antiparkinsonian drug-induced sleepiness: a double-blind placebo-controlled study of L-dopa, bromocriptine and pramipexole in healthy subjects. Br J Clin Pharmacol 2008; **67**: 333–40.

55 Schapira AH. Sleep attacks (sleep episodes) with pergolide. Lancet 2000; **355**: 1332–3.

56 Ferreira JJ, Galitzky M, Montastruc JL, Rascol O. Sleep attacks and Parkinson's disease treatment. Lancet 2000; **355**: 1333–4.

57 Högl B, Seppi K, Brandauer E, et al. Irresistible onset of sleep during acute levodopa challenge in multiple system atrophy: placebo-controlled, polysomnographic case report. Mov Disord 2001; **16**: 1177–9.

58 Parkinson Study Group CALM Cohort Investigators. Long-term effect of initiating pramipexole vs levodopa in early Parkinson's disease. Arch Neurol 2009; **66**: 563–70.

59 Diederich NJ, Vaillant M, Leischen M, et al. Sleep apnea syndrome in Parkinson's disease. A case-control study in 49 patients. Mov Disord 2005; **20**: 1413–18.

60 Cochen De Cock V, Abouda M, Leu S, et al. Is obstructive sleep apnea a problem in Parkinson's disease. Sleep Med 2010; **11**: 247–52.

61 Trotti LM, Bliwise DL. No increased risk of obstructive sleep apnea in Parkinson's disease. Mov Disord 2010; **25**: 2246–9.

62 Yong MH, Fook-Chong S, Pavanni R, Lim LL, Tan EK. Case control polysomnographic studies of sleep disorders in Parkinson's disease. PLoS ONE 2011; **6**: e22511.

63 Nieto FJ, Young TB, Lind BK, et al. Association of sleep-disordered breathing, sleep apnea, and hypertension in a large community-based study. J Am Med Assoc 2000; **283**: 1829–36.

64 Ondo WG, Vuong KD, Jankovic J. Exploring the relationship between Parkinson disease and restless legs syndrome. Arch Neurol 2002; **59**: 421–4.

65 Peralta CM, Frauscher B, Seppi K, et al. Restless legs syndrome in Parkinson's disease. Mov Disord 2009; **24**: 2076–80.

66 Högl B, Kiechl S, Willeit J, et al. Restless legs syndrome. A community-based study of prevalence, severity, and risk factors. Neurology 2005; **64**: 1920–4.

67 Gjerstad MD, Tysnes OB, Larsen JP. Increased risk of leg motor restlessness but not RLS in early Parkinson disease. Neurology 2011; **77**: 1941–6.

68 Verbaan D, van Rooden SM, van Hilten JJ, Rijsman RM. Prevalence and clinical profile of restless legs syndrome in Parkinson's disease. Mov Disord 2010; **13**: 2142–7.

69 Frauscher B, Högl B, Maret S, et al. Association of daytime sleepiness with COMT polymorphism in patients with Parkinson's disease: a pilot study. Sleep 2004; **27**: 733–6.

70 Paus S, Seeger G, Brecht HM, et al. Association study of dopamine D2, D3, D4 receptor and serotonin transporter gene polymorphisms with sleep attacks in Parkinson's disease. Mov Disord 2004; **19**: 705–7.

71 Rissling I, Geller F, Bandmann O, et al. Dopamine receptor gene polymorphisms in Parkinson's disease patients reporting 'sleep attacks'. Mov Disord 2004; **19**: 1279–84.

72 Rissling I, Körner Y, Geller F, et al. Preprohypocretin polymorphisms in Parkinson disease patients reporting 'sleep attacks'. Sleep 2005; **28**: 871–5.

73 Greulich W, Schäfer D, Georg WM, Schläfke ME. Schlafverhalten bei Patienten mit Morbus Parkinson [Sleep behaviour in patients with Parkinson's disease]. Somologie 1998; **2**: 163–71.

74 Wisor J, Nishino S, Sora I, et al. Dopaminergic role in stimulant-induced wakefulness. J Neurosci 2001; **21**: 1787–94.

75 Nieves AV, Lang AE. Treatment of excessive daytime sleepiness in patients with Parkinson's disease with modafinil. Clin Neuropharmacol 2002; **25**: 111–14.

76 Högl B, Saletu M, Brandauer E, et al. Modafinil for the treatment of daytime sleepiness in Parkinson's disease: a double-blind, randomized, crossover, placebo-controlled polygraphic trial. Sleep 2002; **25**: 905–9.

77 Adler CH, Caviness JN, Hentz JG, et al. Randomized trial of modafinil for treating subjective daytime sleepiness in patients with Parkinson's disease. Mov Disord 2003; **18**: 287–93.

78 Ondo WG, Fayle R, Atassi F, Jankovic J. Modafinil for daytime somnolence in Parkinson's disease: double-blind, placebo-controlled parallel trial. J Neurol Neurosurg Psychiatry 2005; **76**: 1636–9.

79 Seppi K, Weintraub D, Coelho M, et al. the Movement Disorder Society evidence-based medicine review update: treatments for the non-motor symptoms of Parkinson's disease. Mov Disord 2011; **26**(Suppl 3): S42–S80.

80 Ondo WG, Perkins T, Swick T, et al. Sodium oxybate for excessive daytime sleepiness in Parkinson disease. An open label polysomnographic study. Arch Neurol 2008; **65**: 1337–40.

81 Postuma RB, Lang AE, Munhoz RP, et al. Caffeine for treatment of Parkinson disease a randomized controlled trial. Neurology 2012; **79**: 651–8.

Chapter 17

Bladder dysfunction in Parkinson's disease

Ryuji Sakakibara and Clare Fowler

Introduction

When reading the literature about bladder dysfunction in Parkinson's disease (PD) one should bear in mind that the importance of a secure neurological diagnosis when considering urinary symptoms, was only recognized within the last decade. The bladder symptoms of multiple system atrophy (MSA) may be similar to PD; urogenital symptoms can be one of the earliest manifestations of MSA and urinary incontinence may be pronounced even with mild disability. As almost 50% of patients with MSA parkinsonism are initially misdiagnosed as having PD, any such misclassified patients may have had a confounding effect on early bladder studies.

Prevalence of lower urinary tract symptoms in PD

The first studies to look at the prevalence of lower urinary tract (LUT) symptoms in PD showed a high incidence of neurogenic detrusor overactivity (DO), although there was probably an element of pre-selection in the patient groups [1]. A study in 2000 found that 27% of those attending a neurology clinic had LUT symptoms [2]. One international survey used the recently devised NMSQuest questionnaire to assess non-motor symptoms of PD in 545 patients with a mean Hoehn and Yahr (HY) stage of 2.5 [3]. This survey found that 56% answered positively to the question 'have you experienced a sense of urgency to pass urine which makes you rush to the toilet', but the most common complaint was nocturia, with 62% answering in the affirmative to the question 'have you experienced getting up regularly at night to pass urine'? It emerged from the study that 'urinary' had the highest percentage of positive answers of all nine symptom domains [4]. An earlier questionnaire study from Japan, which focused on pelvic organ symptoms of 115 patients with PD and a mean HY stage of 3, found that 42% of women and 54% of men complained of urinary urgency, which was significantly higher than an age-matched control group [5] (Figs. 17.1 and 17.2). In a recent study of early untreated PD, the most common LUT symptom in PD was urinary urgency/frequency (64%). In addition, although there are only small post-void residuals in patients, complaints of voiding difficulty are not rare (28%) [6].

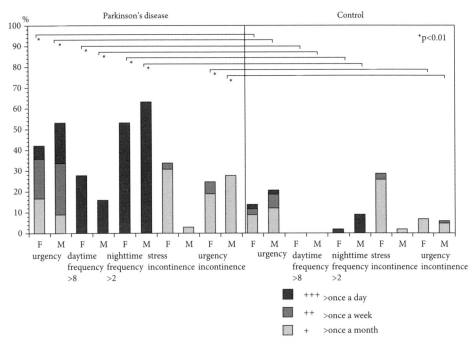

Fig. 17.1 The occurrence of symptoms related to bladder filling [5].
Reproduced with permission from Sakakibara R, Shinotoh H, Uchiyama T, et al. Questionnaire-based assessment of pelvic organ dysfunction in Parkinson's disease. Auton Neurosci 2001; 92: 76–85.

The nature of symptoms and urodynamic assessment in PD

As already mentioned, nocturia is the most common LUT symptom in PD. The reason for the prevalence of this complaint has not been properly elucidated, and possible explanations lie with (1) an increased urine output at night, (2) reduced bladder capacity or (3) impairment of sleep. In addition to nocturia, PD patients often have urinary urgency, suggesting that the patient's bladder is irritable. Urodynamics with a bladder filling rate of 50 ml min^{-1} is a feasible means of reproducing a patient's usual bladder behaviour in the laboratory. Detrusor overactivity (DO) is a urodynamic observation characterized by involuntary detrusor contractions during the filling phase which may be spontaneous or provoked. Various studies have shown that DO occurs in PD in 45 to 93% [6–8] of patients, which correlates well with the results of questionnaires [1–6] and uninhibited external sphincter relaxation in 33% [7] of patients. Therefore, DO could be the major factor contributing to overactive bladder (OAB) symptoms in PD. In addition, a subset (8.1%) of PD patients show increased bladder sensation without DO, which might also underlie OAB in PD [9]. However, the nighttime frequency of patients with PD appears to be disproportionate to their daytime frequency. Nighttime urine output has yet to be fully investigated as a factor, but impairment of sleep, a pronounced problem in patients with PD, may well be a significant additional factor.

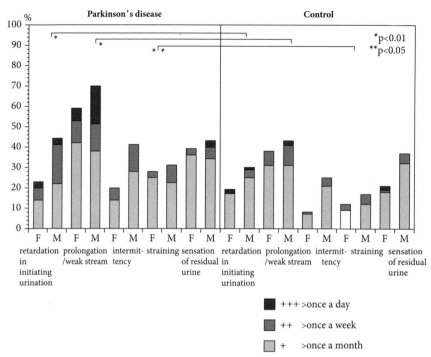

Fig. 17.2 The occurrence of symptoms related to bladder emptying [5].
Reproduced with permission from Sakakibara R, Shinotoh H, Uchiyama T, et al. Questionnaire-based assessment of pelvic organ dysfunction in Parkinson's disease. Auton Neurosci 2001; 92: 76–85.

The explanation for difficulty with voiding is less clear. Pressure-flow analysis of the voiding phase in PD has shown weak detrusor activity (in 40% of men and 66% of women) [7]. A subset of PD patients had DO during storage but weak detrusor activity in voiding. This combination has recently been estimated to occur in 18% of patients with PD [10]. Some older studies described detrusor–external sphincter dyssynergia or 'pseudo-dyssynergia' in PD, and these findings were attributed to PD by analogy with bradykinesia of the limbs. However, in more recent studies, detrusor–external sphincter dyssynergia was found to be rare in PD [7]. Irrespective of voiding symptoms in PD, the average volume of post-void residuals in PD was as small as 18 ml [7].

Correlation with the severity of neurological disease

Several studies have demonstrated a correlation between increasing severity of neurological disease and increasing bladder problems, including both the NMSQuest survey and the Japanese pelvic organ questionnaire [4,5]. In a study that used the International Prostate Symptom Score (IPSS) (and found it to be an equally effective tool in men and women), an almost linear relationship was found between the HY stage (with the introduction of a classification grade 3.5 for patients requiring assistance to walk outside) and the IPSS score [2]. Looking at the urodynamic abnormalities, Araki and colleagues [11] found that the volume of post-void residual was related to a three-grade scale of motor disorder (HY Stages 1–2, 3, 4–5). In a study by Terayama and colleagues [12], no relation was found between filling-phase urodynamics (DO, first sensation and bladder capacity) and detailed video-gait analysis parameters. By contrast, they found a significant relation between voiding-phase urodynamics (Watts factor, reflecting detrusor power) and video-gait analysis parameters (bradykinesia and loss of postural reflex) in PD ($P < 0.01$).

Detailed studies in individual patients using single-photon emission computed tomography (SPECT) imaging of dopamine transporters have shown a correlation between urinary dysfunction and nigrostriatal degeneration. Greater loss was shown in the striatum of patients with bladder symptoms compared with those without [13], while a recent Danish study showed that the severity of bladder dysfunction correlated with the relative degeneration of the caudate nucleus compared with the putamen [14]. Although Braak's hypothesis [15] proposing the progressive spread of a neurodegenerative process in PD starting in the lower brainstem and ascending through the basal forebrain into the cortex has yet to be universally accepted, it serves as a valuable framework for understanding how bladder symptoms occur in the context of a patient with more severe disability than simply motor symptoms. In the present authors' opinion, and based on the demonstrated correlation of severity of neurological deficit and the occurrence of bladder symptoms, it is reasonable to put the clinical threshold for bladder symptomatology above Braak Stage 4, in other words, when the neuropathology is starting to affect the neocortex.

The underlying pathophysiology of symptoms

Data from animal experiments have shown that D1 receptors in the striatum have an inhibitory effect on the pontine micturition centre, whereas D2 receptor activation facilitates the micturition reflex [16]. Both neuronal firing in the substantia nigra pars compacta (SNc) and the released striatal dopamine seem to activate the dopamine D1–GABA-ergic *direct pathway*, which not only inhibits the output nuclei of the basal ganglia but may also inhibit the micturition reflex by GABA-ergic collateral to the periaqueductal grey (PAG) micturition circuit, or by the striatal–frontal pathways [17] (Fig. 17.3). It has thus been proposed that the DO which underlies many of the OAB symptoms that affect patients with PD is due to a failure of D1 activation, with the addition of possible exacerbation by the D2 content of many medications. The pathophysiology is probably more complicated than that, however, as the results of deep brain stimulation have largely shown an improvement in bladder function with the stimulator on [18]. Although high-frequency stimulation of the subthalamic nucleus inhibited the micturition reflex in a cat [19], a human positron emission tomography (PET) study that looked at the ameliorating effect in some detail proposed that it might result from facilitated processing of afferent activity by the basal ganglia [18]. It has been shown that subthalamic nucleus deep brain stimulation leads to improved sensory motor integration and there is evidence that higher-order processing of afferent activity is improved in patients with PD whose bladder symptoms

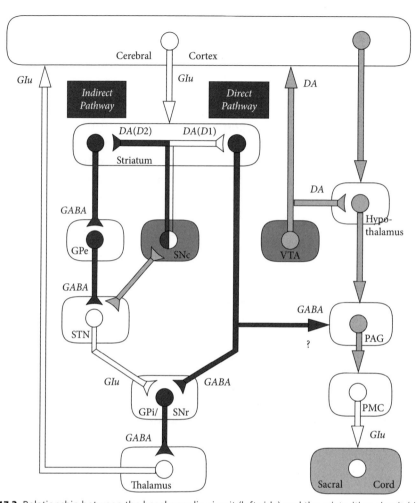

Fig. 17.3 Relationship between the basal ganglia circuit (left side) and the micturition circuit (right side). The micturition reflex (right-side pathway) is under the influences of dopamine (DA) (both inhibitory in D1 and facilitatory in D2) and gamma-aminobutyric acid (GABA) (inhibitory). The neuronal firing in the substantia nigra pars compacta (SNc) and the released striatal dopamine seem to activate the dopamine D1–GABA-ergic direct pathway, which not only inhibits the basal ganglia output nuclei [e.g. the globus pallidus internus (GPi) and the substantia nigra pars reticulata (SNr)], but may also inhibit the micturition reflex via GABA-ergic collateral to the micturition circuit. High frequency stimulation (leading to inhibition) in the subthalamic nucleus (STN) also results in bladder inhibition. Key: SNr, substantia nigra pars reticulata; STN, subthalamic nucleus; GPe, globus pallidus externus; VTA, ventral tegmental area; PAG, periaqueductal grey micturition circuit; PMC, pontine micturition centre; Glu, glutamate; black line, inhibitory neurons; white line, excitatory neurons; hatched line, neurons of undetermined property.
Modified from Sakakibara et al. 2003 [19].

are ameliorated by medication [20]. In addition, not only basal ganglia dopaminergic pathways but also extra-basal ganglia pathways, for example A11 hypothalamospinal dopaminergic pathways and possibly peripheral noradrenergic beta-3 pathways, might have a role in suppressing DO in PD [17].

Bladder symptoms and PD therapies

The effect of antiparkinsonian medication on the bladder is unpredictable. The only agreed finding from various studies is that voiding difficulty is less in all subjects when 'on'. Several studies have shown that levodopa can in individual patients either worsen or (less commonly) ameliorate urgency and other symptoms of DO [21]. In the most recent study, 18 PD patients with median HY scores of 5 during the 'off' phase and 3 during the 'on' phase had urodynamic studies before and about 1 hour after the patients had taken 100 mg of levodopa with dopa-decarboxylase inhibitor. After their treatment, urinary urgency and urge incontinence were unaltered or aggravated in the majority of patients, whereas voiding difficulty was alleviated in all those who had had this as a complaint [23].

One study observed that levodopa alone worsened DO but that L-sulpride (a central and peripheral D2 antagonist) counteracted the worsening in a dose-dependent manner, while domperidone (a peripheral D2 antagonist) failed to show the same counteraction [23]. The study concluded that central acute D2 stimulation appeared to reduce bladder capacity and worsen DO in patients with mild PD. Because of the differential effect of D1 and D2 agonists on bladder control, attempts were made in an animal model to see if pergolide (a D1/2 agonist) has a more beneficial effect on bladder control than other agonists [24].

Management of bladder symptoms in PD

Investigations

A good history, often from the patient's carer, is an essential starting point. If appropriate, the patient and their carer should be asked to keep a 3-day 24-hour bladder diary (Fig. 17.4). This should be used to record the time and volume of each void together with sensation preceding the void (i.e. a strong desire or urgency). Additional useful information about fluid intake and the time the patient went to bed at night and got up in the morning should be recorded. From this it may be possible to establish the possible role of excessive fluid intake, probable DO, nocturnal polyuria or a sleep disorder as aetiological factors in the patient's symptoms.

Medication for bladder symptoms

If symptoms of urgency and frequency suggest DO and a voiding diary confirms frequent, small-volume voids both day and night, a trial of an antimuscarinic is appropriate. However, it is important to balance the therapeutic benefits with the adverse effects of such drugs. A dry mouth due to the blocking of M3 receptors in the salivary glands and constipation due to the blocking of both M2 and M3 receptors in the bowel are common.

Frequency-volume chart
Instructions

Please complete the chart as accurately as possible. Please record the time you have passed water and underneath this, the volume you have passed. Any measuring jug will do for this purpose. If it is inconvenient to measure the volume at a particular instance, record only the time. However, as much as possible, please try to record both. If you are doing intermittent catheterisation, please record the residual urine drained as well. The information should be recorded for any 3 days.

- If you wet yourself at any time, record the time and underneath, the letter "W"
- If you use incontinence pads, please record how may you use per day
- Please remember to record what time you retire in the night for sleep and what time you wake up in morning
- Please record how much fluid you drink each day

PLEASE RETURN TO:

Name/Hospital number-   Any Comments-

		Time / volume (mL)					Fluid intake	Episodes of leakage
Day 1 ___/___/20___	Time							
	volume							
	Time							
Time out of bed (am)-	volume							
Time to bed (pm)-	Time							
	volume							
Day 2 ___/___/20___	Time							
	volume							
	Time							
Time out of bed (am)-	volume							
Time to bed (pm)-	Time							
	volume							
Day 3 ___/___/20___	Time							
	volume							
	Time							
Time out of bed (am)-	volume							
Time to bed (pm)-	Time							
	volume							

Fig. 17.4 A 3-day 24-hour bladder diary.

Adverse cognitive events from antimuscarinics are a concern, particularly in the elderly, and oxybutynin has been demonstrated to have a central nervous system effect, producing changes in quantitative electroencephalography in healthy young volunteers [25] and memory function in the elderly [26]. The cerebral cortex has abundant muscarinic M1 receptors, and factors contributing to the central effects of drugs include receptor subtype selectivity and penetration of the blood–brain barrier [27]. Factors which affect penetration of the blood–brain barrier are diffusion (diffusion of a substance is facilitated by smaller molecular size, <450–500 Da), neutrality or a smaller polar surface area (<90 Å^2) and lipophilicity or a smaller partition coefficient of water versus oil (log P < 3) [28]. Whereas most anticholinergics are neutral, trospium is ionic and less apt to penetrate the blood–brain barrier. Anticholinergics should be used with caution in elderly patients who have hallucinations or cognitive decline (PD with dementia or dementia with Lewy bodies) [29,30].

Whereas nighttime polyuria is a common consequence of postural hypotension in MSA, it is not thought to be a major factor in the nocturia that affects so many patients with PD. The use of desmopressin spray is generally not advised for treating nighttime frequency in patients over the age of 60 in the absence of nocturnal polyuria and, if inappropriately given, any resulting hyponatraemia will exacerbate confusion.

If the chart shows nighttime frequency disproportionate to the number of voids during the day, further investigation of sleep disturbance and appropriate treatment would be indicated.

Flow rate, residual volume and cystometry

As a general rule, it would seem reasonable to restrict the level of investigation to that which would have a determining role in any future management that might be considered. A simple flow rate measurement and determination of the residual volume can exclude major outflow obstruction and show that incomplete bladder emptying is not a factor contributing to urinary frequency and urgency. If these initial investigations do suggest an element of prostatic outflow obstruction, cystometry with insertion of urethral and rectal catheters may be appropriate so that pressure/flow studies can be made. The question of prostatic surgery in men with PD and bladder symptoms is difficult, but a man with advanced PD may not wish to have a transurethral resection of the prostate (TURP) even if pressure/flow studies were to show obstructed outflow. A digital rectal examination of the prostate and blood prostate-specific antigen (PSA) should be carried out if there is any reason to suspect prostate cancer.

Prostate surgery in men with idiopathic PD

TURP in men with PD has a reputation among urologists for poor outcome. A much cited paper has shown that of 36 patients undergoing TURP, six were incontinent prior to surgery and nine were incontinent subsequently [31]. Interestingly, the ability of the patient to voluntarily perform sphincter contraction was examined with needle recordings of EMG, and incontinence was particularly likely in those patients who could not voluntarily perform sphincter contraction prior to surgery. It was also noted that the EMG showed many of the patients had changes of chronic reinnervation, and in retrospect it seems highly likely that some of the patients in fact had a diagnosis of MSA. A recent study which looked at the effect of radical prostatectomy for prostate cancer included 20 men who had PD and demonstrated that the rate of incontinence was the same in that group as in the general population, concluding that those with PD were not at particular risk [32]. Certainly a man with a secure diagnosis of PD with mild disease and confirmed outflow obstruction should be considered for appropriate surgery.

Possible future treatments

In idiopathic PD not only is there loss of dopaminergic pathways but also neuronal cell loss in the serotonergic raphe nucleus [33], and although complex, the main action of serotonergic pathways on the lower urinary tract is facilitation of urine storage [34]. Little is known about the effect of serotonergic drugs in the treatment of OAB symptoms, but this might be a possible therapeutic avenue to explore, especially in those patients with co-morbid depression [35].

Apomorphine induces DO in rats, which was shown to be reversed by intravenous tramadol [36]. Tramadol is a well-established analgesic which combines opioid receptor activation and reuptake inhibition of serotonin and noradrenaline. It is its action on the μ-opioid receptors which is thought to have an inhibitory effect on micturition. It is not of course licensed to treat urinary symptoms.

Detrusor injection of botulinum toxin is shown to be of immense benefit in patients with DO due to spinal cord disease [37], including patients with multiple sclerosis (MS) [38]. Recently its use in patients with PD having intractable DO has been reported [39,40]. Experience with patients with MS has shown that almost all patients have a raised post-micturition residual volume in excess of 100 ml following the treatment and therefore their symptoms only benefited if they performed clean intermittent self-catheterization. In fact, the need to perform clean intermittent self-catheterization was not found to adversely affect quality of life [38]. However, it is important that all patients are warned about this possible need, as those with advanced PD may not be capable of performing clean inter-mittent self-catheterization, and their carers may be unwilling to do this for them.

There have not as yet been any published studies looking at the effect of sacral neuro-modulation in patients with PD, but while the current techniques for this intervention require not inconsiderable surgical procedures, careful patient selection will be necessary if this treatment is to be considered.

Containment or catheterization

Although there are currently various treatment options for mild to moderate bladder dis-orders, the major problem in PD is that continence problems worsen with increasing neu-rological disability and may be part of the severe disability seen in the late stages of the disease. In these circumstances, some of the newer treatments would be inappropriate, and if antimuscarinic medications prove to be inadequate, containment with pads or catheteri-zation may be the only reasonable alternatives.

Much research has been done to maximize the effectiveness and usability of inconti-nence pads, and the quality and therefore the cost of those that are available is quite di-verse. An experienced continence advisor or urology nurse is the best person to advise the patient and their carer as to the suitability of the many varied products available.

A long-term indwelling urethral catheter in either gender is not recommended because of the inevitable urethral trauma and damage to the bladder neck region that will ensue. A suprapubic catheter is usually preferable, and although by no means problem-free, if attached to a free-drainage system it will often provide relief from frequent toileting and incontinence.

The catheter needs to be sited by an experienced urologist, as puncturing a small blad-der may be made easier if the bladder can be distended under a light anaesthetic and a cystoscope used to check correct trochar insertion. Patients should be encouraged to drink plenty once the catheter is *in situ*. Some patients are persistent 'catheter blockers' and require frequent catheter changes. The first change should be done by the expert who inserted the catheter, but after that, if the tract has epithelialized, changes can be done in the community. Infections are almost inevitable and the best advice is not to test the urine routinely but only to give antibiotics if there is evidence of a systemic infection with fever and obviously contaminated urine. Persistent reinfection will require urological intervention to check there is not a focus for infection, such as debris or a urinary tract stone.

Conclusion

If a man has mild symptoms of PD but the diagnosis is secure, consideration of a TURP should be given if cystometry confirms outflow obstruction. Neurogenic bladder symptoms usually occur late in the course of idiopathic PD and often in the context of considerable disability. Antimuscarinic medication is currently the mainstay of treatment, but care should be exercised to avoid exacerbating any existing cognitive impairment by prescribing drugs that have minimal central action. Should this type of medication prove inadequate, newer, more invasive interventions are becoming available. However, it is uncertain if these will be appropriate for patients with advanced disease. Investigations should be appropriate for the type of management that is being considered.

Poor bladder control can be one of the most troublesome non-motor symptoms of PD. Research is much needed to improve understanding of why this occurs and to develop better management options, particularly for patients with advanced disease.

References

1 **Andersen JT, Bradley WE**. Cystometric, sphincter and electromyelographic abnormalities in Parkinson's disease. J Urol 1976; **116**: 75–8.

2 **Araki I, Kuno S**. Assessment of voiding dysfunction in Parkinson's disease by the international prostate symptom score. J Neurol Neurosurg Psychiatry 2000; **68**: 429–33.

3 **Chaudhuri KR, Martinez-Martin P, Schapira AH, et al**. International multicenter pilot study of the first comprehensive self-completed nonmotor symptoms questionnaire for Parkinson's disease: the NMSQuest study. Mov Disord 2006; **21**: 916–23.

4 **Martinez-Martin P, Schapira AH, Stocchi F, et al**. Prevalence of nonmotor symptoms in Parkinson's disease in an international setting; Study using nonmotor symptoms questionnaire in 545 patients. Mov Disord 2007; **22**: 1623–9.

5 **Sakakibara R, Shinotoh H, Uchiyama T, et al**. Questionnaire-based assessment of pelvic organ dysfunction in Parkinson's disease. Auton Neurosci 2001; **92**: 76–85.

6 **Uchiyama T, Sakakibara R, Yamamoto T, et al**. Urinary dysfunction in early and untreated Parkinson's disease. J Neurol Neurosurg Psychiatry 2011; **82**: 1382–6.

7 **Sakakibara R, Hattori T, Uchiyama T, et al**. Videourodynamic and sphincter motor unit potential analyses in Parkinson's disease and multiple system atrophy. J Neurol Neurosurg Psychiatry 2001; **71**: 600–6.

8 **Palleschi G, Pastore AL, Stocchi F, et al**. Correlation between the Overactive Bladder questionnaire (OAB-q) and urodynamic data of Parkinson disease patients affected by neurogenic detrusor overactivity during antimuscarinic treatment. Clin Neuropharmacol 2006; **29**: 220–9.

9 **Tsunoyama K, Sakakibara R, Yamaguchi C, et al**. Pathogenesis of reduced or increased bladder sensation. Neurourol Urodyn 2011; **30**: 339–43.

10 **Yamamoto T, Sakakibara R, Uchiyama T, et al**. Neurological diseases that cause detrusor hyperactivity with impaired contractile function. Neurourol Urodynam 2006; **25**: 356–60.

11 **Araki I, Kitahara M, Oida T, et al**. Voiding dysfunction and Parkinson's disease: urodynamic abnormalities and urinary symptoms. J Urol 2000; **164**: 1640–3.

12 **Terayama K, Sakakibara R, Ogawa A, et al**. Weak detrusor contractility correlates with motor disorders in Parkinson's disease. Mov Disord 2012; **27**: 1775–80.

13 **Sakakibara R, Shinotoh H, Uchiyama T, et al**. SPECT imaging of the dopamine transporter with [(123)I]-beta-CIT reveals marked decline of nigrostriatal dopaminergic function in Parkinson's disease with urinary dysfunction. J Neurol Sci 2001; **187**: 55–9.

14 **Winge K, Friberg L, Werdelin L, et al**. Relationship between nigrostriatal dopaminergic degeneration, urinary symptoms, and bladder control in Parkinson's disease. Eur J Neurol 2005; **12**: 842–50.

15 **Braak H, Ghebremedhin E, Rub U, et al**. Stages in the development of Parkinson's disease-related pathology. Cell Tissue Res 2004; **318**: 121–34.

16 **Seki S, Igawa Y, Kaidoh K, et al**. Role of dopamine D1 and D1 receptors in the micturition reflex in conscious rats. Neurourol Urodyn 2001; **20**: 105–13.

17 **Sakakibara R, Tateno F, Kishi M, et al**. Pathophysiology of bladder dysfunction in Parkinson's disease. Neurobiol Dis 2012; **46**: 565–71.

18 **Herzog J, Weiss PH, Assmus A, et al**. Subthalamic stimulation modulates cortical control of urinary bladder in Parkinson's disease. Brain 2006; **129**: 3366–75.

19 **Sakakibara R, Nakazawa K, Uchiyama T, et al**. Effects of subthalamic nucleus stimulation on the micturition reflex in cats. Neuroscience 2003; **120**: 871–5.

20 **Winge K, Werdelin LM, Nielsen KK, Stimpel H**. Effects of dopaminergic treatment on bladder function in Parkinson's disease. Neurourol Urodyn 2004; **23**: 689–96.

21 **Aranda B, Cramer P**. Effects of apomorphine and L-dopa on the parkinsonian bladder. Neurourol Urodyn 1993; **12**: 203–9.

22 **Uchiyama T, Sakakibara R, Hattori T, Yamanishi T**. Short-term effect of a single levodopa dose on micturition disturbance in Parkinson's disease patients with the wearing-off phenomenon. Mov Disord 2003; **18**: 573–8.

23 **Brusa L, Petta F, Pisani A, et al**. Central acute D2 stimulation worsens bladder function in patients with mild Parkinson's disease. J Urol 2006; **175**: 202–6 [discussion 206–7].

24 **Yoshimura N, Mizuta E, Yoshida O, Kuno S**. Therapeutic effects of dopamine D1/D2 receptor agonists on detrusor hyperreflexia i1-methyl-4-phenyl-1,2,3,6-tetrahydropyridine-lesioned parkinsonian *Cynomolgus* monkeys. Pharmacol Exp Ther 1998; **286**: 228–33.

25 **Todorova A, Vonderheid-Guth B, Dimpfel W**. Effects of tolterodine, trospium chloride, and oxybutynin on the central nervous system. J Clin Pharmacol 2001; **41**: 636–44.

26 **Kay G, Crook T, Rekeda L, et al**. Differential Effects of the antimuscarinic agents darifenacin and oxybutynin ER on memory in older subjects. Eur Urol 2006; **50**: 317–26.

27 **Sakakibara R, Uchiyama T, Yamanishi T, et al**. Dementia and lower urinary dysfunction: with a reference to anticholinergic use in elderly population. Int J Urol 2008; **15**: 778–88.

28 **Andersson KE**. New pharmacologic targets for the treatment of the overactive bladder: an update. Urology 2004; 63(3 Suppl 1): **32**–41.

29 **McKeith IG, Dickson DW, Lowe J, et al**. Diagnosis and management of dementia with Lewy bodies: third report of the DLB Consortium. Neurology 2005; **65**: 1863–72.

30 **Sakakibara R, Ito T, Uchiyama T, et al**. Lower urinary tract function in dementia of Lewy body type. J Neurol Neurosurg Psychiatry 2005; **76**: 729–32.

31 **Staskin DS, Vardi Y, Siroky MA**. Post-prostatectomy incontinence in the parkinsonian patient: the significance of poor voluntary sphincter control. J Urol 1988; **140**: 117–18.

32 **Routh JC, Crimmins CR, Leibovich BC, Elliott DS**. Impact of Parkinson's disease on continence after radical prostatectomy. Urology 2006; **68**: 575–7.

33 **Halliday GM, Blumbergs PC, Cotton RG, et al**. Loss of brainstem serotonin- and substance P-containing neurons in Parkinson's disease. Brain Res 1990; **510**: 104–7.

34 **Ito T, Sakakibara R, Nakazawa K, et al**. Effects of electrical stimulation of the raphe area on the micturition reflex in cats. Neuroscience 2006; **142**: 1273–80.

35 **Andersson KE**. Treatment of overactive bladder: other drug mechanisms. Urology 2000; 55(5A Suppl): 51–7.

36 **Pehrson R, Andersson KE**. Tramadol inhibits rat detrusor overactivity caused by dopamine receptor stimulation. J Urol 2003; **170**: 272–5.

37 **Schurch B, Hauri D, Rodic B, et al**. Botulinum-A toxin as a treatment of detrusor-sphincter dyssynergia: a prospective study in 24 spinal cord injury patients. J Urol 1996; **155**: 1023–9.

38 **Kalsi V, Gonzales G, Popat R, et al**. Botulinum injections for the treatment of bladder symptoms of multiple sclerosis. Ann Neurol 2007; **62**: 452–7.

39 **Kulaksizoglu H, Parman Y**. Use of botulinim toxin-A for the treatment of overactive bladder symptoms in patients with Parkinson's disease. Parkinsonism Relat Disord 2010; **16**: 531–4.

40 **Conte A, Giannantoni A, Proietti S, et al**. Botulinum toxin A modulates afferent fibers in neurogenic detrusor overactivity. Eur J Neurol 2012; **19**:725–32.

Chapter 18

Sexuality in Parkinson's disease

Orna Moore, Gila Bronner, Sharon Hassin-Baer
and Nir Giladi

Introduction

Sexuality is a key aspect of the personality and behaviour of every human being, encompassing basic needs for contact, intimacy, emotional expression, pleasure, tenderness and love.

Parkinson's disease (PD) is a common multisystem disorder that is frequently associated with sexual dysfunction (SD) [1,2]. In a life restricted by illness, sexuality can be a powerful source of comfort and pleasure and an affirmation of gender when other gender roles have been stripped away.

Given the high prevalence of SD among couples living with PD, healthcare providers should play a major role in advocating sexual health rights and treat sexual health issues as part of the holistic management of PD.

In this chapter we will review the effects of PD on the sexuality of patients and their partners, and present various treatment options. We will also describe our experience with the implementation of sexual counselling services within the framework of a PD centre.

Epidemiology of sexual dysfunction in PD

Sexual function is a complex process that depends on neurological, vascular and endocrine systems that can be altered by ageing, life experiences and exposures, psychosocial factors and various medical disorders and interventions [3].

Results from a national probability sample among 2522 men and 2523 women between 18 and 92 years of age showed that masturbation, oral sex and vaginal intercourse are widely practised in the United States. Intercourse was more common among in men in their 20s and 30s than in the other age groups, although about 50% of men in their 60s and 70s were still sexually active [4,5].

Several epidemiological studies have shown that the most important factor in the development of SD is ageing [6]. Sexual activity declined with age (prevalence of 73% at 57–64 years, 53% at 65–74 years and 26% at 75–85 years) in a national sample of 3005 healthy US adults. The most common problems among ageing women were low desire (43%), difficulty with vaginal lubrication (39%) and inability to climax (34%), and among men erectile dysfunction (ED; 37%) [7]. Other studies have shown that many older adults continue be sexually active well into advanced age (80+ years), with sexual activity reported by 63.6% of men and 42% of women aged 50–107 years. Intercourse and masturbation were still common at the age of 70–79+ among both men (46.2 and 54.2%, respectively) and women (26.8 and 36.0%, respectively) [8]. As expected, SD was more common among women and men with poor physical and emotional health.

Neurological disease frequently alters sexual function, and some patients regard this as the most devastating consequence of their illness [9]. SD is common among patients with PD [10,11] and it is associated with depression and dissatisfaction with relationships [12] (Table 18.1). Concern over sexual function was reported in 22 of 88 PD patients (25%), with men and younger people being significantly more likely to report these problems [13]. Bronner et al. [10] found that many patients (41.9% of men and 28.2% of women) refrained from sexual activity because of their state of health. In that study general dissatisfaction with their sexual life (65.1% of men and 37.5% of women) and a high prevalence of SD in all six measured aspects (intimacy, sexual desire, orgasm, painful sex, erectile dysfunction and premature ejaculation) were found among 75 PD patients (32 women and 43 men). In addition to factors directly related to the disease itself, pre-morbid SD may also contribute to cessation of sexual activity and the development of SD as PD progresses.

The impact of intimacy and sexuality on quality of life in PD

Studies on people with PD have indicated that the need for intimacy and sexual expression is of major importance and contributes to their quality of life (QoL) [13,14]. It has been suggested that a satisfying sex life is one way of feeling 'normal' when many other aspects of life have changed for the worse.

Table 18.1 Sexual problems in Parkinson's disease

General	Hypoactive sexual desire disorders
	Increased sexual desire or hypersexuality
	Arousal problems
	Orgasmic problems
	Sexual dissatisfaction
	Role changes in sexual activity (active to passive and vice versa)
	Inability or limitation in intimate touching
	Limited choice of sexual positions
	Difficulties in sexual communication
	Need for adequate planning of sexual activity (time, location, position, sexual aids)
Men	Erectile dysfunction
	Premature ejaculation
	Difficulties reaching orgasm and ejaculation
	Delayed ejaculation
Women	Lack of or reduced vaginal lubrication
	Painful intercourse or secondary vaginismus
	Difficulties reaching orgasm

Sexual problems are common in PD, and these commonly influence the QoL of both patients and their partners [14]. Moore et al. [15] showed that the health-related QoL together with the quality of sexual life (QoSL) in PD are significantly correlated with patients' general satisfaction with life. They found that the QoSL was often related to age and disease severity, as previously reported by others [1,15]. This observation is of clinical significance if one considers that sexual interest often remains intact in older age. Indeed, the participants in that study [15] were more open to discussing their sexual problems with the neurological staff and to seek sexual counselling outside the PD clinic.

Recognizing the importance of enhancing the PD patient's QoSL, it was proposed that sexual assessment should be an integral part of the general and neurological interview [9,15], and that sexual health and related issues should be addressed. Moreover, it was recommended that patients' partners should be present during the interview as well as during any interventions.

Specific aspects of sexuality in PD

Motor impairment such as rigidity, tremor and immobility in bed or decreased fine finger movements may affect the intimate touching needed for pleasure and sexual arousal. Moreover, altered appearance, excessive sweating, drooling and gait disturbances make patients less attractive. Similarly, masked faces can be interpreted as showing lack of affection and desire. The hypokinetic movements make patients more passive sexually, thus imposing a more active role on the partner. Sleep disturbances may lead to the choice of separate beds, thus decreasing opportunities for intimate contact [2,16]. According to Kotkova and Weiss [17], depression, which is very common in PD, is the most significant factor to affect sexuality in families with PD, while anxiety is of special importance among women with PD. In another study, depression was found in about 30% of patients with advanced PD and was more common among younger patients (under the age of 51 years) [18]. Contrary to commonly held beliefs, sexual dissatisfaction in young PD patients did not correlate with disease duration or severity but with unemployment and depression, thus further demonstrating the significance of depression when assessing and treating sexual difficulties among families with PD [2].

Sexual dysfunction in men with PD

Difficulties with sexual arousal, sexual drive and ability to reach an orgasm have been demonstrated in most men with PD (both young and old), and were positively correlated with longer disease duration [19]. Furthermore, sexual difficulties were significantly more frequent in young couples, and especially when the partner with PD was the man [20].

Deterioration in their sexual life was reported by 76.7% of men with PD [10]. In another study, 88% of the participants described a decrease in the frequency of sexual intercourse [21]. Decreased sexual drive was reported by a wide range of the patients (from 23 to 88% in different studies), thus reflecting the difficulties in defining and measuring sexual drive. ED has been commonly reported, affecting 54–79% of survey participants, with premature ejaculation in 40% and difficulties reaching orgasm in 40–87% [2,10,17,21,22].

Another aspect of sexual dysfunction in men is a suggestion that its onset is in the premotor and pre-diagnosis phase of the PD, along with other autonomic dysfunctions. A single retrospective large-scale study assessed this issue and demonstrated that idiopathic ED in mid life was associated with a higher risk of developing PD. Healthy men ($n = 32\ 616$) aged 40–75 years who reported ED before 1986 were 3.8 times more likely to develop PD by 2000 than men without ED [23].

In a randomized multicentre study of couples without PD, a decrease in sexual function was reported by women in association with their partner's ED. When the men were effectively using phosphodiesterase type 5 (PDE5) inhibitor, the women reported improved satisfaction from their sexual life [24]. Seventeen female partners of men with PD reported that their sexual function had become severely compromised, specifically with regard to sexual arousal, behaviour, orgasm, fantasy and drive [19]. The effect of PD on the couple's sexual function seems to be greater when the partner with PD is the man [25].

Sexual dysfunction in women with PD

The female sexual response is initiated by neurotransmitter-mediated vascular and non-vascular smooth muscle relaxation resulting in increased pelvic blood flow, vaginal lubrication and clitoral and labial engorgement. Due to this highly complicated mechanism, women with neurological diseases are at high risk for developing SD (Table 18.1). SD among women is typically associated with decreased libido and arousal as well as decreased vaginal lubrication, genital sensation and difficulties in achieving orgasm [26]. None of these issues have ever been studied in depth in women with PD.

A general deterioration in sexual life was reported by 78.1% of women with PD in one study. Their most frequently mentioned problems were related to arousal (87.5%), orgasm (75.0%) and desire (50%) [10]. A significant decrease in the frequency of intercourse was reported among 43–82% of female PD patients, 35% of whom also reported associated vaginal dryness. Women with PD reported a significant increase in vaginal tightness, involuntary urination during intercourse, anxiety, depression and sexual dissatisfaction when compared with age-matched healthy women [2,10]. Those difficulties worsened as the disease progressed.

Younger women diagnosed with PD reported more menstrual problems since the appearance of PD motor symptoms, specifically excessive bleeding and pain. Additionally, more than half of menstruating women with PD reported a significant worsening of parkinsonian symptoms just prior to menstruation, more so in those women with more advanced PD and in those with clinically significant motor response fluctuations [27].

Women with PD expressed some concern regarding their changing body image, which led to their feeling unattractive and to changes in apparel in order to cope better with their general appearance and the emergence of specific parkinsonian signs [28]. The issue of body and sexual image is frequently discussed in support groups for young women with

PD (age 35–59 years) [29], and is a cause of distress and discomfort for most of them. Interestingly, these issues are rarely addressed by doctors or nurses, even in PD centres [28].

The effect of PD on couple relationships

Sexual and relationship dysfunction is a problem for people of both genders and all age groups with PD, and can occur regardless of marital status. Marital problems tend to worsen with increasing disease severity and functional decline [13].

Men with PD and their partners have greater marital and sexual problems than women with PD and their partners. Hand et al. [13] reported that both gender and the Unified Parkinson's Disease Rating Scale (UPDRS) score were independent predictors of relationship difficulties. Men with PD and those with increasing functional problems (according to the UPDRS) were more likely to report problems in their relationship. It is notable that disease duration and levels of anxiety or depression were not associated with sexual or relationship difficulties in that study.

Beier et al. [11] investigated the influence of PD on sexuality and partnership in 330 women and 1008 men in the German Parkinson Organization. Besides SD and sexual dissatisfaction, couples' general relationship was negatively affected by the disease. There was less communication, especially physical touching and expression of feelings, after PD had been diagnosed, whereas desire for mutual intimacy remained on the same level as before. In spite of the high frequency of SD, only 34.2% of the patients reported discussing sexual issues with their partners [10].

Our clinical experience is that couples affected by PD describe a major reduction in emotional and physical expressions of intimacy, and that the reduced frequency of intimate touching had a detrimental effect on their self-esteem in addition to increasing marital tension. We found that restoration of intimacy resulted in an improvement in the relationship.

Medical and other treatments for sexual function in PD

While medications used for the treatment of PD have a significant effect on sexual function and can cause reduced libido, ED, premature ejaculation, delayed (retarded) ejaculation and anorgasmia [2,25], it seems that increases in sexual desire (1–50%) associated with dopaminergic therapy and a resumption of sexual activity is a more common and usually positive effect of treatment [30]. The role of dopamine and dopamine agonists (DAs) in reward-seeking behaviour and in pathological hypersexuality (HS) [31–33] will be discussed in the section on Hypersexuality or compulsive sexual behaviour.

In animal models dopamine has been shown to promote sexual motivation, copulatory competence and genital reflexes, probably by acting in brain integrative areas, including the medial preoptic area. The nucleus accumbens that mediates the pleasurable effects of natural rewards (e.g. food and sex) receives mesolimbic dopaminergic nerve endings and in addition dopamine both reduces the release of prolactin, a hormone that may interfere with libido, and is associated with increased plasma levels of oxytocin which has erecto-genic effects [34].

Ingestion of levodopa can either decrease or increase the latency of ejaculation and orgasm and may even cause an absence of ejaculation [35], but chronic therapy has been associated with a resumption of sexual activity in 8% of PD patients treated with levodopa [36].

DA therapy has been more commonly associated with enhanced sexual desire and function. Bromocriptine was reported to decrease the latency to ejaculation and pergolide has been shown to induce spontaneous ejaculation [35]. Pergolide was associated with a long-term beneficial effect on sexual function in young men with advanced, fluctuating PD [37]. Several studies demonstrated that apomorphine can induce penile erections in both healthy men and in men with ED [38], and it has been licensed for the treatment of ED following successful studies [39]. Neither the effects of nor the use of apomorphine for SD in PD have ever been reported. Amantadine has not been reported to cause SD but has been found useful in treatment of neuroleptic and antidepressant-induced SD [40,41].

Psychoactive medications frequently cause adverse effects on sexual function, more frequently than dopaminergic medications [42]. Tricyclic antidepressants (TCAs) have been associated with SD, especially anorgasmia, which occurs in 20–30% or 90% of patients treated with imipramine and clomipramine, respectively. Selective serotonin reuptake inhibitors (SSRIs), paroxetine, sertaline, fluvoxamine, citalopram, (S)-citalopram and fluoxetine, as a class, are all associated with SD, with paroxetine having the highest and fluvoxamine the lowest rate of effects. The major side effect is anorgasmia or delayed orgasm, which seems to occur in 30–40% of patients, depending on the threshold set for the diagnosis in the different studies. While venlafaxine, a mixed serotonin and norepinephrine reuptake inhibitor (SNRI), has a similar rate of SD as the SSRIs, other antidepressants commonly used for PD, namely duloxetine (SNRI), mirtazapine (a drug with α_2-antagonism combined with blockade of serotonin 5-HT2 and 5-HT3 receptors) and bupropion (which affects norepinephrine and dopamine reuptake), are associated with a lower incidence of SD.

Other medications used to treat behavioural symptoms in PD (such as anxiety, agitation insomnia and psychosis) are also associated with SD. Benzodiazepines may independently cause anorgasmia, and antipsychotic agents may also cause SD. Risperidone, typical antipsychotics and clozapine seem to involve a much higher rate of SD (namely, delayed ejaculation) than aripiprazole, olanzapine and quetiapine [35,43].

Deep brain stimulation (DBS) of the subthalamic nucleus (STN) appears to affect sexual functioning in a small but positive way. Only younger male patients with PD (age < 60 years) appeared more sexually satisfied over a short-term follow-up period, implying that dopaminergic treatment and disease severity were not discriminating factors in sexual satisfaction [44].

Hypersexuality or compulsive sexual behaviour

Hypersexuality (HS) or compulsive sexual behaviour (CSB) is part of the spectrum of impulse control disorders (ICDs) in PD patients treated with dopaminergic agents and one that has attracted the attention of healthcare professionals due to its impact on patients and their families [32,45,46].

ICDs result from a failure to resist an urge, drive or temptation to perform an act considered to be harmful to the patient or to others [33,47]. They occur in 13.6% of patients with treated PD, more commonly in those taking DAs [46]. Different terms are used to describe the hypersexual disorder in PD, among which are 'CSB' 'sexual addiction', 'sexual compulsivity', 'sexual impulsivity' 'excessive sexual behaviour', 'pathological hypersexuality' and 'increased interest in sex'. For example, CSB was reported in 1.7–3.5% of PD patients [46,48]. There are only a few validated tools for assessing HS in PD patients. A shortened form of the Sexual Addiction Screening Test (SAST), covering multidimensional aspects of HS, was recently tested in 159 PD patients (PD-SAST) and shown to be acceptable to patients in addition to performing well as a screening instrument [49].

PD patients may present with behaviours that appear to be hypersexual and are mistakenly diagnosed as having CSB induced by medications while actually they suffer from a distinct SD. A wide array of SDs may cause frustration and sexual dissatisfaction, leading to preoccupation and repeated attempts to engage in sex. A comprehensive diagnostic and management algorithm for hypersexual behaviour is suggested by Bronner and Hassin-Baer [45] with the aim of assisting professionals in this differential diagnosis.

Patients with true HS and CSB present with increased libido and an increased frequency of erections as well as preoccupation with sexual thoughts, increased sexual demands and acts (including promiscuity, obsessive masturbation, habitual use of telephone sex lines, internet pornography or contact with sex workers). There have also been reports of paraphilia, such as sexual exhibitionism, sadomasochism, paedophilia and zoophilia [32,50,51].

HS in PD has been associated with male gender, earlier onset of PD, DA therapy and depression. Furthermore, hypersexual patients showed more significant cognitive impairment, including lower scores on learning tests and poorer inhibitory control, in comparison with PD patients with other ICDs (e.g. pathological gambling and compulsive eating). A temporal association was found between the initiation of DA therapy and the onset of HS. HS has been reported to occur with all dopaminergic medications [50–52].

Controversies exist concerning the role of dopamine in sexual function. This issue has been reviewed by Paredes and Agmo [53]. Following several years of physiological and pharmacological studies in animals, those authors concluded that dopamine is important for motor functions and general arousal and that these actions could, in fact, explain most of the effects seen on sexual behaviour. The release of dopamine in the nucleus accumbens has been associated with all kinds of aversive or appetitive events, but it was not found to have any specific effect on sexual behaviour other than by promoting arousal and activation of non-specific motor patterns. It is plausible that release of dopamine preoptically and by the paraventricular nucleus may have some relationship to mechanisms of ejaculation or the neuroendocrine consequences of sexual activity, but there is no compelling indication in existing experimental data that dopamine is of any particular importance for sexual motivation.

The most accepted approach to understanding HS in PD is to regard it as one of the ICDs provoked by dopamine replacement therapy (DRT). In order to treat the motor symptoms that are associated with dopaminergic deficiency of the dorsal motor striatum we 'overdose' with non-physiological dopaminergic stimulation in the mesolimbic and mesocortical pathways of the ventral corticostriatal circuitry, and this leads to ICDs. These central dopaminergic pathways are intricately linked to the brain's reward system which is implicated in various states of addiction. Activation of these systems is thought to be mediated by stimulation of D3 receptors which are predominantly expressed in the ventral striatum and which mediate reward, emotional and cognitive processes. The newer non-ergot DA currently used in PD has a high affinity for the D2/D3 receptors compared with D1 receptors [54].

Functional imaging studies have strengthened the links between the ICDs seen in PD and addiction in general, demonstrating abnormalities of the reward pathways including the ventral striatum, the cingulate gyrus and the orbitofrontal cortex [55,56].

In our experience, it is not uncommon to encounter an increase in libido following initiation or augmentation of medical treatment in a patient with PD. The first step in dealing with the impression of increased libido is to differentiate between a state where there is restoration of the patient's sexual interest with DRT but differences in sexual interest within a couple and true, compulsive HS [45]. While the former requires sexual counselling and intervention, the latter calls for medical advice and possibly a change of pharmacological treatment, namely DRT. Patients with HS tend to deny the problem, and it is their spouses who often inform the health professional, usually the neurologist. HS is generally under-reported [32], but it is important to rapidly diagnose and treat it as early as possible in order to prevent social and psychologically harmful consequences as well as tension within a family that is already dealing with the difficult consequences of PD [33,45].

Patient assessment—or how to talk about sex with your patient

A deterioration in sexual life along the course of PD and an inability to discuss sexual issues commonly coexist, emphasizing the need for assistance in coping with these changes. Healthcare professionals may assist by initiating a discussion on sexual issues on a routine basis [57,58]. The availability of effective treatments for sexual problems, particularly in the case of ED, provides powerful justification for a comprehensive assessment of sexual functioning [57].

In spite of their distress, patients and partners find it difficult to initiate discussions about their sexuality [10]. In one survey only 21% of 1940 men and women with sexual problem sought medical help [59]. The difficulties in seeking medical help originate in shame with respect to discussing sex and in admitting that they have a sexual problem, low self-esteem and fear of appearing foolish. In addition, many patients are not aware of new treatments and have difficulties in discussing sexual issues with their partners [10].

Inquiry about sexual functioning may be neglected by neurologists due to the complexity of the illness, time constraints, confusion about how to open the conversation and a lack of proper training [45]. Most patients and their partners, however, value opportunities to discuss issues of sexuality and intimacy with trusted health professionals, and they would prefer that the physician or the nurse initiate the discussion [28,60]. When asked about the preferred source of information, more than half of PD patients responded that would like to receive information directly from their physician and more than one-third would prefer to receive it together with their partner. Most of them would like to have written material on the effects of PD on their sexuality [11].

Treatment options for sexual problems in PD

The behavioural therapeutic approach assumes that SD is a learned maladaptive behaviour and prescribes specific exercises for the couple in order for them to experience and adapt to new sexual habits. The two aspects of pharmacological treatment are the elimination or adjustment of drugs that compromise sexual function and the introduction of drugs that improve sexual function.

The patient's list of medications has to be reviewed in cases of ED, delayed ejaculation and anorgasmia. The need for continued use of antidepressants should be weighed by the psychiatrist, who should consider the possibility of a decreased dose or switching to an antidepressant that does not lead to SD.

Neurogenic ED is due to an imbalance between neurotransmitters favouring erection (notably nitric oxide, NO) and those favouring flaccidity (notably norepinephrine) [16]. Therefore, PDE5 inhibitors and NO-enhancing drugs are likely to be effective in PD. Zesiewicz et al. [61] reported that sildenafil citrate (Viagra®) significantly improved erections in 28 (84.8%) depressed patients with idiopathic PD and was well tolerated. The better erections increased libido, sexual satisfaction and ability to reach orgasm, and decreased depressive symptoms in 75% of patients [62]. A single Class II study evaluated the efficacy of sildenafil citrate in treating ED in 12 patients with PD [63]. There was increased ability to achieve and maintain an erection with an improved sex life compared with placebo, with minimal changes in blood pressure. The Quality Standards Subcommittee of the American Academy of Neurology considered treatment options for non-motor symptoms of PD and determined that sildenafil citrate (50 mg) is possibly efficacious in the treatment of ED in PD (one Class II study) [64]. Neurogenic ED, in contrast to vasculogenic ED, enables the use of a lower dosage of intracavernosal injection of prostaglandin E1 (PGE1) to relax smooth muscle around the sinusoids to cause erection.

When pathological HS is suspected the patient should be reviewed for the presence of other ICDs and additional psychiatric symptoms as well as concomitant dopamine dysregulation syndrome with abuse of DRT. Changes in the medication regimen should be considered, including reduction of the DA dose or discontinuation of DA treatment entirely, along with an increase in the levodopa dose in order to prevent worsening of motor symptoms. The role of antidepressants and other psychoactive medication in HS or ICD is not clear, and their use should be considered individually.

Consultation with a PD nurse or sex therapist is recommended in order to discuss the association between therapy and CSB, to prevent sexual health problems and to enhance spousal support and understanding. In specific cases where decreasing dopaminergic therapy is expected to worsen motor symptoms surgical interventions, such as DBS or duodenal infusion with an intestinal levodopa gel should be considered.

Integration of treatment methods into the sex lives of couples with PD

Deciding which treatment is best for an individual depends on many factors, among them medical condition, interaction with other medication and patient and partner preferences (Table 18.2). For example, patients with ED should undergo medical evaluation to detect possible associated conditions that might induce ED and to exclude contraindications to treatment (Box 18.1). The urologist may offer intracavernosal injection, which can be effective in producing erection independent of the man's arousal level. A discussion of the proposed treatment can help the couple integrate the injection into their existing sexual habits. They can prepare a pre-loaded syringe and place it at the bedside, and the partner can help with the injection.

When a PDE5 inhibitor is recommended, patients should be informed that the drug enhances penile erection only in response to sexual arousal. Patients and physicians should be aware of the time required after dosing to attain penile erection sufficient for successful sexual intercourse. Men are usually instructed to wait for between 30 and 60 minutes after the drug is taken before engaging sexual activity [65]. There may be delayed absorption of the PDE5 inhibitor due to impaired gastrointestinal motility in some male PD patients [66]. Informing patients about the possibility of a delay and assisting them in planning better timing for sexual activities in relation to drug use will spare the couple from unnecessary sexual failure.

Our clinical experience

Our approach to treating the sexual problems of PD patients is based on practical solutions to preserve the couple's intimate relationship and to adapt their sexual activities to the limitations imposed by the disease. We combine tips on timing of engaging in sex, methods of stimulation to enhance arousal, planning of sexual positions, instruction for proper use of PDE5 inhibitors, use of lubricants to enable intercourse and finding pleasurable alternatives to intercourse. The intercourse–outercourse approach [58] is one of the useful sexual alternatives. The couple can have intercourse or alternatively enjoy a variety of erotic activities without inserting the penis into the vagina (outercourse). If they wish, they can reach orgasm through genital rubbing, oral stimulation or manual stimulation. Our counselling also involves re-evaluation of attitudes towards sex, and challenges maladaptive beliefs, for example 'sex is only intercourse' or 'sex must always end with orgasm'.

Our clinical experience was that most of patients were satisfied after a short intervention (two to four sessions) of counselling despite the fact that only half of them reported

Table 18.2 Treatments of sexual dysfunction in Parkinson's disease (PD)

Medical treatment for erectile dysfunction	(1) Oral medications:
	    sildenafil (Viagra)
	    tadalafil (Cialis)
	    vardenafil (Levitra)
	(2) Others:
	    direct injections into the penis (intracavernosal injections)
	    intraurethral applications—MUSE (alprostadil)
	    vacuum constrictor pump
	    surgical placement of intrapenile prosthesis

Medical treatment for premature ejaculation	Antidepressant drugs—selective serotonin reuptake inhibitors (SSRIs) Topical anaesthetic cream
Medical treatment for female arousal problems	Lubrications agents Hormonal replacement therapy (systemic or local)
Medical treatment for desire problems (decreased libido)	Hormonal treatment (androgen, oestrogen)
Sex therapy, couple therapy, and behavioural therapy	Increasing open sexual communication among the sexual partners Planning the setting of sexual activity (time, location, position, roles, aids) Practising comfortable positions Adapting new sexual roles according to the couple's abilities Finding new solutions for physical limitation (e.g. touch, arousal, orgasm) Intimacy training Practising sensate focus—a process of relearning of body sensations and erotic tasks Practising the intercourse–outercourse approach [58] Consulting the neurologist on how to reduce the effect of medications on sexual function
Sex education	Genital anatomy and sexual response cycle Differences between male and female sexual response Impact of PD or PD treatment on sexual function Sexual changes with normal ageing in men and women
Attitude change	Positive attitude towards sexual activities Challenge of maladaptive beliefs (e.g. 'sex is unhealthy', 'sex should always be spontaneous', 'intercourse is the only normal type of sex')

improvement in sexual function. They reported reduced anxiety and tension when they received 'permission' to be intimate without the need to have intercourse. In addition, the combination of intercourse–outercourse training with the use of a PDE5 inhibitor was highly effective: 90% were satisfied with the combined treatment and 64% of them experienced an improvement in their sexual functioning. The presence of a sex therapist in the neurology clinic increased the awareness of other professionals and improved the sexual

Box 18.1 Diagnosis and evaluation of sexual problems

1. Sexual history

Discuss onset and progression of sexual problem

Evaluate if sexual problem is generalized or specific to:

Timing of sexual activity (morning, evening, weekend, etc.)

Type of activity (self-stimulation, manual or oral stimulation, masturbation)

Partner (steady, occasional, present or past)

Ask about sexual function and satisfaction before onset of Parkinson's

Consider psychological or interpersonal factors and relationship conflict

Ask which problem is the most bothersome: desire, arousal, erectile, early or delayed ejaculation, orgasm, pain, frequency of sexual activity

Check the sequence of appearance of the sexual problems

Ask about sexual problems of the partner

2. Medical history and lifestyle

Evaluate co-morbid illness (cardiovascular, neurological, genitourinary system, diabetes, hyperlipidaemia, blood pressure, hypertension, depression), trauma, surgery and medication use.

Psychiatric evaluation (e.g. depression)

Ask about habits: smoking, coffee and alcohol consumption, substance abuse, work, sleep and sport

Focused physical examination

3. Diagnostic testing

Urogynaecological examination

Basic laboratory work-up based on patient complaints, including glucose, lipid profile

Endocrine tests: total and free testosterone, oestradiol, prolactin, luteinizing hormone, follicle-stimulating hormone, androstenedione, dehydroepiandrosterone (DHEA), DHEA-sulphate (DHEAS), total and free thyroxine, triiodothyronine, thyroid-stimulating hormone

Neurological tests: electromyography, nerve conduction studies, thermal or vibratory thresholds, bulbocavernosus latency

Vascular diagnostics for erectile dysfunction: nocturnal penile tumescence and rigidity, penile injection pharmacotesting; penile Doppler ultrasound; dynamic infusion pharmacocavernosometry, pharmacocavernosography, penile arteriography, computed tomography and magnetic resonance imaging (to evaluate trauma and infection), nuclear imaging

4. Referral to specialist

For example, specialist in sexual medicine, sex therapist, marital therapist well-being of PD patients and their partners. The take-home message for everyday clinical practice should be that there is a definite need for sexual counselling for PD patients.

Conclusion

The physical and emotional changes associated with PD as well as with the treatment of the disease have a profound effect on the sexual functioning of patients and their partners. They experience problems of desire, arousal, orgasm and satisfaction as well as of low self-esteem, depression and tension between partners. As such, patients may experience some kind of impairment of their sexual function and decreased QoL. Physicians and other healthcare providers must proactively address sexual health issues within the routine treatment of their PD patients and should be aware of the common SDs in PD and the basic approach to their management. Adjustment of current medications should be considered as well as introduction of medications targeted at improving sexual functioning. Intervention should include providing information on sexual issues, thus recognizing the sexual needs of PD patients and their partners and giving them the opportunity to express their difficulties, and referral to specialists.

References

1 Lipe H, Longstreth WT, Bird TD, Linde M. Sexual function in married men with Parkinson's disease compared to married men with arthritis. Neurology 1990; **40**: 1347–9.

2 Koller WC, Vetere-Overfield B, Williamson A, et al. Sexual dysfunction in Parkinson's disease. Clin Neuropharmacol 1990; **13**: 461–3.

3 Verschuren JE, Enzlin P, Dijkstra PU, Geertzen JH, Dekker R. Chronic disease and sexuality: a generic conceptual framework. J Sex Res 2010; **47**: 153–70.

4 Reece M, Herbenick D, Schick V, Sanders SA, Dodge B, Fortenberry JD. Sexual behaviors, relationships, and perceived health among adult men in the United States: results from a national probability sample. J Sex Med 2010; **7**(Suppl 5): 291–304.

5 Herbenick D, Reece M, Schick V, Sanders SA, Dodge B, Fortenberry JD. Sexual behaviors, relationships, and perceived health status among adult women in the United States: Results from a national probability sample. J Sex Med 2010; **7**(Suppl 5): 277–90.

6 Bancroft JH. Sex and aging. N Engl J Med 2007; **357**: 820–2.

7 Lindau ST, Schumm LP, Laumann EO, et al. A study of sexuality and health among older adults in the United States. N Engl J Med 2007; **357**: 762–74.

8 Schick V, Herbenick D, Reece M, et al. Sexual behaviors, condom use, and sexual health of Americans over 50: implications for sexual health promotion for older adults. J Sex Med 2010; **7**(Suppl 5): 315–29.

9 Rees PM, Fowler CJ, Maas CP. Sexual dysfunction 2: sexual function in men and women with neurological disorders. Lancet 2007; **369**: 512–25.

10 Bronner G, Royter V, Korczyn AD, Giladi N. Sexual dysfunction in Parkinson's disease. J Sex Marital Ther 2004; **30**: 95–105.

11 Beier KM, Luders M, Boxdorfer SA. Sexuality and partnership aspects of Parkinson's disease: results of an empirical study of patients and their partners. Fortschr Neurol Psychiatr 2000; **68**: 564–75.

12 Wielinski CL, Varpness SC, Erickson-Davis C, Paraschos AJ, Parashos SA. Sexual and relationship satisfaction among persons with young-onset Parkinson's disease. J Sex Med 2010; **7**: 1438–44.

13 **Hand A, Gray WK, Chandler BJ, Walker RW**. Sexual and relationship dysfunction in people with Parkinson's disease. Parkinsonism Relat Disord 2010; **16**: 172–6.

14 **Bronner G**. Sexual problems in Parkinson's disease: the multidimensional nature of the problem and of the intervention. J Neurol Sci 2011; **310**: 139–43.

15 **Moore O, Gurevich T, Korczyn AD, et al**. Quality of sexual life in Parkinson's disease. Parkinsonism Relat Disord 2002; **8**: 243–6.

16 **Basson R**. Sex and idiopathic Parkinson's disease. Adv Neurol 2001; **86**: 295–300.

17 **Kotkova P, Weiss P**. Psychiatric factors related to sexual functioning in patients with Parkinson's disease. Clin Neurol Neurosurg 2013; **115**: 419–24.

18 **Giladi N, Treves TA, Paleacu D, et al**. Risk factors for dementia, depression, and psychosis in long-standing Parkinson's disease. J Neural Transm 2000; **107**: 59–71.

19 **Yu M, Roane DM, Miner CR, et al**. Dimensions of sexual dysfunction in Parkinson disease. Am J Geriatr Psychiatry 2004; **12**: 221–6.

20 **Jacobs H, Vieregge A, Vieregge P**. Sexuality in young patients with Parkinson's disease: a population based comparison with healthy controls. J Neurol Neurosurg Psychiatry 2000; **69**: 550–2.

21 **Sakakibara R, Shinotoh H, Uchiyama T, et al**. Questionnaire-based assessment of pelvic organ dysfunction in Parkinson's disease. Auton Neurosci 2001; **92**: 76–85.

22 **Lucon M, Pinto AS, Simm RF, et al**. Assessment of erectile dysfunction in patients with Parkinson's disease. Arq Neuropsiquiatr 2001; **59**: 559–62.

23 **Gao X, Chen H, Schwarzschild MA, et al**. Erectile function and risk of Parkinson's disease. Am J Epidemiol 2007; **166**: 1446–50.

24 **Fisher WA, Rosen RC, Eardley I, et al**. Sexual experience of female partners of men with erectile dysfunction: the female experience of men's attitudes to life events and sexuality (FEMALES) study. J Sex Med 2005; **2**: 675–84.

25 **Brown RG, Jahanshahi N, Quinn N, Marsden CD**. Sexual function in patients with Parkinson's disease and their partners. J Neurol Neurosurg Psychiatry 1990; **53**: 480–6.

26 **Berman JR, Adhikari SP, Goldstein I**. Anatomy and physiology of female sexual function and dysfunction: classification, evaluation, and treatment options. Eur Urol 2000; **38**: 20–9.

27 **Rubin SM**. Parkinson's disease in women. Dis Mon 2007; **53**: 206–13.

28 **Schartau E, Tolson D, Fleming V**. Parkinson's disease: the effects on womanhood. Nurs Stand 2003; **17**: 33–9.

29 **Posen J, Moore O, Tassa D, et al**. Young women with PD: a group work experience. Soc Work Health Care 2000; **32**: 77–91.

30 **Meco G, Rubino A, Caravona N, Valente M**. Sexual dysfunction in Parkinson's disease. Parkinsonism Relat Disord 2008; **14**: 451–6.

31 **Damino AM, Snyder C, Strausser B, Willian MK**. A review of health-related quality of life concepts and measures for Parkinson's disease. Qual Life Res 1999; **8**: 235–43.

32 **Giladi N, Weitzman N, Schreiber S, et al**. New-onset heightened interest or drive for gambling, eating, shopping or sexual activity in patients with Parkinson's disease: the role of dopamine agonist treatment and age at motor symptoms onset. J Psychopharmacol 2007; **21**: 501–6.

33 **Merims D, Giladi N**. Dopamine dysregulation syndrome, addiction and behavioral changes in Parkinson's disease. Parkinsonism Relat Disord 2008; **14**: 273–80.

34 **Succu S, Sanna F, Melis T, Boi A, Argiolas A, Melis MR**. Stimulation of dopamine receptors in the paraventricular nucleus of the hypothalamus of male rats induces penile erection and increases extra-cellular dopamine in the nucleus accumbens: involvement of central oxytocin. Neuropharmacology 2007; **52**: 1034–43.

35 McMahon CG, Abdo C, Incrocci L, et al. Disorders of orgasm and ejaculation in men. J Sex Med 2004; **1**: 58–65.

36 Yahr MD, Duvoisin RC. Drug therapy of parkinsonism. N Engl J Med 1972; **287**: 20–4.

37 Pohanka M, Kanovský P, Bares M, Pulkrábek J, Rektor I. The long-lasting improvement of sexual dysfunction in patients with advanced, fluctuating Parkinson's disease induced by pergolide: evidence from the results of an open, prospective, one-year trial. Parkinsonism Relat Disord 2005; **11**: 509–12.

38 Lorrain DS, Riolo JV, Matuszewich L, et al. Lateral hypothalamic serotonin inhibits nucleus accumbens dopamine: implication for sexual satiety. J Neurosci 1999; **19**: 7648–53.

39 Mohee A, Bretsztajn L, Eardley I. The evaluation of apomorphine for the treatment of erectile dysfunction. Expert Opin Drug Metab Toxicol 2012; **8**:1447–53.

40 Valevski A, Modai I, Zbarski E, et al. Effect of amantadine on sexual dysfunction in neuroleptic-treated male schizophrenic patients. Clin Neuropharmacol 1998; **21**: 355–7.

41 Michelson D, Bancroft J, Targum S, et al. Female sexual dysfunction associated with antidepressant administration: a randomized, placebo-controlled study of pharmacologic intervention. Am J Psychiatry 2000; **157**: 239–43.

42 Serretti A, Chiesa A. Sexual side effects of pharmacological treatment of psychiatric diseases. Clin Pharmacol Ther 2011; **89**: 142–7.

43 Segraves RT. Sexual dysfunction associated with antidepressant therapy. Urol Clin North Am 2007; **34**: 575.

44 Castelli L, Perozzo P, Genesia ML, et al. Sexual well being in parkinsonian patients after deep brain stimulation of the subthalamic nucleus. J Neurol Neurosurg Psychiatry 2004; **75**: 1260–4.

45 Bronner G, Hassin-Baer S. Exploring hypersexual behavior in men with Parkinson's disease: is it compulsive sexual behavior? J Parkinson's Dis 2012; **2**: 225–34.

46 Weintraub D, Koester J, Potenza MN, et al. Impulse control disorders in Parkinson disease: a cross-sectional study of 3090 patients. Arch Neurol 2010; **67**: 589–95.

47 Lyons KE, Pahwa R. The impact and management of nonmotor symptoms of Parkinson's disease. Am J Manag Care 2011; **17**(Suppl 12): S308–S314.

48 de Chazeron I, Llorca PM, Chéreau-Boudet I, et al. Hypersexuality and pathological gambling in Parkinson's disease: a cross-sectional case-control study. Mov Disord 2011; **26**: 2127–30.

49 Pereira B, Llorca PM, Durif F, et al. Screening hypersexuality in Parkinson's disease in everyday practice. Parkinsonism Relat Disord 2013; **19**: 242–6.

50 Evans AH, Lees AJ. Dopamine dysregulation syndrome in Parkinson's disease. Curr Opin Neurol 2004; **17**: 393–8.

51 Klos KJ, Bower JH, Josephs KA, et al. Pathological hypersexuality predominantly linked to adjuvant dopamine agonist therapy in Parkinson's disease and multiple system atrophy. Parkinsonism Relat Disord 2005; **11**: 381–6.

52 Harvey NS. Serial cognitive profiles in levodopa-induced hypersexuality. Br J Psychiatry 1988; **153**: 833–6.

53 Paredes RG, Agmo A. Has dopamine a physiological role in the control of sexual behavior? A critical review of the evidence. Prog Neurobiol 2004; **73**: 179–226.

54 Weintraub D. Dopamine and impulse control disorders in Parkinson's disease. Ann Neurol 2008; **64**(Suppl): S93–S100.

55 Vilas D, Pont-Sunyer C, Tolosa E. Impulse control disorders in Parkinson's disease. Parkinsonism Relat Disord 2012; **18**(Suppl 1): S80–S84.

56 Djamshidian A, Averbeck BB, Lees AJ, O'Sullivan SS.Clinical aspects of impulsive compulsive behaviours in Parkinson's disease. J Neurol Sci 2011; **310**: 183–8.

57 Frohman EM. Sexual dysfunction in neurologic disease. Clin Neuropharmacol 2002; **25**: 126–32.

58 **Bronner G**. Practical strategies for the management of sexual problems in Parkinson's disease. Parkinsonism Relat Dis 2009; **15**(Suppl 3): S96–S100.

59 **Nicolosi A, Glasser DB, Kim SC, et al**. GSSAB Investigators' Group. Sexual behavior and dysfunction and help-seeking patterns in adults aged 40–80 years in the urban population of Asian countries. Br J Urol Int 2005; **95**: 609–14.

60 **Aschka C, Himmel W, Ittner E, Kochen MM**. Sexual problems of male patients in family practice. J Fam Pract 2001; **50**: 773–8.

61 **Zesiewicz TA, Helal M, Hauser MD**. Sildenafil citrate (Viagra) for the treatment of erectile dysfunction in men with Parkinson's disease. Mov Dis 2000; **15**: 305–8.

62 **Raffaele R, Vecchio I, Giammusso B, et al**. Efficacy and safety of fixed-dose oral sildenafil in the treatment of sexual dysfunction in depressed patients with idiopathic Parkinson's disease. Eur Urol 2002; **41**: 382–6.

63 **Hussain IF, Brady CM, Swinn MJ, Mathias CJ, Fowler CJ**.Treatment of erectile dysfunction with sildenafil citrate (Viagra) in parkinsonism due to Parkinson's disease or multiple system atrophy with observations on orthostatic hypotension. J Neurol Neurosurg Psychiatry 2001; **71**: 371–4.

64 **Zesiewicz TA, Sullivan KL, Arnulf I, et al.**; Quality Standards Subcommittee of the American Academy of Neurology. Practice Parameter: treatment of nonmotor symptoms of Parkinson disease: report of the Quality Standards Subcommittee of the American Academy of Neurology. Neurology 2010; **74**: 924–31.

65 **Montorsi F, Padma-Nathan H, Buvat J, et al.** for the Vardenafil Study Group. Earliest time to onset of action leading to successful intercourse with vardenafil determined in an at-home setting: a randomized, double-blind, placebo-controlled trial. J Sex Med 2004; **1**: 168–78.

66 **Hardoff R, Sula M, Tamir A, et al**. Gastric emptying time and gastric motility in patients with Parkinson's disease. Mov Disord 2001; **16**: 1041–7.

Chapter 19

Gastrointestinal dysfunctions in Parkinson's disease

Fabrizio Stocchi and Margherita Torti

Introduction

In his classic 1817 monograph, Sir James Parkinson [1] described gastrointestinal dysfunction in patients with the shaking palsy:

> . . . food is with difficulty retained in the mouth until masticated; and then as difficulty swallowed . . . the saliva fails of being directed to the back part of the fauces, and hence is continually draining from the mouth . . . the bowels which all along had been torpid, now in most cases, demand stimulating medicines of very considerable power: the expulsion of the faeces from the rectum sometimes requiring mechanical aid.

Gastrointestinal dysfunctions and constipation are now recognized as symptoms of the disease and can even precede the motor symptoms [2]. The Braak model for the pathodynamics of Lewy pathology in Parkinson's disease (PD), with early involvement of the enteric nervous system (ENS) and dorsal motor nucleus of the vagus (DMV), has led to the interpretation of the gastrointestinal symptoms as pre-motor manifestations of PD [3]. Studies suggest that gastrointestinal symptoms are one of the most common non-motor symptoms in PD patients [4–8]. These symptoms and dysfunctions are not only very distressing for patients but also interfere with treatment. The prevalence of gastrointestinal symptoms was recently evaluated in a questionnaire-based study of 120 parkinsonian patients and matching controls. Gastrointestinal dysfunctions were significantly more prevalent in PD patients, the most frequent complaints being dry mouth, drooling, dysphagia, constipation and defaecatory dysfunction. Constipation and defaecatory dysfunction preceded the motor manifestations [9].

The mobility and activities of daily living of parkinsonian patients depend on the blood level of levodopa. Levodopa (L-dihydroxyphenilalanine) is a large neutral amino acid (LNAA) and is absorbed only from the small bowel (mostly in the duodenum, with some absorption in the jejunum and ileum) which contains LNAA transporters. These drugs have a short half-life, therefore any factor which limits or delays absorption of levodopa results in a reappearance of parkinsonian symptoms.

Pathophysiology

The pathophysiological mechanisms of these gastrointestinal manifestations are multifactorial. Many disturbances of gastrointestinal motility reflect early involvement of both extrinsic and intrinsic innervation of the gut. An autopsy survey published by the Arizona PD Consortium has shown the occurrence of Lewy pathology in the peripheral nervous system, especially in the ENS, in almost all patients with PD [10]. In PD there is accumulation of α-synuclein immunoreactive Lewy bodies and Lewy neurites in the DMV, the sacral parasympathetic nuclei, the sympathetic ganglia and the ENS [3,11–13] Transgenic mice, recently developed as model of PD, show α-synuclein aggregates within their enteric ganglia which are clinically associated with reduced colonic motility and prolonged gut transit time in the absence of any pathological changes in the DMV or any autonomic cardiovascular dysfunction. These findings suggest that ENS dysfunction may be intrinsic in origin and does not develop as a result of central denervation of the gut [14].

α-Synuclein staining has been reported in biopsies of the submucosa of the ascending colon taken during routine screening of patients with mild to moderate PD. A recent study performed on 10 *de novo* PD patients has demonstrated staining for α-synuclein in the lamina propria of the colonic submucosa. 3-Nitrotyrosine staining, a marker of oxidative stress, was also seen in the majority of subjects even though it was not specific for PD. [15].

The DMV is affected at the earliest stage of Lewy body pathology in PD [13,16]. In PD, there is also prominent Lewy body pathology in both the Auerbach and Meissner plexuses along the entire gastrointestinal tract, particularly in neurons of the Auerbach plexus in the lower oesophagus and in the submucosal plexus in the stomach [11]. In contrast, there is sparing of neurons of the compact portion of the nucleus ambiguus (NAmb) involved in control of the pharyngeal and upper oesophageal phases of swallowing. In PD there is also involvement of the pedunculopontine tegmental nucleus (PPT) and medullary raphe, which may affect supraspinal control of swallowing and defaecation, respectively [17–19].

Swallowing abnormalities and oesophageal alterations

Swallowing is a complex and stereotyped sequential motor event that includes an oropharyngeal stage and a subsequent oesophageal stage. The main motor nuclei involved in swallowing are the hypoglossal nucleus (innervating the tongue muscles) and the NAmb (innervating the pharynx, larynx and oesophagus). Pre-ganglionic neurons of the DMV control the activity of the smooth muscle of the oesophagus. Swallowing is initiated by a medullary motor pattern generator. The interneurons of this central pattern generator are located in two main regions, the nucleus of the solitary tract (NTS) and adjacent reticular formation (dorsal swallowing group) and the ventrolateral medullary reticular formation, just above the NAmb (ventral swallowing group). Neurons of the NTS organize the sequential motor pattern for swallowing, whereas the neurons in the ventrolateral medulla may act as switching neurons that coordinate and distribute the drive generated in the NTS to the various pools of motor neurons [20].

Dysphagia and a variety of swallowing abnormalities are well-recognized complications of PD. Logemann et al. [21] reported abnormal lingual control of swallowing. Blonsky et al. [22] described lingual festination in which the elevated tongue prevented passage of the bolus into the pharynx. Longemann et al. [23] discussed a delayed swallowing reflex and noted aspiration. Bushmann et al. [24] reported a repetitive and involuntary reflux from the vallecula and piriform sinuses into the oral cavity. They also observed that some patients have great difficulty swallowing pills, with retention in the vallecula for long periods of time. This problem has also been observed by us with videofluoroscopy (Fig. 19.1 and Plate 4). Another abnormality that has recently been demonstrated is the tendency of parkinsonian patients to swallow during the inspiration phase, increasing the possibility of aspiration [25,26]. Dopaminergic drugs may improve swallowing, although a recent meta-analysis has demonstrated that levodopa does not improve dysphagia in PD patients [27].

Dry mouth and drooling

Excessive drooling is a frequent complaint in PD patients [28]. Drooling is due to reduced swallowing frequency, allowing excess saliva to accumulate in the mouth. Drooling saliva is usually more severe in the 'off' condition and improves during the 'on' state. Salivary production is reduced in PD, in both 'off' and 'on' states [29]. This may reflect the involvement of the salivary nucleus and the submandibular ganglion. Recent studies have shown α-synuclein inclusions in minor salivary glands and Lewy pathology in submandibular glands [10,30]. Levodopa increases both the basal and reflex-activated salivary flow rate even in PD patients pre-treated with the peripheral D2 antagonist domperidone [31]. Anticholinergics may improve drooling saliva by reducing the production of saliva, but they impair swallowing mechanisms. Glycopyrrolate is an anticholinergic drug that doesn't cross the blood–brain barrier, thus producing fewer central nervous system (CNS)-related side effects [32]. Sublingual administration of 1% atropine can reduce the production of saliva without causing systemic anticholinergic effects. Botulinum toxin injected into the four salivary glands improves drooling of saliva by reducing saliva production [33].

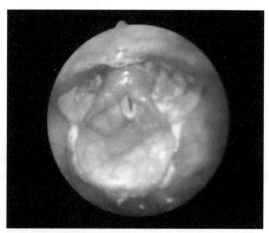

Fig. 19.1 Retention of a melted tablet in the low back part of the mouth. The tablet was taken 90 minutes before the fluoroscopy. (See also Plate 4.)

Dental deterioration

A variety of oral health problems have been described in association with PD. An increased incidence of tooth loss, periodontal pathology, denture discomfort, bruxism and temporo-mandibular joint dysfunction has been reported [34,35].

Oesophageal alterations

The lower oesophageal sphincter (LES) is composed of tonically active smooth muscles with intrinsic myogenic properties that maintain the sphincter closed in basal conditions. Both the vagal excitatory and the vagal inhibitory pathway from the DMV exert a tonic influence on the LES and are selectively activated in several motor reflexes involving the LES. For example, selective activation of the inhibitory pathway is critical for reflex relaxation of the LES associated with swallowing. Coordinated activity of vagal excitatory and inhibitory motor pathways triggered by vago-vagal reflexes via the NTS is also critical for control of the motor function of the stomach [36]. The vagal inhibitory pathway is essential for the reflex receptive relaxation of the proximal stomach (fundus) that is necessary to accommodate ingested food, whereas the vagal excitatory pathway activates the contraction of the distal two-thirds of the corpus and the antrum, which is critical for gastric emptying. Both the vagal excitatory and the vagal inhibitory pathways regulate the pyloric sphincter. Vagotomy impairs antropyloric coordination and delays gastric emptying.

The main oesophageal alterations in parkinsonian patients are non-peristaltic swallows, belching, segmental spasms, oesophageal dilatation and gastro-oesophageal reflux [37]. Belching can be related to 'on/off' fluctuations [38] and therefore disappears when patients turn 'on' (mobile state). Bramble et al. [39] suggested that cholinergic rather than dopaminergic mechanisms are more important in the control of oesophageal motility in parkinsonian patients. They showed that intravenous atropine produced a marked disruption of coordination in response to swallows in patients with PD compared with control subjects. Anticholinergic drugs may therefore worsen coordination in response to swallows.

Patients with swallowing and/or oesophageal alterations may benefit from the use of a liquid formulation of levodopa (levodopa methyl-ester, dispersible Madopar) [40] or from subcutaneous injections of the dopamine receptor agonist apomorphine [41]. Anticholinergic drugs should be withdrawn, but in some patients with severe drooling saliva, peripheral anticholinergic belladonna folium may be useful. Some patients suffer from achalasia, which can be treated with injection of botulinum toxin into the cardia. Significant improvement in the pharyngeal composite score and pharyngeal transit time in patients with deep brain stimulation (DBS) of the subthalamic nucleus (STN) in the DBS 'on' condition compared with the DBS 'off' condition has been reported [42].

Stomach

Gastroparesis, or delayed gastric emptying, can occur in PD [43,44] and other parkinsonian disorders and can produce a variety of symptoms such as early satiety, abnormal discomfort with bloating, nausea, vomiting, weight loss and even malnutrition. Several studies have concluded that gastric emptying and bowel movements are slow in PD [45,46] and can be present even in early and untreated PD patients. A study performed using electrogastrography revealed that 24 out of 36 PD patients had impaired gastric emptying, typically due to pre-prandial dysrhythmia [47]. A multiple regression analysis showed that delayed gastric emptying is significantly associated with severity of motor impairment [48].

In addition to being a LNAA, levodopa is not absorbed from the stomach, although the stomach plays an important role in controlling the access of levodopa to its absorptive sites in the small bowel. Baruzzi et al. [49] showed that delayed gastric emptying also delays and blunts peak plasma levodopa levels and may cause a reduced or a complete failure of the clinical response to the dose. Levodopa taken after meals may be poorly absorbed, probably due to the delay in gastric emptying related to characteristics of the meal such as bulk, tonality and composition [50,51]. Lipid and carbohydrates, but also some drugs like dopamine agonists or anticholinergics, also delay gastric emptying. Excessive gastric acidity also delays gastric emptying, but excessive neutralization of stomach contents may lead to incomplete dissolution of the levodopa tablets and thus incomplete absorption [52]. Gastric emptying may be also delayed by PD itself or by constipation because of the colon–gastric reflex. A levodopa tablet may remain in the stomach of a parkinsonian patient for a very long time, delaying the levodopa from reaching intestinal absorptive sites and the subsequent response time following dose ingestion. Moreover, the enzyme DOPA-decarboxylase is present in the gastric mucosa and can convert levodopa trapped in the stomach due to gastroparesis into dopamine, making it unavailable for CNS delivery and utilization [53]. Furthermore, the dopamine formed in the stomach may stimulate gastric dopamine receptors, which promote stomach relaxation and inhibit gastric motility, with the potential consequence of worsening the gastroparesis [54,55].

Many authors have shown that the direct infusion of liquid levodopa into the duodenum ensures a more reliable and predictable response to the drug [56]. Moreover, the levels of levodopa in the plasma after intraduodenal infusion are much more stable than after intragastric infusion [57]. These studies indicate the role of the stomach in the pathophysiology of motor fluctuations in parkinsonian patients. Levodopa is absorbed only from the small bowel (mostly in the duodenum, but there is some absorption in the jejunum and ileum), which contains LNAA transporters; because of their high capacity, competition between levodopa and other dietary LNAAs (e.g. valine, leucine and isolucine) is not common, although it may occur [58].

Other common gastric symptoms in parkinsonian patients include epigastric fullness and bloating and vomiting.

Liquid levodopa may improve patients with motor fluctuations, ensuring better absorption. Levodopa methyl-ester and dispersible Madopar are absorbed more quickly than standard levodopa preparations, especially when the drug is taken after meals [40,41]. Subcutaneous infusion of dopamine agonists (apomorphine and lisuride) [59] is very effective in controlling motor fluctuations as it by-passes the gastrointestinal tract. Parkinsonian patients should be taught to eat small meals and avoid protein during the day and to take the drugs when fasting. Dopaminergic D2 receptor antagonists such as domperidone

[60] improve gastric emptying in PD. A similar effect can be induced by the 5-HT4 receptor agonist mosapride [61], presumably by increasing local acetylcholine (ACh) release. Erythromycin is an antibiotic that has been found to be effective in accelerating gastric emptying due to its being a motilin receptor agonist, and it has recently been demonstrated that azithromycin is even more effective than erythromycin in improving gastric emptying in PD patients with gastroparesis [62–64].

Helicobacter pylori may interfere with levodopa absorption, probably as a consequence of gastroduodenitis; eradication of this infective agent resulted in effective improvement in the pharmacokinetic and clinical response to levodopa in patients with PD and motor fluctuations [65].

The small bowel

The literature contains references to both symptoms and radiological signs suggestive of small intestine motor dysfunction in PD. However, the frequency and the functional significance of some of these findings remain uncertain.

Weight loss is a frequent finding in elderly patients with PD [66,67], although the reasons have not been fully explained. An increase in energy expenditure has been shown in two studies [66,68], while other possible contributing factors include dietary deficiency or malabsorption due to bacterial overgrowth in the small bowel. Dietary deficiency is unlikely to be the cause [69]. Davies et al. [70] showed a reduced absorption of mannitol with an increase in the lactulase:mannitol ratio, suggesting a reduction in the absorptive surface area of the small intestine in parkinsonian patients. The authors explained these results as being due to a specific alteration in the enterocyte brush border membrane. The same authors did not find any evidence of bacterial contamination of the small bowel, whereas other studies have suggested that bacterial overgrowth in the small bowel is implicated in malabsorption, even when the small bowel is anatomically normal [71,72].

Weight gain can occur in parkinsonian patients treated with dopamine agonists as a result of increased fluid retention or an impulse control disorder with compulsive eating [73]. Important weight gain has also been noted after DBS, probably related to decreased energy expenditure resulting from reduced rigidity, tremor and dyskinesias, improved alimentation or direct influence on the lateral hypothalamus from DBS stimulation.

Davies et al. [70] also found a significantly prolonged orocaecal transit time in patients with PD compared with healthy elderly subjects, which was not related to the severity or duration of the disease. This phenomenon may be due to disordered autonomic function of the gastrointestinal tract. Lewy bodies have been found in the sympathetic vertebral chain and in the coeliac ganglion of patients with PD [74,75]. Thus, dysfunction of the autonomic or enteric nervous system may be responsible for the prolonged orocaecal transit time.

As already mentioned, levodopa is absorbed in the small bowel. Despite the high capacity of the LNAA transporters contained in the small bowel, competition between levodopa and other LNAAs (e.g. valine, leucine and isoleucine) may occur [58]. Moreover, other dysfunctions occurring in this area may influence the effectiveness of levodopa.

The large bowel

Large bowel symptoms are clearly defined and their frequency is high in people with PD [7,76,77]. Constipation is by far the most frequent symptom cited by patients. According to the Rome criterion, which is a validated objective measure, constipation is nearly three times more prevalent (59% versus 21%) among people with PD than controls [78]. In a questionnaire study of a group of PD patients, 76.5% reported a bowel frequency of fewer than three evacuations per week, 94% reported hard stools and straining for difficult defaecation and 88% reported continuous use of laxatives or enemas or both. In our series, 24% of patients reported faecal incontinence, six for liquid stools and one for solid faeces. Seventy-six per cent of the patients reported that the onset, or the worsening, of bowel dysfunctions followed the onset of neurological symptoms [79]. However, constipation may precede the motor symptoms of PD [2] and has recently been identified as a risk factor for PD. In one study individuals with less than one bowel movement a day have been found to have a 2.7 times greater risk of developing PD than individuals with one bowel movement per day and more than a four-fold greater risk than those having two or more evacuations per day [2].

Constipation is variously defined in terms of number of bowel movements and other indicators of defaecatory dysfunction such as straining or hard stools. Infrequent bowel action in the absence of other symptoms can be regarded as within the normal spectrum [4]. The Rome criterion is an internationally recognized objective definition of constipation. Its earliest version focused on four symptoms (straining, lumpy and/or hard stools, incomplete evacuation and two or fewer bowel movements per week) and associated a positive diagnosis of constipation with two or more symptoms being present for at least one-quarter of the time over a period of at least 3 months. An updated version added two further symptoms: sensation of anorectal obstruction or blockage and manual manoeuvres to facilitate evacuation [80]. The stools may be hard and pellet-like or large and difficult to pass. Constipation may be caused by one or several mechanisms: (1) functional obstruction due to an increase in segmenting contractions; (2) poor colonic contractions (colonic inertia or pseudo-obstruction); or (3) functional outlet obstruction [81]. Specific symptoms may suggest the underlying aetiology of the constipation. Patients usually have abdominal pain, although patients with increased segmental contractions are more likely to have lower abdominal cramps associated with irritable bowel syndrome. In contrast, patients with nausea and vomiting are more likely to have an absence of post-prandial colonic contractions [82]. Straining with stool and incomplete evacuation may suggest an outlet obstruction.

Constipation in PD can, however, result from several causes. For stool expulsion to occur, faecal material must first be propelled through the colon by colonic muscle contraction and then be expelled through the coordinated actions of the rectum, anal sphincters and pelvic floor muscles, as well as the musculature of the abdominal wall and diaphragm [83]. In parkinsonism, constipation is due to colonic inertia or to outlet-type dysfunction or both [58–86]. With colonic inertia, the problem seems to be in the colonic musculature, which induces slow transit of faeces through the colon [86,87].

Many authors have shown that the mean colon transit time is considerably prolonged in PD patients [88–90]. Thus, slow colon transit is clearly a component of disturbed bowel function in PD patients. Early involvement of enteric neurons may explain the finding that constipation is a very early sign of PD [2]. There is an accumulation of Lewy bodies in vasoactive intestinal polypeptide (VIP)-ergic neurons of the ENS [11], suggesting that slow intestinal transit in PD may result primarily from impaired reflex relaxation of the distal smooth muscle due to loss of inhibitory motor neurons. However, there is also age-related loss of excitatory cholinergic neurons in the colon [91,92], and impaired cholinergic function is likely to contribute to slow colonic transit time in PD. The 5-HT4 agonists mosapride [93] and tegaserod [94,95] improve constipation in patients with PD, presumably by promoting the release of ACh from myenteric neurons. Loss of enteric dopamine neurons has also been reported in PD [96] but the functional significance of this is uncertain. Dopamine cells constitute only 1–2% of the total population of ENS neurons in humans, and dopamine, acting via pre-synaptic D2 receptors, inhibits the release of ACh and intestinal motility. There is selective loss of enteric dopaminergic neurons in the MPTP (1-methyl-4-phenyl-1,2,3,6-tetrahydropyridine) mouse model of PD [97]. Electrophysiological recording of neural-mediated muscle contraction in isolated colon from MPTP-treated animals showed a defect in relaxation. These animals exhibit a transient increase in colon motility, but no changes in gastric emptying or small intestine transit [97].

Other authors [98,99] have shown most Lewy bodies in the gut to be in VIP-immunoreactive neurons, whereas in the sympathetic ganglia all neurons containing Lewy bodies were immunoreactive for tyrosine hydroxylase. These findings suggest that slow colonic transit may be related to a direct involvement of the colonic myenteric plexus in the PD process.

Outlet obstruction has been attributed to a focal dystonia of the pelvic floor sustained by a failure of the puborectalis muscle to relax during efforts to defaecate, or by its paradoxical contraction. It is characterized by excessive recruitment of synergistic and antagonistic muscle groups during voluntary activity and lack of reciprocal inhibition [99,100].

Normal defaecation occurs at a socially convenient time after rectal distension by faecal material is perceived. Tonic-resting activity in the striated sphincter musculature is inhibited and relaxation of the puborectalis muscle sling permits straightening of the rectoanal angle, allowing access of the rectal contents to the anal canal. Simultaneously, relaxation occurs in the external anal sphincter muscle. During defaecation straining there is co-contraction of glottic, diaphragmatic and abdominal wall muscles, and rectal evacuation is achieved by a combination of raised intra-abdominal pressure and relaxation of the anal sphincter muscles, often aided by colonic pressure waves. Previous descriptions of electromyographic (EMG) activity during simulated defaecation straining have confirmed that, in normal subjects, there is inhibition of the external anal sphincter (EAS) and puborectalis muscles [101]. In subjects with normal EMG sphincter muscle relaxation, activity in the adjacent gluteal muscles does not change when recorded under the laboratory conditions of this study [102]. Mathers et al. [83] showed that the selective pattern of muscle contraction and inhibition that accompanies defaecation straining is disturbed in some parkinsonian patients suffering from constipation. Paradoxical activation of the puborectalis and EAS muscles occurred and some patients also showed a tendency to recruit gluteal muscles during simulated defaecation straining.

During defaecation the puborectalis muscle normally relaxes, opening the anorectal angle to promote outward passage of stool. When the puborectalis fails to relax or contracts during defaecation, as seen in some PD patients, the forward passage of stool is impaired and defecation obstructed. Sometimes paradoxical anal sphincter muscle contraction resembling anismus-type pelvic outlet obstruction may also occur [100].

Anorectal manometry has revealed several abnormalities in parkinsonian patients, including low basal and impaired squeeze pressures, prominent phasic fluctuations during squeeze and a hyper-contractile response to rectosphinteric reflex [65].

We studied the anorectal function in 17 patients [79]. Four hours after receiving a fleet enema patients underwent anorectal manometry with a multilumen catheter (outer diameter 4 mm) with distal side openings spaced 5 mm apart. Three lumens were continuously perfused (0.5 ml/min) with bubble-free distilled water by means of a low-compliance pneumohydraulic capillary-infusion system and were connected through P23 Db Statham external transducers to a multichannel polygraph. A latex balloon was attached to the tip of the catheter, 50 mm from the nearest recording side hole. When suspended in air and inflated with 50 ml of air, the balloon was 65 mm long and 40 mm wide. Intraballoon pressures were recorded and transmitted to the polygraph via a fourth lumen. With the subject lying on his or her left side, the manometric probe was introduced through the anus so that all recording holes were positioned within the rectal ampulla. The manometric catheter was then withdrawn through the anal canal with a station pull-through technique. The probe was then reintroduced into the rectum and withdrawn to be positioned in the anal canal, with the recording sensors at 10, 15 and 20 mm from the anal verge. The operator kept the manometric probe firmly in place throughout the study period. The protocol included three tasks: act of squeezing; progressive intermittent distension of the intrarectal balloon; and straining on two separate occasions.

Resting anal pressure was 49 ± 19 mmHg and the maximal contraction pressure was 99 ± 40 mmHg, lasting 15.6 ± 6.8 seconds, all remaining under the normal value. Three patients were unable to contract the anus. Resting and squeezing anal pressures showed an inverse direct relationship with disease duration. Maximal anal contraction pressure was higher in patients with a lower degree of disability (Hoen and Yahr Stage 2–3) than in the patients with more severe disease (Hoen and Yahr Stage 4–5). A significant relationship between anal pressure and the age of the patients and disease duration was found. The threshold of the inhibitory anal reflex and rectal compliance were within the normal range and the mean threshold of rectal sensitivity (70 ± 58 ml air) was in the upper range of normal values. Manometric recordings during straining showed a lack of anal inhibition in 11 patients (65%).

Altered voluntary anal contraction and paradoxical anal contraction during straining have been repeatedly reported in PD patients [90]. In our study we also found an insufficient relaxation of the anal canal during straining. A possible explanation is a manometric expression of the abdomino-pelvic dyssynergia, recorded with EMG in other studies [103] manifesting as an insufficient decrease in anal pressure accompanied by a paradoxical contraction.

In PD and in multiple system atrophy (MSA) the manometric finding of a paradoxical contraction or insufficient inhibition of the anal canal during straining could reflect the generalized extra-pyramidal motor disorder and hence be unrelated to degeneration of the sacral nuclei. Its frequent occurrence in patients with idiopathic constipation [104] and in children with functional megarectum [105] indicates that the abnormality is strictly related not to the specific neurological alterations of idiopathic PD or MSA but rather to a focal dystonic condition [100] of the abdomino-pelvic muscles facilitated by PD.

The finding of a low resting anal tone has not been consistently reported in PD patients; our investigation confirmed that although resting anal pressure may range within normal values in PD some patients have marked hypotonia. Because the resting anal pressure is essentially due to the contractile activity of the internal anal sphincter—a function mainly regulated by the orthosympathetic nervous system—this abnormality may reflect a degenerative lesion of the intermediolateral columns of the spinal cord or autonomic ganglia, or both [74].

Alternative explanations for the reduced anal pressure in resting conditions and during voluntary contraction can be found in the possible presence of anatomical changes in the internal and external anal sphincters consequent to age-related degeneration or continuous straining efforts, or both, which, in the attempt to overcome the difficulties in defaecation may lead to traction neuropathy involving the distal fibres of the pudendal nerves.

Irrespective of its pathophysiological mechanism, the reduced anal tone during resting conditions and voluntary contraction could explain the relatively high frequency of episodes of faecal incontinence for liquid stools frequently reported by PD patients, especially after laxative intake.

The inefficient voluntary anal contraction found in PD patients may be due to their inability to recruit properly the muscle fibres of the EAS.

Treatment of constipation

While many therapies have been advocated for the treatment of constipation in PD, few have been subjected to clinical trial. Ashraf et al. [106] reported that psyllium increased stool frequency and weight but did not alter colonic transit or anorectal function in PD patients with confirmed constipation. Astarloa et al. [107] reported that a diet rich in insoluble fibre produced a significant improvement in constipation, as indicated by an increase in stool frequency and an improvement in stool consistency. A fascinating observation in this study was a parallel improvement in extra-pyramidal function, which in turn appeared to be related to an increase in the bioavailability of orally administered levodopa. The authors suggested that this increase in levodopa absorption and resultant improvement in clinical status were related to an augmentation in gastrointestinal motility and therefore drug delivery. Suppression of defaecation can result in delayed gastric emptying, perhaps through a cologastric reflex [108,109]. This could explain the beneficial effect on extra-pyramidal symptoms of treatments that improve constipation.

Mosapride citrate, a selective 5-HT4 receptor agonist which facilitates the release of ACh from the enteric cholinergic neurons was shown to ameliorate constipation in PD patients. The drug augmented lower gastrointestinal tract motility, as shown in a colonic transit time study and videomanometry, without serious adverse events [110].

Prucalopride, another selective high-affinity 5-HT4 receptor agonist, has been marketed in the last years and approved for chronic constipation. It has greater selectivity for KCHN2 channels, improving gastric mobility and colonic transit time and increasing bowel movement [111]. Prucalopride has never been tested in PD. In a double-blind controlled trial Zangaglia et al. [112] showed that an isosmotic macrogol electrolyte solution improved constipation in PD patients. The drug was well tolerated and did not affect PD motor symptomatology

The difficulties in relaxing the pelvic floor and paradoxical puborectalis contraction generally respond dramatically to dopaminergic drugs [83]. Paradoxical EMG activity in anal sphincter muscles tends to persist even in the 'on' phase. However, a definite improvement in pelvic outlet obstruction has been demonstrated with proctography after the administration of apomorphine [83]. This evidence extends the concept of an 'off'-period pelvic floor dystonia in PD, as advanced by Mathers and colleagues [100].

Patients should therefore try to pass faeces when 'on' or take a quick-acting drug (soluble levodopa [40] or apomorphine [83]) before starting to defaecate. Unfortunately, some patients still experience difficulty defaecating when motor disability has otherwise been reversed by dopaminergic drugs. In these patients, the injection of botulinum toxin into the puborectalis muscle and/or the EAS may be useful. Injection of botulinum toxin may also be used in those patients with painful anismus-type dystonia [101].

Laxatives are useful in patients with normal pelvic floor relaxation. On the other hand, continuing to give laxatives to patients who cannot achieve effective defaecation due to pelvic floor dystonia will only produce adverse effects from the laxatives and further increase patients' frustration.

Megacolon and even sigmoid volvulus may be a complication of impaired colonic motor function in PD. Although uncommon, these complications may be life-threatening, and volvulus should certainly be considered in any PD patient who presents with an acute abdomen.

References

1 Parkinson J. An essay on the shaking palsy. London: Sherwood, Neely, and Jones, 1817.

2 Abbott RD, Petrovitch H, White LR, et al. Frequency of bowel movements and the future risk of Parkinson's disease. Neurology 2001; **57**: 456–62.

3 Braak H, de Vos RA, Bohl J, Del Tredici K. Gastric alpha-synuclein immunoreactive inclusions in Meissner's and Auerbach's plexuses in cases staged for Parkinson's disease-related brain pathology. Neurosci Lett 2006; **396**: 67–72.

4 Edwards LL, Quigley EMM, Pfeiffer RF. Gastrointestinal dysfunction in Parkinson's disease: frequency and pathophysiology. Neurology 1992; **42**: 726–32.

5 **Edwards LL, Pfeiffer RF, Quigley EMM, et al**. Gastrointestinal symptoms in Parkinson's disease. Mov Disord 1991; **6**: 151–6.

6 **Edwards LL, Quigley EMM, Hofman R, et al**. Gastrointestinal symptoms in Parkinson's disease: 18-month follow-up study. Mov Disord 1993; **8**: 83–6.

7 **Martinez-Martin P, Schapira AH, Stocchi F, et al**. Prevalence of nonmotor symptoms in Parkinson's disease in an international setting; study using nonmotor symptoms questionnaire in 545 patients. Mov Disord 2007; **22**: 1623–9.

8 **Verbaan D, Marinus J, Visser M, et al**. Patient-reported autonomic symptoms in Parkinson disease. Neurology 2007; **69**: 333–41.

9 **Cersosimo MG, Raina GB, Pecci C, et al**. Gastrointestinal manifestations in Parkinson's disease: prevalence and occurrence before motor symptoms. J Neurol 2013; **260**:1332–8.

10 **Beach TG, Adler CH, Sue LI, et al**. Multi-organ distribution of phosphorylated alpha-synuclein histopathology in subjects with Lewy body disorders Acta Neuropathol 2009; **119**: 689–702.

11 **Wakabayashi K, Takahashi H, Ohama E, et al**. Lewy bodies in the visceral autonomic nervous system in Parkinson's disease. Adv Neurol 1993; **60**: 609–12.

12 **Braak H, Bohl JR, Müller CM, et al**. Stanley Fahn Lecture 2005: the staging procedure for the inclusion body pathology associated with sporadic Parkinson's disease reconsidered. Mov Disord 2006; **21**: 2042–51.

13 **Braak H, Müller CM, Rüb U, et al**. Pathology associated with sporadic Parkinson's disease—where does it end? J Neural Transm 2006; 70(Suppl): 89–97.

14 **Kuo YM, Li Z, Jiao Y, et al**. Extensive enteric nervous system abnormalities in mice transgenic for artificial chromosomes containing Parkinson's disease -associated alpha-synuclein gene mutations precede central nervous system changes. Hum Mol Genet 2010; **19**: 1633–50.

15 **Shannon KM, Kesharvarzian A, Mutlu E, et al**. Alpha-synuclein in colonic submucosa in early untreated Parkinson's disease. Mov Disord 2012; **6**: 709–15.

16 **Gai WP, Blumbergs PC, Geffen LB, Blessing WW**. Age-related loss of dorsal vagal neurons in Parkinson's disease. Neurology 1992; **42**: 2106–11.

17 **Pahapill PA, Lozano AM**. The pedunculopontine nucleus and Parkinson's disease. Brain 2000; **123**: 1767–83.

18 **Jellinger KA**. Pathology of Parkinson's disease. Changes other than the nigrostriatal pathway. Mol Chem Neuropathol 1991; **14**: 153–97.

19 **Del Tredici K, Rüb U, De Vos RA, et al**. Where does Parkinson disease pathology begin in the brain? J Neuropathol Exp Neurol 2002; **61**: 413–26.

20 **Cersosimo MG, Benarroch EE**. Neural control of the gastrointestinal tract: implications for Parkinson disease. Mov Disord 2008; **23**: 1065–75.

21 **Logemann JA, Blonsky ER, Boshes B**. Lingual control in Parkinson's disease. Trans Am Neurol Assoc 1973; **98**: 276–8.

22 **Blonsky ER, Logemann JA, Boshes B, et al**. Comparison of speech and swallowing function in patients with tremor disorders and in normal geriatric patients: a cinefluorographic study. J Gerontol 1975; **30**: 299–303.

23 **Logemann JA, Boshes B, Blonsky ER, Fisher HB**. Speech and swallowing evaluation in the differential diagnosis of neurologic disease. Neurol Neurocir Psiquiatr 1977; 18(2–3 Suppl): 71–8.

24 **Bushmann M, Dobmeyer SM, Leeker L, et al**. Swallowing abnormalities and their response to treatment in Parkinson's disease. Neurology 1989; **39**: 1309–14.

25 **Gross RD, Atwood CWJR, Ross SB, et al**. The coordination of breathing and swallowing in Parkinson's disease. Dysphagia 2008; **23**: 136–45.

26 **Troche MS, Huebner I, Rosembeck JC, et al**. Respiratory-swallowing coordination and swallowing safety in patients with Parkinson's disease. Dysphagia 2011; **26**: 218–24.

27 Menezes C, Melo A. Does levo-dopa improve swallowing dysfunction in Parkinson's disease patients? J Clin Pharm Ther 2009; **34**: 673–6.

28 Calne DB, Shaw DG, Spiers ASD, et al. Swallowing in parkinsonism. Br J Radiol 1970; **43**: 456–7.

29 Proulx M, de Courval FP, Wiseman MA, Panisset M. Salivary production in Parkinson's disease. Mov Disord 2005; **20**: 204–7.

30 Cersosimo MG, Perandones C, Micheli FE, et al. Alpha-synuclein immunoreactivity in minor salivary gland biopsies of Parkinson's disease patients. Mov Disord 2011; **26**: 188–90.

31 Tumilasci OR, Cersosimo MG, Belforte JE, Micheli FE, Benarroch EE, Pazo JH. Quantitative study of salivary secretion in Parkinson's disease. Mov Disord 2006; **21**: 660–7.

32 Arbouw ME, Movig KL, Koopman M, et al. Glycopyrrolate for sialorrhea in Parkinson's disease: a randomized, double blind, cross-over trial. Neurology 2010; **74**: 1203–7.

33 Porta M, Gamba M, Bertacchi G, Vaj P. Treatment of sialorrhoea with ultrasound guided botulinum toxin type A injection in patients with neurological disorders. J Neurol Neurosurg Psychiatry 2001; **70**: 538–40.

34 Nakayama Y, Washio M, Mori M. Oral health conditions in patients with Parkinson's disease. J Epidemiol 2004; **14**: 143–50.

35 Schwarz J, Heimhilger E, Storch A. Increased periodontal pathology in Parkinson's disease. J Neurol 2006; **253**: 608–11.

36 Travagli RA, Hermann GE, Browning KN, Rogers RC. Brainstem circuits regulating gastric function. Ann Rev Physiol 2006; **68**: 279–305.

37 Gibberd FB, Gleeson JA, Gossage AAR, et al. Oesophageal dilatation in Parkinson's disease. J Neurol Neurosurg Psychiatry 1974; **37**: 938–40.

38 Kempster PA, Lees AJ, Crichton P, et al. Off-period belching due to a reversible disturbance of oesophageal motility in Parkinson's disease and its treatment with apomorphine. Mov Disord 1989; **4**: 47–52.

39 Bramble MG, Cunliffe J, Dellipiani W. Evidence for a change in neurotransmitter affecting oesophageal motility in Parkinson's disease. J Neurol Neurosurg Psychiatry 1978; **41**: 709–12.

40 Stocchi F, Barbato L, Bramante L, et al. Fluctuating parkinsonism: a pilot study of a single afternoon dose of levodopa methyl ester. J Neurol 1996 **243**: 377–80.

41 Stocchi F. Prevention and treatment of motor fluctuations. Parkinsonism Relat Disord 2003; **9**(Suppl 2): 73–81.

42 Ciucci MR, Barkmeier-Kraemer JM, Sherman SJ. Subthalamic nucleus deep brain stimulation improves deglutition in Parkinson's disease. Mov Disord 2008; **23**: 676–83.

43 Sulla M, Hardoff R, Gilardi N, et al. Gastric emptying time and gastric motility in patients with untreated Parkinson's disease [abstract]. Mov Disord 1996; **11**(Suppl 1): 167.

44 Djaletti R, Baron J, Ziv I, et al. Gastric emptying in Parkinson's disease: patients with and without response fluctuations. Neurology 1996; **46**: 1051–4.

45 Hardoff R, Sula M, Tamir A, et al. Gastric emptying time and gastric motility in patients with Parkinson's disease [abstract]. Mov Disord 2001; **16**: 1041.

46 Goetze O, Wieczorek J, Mueller T, et al. Impaired gastric emptying of a solid test meal in patients with Parkinson's disease using 13C-sodium octanoate breath test. Neurosci Lett 2005; **375**: 170–3.

47 Naftali T, Gadoth N, Huberman M, Novis B. Electrogastrography in patients with Parkinson's disease. Can J Neurol Sci 2005; **32**: 82–6.

48 Goetze O, Nikodem AB, Wiezcorek J, et al. Predictors of gastric emptying in Parkinson's disease. Neurogastroenterol Motil 2006; **18**: 369–75.

49 Baruzzi A, Contin M, Riva R, et al. Influence of meal ingestion time on pharmacokinetics of orally administered levodopa in parkinsonian patients. Clin Neuropharmacol 1987; **10**: 527–37.

50 **Dubois A**. Diet and gastric digestion. Am J Clin Nutr 1985; **42**: 1002–5.

51 **Kelly KA**. Motility of the stomach and gastroduodenal junction. In: LR Johnson (ed.) Physiology of the gastrointestinal tract, pp. 393–410. New York: Raven Press, 1981.

52 **Leon AS, Speigel H**. The effect of antacid administration on the absorption and metabolism of levodopa. J Clin Pharmacol 1972; **12**: 263–7.

53 **Evans MA, Broe GA, Triggs EJ, et al**. Gastric emptying rate and the systemic availability of levodopa in the elderly parkinsonian patients. Neurology 1981; **31**: 1288–94.

54 **Valenzuala JE**. Dopamine as a possible neurotransmitter in gastric relaxation. Gastroenterology 1976; **71**: 1019–22.

55 **Berkowitz DM, McCallum RW**. Interaction of levodopa and metoclopramide on gastric emptying. Clin Pharmacol Ther 1980; **27**: 414–20.

56 **Ruggieri S, Stocchi F, Carta A, et al**. Jejunal delivery of L-dopa methyl ester. Lancet 1989; **2**: 45–6.

57 **Kurlan R, Rothfield KP, Woodward WR, et al**. Erratic gastric emptying of levodopa may cause 'random' fluctuations of parkinsonian mobility. Neurology 1988; **38**: 419–21.

58 **Wade DN, Mearrik PT, Birkett DJ, et al**. Active transport of L-dopa in the intestine. Nature 1973; **242**: 463–5.

59 **Olanow C, Obseo J, Stocchi F**. Drug insight: continuous dopaminergic stimulation in the treatment of Parkinson's disease. Nat Clin Pract Neurol 2006; **2**: 382–92.

60 **Sarosiek I, Shifflett J, Wooten GF, McCallum RW**. Effect of chronic oral domperidone therapy on gastrointestinal symptoms and gastric emptying in patients with Parkinson's disease. Mov Disord 1997; **12**: 952–7.

61 **Hirohide A, Fukashi U, Makito H, et al**. Increased gastric motility during 5-HT4 agonist therapy reduces response fluctuations in Parkinson's disease. Parkinsonism Relat Disord 2005; **11**: 499–502.

62 **Weber FH Jr, Richards RD, McCallum RW**. Erythromycin: a motilin agonist and gastrointestinal prokinetic agent. Am J Gastroenterol 1993; **88**: 485–90.

63 **Maganti K, Nyemere K, Jones MP**. Oral erythromycin and symptomatic relief of gastroparesis: a systematic review. Am J Gastroenterol 2003; **98**: 259–63.

64 **Larson JM, Tavakkoli A, Drane WE, et al**. Advantages of azithromycin over erythromycin in improving the gastric emptying half-time in adult patients with gastroparesis. J Neurogastroenterol Motil. 2010; **16**: 407–13.

65 **Pierantozzi M, Pietroiusti A, Brusa L, et al**. Helicobacter pylori eradication and l-dopa absorption in patients with PD and motor fluctuations. Neurology 2006; **66**: 1824–9.

66 **Levi S, Cox M, Lugon M, et al**. Increased energy expenditure in Parkinson's disease. Br Med J 1990; **301**: 1256–7.

67 **Yapa RSS, Playfer JR, Lye M**. Anthropometric and nutritional assessment of elderly patients with Parkinson's disease. J Clin Exp Geront 1989; **11**: 155–64.

68 **Markus HS, Cox M, Tomkins AM**. Raised energy expenditure in Parkinson's disease and its relationship to muscular rigidity. Clin Sci 1992; **83**: 199–204.

69 **Davies KN, King D, Davies H**. A study of the nutritional status of elderly patients with Parkinson's disease. Age Ageing 1994; **23**: 142–5.

70 **Davies KN, King D, Billington D, Barrett JA**. Intestinal permeability and orocaecal transit time in elderly patients with Parkinson's disease. Postgrad Med J 1996; **72**: 164–7.

71 **McEvoy A, Dutton J, James OFW**. Bacterial contamination of the small intestine is an important cause of malabsorption in the elderly. Br Med J 1983; **287**: 789–93.

72 **Montgomery RD, Haboubi NY, Mike NH, et al**. Cause of malabsorption in the elderly. Age Ageing 1986; **15**: 235–40.

73 Niremberg MJ, Waters C. Compulsive eating and weight gain related to dopamine agonist use. Mov Disord 2006; **21**: 524–9.

74 Den Hartog Jager WA, Bethlem J. The distribution of Lewy bodies in the central and autonomic nervous system in idiopathic paralysis agitans. J Neurol Neurosurg Psychiatry 1960; **23**: 283–90.

75 Ohama E, Ikuta F. Parkinson's disease: distribution of Lewy bodies and monoamine neuron system. Acta Neuropathol 1976; **34**: 311–19.

76 Kupsky WJ, Grimes MM, Sweeting J, et al. Parkinson's disease and megacolon: concentric hyaline inclusions (Lewy bodies) in enteric ganglionic cells. Neurology 1987; **37**: 1253–5.

77 Ashraf W, Pfeiffer RF, Park F, Lof J, Quigley EM. Constipation in Parkinson's disease: objective assessment and response to psyllium. Mov Disord 1997; **12**: 946–51.

78 Kaye J, Gage H, Kimber A, et al. Excess burden of constipation in Parkinson's disease: a pilot study. Mov Disord 2006; **21**: 1270–3.

79 Stocchi F, Badiali D, Vacca L, et al. Anorectal function in multiple system atrophy and Parkinson's disease. Mov Disord 2000; **15**: 71–6.

80 Thompson WG, Longstreth GF, Drossman DA, et al. Functional bowel disorders and functional abdominal pain. Gut 1999; 45(Suppl. 2): II43–II47.

81 Reynolds JC, Ouyang A, Lee C, et al. Chronic severe constipation. Gastroenterology 1987; **92**: 414–42.

82 Bazzocchi G, Ellis J, Villanueva-Meyer J, et al. Postprandial colonic transit and motor activity in chronic constipation. Gastroenterology 1990; **98**: 686–9.

83 Mathers SE, Kempster PA, Law PJ, et al. Anal sphincter dysfunction in Parkinson's disease. Arch Neurol 1989; **46**: 1061–4.

84 Lubowski DZ, Swash M, Henry M. Neural mechanisms in disorders of defecation. Baillieres Clin Gastroenterol 1988; **2**: 210–23.

85 Martelli H, Devroede G, Arhan P, et al. Mechanisms of idiopathic constipation: outlet obstruction. Gastroenterology 1978; **75**: 623–31.

86 Arhtan P, Devroede G, Jehannin B, et al. Segmental colon transit time. Dis Colon Rectum 1981; **24**: 625–9.

87 Sakakibara R, Odaka T, Uchiyama T, et al. Colonic transit time and rectoanal videomanometry in Parkinson's disease. J Neurol Neurosurg Psychiatry 2003; **74**: 268–72.

88 Metcalf AM, Phillips SF, Zinsmeister AR, et al. Simplified assessment of segmental colonic transit. Gastroenterology 1987; **92**: 40–7.

89 Jost WH, Schimrigk K. Constipation in Parkinson's disease. Klin Wochenschr 1991; **69**: 906–9.

90 Edwards LL, Quigley EMM, Harned RK, et al. Characterisation of swallowing and defecation in Parkinson's disease. Am J Gastroenterol 1994; **89**: 15–25.

91 Phillips RJ, Powley TL. Innervation of the gastrointestinal tract: patterns of aging. Auton Neurosci 2007; **136**: 1–19.

92 Wade PR, Hornby PJ. Age-related neurodegenerative changes and how they affect the gut. Sci Aging Knowledge Environ 2005; **2005**(12): pe8.

93 Liu Z, Sakakibara R, Odaka T, et al. Mosapride citrate, a novel 5-HT4 agonist and partial 5-HT3 antagonist, ameliorates constipation in parkinsonian patients. Mov Disord 2005; **20**: 680–6.

94 Morgan JC, Sethi KD. Tegaserod in constipation associated with Parkinson disease. Clin Neuropharmacol 2007; **30**: 52–4.

95 Sullivan KL, Staffetti JF, Hauser RA, et al. Tegaserod (Zelnorm) for the treatment of constipation in Parkinson's disease. Mov Disord 2006; **21**: 115–16.

96 Singaram C, Ashraf W, Gaumnitz EA, et al. Dopaminergic defect of enteric nervous system in Parkinson's disease patients with chronic constipation. Lancet 1995; **346**: 861–4.

97 Anderson G, Noorian AR, Taylor G, et al. Loss of enteric dopaminergic neurons and associated changes in colon motility in an MPTP mouse model of Parkinson's disease. Exp Neurol 2007; **207**: 4–12.

98 Wakabayashi K, Takahachi H, Ohama E, Ikuta F. Tyrosine hydroxylase-immunereactive intrinsic neurons in the Auerbah's and Meissner's plexuses of humans. Neurosci Lett 1989; **96**: 259–63.

99 Wakabayashi K, Takahachi H, Ohama E, Ikuta F. Parkinson's disease: an immunohistochemical study of Lewy body-containing neurons in the enteric nervous system. Acta Neuropathol 1990; **79**: 581–3.

100 Mathers SE, Kempster PA, Swash M, Lees AJ. Constipation and paradoxical puborectalis contraction in anismus and Parkinson's disease: a dystonic phenomenon? J Neurol Neurosurg Psychiatry 1988; **51**: 1503–7.

101 Albanese A, Brisinda G, Bentivoglio AR, Maria G. Treatment of outlet obstruction constipation in Parkinson's disease with botulinum neurotoxin A. Am J Gastroenterol 2003; **98**: 1439–40.

102 Floyd WF, Walls EW. Electromyography of the sphincter ani externus in man. J Physiol 1953; **122**: 599–609.

103 Ger G-C, Wexner SD, Jorge JMN, Salanga VD. Anorectal manometry in the diagnosis of paradoxical puborectalis syndrome. Dis Colon Rectum 1993; **36**: 816–25.

104 Whitehead WE, Devroede G, Habib FI, et al. Functional disorders of the anorectum. Gastroenterol Int 1992; **5**: 92–108.

105 Loening-Baucke VA, Cruikshank BM. Abnormal defecation dynamics in chronic constipated children with encopresis. J Pediatr 1986; **108**: 562–6.

106 Ashraf W, Pfeiffer RP, Park F, et al. Constipation in Parkinson's disease: objective assessment and response to psyllium. Mov Disord 1997; **6**: 946–51.

107 Astarloa R, Mena MA, Sanchez V, et al. Clinical and pharmacological effects of a diet rich in insoluble fiber on Parkinson's disease. Clin Neuropharmacol 1992; **15**: 375–80.

108 Kellow JE, Gill RC, Wingate DL. Modulation of human upper gastrointestinal motility by rectal distension. Gut 1987; **28**: 864–8.

109 Tjeerdsma HC, Smout AJPM, Akkermans LMA. Voluntary suppression of defecation delays gastric emptying. Dig Dis Sci 1993; **38**: 832–6.

110 Zhi L, Sakakibara R, Odaka T, et al. Mosapride citrate, a novel 5-HT4 agonist and partial 5-HT3 antagonist, ameliorates constipation in parkinsonian patients. Mov Disord 2005; **20**: 680–6.

111 Bouras EP, Camilleri M, Burton DD, et al. Prucalopride accelerates gastrointestinal and colonic transit in patients with constipation without a rectal evacuation disorder. Gastroenterology 2001; **120**: 354–60.

112 Zangaglia R, Martignoni E, Glorioso M, et al. Macrogol for the treatment of constipation in Parkinson's disease. A randomized placebo-controlled study. Mov Disord 2007; **22**: 1239–44.

Chapter 20

Postural hypotension in Parkinson's disease

Italo Biaggioni and Horacio Kaufmann

Background

Parkinson's disease (PD) is a movement disorder characterized by abnormal intraneuronal aggregates of misfolded proteins, known as Lewy bodies. Lewy bodies are found throughout the central nervous system (CNS) of patients with PD, most notably in the dopaminergic neurons of the substantia nigra, a finding that explains the movement disorder. It is less well known that patients with PD also suffer from varying degrees of autonomic impairment. Paradoxically, autonomic impairment is mainly due to the degeneration of peripheral, rather than central, autonomic neurons. Indeed, Lewy bodies identical to those found in the CNS are found in peripheral autonomic neurons of PD patients. The main component of Lewy bodies is the protein α-synuclein. Abnormal metabolism of α-synuclein is probably at the core of the neurodegenerative process of PD, and leads to the term ' α-synucleinopathy' to describe this disease. There are two types of α-synucleinopathy: (1) the Lewy body diseases [e.g. PD, dementia with Lewy bodies (DLB) and pure autonomic failure (PAF)], in which α-synuclein accumulates in the Lewy bodies, and (2) multiple system atrophy (MSA), in which α-synuclein accumulates in glial cytoplasmic inclusions. Other neurodegenerative disorders are classified as tauopathies because filaments of the protein tau aggregate in the CNS (e.g. Alzheimer's disease, progressive supranuclear palsy, Pick's disease, corticobasal degeneration and amyotrophic lateral sclerosis). Whereas autonomic failure is a prominent feature of the synucleinopathies, it is rarely clinically significant in the tauopathies.

This chapter focuses on the autonomic cardiovascular abnormalities present in PD patients, which are clinically evidenced as orthostatic hypotension.

The pathophysiology of orthostatic hypotension

When a normal individual stands, approximately 700 ml of blood pools in their legs and lower abdominal veins. Venous return to the heart decreases, resulting in a transient decline in cardiac output. The reduction in central blood volume and arterial pressure is sensed by pressure-sensitive cardiopulmonary volume receptors and arterial baroreceptors. This leads to baroreflex-mediated sympathetic activation with an increase in stroke volume and peripheral vasoconstriction, and consequently to parasympathetic withdrawal with an increase in heart rate. These rapid haemodynamic changes prevent blood pressure from falling; their failure causes orthostatic hypotension.

When arterial blood pressure falls below a critical level, cerebral blood flow also falls. When systolic blood pressure is around 50 mmHg at the level of the brain (which corresponds to a systolic blood pressure of around 70 mmHg at cardiac level when a person is standing), the autoregulatory capacity of cerebral blood flow reaches maximum vasodilation and is unable to compensate for a further fall in blood pressure.

Patients with autonomic impairment are unable to buffer these haemodynamic changes imposed by gravitational forces during upright posture. The clinical translation of this derangement is orthostatic hypotension, which is defined as a fall in systolic blood pressure of at least 20 mmHg and/or diastolic blood pressure of at least 10 mmHg within 3 minutes of standing [1] in conjunction with symptoms of cerebral hypoperfusion. These patients often suffer classic symptoms of pre-syncope within minutes of standing. Symptoms may include light-headedness, blurred vision, weakness, fatigue, cognitive impairment and pain in the back of the neck, finally leading to transient loss of consciousness. Symptoms never occur while supine but usually happen shortly after standing and are always relieved immediately on sitting or lying down. Failure to meet these criteria should make the physician rule out other causes of transient loss of consciousness (e.g. hypoglycaemia, arrhythmias, disturbance in the vestibular system or transient ischaemic attack). Severely affected patients can stand up for only a few seconds, resulting in disability and poor quality of life.

Prevalence

Orthostatic hypotension in PD

Mild orthostatic hypotension is not infrequent in patients with PD, but symptomatic and disabling orthostatic hypotension only occurs in a minority of patients. The incidence of documented orthostatic hypotension in PD, in community-based studies, ranges from 10 to 40%. Other synucleinopathies (e.g. PAF and MSA) are more readily associated with orthostatic hypotension but are relatively rare diseases. Simply because of its higher prevalence, orthostatic hypotension in PD is likely to cause a greater healthcare burden. For example, in 2004 the incidence of hospitalization related to orthostatic hypotension was 36 per 100 000 US adults. Of these, 4% had PD. The percentage of these hospitalizations related to PD increased with age; in patients over 75 years old, it was 5.8% [2].

In a study of 116 patients with typical PD, almost two-thirds had orthostatic hypotension with symptoms of cerebral hypoperfusion, including syncope, when tested using a tilt table for 40 minutes or until symptoms developed [3]. Antiparkinsonian drugs were not the main cause of orthostatic hypotension because these patients were on similar drug regimens to those with normal blood pressure responses to prolonged head-up tilt.

In another study [4], a fall in systolic blood pressure of at least 20 mmHg was found in almost 60% of patients with PD. Orthostatic hypotension was symptomatic in 20% of these patients. Orthostatic hypotension was related to the duration and severity of the disease and with the use of higher daily doses of levodopa and bromocriptine [4].

Bonuccelli et al. [5] evaluated 60 patients newly diagnosed as having idiopathic PD who had never been treated with antiparkinsonian agents. The investigators performed autonomic function tests at study entry, and followed patients for at least 7 years to ensure diagnosis. During the follow-up period, nine (15%) of the 60 patients were reclassified as having either MSA ($n = 5$) or progressive supranuclear palsy ($n = 4$) rather than PD. This highlights the clinical difficulty in making an accurate diagnosis early in the disease process. Seven (14%) of 51 patients with PD and three (60%) of the five patients who had been reclassified as having MSA had orthostatic hypotension during their initial evaluation. PD patients also had impaired sinus arrhythmia compared with controls, suggesting sympathetic and parasympathetic failure in patients with *de novo* PD.

Symptomatic orthostatic hypotension was seen in 18% of 1125 PD patients in a specialized clinic. Patients with orthostatic hypotension were older and had a more advanced Hoehn and Yahr stage and longer disease duration [6]. Orthostatic hypotension was detected in 37% of 103 patients seen in a referral centre, and its presence was associated with age, polypharmacy, amantadine or diuretics, whereas the administration of the catechol-*O*-methyltransferase (COMT) inhibitor entacapone was protective [7]. These studies underscore the variability in the prevalence estimation, probably due to referral patterns, and the impact that medications have in the worsening of orthostatic hypotension.

Orthostatic hypotension is clinically associated with cognitive impairment and white matter abnormalities in brain magnetic resonance imaging (MRI) [8] but the underlying explanation for this association is not known [9].

In addition to orthostatic hypotension, post-prandial hypotension is a common problem in PD patients with autonomic impairment. The pathophysiology of post-prandial hypotension is similar to that of orthostatic hypotension and unmasks the patient's inability to compensate for splanchnic venous pooling after the ingestion of food [10]. Not infrequently, post-prandial hypotension is the initial sign of autonomic impairment [11].

Parkinson's disease, a peripheral autonomic neuronopathy

Orthostatic hypotension in PD is commonly believed to be drug induced, attributed to the known side effects of dopaminergic drugs. Dopaminergic agents and other medications commonly used by PD patients (e.g. antihypertensives, diuretics and alpha-blockers used to treat benign prostatic hypertrophy) can induce or worsen orthostatic hypotension. More often, however, the hypotensive effects of these drugs are unmasked by the presence of an underlying autonomic neuropathy. Indeed, there is increasing evidence that peripheral autonomic nerves are compromised in PD and that this explains the orthostatic hypotension. Lewy body inclusions containing α-synuclein have been found in peripheral autonomic neurons in autopsies of patients with classic PD [12]. Eosinophilic ubiquitin and α-synuclein-positive Lewy bodies were widespread in ganglion cells and axons of the paravertebral and pre-vertebral mesenteric sympathetic chain, stellate ganglia and cardiac plexus, indicating that there is a likely loss of sympathetic neurons innervating the peripheral vasculature and the heart of patients with PD. Indeed, *in vivo* imaging studies have shown that patients with PD frequently have a loss of sympathetic innervation of the heart. Impaired catecholamine uptake by post-ganglionic sympathetic neurons innervating the heart was demonstrated by low myocardial concentrations of radioactivity after injection of the sympathoneural imaging agents ^{123}I-metaiodobenzylguanidine (MIBG) [13–15], 6-[^{18}F]-fluorodopamine and ^{11}C-metahydroxyephedrine. This imaging abnormality was confirmed by post-mortem pathology studies [16]. Tyrosine hydroxylase immunoreactive axons had nearly disappeared in the left ventricular anterior wall of the heart of patients with PD [17]. A report [18] using ^{11}C-metahydroxyephedrine found cardiac sympathetic denervation not only in PD but also in patients with MSA and progressive supranuclear palsy. This finding questions the use of scintigraphic detection of cardiac sympathetic denervation as an independent test to discriminate PD from other movement disorders,

It is not surprising that PD is associated with autonomic impairment considering that this is also seen in other α-synucleinopathies (Table 20.1). α-Synuclein deposits forming Lewy bodies in peripheral sympathetic neurons are found in patients with PAF, the archetypical disorder of autonomic function, and in patients with DLB, another disorder with frequent symptomatic autonomic impairment. α-Synuclein deposits are also the hallmark of MSA, a neurodegenerative disorder with prominent autonomic involvement and parkinsonian or cerebellar features. In MSA, α-synuclein deposits do not form Lewy bodies but are present in glial cytoplasmic inclusions instead. The one feature that all these α-synucleinopathies have in common is the increased risk of developing symptomatic autonomic failure.

Studies suggest that sympathetic involvement can be documented in PD patients even in the absence of overt orthostatic hypotension. Barbic et al. [19] found that PD patients had a reduction in the high-frequency variability of heart rate, which reflects parasympathetic modulation of sinus node function, and in the low-frequency variability of blood pressure, which reflects sympathetic modulation of vascular tone [20]. The patients studied in this series had an average disease duration of 7.5 years but had otherwise mild disease, and importantly they included a group of patients who had no clinical evidence of orthostatic hypotension. A limitation in this study was that the patients were being treated with dopaminergic agents. It is doubtful, however, that this explains the abnormalities observed.

Table 20.1 Clinical presentation and pathological findings of the synucleinopathies

	DLB	PD	PAF	MSA
Autonomic failure	+	+/−	+ + +	+ + +
Movement disorder	+	+ +	−	+ + +
Cognitive impairment	+ + +	+	−	−/?
Lewy bodies	+	+	+	−
Glial cytoplasmic inclusions	−	−	−	+

+, present; −, absent. Number of + symbols indicates severity.

DLB, dementia with Lewy bodies; PD, Parkinson's disease; PAF, pure autonomic failure; MSA, multiple system atrophy.

These results provide additional evidence supporting the concept that PD, in addition to central degeneration of dopaminergic neurons, is also characterized by peripheral degeneration of autonomic nerves involved in cardiovascular regulation. Anecdotal reports indicate that these abnormalities can be seen very early in the disease, but the incidence of subclinical autonomic abnormalities has not been determined in patients with otherwise classic PD.

Signs and symptoms

Identifying the presence of autonomic failure

The most important and easiest test for assessing autonomic function is the orthostatic stress or posture study. It consists of measuring blood pressure and heart rate after the subject has been supine for at least 10 minutes, and 1–3 minutes after standing. Blood pressure falls almost immediately after assuming an upright posture in patients with severe autonomic failure. Figure 20.1 shows the haemodynamic changes during orthostatic stress on a tilt table in a patient with severe autonomic failure and supine hypertension. It is important to consider the compensatory changes in heart rate for the overall interpretation

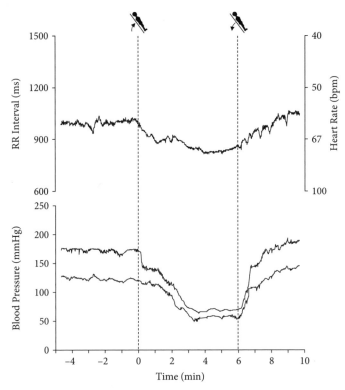

Fig. 20.1 Blood pressure and heart rate in an 83-year old man with Parkinson's disease before, during and after a 60° passive head-up tilt. Note supine hypertension (175/122 mmHg), orthostatic hypotension (65/52 mmHg) and only a small increase in heart rate (from 60 to 72 beats per minute) despite hypotension.

of this test. An intact autonomic nervous system will increase heart rate in response to a fall in blood pressure. A pronounced increase in heart rate suggests that orthostatic hypotension may be related to volume depletion or medications. In patients with autonomic failure there is only a modest response in heart rate despite their profound orthostatic hypotension. Other autonomic tests, including assessment of heart rate variability and beat-to-beat blood pressure during Valsalva manoeuvre, are useful to ascertain the degree of autonomic impairment.

Differential diagnosis of synucleinopathies based on pathophysiology

Among the synucleinopathies, the anatomical location and distribution of the α-synuclein accumulation and the associated neurodegeneration determines not only the presence or absence of cognitive impairment and movement disorder but also the characteristics of the autonomic cardiovascular abnormality. PD and PAF share the same pathophysiology, namely α-synuclein deposits in peripheral autonomic nerves. This differs from the pathophysiology in MSA, which is characterized by the involvement of central autonomic pathways while peripheral autonomic nerves remain intact.

Most of our understanding of the autonomic abnormalities present in PD is based on studies in patients with PAF, which has been studied more extensively, particularly in regard to its differentiation from MSA. Based on the similarities in their pathophysiology, it is therefore likely that the autonomic abnormalities described in PAF will apply to PD. Patients with PAF can be distinguished from those with MSA based on their intact afferent-central pathways. Conversely, only patients with MSA have intact peripheral adrenergic fibres.

Brain imaging

MRI may be helpful in the differential diagnosis of parkinsonism and autonomic failure. In PD, brain MRI shows only mild putaminal abnormalities with few changes to the brainstem or cerebellum. In MSA, brain MRI shows severe putaminal abnormalities and these are frequently accompanied by changes to the brainstem and cerebellum [21]. However, MRI abnormalities in MSA frequently occur late in the disease process. In patients with short disease duration, MRI is not very sensitive but has good specificity. In patients with MSA, MRI of the brain can frequently detect abnormalities of the striatum, cerebellum and brainstem [22–26]. Striatal abnormalities in MSA include putaminal atrophy and putaminal hypointensity (relative to the pallidum) on T_2-weighted images, as well as slit-like signal change at the posterolateral putaminal margin. The striking slit-like signal change in the lateral putamen corresponds to the area showing the most pronounced microgliosis and astrogliosis as well as the greatest amount of ferric iron at autopsy. This abnormal intensity is frequently asymmetric.

Infratentorial abnormalities in patients with MSA seen on MRI include atrophy and signal change in the pons and middle cerebellar peduncle. The pontine base and the middle cerebellar peduncle may appear as areas of high signal intensity on T_2-weighted images and as low-intensity areas on T_1, suggesting degeneration and demyelination.

Neuroendocrine testing

The presence of intact central neuroendocrine pathways in PD and PAF can be revealed clinically and used in the diagnosis of these disorders. For example, tilt-induced hypotension leads to the release of vasopressin in PAF and presumably in PD, but is blunted in MSA [27]. This finding implies that baroreflex afferents, their synapses in the nucleus tractus solitarii and projections from this nucleus to the hypothalamus are intact in PAF but impaired in MSA.

Intravenous clonidine, a centrally active α_2-adrenoceptor agonist that stimulates the secretion of growth hormone, also tests the function of hypothalamic–pituitary pathways. Clonidine increased serum growth hormone in patients with PD and patients with PAF but not in those with MSA. This finding suggests that the responses of growth hormone to intravenous clonidine can distinguish MSA from PD and PAF, and suggest a specific α_2-adrenoceptor–hypothalamic deficit in MSA [28]. It is not clear, however, if the specificity of this response allows it to be used as a diagnostic test [29].

Cardiac imaging

Whereas some central autonomic pathways are intact in PD and PAF and impaired in MSA, the opposite is true in the periphery; post-ganglionic efferent autonomic fibres are intact in MSA but impaired in PD and PAF. These differences can be readily apparent in the heart because of its rich sympathetic innervation, and this can be revealed using isotope-labelled catechols that are taken up by adrenergic nerve terminals if these fibres are intact.

Several studies using single-photon emission computed tomography (SPECT) imaging with MIBG [14,15] and positron emission tomography (PET) with 6-[^{18}F]-fluorodopamine have shown abnormal cardiac sympathetic innervation in patients with PD while it was normal in patients with MSA [30].

Cardiac imaging of sympathetic neurons using fluorodopamine and MIBG uptake are advocated as sensitive methods for diagnosing early cardiac sympathetic denervation, but this approach requires imaging techniques that are expensive, available mostly in research institutions and difficult to apply to a large number of patients.

Olfactory testing

Olfactory dysfunction is increasingly being recognized as another manifestation of peripheral autonomic impairment; patients with pure autonomic failure and loss of peripheral autonomic fibres have impaired odour identification whereas smell function is intact in patients with MSA [31]. The presence of anosmia in PD correlates with impaired autonomic reflexes, blunted plasma norepinephrine and lower cardiac catechol uptake [32].

Plasma catecholamines

The presence of intact post-ganglionic adrenergic fibres in MSA means that it can also be distinguished biochemically from PAF: plasma norepinephrine is normal or only slightly decreased in MSA and very low in PAF [33].

Spectral analysis

Spectral analysis of heart rate (reflecting mostly vagal regulation of sinus node function) and of blood pressure (reflecting sympathetic vascular regulation) shows that they are both reduced in PD [19]. High-frequency variability of the heart rate is also decreased in PAF and in MSA [20]. Of greater usefulness in the differentiation between these disorders is the low-frequency variability of the blood pressure, which is low in PAF but preserved in MSA [20]. There is, however, significant interindividual variability in spectral measurements, which limits their use in the diagnosis of individual patients.

It should be noted that most of the studies reporting differences between PAF and MSA using the above-mentioned diagnostic tests mostly included patients with severe autonomic impairment. It is not known if the reported differences will also be apparent in patients with milder forms of autonomic impairment, or in patients at an initial stage of disease when the differential diagnosis would be more important.

Treatment

There is no known effective disease-modifying treatment for the autonomic abnormalities in PD. One would question, therefore, the usefulness of early recognition of subclinical autonomic impairment in individual patients. It is important to recognize patients who are at risk of orthostatic hypotension, particularly in the post-prandial period when they are at a higher danger of falls. It may be that a reduction in dopaminergic treatment may be required in some patients to prevent falls in blood pressure, at the expense of worsening their movement disorder. This, however, may not be necessary if treatment of their orthostatic hypotension with a short-acting pressor agent and a volume regulator is tried first. A list of potential treatments is shown in Table 20.2, but it should be recognized that controlled studies for the treatment of orthostatic hypotension are lacking in patients with autonomic failure in general, and in PD patients in particular.

Maintenance of blood pressure in the standing position requires a sustained increase in peripheral vascular resistance (i.e. vasoconstriction) and adequate intravascular volume to ensure appropriate venous return to the heart. These mechanisms are impaired in patients with chronic autonomic failure, and the treatment to improve orthostatic tolerance should therefore be dedicated to counteracting these deficiencies.

In general, a stepwise approach to treatment according to the severity of the symptoms is preferable (Table 20.2). These should be considered as general guidelines, and treatment should be individualized. Some recommendations may actually be contraindicated in a given patient. Patients should avoid standing motionless, as this will reduce the lower limb muscle pump that normally improves venous return. They should also avoid standing up quickly, particularly from a squatting position. They should be warned that orthostatic symptoms tend to be worse early in the morning, after meals and if the arms are raised above heart level. Hot baths should be avoided, and patients should be especially careful during warm weather. This is because heat-induced vasodilation still occurs but sympathetic vasoconstriction is impaired. Straining at stool with a closed glottis (i.e. producing a

Table 20.2 Stepwise approach to the management of orthostatic hypotension

1. Remove aggravating factors:
   - Volume depletion
   - Prolonged bed rest/deconditioning
   - Alcohol
   - Diuretics
   - Tricyclic antidepressants
   - Venodilators (nitrates)
   - Antihypertensives (alpha-blockers, guanethidine)
   - Alpha-blockers used to treat prostatic hypertrophy

2. Medical non-pharmacological treatment:
   - Liberalize salt intake, salt supplements
   - Head-up tilt during the night
   - Waist-high support stockings
   - Exercise as tolerated, preferable in-water exercises

3. Pharmacological treatment:
   - Sodium chloride 1 g/meal
   - Fludrocortisone 0.1–0.3 mg/day
   - Short-acting pressor agent: midodrine, 5–10 mg[a]

[a]A short-acting pressor agent should be used as needed to improve orthostatic tolerance on an as-required basis rather than at fixed doses. A dose given before exertion will improve orthostatic symptoms for 2–3 h. In general, administration of more than three doses per day is discouraged to avoid side effects and the development of tolerance.

Valsalva manoeuvre) can induce syncope due to reduced venous return. A high-fibre diet is encouraged to prevent constipation.

Patients with autonomic failure may be unable to conserve sodium, and liberalization of sodium intake is generally recommended. These patients have exaggerated nocturnal diuresis with relative hypovolaemia and worsening of orthostatic hypotension early in the morning. Nocturnal diuresis can be reduced by elevating the head of the bed with 15–23-cm (6–9-inch) blocks.

During the day, patients should wear waist-high custom-fitted elastic support stockings that will exert pressure on the legs and reduce venous pooling. Most patients, however, find these cumbersome to wear. Considering that most of the venous pooling occurs in the lower abdomen, abdominal binders, which are easier to use, can be tried first. Patients should avoid wearing support stockings while supine because they may contribute to diuresis and supine hypertension.

In patients with autonomic failure, eating can significantly lower blood pressure because the splanchnic vasodilation induced by food is not appropriately compensated by vasoconstriction in other vascular beds. Post-prandial hypotension may be apparent in some PD patients before orthostatic hypotension becomes evident [11]. Thus, patients should eat frequent, small meals with a low carbohydrate content; alcohol intake should be minimized. Caffeine taken with meals may be helpful in blunting post-prandial hypotension, presumably by blocking splanchnic vasodilation [34]. Acarbose, an α-glucosidase inhibitor, attenuates post-prandial hypotension in autonomic failure by delaying the absorption of glucose by the gut [35]. This medication can be used to treat post-prandial hypotension, starting at a dose of 50 mg taken with meals.

Pharmacological treatment

Two general approaches are available to increase the abnormally low blood pressure these patients have on standing: improve intravascular volume and increase vascular resistance. The goal of treating orthostatic hypotension is twofold: to reduce symptoms and improve quality of life, and to prevent falls. Thus, only patients with symptomatic orthostatic hypotension should be treated pharmacologically. Some patients with autonomic failure tolerate very low arterial pressures when standing without experiencing symptoms of cerebral hypoperfusion, perhaps because of adaptive cerebral autoregulatory changes, and they may require less aggressive treatment. Blood pressure levels change throughout the day, and from one day to another. Thus, the patient's normal cycle of blood pressure and orthostatic symptoms should be identified before treatment is initiated. For example, patients may require treatment only in the morning, when symptoms of orthostatic hypotension are worse. A short-acting pressor agent in particular is best prescribed on an as-required basis, rather than at fixed intervals throughout the day without consideration of the patient's symptoms.

Fludrocortisone

Fludrocortisone (Florinef®), a synthetic mineralocorticoid practically devoid of glucocorticoid effect [36], can be given initially at a dose of 0.1 mg per day. At least 4 or 5 days of treatment are necessary for a therapeutic effect to be evident. Special attention should be given to the development of hypokalaemia. Fludrocortisone increases extracellular and intravascular volume by increasing sodium reabsorption by the kidney, thus increasing cardiac output and standing blood pressure. It is therefore important to ensure adequate dietary sodium intake. The dose of fludrocortisone should be increased slowly. Doses greater than 0.3 mg per day are probably no more effective than lower doses and carry the risk of losing the mineralocorticoid selectivity. Body weight, blood pressure and the possible development of heart failure due to volume overload should be monitored. The latter is more frequent at the start of treatment. Weight gain is expected. A certain degree of pedal oedema should not be of concern. Indeed, it may be necessary to support the venous capacitance bed (a 'water jacket' effect). The long-term effectiveness of fludrocortisone may be unrelated to fluid retention, but rather to potentiation of the pressor effects of pressor substances.

Desmopressin acetate

Desmopressin acetate (DDAVP) is a synthetic vasopressin analogue which acts specifically on the V2 receptors (renal tubular cells) responsible for the antidiuretic effect of the hormone. DDAVP has no vasoconstrictor effect at recommended doses because it does not activate the V1 receptor expressed in vascular smooth muscle. Nocturnal intranasal administration of DDAVP reduces nocturnal polyuria and raises standing blood pressure in the morning without worsening supine hypertension. A problem with the use of DDAVP is the potential development of hyponatraemia. Treatment with this drug should therefore always be started with the patient in hospital and serum sodium should be monitored.

Midodrine

When volume expansion is not sufficient to control symptoms, a pressor agent should be added. The only drug currently approved in the United States for the treatment of ortho-static hypotension is midodrine, a selective α_1-adrenergic agonist which is well absorbed after oral administration and does not cross the blood–brain barrier [37,38]. A 10 mg dose of midodrine is effective in increasing orthostatic blood pressure and ameliorating symp-toms in patients with orthostatic hypotension [39]. Because this dose increases pressure for only 4 hours, it can be prescribed two or three times daily, depending upon the physical activity of the patient, and can be avoided later in the day as it increases supine blood pres-sure. An advantage of a pressor agent over fludrocortisone is that its blood pressure-raising effect lasts only a few hours. Thus, it can be administered specifically when the patient needs it; typically before breakfast and before lunch and preceding physical activity [39]. Recumbent hypertension is a common side effect but standing up readily lowers blood pressure. The dose of midodrine should be titrated slowly, starting with 2.5 mg. The dose can be quickly increased to 10 mg two or three times a day based on the blood pressure response. Most patients with orthostatic hypotension require chronic treatment with fl-udrocortisone; it is likely that by adding midodrine to fludrocortisone, the dose of the lat-ter can be reduced. This combination treatment may reduce the long-term complications associated with chronic mineralocorticoid administration.

Yohimbine

Yohimbine is a selective α_2-antagonist, and as such it is the pharmacological counterpart to the partial α_2-agonist clonidine and has opposite cardiovascular effects. Yohimbine acts centrally to stimulate sympathetic outflow. In the periphery, it enhances the release of nor-epinephrine from adrenergic nerve fibres by antagonizing the pre-synaptic α_2-adrenergic receptors that normally inhibit norepinephrine release. Yohimbine produces a significant increase in blood pressure in patients with autonomic failure and attenuates orthostatic hypotension at doses that would have negligible effects in normal subjects [40]. Yohim-bine was removed from the market for commercial reasons, but can be obtained through compounding pharmacies.

Pyridostigmine

Pyridostigmine is an inhibitor of cholinesterase, the enzyme that catalyses the hydrol-ysis of the neurotransmitter acetylcholine into choline and acetic acid, a reaction that essentially terminates the actions of acetylcholine. Pyridostigmine therefore potentiates tonic cholinergic neurotransmission. In the case of sympathetic ganglia, pyridostigmine has less of an effect in the supine position, when sympathetic tone is low. In contrast, its effect is greatly increase with standing, when traffic through sympathetic ganglia is increased. This offers the theoretical advantage of preferentially increasing sympathetic neurotransmission and upright blood pressure in patients with autonomic failure, and in proportion to their orthostatic needs. Furthermore, the worsening of supine hypertension, which occurs with most other pressor agents, is avoided. In an initial study of 15 patients with neurogenic orthostatic hypotension due to a variety of diseases (PAF, MSA, PD and others), 60 mg of pyridostigmine taken orally produced only a non-significant increase in supine blood pressure. In contrast, acetylcholinesterase inhibition significantly increased orthostatic blood pressure and reduced the fall in blood pressure during head-up tilt. The improvement in orthostatic blood pressure was associated with a significant improvement in orthostatic symptoms [41]. In theory, patients with residual sympathetic tone (i.e. MSA) should be more responsive to enhancement of the neurotransmission of sympathetic ganglia compared with patients with peripheral neuropathy (i.e. PAF or PD). This, however, was not found, possibly because of the small number of patients in each group. Nonetheless, patients with relatively preserved baroreflex gain had a greater response [41], supporting the notion that the response to pyridostigmine is proportional to the degree of residual sympathetic tone. A subsequent double-blind study involving 58 patients with diverse forms of neurogenic orthostatic hypotension confirmed that 60 mg of pyridostigmine preferentially prevented the orthostatic fall in blood pressure without worsening supine hypertension [41]. The pressor effect of pyridostigmine, however, was rather modest; 2 hours after drug administration, upright systolic blood pressure was only 4 mmHg higher in the pyridostigmine group compared with the placebo group. A combination of 5 mg midodrine with 60 mg pyridostigmine was slightly more effective than pyridostigmine alone. As in the previous study, pyridostigmine did not produce a greater pressor effect in MSA patients compared with those with peripheral forms of autonomic failure. A follow-up study suggested continuous improvement of symptoms with pyridostigmine therapy [42]. Pyridostigmine is not as potent as other pressor agents [43] and it is likely to be less useful in patients with severe symptoms.

Droxidopa (DOPS)

L-Threo-dihydroxyphenylserine (L-threo-DOPS) is an unnatural amino acid that is converted to norepinephrine through a single decarboxylation step by the enzyme DOPA decarboxylase (aromatic L-amino acid decarboxylase). In patients with autonomic failure due to congenital deficiency of dopamine beta-hydroxylase (the enzyme that converts dopamine to norepinephrine), L-Threo-DOPS is extremely efficacious in relieving orthostatic hypotension [44,45]. In patients with PAF and MSA L-DOPS (given in a racemic mixture) [46] showed a significant pressor effect and significantly ameliorated orthostatic hypotension. DOPS is only available in Asia, but clinical trials to gain approval in the United States for the treatment or orthostatic hypotension are ongoing [47].

Other agents

Several other agents have been used in the treatment of orthostatic hypotension in autonomic failure. Inhibitors of prostaglandin synthesis (indomethacin, ibuprofen) [48,49] and the somatostatin analogue octreotide [50] are sometimes effective in reducing post-prandial hypotension, but both agents may induce intolerable gastrointestinal side effects. The dopaminergic blocker metoclopramide increases blood pressure in some patients with autonomic failure but may aggravate or induce extra-pyramidal symptoms and is therefore contraindicated in PD. Beta-blockers with and without intrinsic sympathomimetic activity (propranolol and pindolol) can be effective in some patients. Ergotamine has also been reported to be effective [51]. The norepinephrine reuptake inhibitor atomoxetine increases upright blood pressure in patients with autonomic failure [35]. Patients with central forms of autonomic failure with residual sympathetic tone (MSA) have significantly greater pressor responses, as a group, than those with peripheral autonomic failure (PAF and PD). Nonetheless, individual patients with peripheral autonomic failure may have significant improvement in upright blood pressure and symptoms.

References

1 Consensus statement on the definition of orthostatic hypotension, pure autonomic failure, and multiple system atrophy. The Consensus Committee of the American Autonomic Society and the American Academy of Neurology. Neurology 1996; **46**: 1470.

2 Shibao C, Grijalva CG, Raj SR, Biaggioni I, Griffin MR. Orthostatic hypotension-related hospitalizations in the United States. Am J Med 2007; **120**: 975–80.

3 Kaufmann H, Nouri S, Olanow W, Yahr M. Orthostatic Intolerance in Parkinson's disease [abstract]. Neurology 1997; **48**(Suppl 2): 149.

4 Senard JM, Rai S, Lapeyre-Mestre M, et al. Prevalence of orthostatic hypotension in Parkinson's disease. J Neurol Neurosurg Psychiatry 1997; **63**: 584–9.

5 Bonuccelli U, Lucetti C, Del Dotto P, et al. Orthostatic hypotension in de novo Parkinson disease. Arch Neurol 2003; **60**: 1400–4.

6 Ha AD, Brown CH, York MK, Jankovic J. The prevalence of symptomatic orthostatic hypotension in patients with Parkinson's disease and atypical parkinsonism. Parkinsonism Relat Disord 2011; **17**: 625–8.

7 Perez-Lloret S, Rey MV, Fabre N, et al. Factors related to orthostatic hypotension in Parkinson's disease. Parkinsonism Relat Disord 2012; **18**: 501–5.

8 Kim JS, Oh YS, Lee KS, Kim YI, Yang DW, Goldstein DS. Association of cognitive dysfunction with neurocirculatory abnormalities in early Parkinson disease. Neurology 2012; **79**: 1323–31.

9 Pilleri M, Facchini S, Gasparoli E, et al. Cognitive and MRI correlates of orthostatic hypotension in Parkinson's disease. J Neurol 2013; **260**: 253–9.

10 Robertson D, Wade D, Robertson R. Post-prandial alterations in cardiovascular hemodynamics in autonomic dysfunction states. Am J Cardiol 1981; **48**: 1048–52.

11 Mehagnoul-Schipper DJ, Boerman RH, Hoefnagels WH, Jansen RW. Effect of levodopa on orthostatic and postprandial hypotension in elderly Parkinsonian patients. J Gerontol A Biol Sci Med Sci 2001; **56**: M749–M755.

12 Kaufmann H, Nahm K, Purohit D, Wolfe D. Autonomic failure as the initial presentation of Parkinson disease and dementia with Lewy bodies. Neurology 2004; **63**: 1093–5.

13 Takatsu H, Nishida H, Matsuo H, et al. Cardiac sympathetic denervation from the early stage of Parkinson's disease: clinical and experimental studies with radiolabeled MIBG. J Nucl Med 2000; **41**: 71–7.

14 Orimo S, Ozawa E, Nakade S, et al. (123)I-metaiodobenzylguanidine myocardial scintigraphy in Parkinson's disease. J Neurol Neurosurg Psychiatry 1999; **67**: 189–94.

15 Braune S, Reinhardt M, Schnitzer R, et al. Cardiac uptake of [123I]MIBG separates Parkinson's disease from multiple system atrophy. Neurology 1999; **53**: 1020–5.

16 Orimo S, Uchihara T, Nakamura A, et al. Axonal alpha-synuclein aggregates herald centripetal degeneration of cardiac sympathetic nerve in Parkinson's disease. Brain 2008; **131**: 642–50.

17 Amino T, Orimo S, Itoh Y, Takahashi A, Uchihara T, Mizusawa H. Profound cardiac sympathetic denervation occurs in Parkinson disease. Brain Pathol 2005; **15**: 29–34.

18 Raffel DM, Koeppe RA, Little R, et al. PET measurement of cardiac and nigrostriatal denervation in Parkinsonian syndromes. J Nucl Med 2006; **47**: 1769–77.

19 Barbic F, Perego F, Canesi M, et al. Early abnormalities of vascular and cardiac autonomic control in Parkinson's disease without orthostatic hypotension. Hypertension 2007; **49**: 120–6.

20 Diedrich A, Jordan J, Tank J, et al. The sympathetic nervous system in hypertension: assessment by blood pressure variability and ganglionic blockade. J Hypertens 2003; **21**: 1677–86.

21 Bhattacharya K, Saadia D, Eisenkraft B, et al. Brain magnetic resonance imaging in multiple-system atrophy and Parkinson disease: a diagnostic algorithm. Arch Neurol 2002; **59**: 835–42.

22 Yagishita T, Kojima S, Hirayama K. MRI study of degenerative process in multiple system atrophy [in Japanese]. Rinsho Shinkeigaku 1995; **35**: 126–31.

23 Testa D, Savoiardo M, Fetoni V, et al. Multiple system atrophy. Clinical and MR observations on 42 cases. Ital J Neurol Sci 1993; **14**: 211–16.

24 Schwarz J, Weis S, Kraft E, et al. Signal changes on MRI and increases in reactive microgliosis, astrogliosis, and iron in the putamen of two patients with multiple system atrophy. J Neurol Neurosurg Psychiatry 1996; **60**: 98–101.

25 Schrag A, Good CD, Miszkiel K, et al. Differentiation of atypical parkinsonian syndromes with routine MRI. Neurology 2000; **54**: 697–702.

26 Konagaya M, Konagaya Y, Honda H, Iida M. A clinico-MRI study of extrapyramidal symptoms in multiple system atrophy—linear hyperintensity in the outer margin of the putamen [in Japanese]. No To Shinkei 1993; **45**: 509–13.

27 Kaufmann H, Oribe E, Miller M, et al. Hypotension-induced vasopressin release distinguishes between pure autonomic failure and multiple system atrophy with autonomic failure. Neurology 1992; **42**: 590–3.

28 Kimber JR, Watson L, Mathias CJ. Distinction of idiopathic Parkinson's disease from multiple-system atrophy by stimulation of growth-hormone release with clonidine. Lancet 1997; **349**: 1877–81.

29 Tranchant C, Guiraud-Chaumeil C, Echaniz-Laguna A, Warter JM. Is clonidine growth hormone stimulation a good test to differentiate multiple system atrophy from idiopathic Parkinson's disease? J Neurol 2000; **247**: 853–6.

30 Goldstein DS, Holmes C, Li ST, et al. Cardiac sympathetic denervation in Parkinson disease. Ann Intern Med 2000; **133**: 338–47.

31 Garland EM, Raj SR, Peltier AC, Robertson D, Biaggioni I. A cross-sectional study contrasting olfactory function in autonomic disorders. Neurology 2011; **76**: 456–60.

32 Goldstein DS, Sewell L, Holmes C. Association of anosmia with autonomic failure in Parkinson disease. Neurology 2010; **74**: 245–51.

33 Goldstein DS, Polinsky RJ, Garty M, et al. Patterns of plasma levels of catechols in neurogenic orthostatic hypotension. Ann Neurol 1989; **26**: 558–63.

34 Onrot J, Goldberg MR, Biaggioni I, et al. Hemodynamic and humoral effects of caffeine in autonomic failure. Therapeutic implications for postprandial hypotension. N Engl J Med 1985; **313**: 549–54.

35 Shibao C, Gamboa A, Diedrich A, et al. Acarbose, an alpha-glucosidase inhibitor, attenuates postprandial hypotension in autonomic failure. Hypertension 2007; **50**: 54–61.

36 **Hickler R**. Successful treatment of orthostatic hypotension with 9-alpha fluorohydrocortisone. N Eng J Med 1959; **261**: 788–91.

37 **Kaufmann H**. Treatment of patients with orthostatic hypotension and syncope. Clin Neuropharmacol 2002; **25**: 133–41.

38 **Jankovic J, Gilden JL, Hiner BC, et al**. Neurogenic orthostatic hypotension: a double-blind, placebo-controlled study with midodrine. Am J Med 1993; **95**: 38–48.

39 **Wright RA, Kaufmann HC, Perera R, et al**. A double-blind, dose-response study of midodrine in neurogenic orthostatic hypotension. Neurology 1998; **51**: 120–4.

40 **Biaggioni I, Robertson R, Robertson D**. Manipulation of norepinephrine metabolism with yohimbine in the treatment of autonomic failure. J Clin Pharmacol 1994; **34**: 418–23.

41 **Singer W, Opfer-Gehrking TL, McPhee BR, et al**. Acetylcholinesterase inhibition: a novel approach in the treatment of neurogenic orthostatic hypotension. J Neurol Neurosurg Psychiatry 2003; **74**: 1294–8.

42 **Sandroni P, Opfer-Gehrking TL, Singer W, Low PA, et al**. Pyridostigmine for treatment of neurogenic orthostatic hypotension [correction of hypertension]—a follow-up survey study. Clin Auton Res 2005; **15**: 51–3.

43 **Shibao C, Okamoto LE, Gamboa A, et al**. Comparative efficacy of yohimbine against pyridostigmine for the treatment of orthostatic hypotension in autonomic failure. Hypertension 2010; **56**: 847–51.

44 **Man in't Veld AJ, Boomsma F, Moleman P, Schalekamp MA**. Congenital dopamine-beta-hydroxylase deficiency. A novel orthostatic syndrome. Lancet 1987; **1**: 183–8.

45 **Biaggioni I, Robertson D**. Endogenous restoration of noradrenaline by precursor therapy in dopamine-beta-hydroxylase deficiency. Lancet 1987; **2**: 1170–2.

46 **Kaufmann H, Saadia D, Voustianiouk A, et al**. Norepinephrine precursor therapy in neurogenic orthostatic hypotension. Circulation 2003; **108**: 724–8.

47 **Kaufmann H, Freeman R., Biaggioni I, Low P, Pedder S, Hewitt A, Mathias C**. Treatment of neurogenic orthostatic hypotension with droxidopa: results from a multi-center, double-blind, randomized, placebo-controlled, parallel group, induction design study. Neurology 2012; **78**(Suppl 1): PL02.001.

48 **Kochar M, Itskowitz H, Albers J**. Treatment of orthostatic hypotension with indomethacin. Am Heart J 1979; **98**: 271–80.

49 **Jordan J, Shannon JR, Biaggioni I, et al**. Contrasting actions of pressor agents in severe autonomic failure. Am J Med 1998; **105**: 116–24.

50 **Hoeldtke R, Israel B**. Treatment of orthostatic hypotension with octreotide. J Clin Endocrinol Metab 1989; **68**: 1051–9.

51 **Biaggioni I, Zygmunt D, Haile V, Robertson D**. Pressor effect of inhaled ergotamine in orthostatic hypotension. Am J Cardiol 1990; **65**: 89–92.

Chapter 21

Sialorrhoea in Parkinson's disease

Julia Johnson, Marian L. Evatt and K. Ray Chaudhuri

Introduction

Sialorrhoea is a common symptom in neurodegenerative conditions such as Parkinson's disease (PD). The term sialorrhoea is defined as an inability to control salivary secretion which results in pooling of saliva in the oral cavity [1]. This pooling is susceptible to both anterior and posterior spillage. Anterior spillage is commonly known as drooling of saliva, which causes a significant degree of social embarrassment and psychosocial difficulty for patients and their caregivers and leads to a risk of dehydration. It can also cause soiling of clothes and perioral dermatitis/angular chelitis due to oral candidiasis [2, 3]. Posterior spillage involves saliva trickling into the pharynx, and if it is not safely swallowed it may penetrate the airway and be aspirated, as described by Rodrigues et al. [4] in a study using fibreoptic endoscopic evaluation of swallowing (FEES). Aspirated saliva may lead to pneumonia, especially if oral infections are present in the mouth which infiltrate the saliva. Despite its negative impact on quality of life, the literature contains limited data on sialorrhoea in PD. In a prevalence study of gastrointestinal symptoms in PD, abnormal salivation was reported as one of the most common gastrointestinal symptoms in patients with PD (70%) compared with controls (6%) [5]. A prevalence of up to 75% has been reported in other studies [5,6]. A significant proportion of patients with sialorrhoea (86%) also present with swallowing abnormalities [7]. Dysphagia can lead to aspiration pneumonia, which is the major source of morbidity and mortality in PD. Videofluoroscopic studies of people with PD have demonstrated motility disorders in all phases of the swallow. Many of those assessed showed silent aspiration with no overt signs such as coughing or choking. According to the literature, patients also tend not to report a swallowing difficulty until it becomes severe [8–11].

Mechanism of sialorrhoea in Parkinson's disease

Normal production of saliva in a healthy adult is approximately 1.5 litres per day, mainly from the parotids, submandibular and sublingual glands which are controlled by the parasympathetic nervous system. In people without neurological illness saliva is generally cleared from the mouth by spontaneous swallowing (SS), which occurs without awareness about every 60 seconds while awake and less often during sleep. Voluntary swallowing (VS) occurs when awake and is part of normal eating and drinking behaviour [12]. VS and

SS are similar regarding their dependence on the swallowing central pattern generator at the brainstem, which receives sensory feedback from the oropharynx. Sensory triggers for swallowing are cutaneous pressure, i.e. the weight of the bolus on sensory receptors in the mouth, taste and thermal quality. There is no taste or thermal trigger in saliva so the swallow is reliant on cutaneous pressure. There is some evidence that the bolus size required to trigger a swallow in elderly subjects and those with a neurological illness such as PD is larger than in younger people and those without neurological problems, and this risks a build-up of excess saliva in the mouth.

The exact mechanism of sialorrhoea in PD is unclear. Excessive production of saliva can cause sialorrhoea, but studies have shown a significantly lower rate of secretion in advanced PD [8,10,13,14]. One study compared rates of secretion among 30 PD patients and 585 controls, and reported similar rates between the two groups. Stimulated salivary secretion decreased with increasing disease severity [7]. In another study, Bagheri et al. [15] demonstrated decreased salivary secretion in both drug naïve and treated PD patients compared with controls. These studies tend to contradict the notion of hypersecretion as a mechanism for sialorrhoea in PD. A more acceptable theory for sialorrhoea in PD is dysphagia, with muscle rigidity and bradykinesia of the oropharyngeal muscles also making a contribution. This view is supported by Kalf et al. [16] who compared 15 PD patients who drooled with 15 PD patients who did not and found that hypomimia correlated best with drooling. PD patients often have a stooped posture, and this may also contribute to drooling of saliva as, when the head is tilted down to the chest, the effect of gravity may make anterior loss of oral secretions more likely [1].

The literature on the influence of dopaminergic treatment is inconclusive. Some studies have implicated dopaminergic treatment in increasing salivary flow, while other studies have shown decreased salivary production with levodopa [8]. Sialorrhoea is a well-known side effect of some atypical antipsychotics such as clozapine, which is recommended in the National Institute of Health and Care Excellence (NICE) guidelines as a treatment for psychotic symptoms in PD [17,18].

Nobrega et al. [14] assessed the severity of drooling using the Dribbling of Saliva Scale (DSS) and swallowing function using videofluoroscopy in 16 patients with PD. The authors reported a significant correlation between the degree of dysphagia and the drooling score. Sixteen patients had dysphagia, providing evidence for an association between dysphagia and drooling. However, the study did not take into account the posture of patients studied and used a non-validated drooling scale. Several authors have cited an increased likelihood of drooling in men. Kalf et al. [16] identified disease severity, dysphagia and male sex as significant explanatory factors in a linear regression with hypomimia as the dependent variable. The preliminary analysis at baseline of the first 425 patients in the French COPARK study reported 37% with sialorrhoea, and multivariate analysis showed this was related to male gender, the presence of depressive symptoms and motor fluctuations along with dysarthria and dysphagia [19]. A correlation has also been shown between drooling and dementia in PD, which was more significant in males than in females [20].

Rating scales

Several scales, including the Drooling Severity and Frequency Scale (DSFS), the Drooling Rating Scale, Unified Parkinson's Disease Rating Scale (UPDRS) item 6, the Sialorrhoea Clinical Scale for PD (SCS-Pd), the PD Non-Motor Symptoms Scale (NMSS) and the Non-Motor Symptoms Questionnaire (NMSQuest) can be used in clinical practice for assessing sialorrhoea [1]. These have been reviewed by Evatt et al. [21]. The DSFS, first published by Thomas-Stonell and Greenberg in children with drooling, has also been used in other population groups including people with PD [22,23]. However, this scale has not been validated for use in these groups. The DSFS assesses the frequency and severity of drooling. The scale is easy to administer and takes less than 10 minutes. It has the disadvantage of not addressing the psychosocial impact of drooling on patients, and furthermore has not undergone specific clinimetric validation for PD [1].

The Drooling Rating Scale was developed to assess the severity of drooling in PD. However, its clinimetric properties have not been evaluated. It assesses drooling severity in certain situations, for example sitting, standing, talking, in bed and eating or drinking, and a score of 0–3 is given for each situation. The SCS-Pd was first developed and validated in Spanish and has now been translated into English [24]. It has been validated for use in PD to assess the severity and frequency of drooling. It also evaluates other aspects such as social and functional impairment. The scale consists of seven questions addressing these issues. It is easy to use and takes about 10 minutes to complete. Despite these advantages, the results of the validation study should be extrapolated with caution to other population groups as the sample size was small.

UPDRS item 6 is also used but has not been validated for measuring sialorrhoea in PD [25].

Finally, the combined tools of the self-rated NMSQuest and NMSS have both been validated in PD and both address sialorrhoea, the NMSS allowing a score for frequency and severity [25,26].

Other objective measures include spit collection techniques such as using suctioning, a Lashley disc and dental cotton pads, as well as swallowing counts [1]. However, these methods do not assess functional or social disability due to drooling and may be logistically difficult to use in the clinical setting [1].

Treatment

Management of sialorrhoea requires a multidisciplinary approach, including neurologists, speech and language therapists and occupational therapists [26]. Referral to a speech and language therapist for assessment of swallowing function is recommended by the NICE guidelines [17]. Initial assessment of the severity of drooling and its impact on the patient's life is essential in determining the appropriate management. Anecdotal reports have shown that simple methods such sucking sweets or chewing gum seem to give temporary relief in some patients. A study by South et al. [28] of 20 PD patients at Hoehn and Yahr Stages 2 to 4 showed that chewing gum increased swallow frequency and may therefore be an effective strategy for secretion management. Behavioural modification and the use of cueing techniques that remind a person to swallow the saliva as it builds up in their mouths have been found of benefit in some people [29]. A small study by Marks et al. [29] showed a reduction in dribbling of saliva at 1 and 3 months in six patients who took part in their study using a metronome brooch timed to let off a beeping sound every 20 seconds or so as a swallow reminder cue. These reminder functions are now available as smart phone apps such as 'Swallow Now' from the Apple App Store and as settings within watches. Other behavioural techniques include lip seal strengthening and swallowing exercises [2]. Cognitive dysfunction may make the use of behavioural methods challenging.

Occupational therapists or physiotherapists can provide devices to improve the stooped or flexed head posture in some patients [17]. Speech therapy interventions shown to be effective in other conditions such as cerebral palsy include oral motor therapy and orofacial regulation therapy, and these may be considered [17,30,31]. The adaptation of clothing to incorporate a discreet waterproof-backed insert has also been recommended.

Some natural products and homeopathic remedies have been advocated, such as dark grape juice, pineapple and paw-paw juice as well as sage caps, tablets or powder. There are no randomized control trial data to support these products. Identifying and treating dysphagia is crucial in the management of drooling as this may be a contributing factor and may help avoid aspiration pneumonia.

Anticholinergics

Salivary production is mediated via parasympathetic fibres. Anticholinergic drugs may improve sialorrhoea by decreasing salivary production, but their use is limited by side effects. These include confusion, hallucinations, memory problems, blurred vision, urinary retention, constipation and cardiac arrhythmias. The risk of side effects is even higher in elderly patients who form the majority of PD patients. Only a few anticholinergics have been evaluated in PD. Sublingual atropine was used to treat sialorrhoea in seven patients, six with PD and one with progressive supranuclear palsy. Salivary production and severity was decreased significantly within 1 week of follow-up; one patient developed delirium and two hallucinations. In another double-blind randomized study, ipatropium bromide spray was compared with placebo in 17 PD patients [32]. No improvement in objective measures of salivary production was noted, but ipatropium bromide was well tolerated. Other anticholinergic drugs, including glycopyrrolate, benzatropine, trihexylphenidyl, pirenzepine and diphenhydramine, have been studied in other conditions in which use is limited by emergence of side effects [33]. Glycopyrrolate is thought to decrease the effectiveness of levodopa.

Botulinum toxin

Injection of botulinum toxin type A and type B into the salivary glands has been shown to improve sialorrhoea in PD and other conditions [1]. Botulinum toxin inhibits parasympathetic (cholinergic) and post-ganglionic sympathetic fibres, thus reducing salivary production [1]. Blind injection and ultrasound-guided injection into the parotids or submandibular glands have been reported [25,34–37], and the results show that botulinum toxin is an effective and well-tolerated treatment for sialorrhoea. In a double-blind randomized placebo-controlled study Lagalla et al. [38] enrolled 32 patients with excessive drooling. Fifty mouse units of botulinum toxin type A was injected blindly into the parotid glands. A significant reduction in saliva production, drooling frequency and disability was reported and no adverse effects were reported. In a more recent study by Chinnapongse et al. [39], 54 PD patients with troublesome sialorrhoea were randomized in a double-blind study with a sequential-dose escalation design using botulinum toxin type B injected first into the submandibular glands, followed by the parotid glands. Injections were guided by external anatomical landmarks not supported by ultrasound. Efficacy was assessed by the DSFS and a subject-rated salivation item on the modified UPDRS Section II (ADL) on a scale ranging from 0 (No. I do not have too much saliva and I never drool) to 4 (Yes. I have so much drooling that I often carry a tissue or handkerchief). Saliva production was quantified via salivary flow rate, i.e. the amount of saliva collected over a 5-minute interval and reported as weight of saliva per minute. Patients were followed for up to 20 weeks and all active dosage groups showed a significant reduction in saliva flow and drooling when compared with those taking placebo.

At present, no studies have compared the superiority of one botulinum toxin type over the other for the treatment of sialorrhoea, nor have the optimum dosage and injection site been established [1]. However, some studies suggest that ultrasound-guided injection is superior to blind injection [34–37]. If improvement is noted, the injections need to be repeated at 3–6-monthly intervals to maintain the beneficial effect. There is a risk that the botulinum toxin may spread to the pharyngeal musculature and affect swallow efficiency.

There are currently many studies that have been published in relation to the use of botulinum toxin and treatment of sialorrhoea, but there are no formal indication guidelines and, as yet, sialorrhoea is not an approved indication for treatment with botulinum toxin. Even though there is a lack of double-blind studies, literature review would suggest that this treatment is worth considering and is an attractive, if expensive, alternative because of lack of central nervous system side effects.

Radiotherapy

Evidence for the use of radiation therapy in neurological illness comes from several studies in patients with amyotrophic lateral sclerosis [40,41]. Side effects include dry mouth and loss of taste but the risk is reduced by using small radiation doses. Studies in PD are limited. A retrospective study involving 28 patients with parkinsonism treated with radiotherapy between 2001 and 2006 showed a significant improvement in sialorrhoea 1 month after radiation therapy, and the effect lasted for at least a year [42]. Quality-of-life and clinical global impression scores also improved significantly. Before considering this treatment option, one must consider the possible long-term risk of radiation as available data remain anecdotal.

Surgery

Invasive procedures such as submandibular gland excision and parotid duct ligation are effective and have been used with success in children with neurological disabilities such as cerebral palsy [43,44]. Other surgical options include duct relocation and neuroctomy [1]. Although these interventions are effective, surgery has not been evaluated in PD and may be considered unacceptable by patients and their caregivers.

Conclusion

Drooling of saliva is a common problem in PD which may contribute to social embarrassment and isolation. Despite the negative impact on patients' quality of life, studies on sialorrhoea in PD and its effects are limited. Evidence suggests that bradykinesia and rigidity of the oropharyngeal muscles result in dysphagia which is considered to be one of the main causes of sialorrhoea. Several clinical scales are used for assessing sialorrhoea but very few of these have been validated in PD. Pharmacological interventions such as botulinum toxin injection and anticholinergics are useful in the management of drooling but their use is limited by side effects, lack of good quality studies with a double-blind placebo-controlled design and cost, particularly related to botulinum toxin therapy. The role of surgery and radiotherapy is unclear as evidence for their use in PD is limited. The consequences of excessive fluid loss also need to be considered and fluid intake should be increased to guard against constipation and dehydration.

A multidisciplinary approach involving the patient, clinician, nurse specialist, therapists and the patient's caregiver is essential in deciding on the most appropriate treatment.

References

1 **Chou K, Evatt M, Hinson V, et al**. Sialorrhoea in Parkinson's disease: a review. Mov Disord 2007; **22**: 2306–13.

2 **Playfer J, Hindle J**. Parkinson's disease in the older patient, 2nd edn, pp. 175–6. Oxford: Radcliffe Publishing, 2008.

3 **Bloem BR, Kalf JG, Van de Kerkhof PC, Zwarts MJ**. Debilitating consequences of drooling. J Neurol 2009; **256**: 1382–3.

4 **Rodrigues B, Nóbrega AC, Sampaio M, Argolo N, Melo A**. Silent saliva aspiration in Parkinson's disease. Mov Disord 2011; **26**: 138–41.

5 **Edwards LL, Pfeiffer RF, Quigley EM, et al**. Gastrointestinal symptoms in Parkinson's disease. Mov Disord 1991; **6**: 151–6.

6 **Johnston BT, Li Q, Castell JA, Castell DO**. Swallowing and esophageal function in Parkinson's disease. Am J Gastroenterol 1995; **90**: 1741–6.

7 **Eadie MJ, Tyrer JH**. Alimentary disorder in parkinsonism. Aust Ann Med 1965; **14**: 13–22.

8 **Proulx M, de Courval FP, Wiseman MA, Panisset M**. Salivary production in Parkinson's disease. Mov Disord 2005; **20**: 204–7.

9 **Bird MR, Woodward MC, Gibson EM, et al**. Asymptomatic swallowing disorders in elderly patients with Parkinson's disease: a description of findings on clinical examination and videofluoroscopy in sixteen patients. Age Ageing 1994; **23**: 251–4.

10 Bateson MC, Gibberd FB, Wilson RS. Salivary symptoms in Parkinson disease. Arch Neurol 1973; **29**: 274–5.

11 Nilsson H, Ekberg O, Olsson R, et al. Quantitative assessment of oral and pharyngeal function in Parkinson's disease. Dysphagia 1996; **11**: 144–50.

12 Ertekin C. Voluntary versus spontaneous swallowing in man. Dysphagia 2011; **26**: 183–92.

13 Persson M, Osterberg T, Granerus AK, Karlsson S. Influence of Parkinson's disease on oral health. Acta Odontol Scand 1992; **50**: 37–42.

14 Nobrega A, Rodrigues B, Torres AC, et al. Is drooling secondary to a swallowing disorder in patients with Parkinson's disease? Parkinsonism Relat Disord 2008; **14**: 243–5.

15 Bagheri H, Damase-Michel C, Lapeyre-Mestre M, et al. A study of salivary secretion in Parkinson's disease. Clin Neuropharmacol 1999; **22**: 213–15.

16 Kalf JG, Munneke M, van den Engel-Hoek L, et al. Pathophysiology of Diurnal Drooling in Parkinson's Disease Mov Disord. 2011; **26**: 1670–6.

17 National Institute for Health and Care Excellence. Guidelines on the diagnosis and management of Parkinson's disease in primary and secondary care. NICE clinical guideline CG035. London: NICE, 2006.

18 Sockalingam S, Shammi C, Remington G. Treatment of clozapine-induced hypersalivation with ipratropium bromide: a randomized, double-blind, placebo-controlled crossover study. J Clin Psychiatry 2009; **70**: 1114–19.

19 Perez-Lloret S, Nègre-Pagès L, Ojero-Senard A, et al.; COPARK Study Group. Oro-buccal symptoms (dysphagia, dysarthria, and sialorrhea) in patients with Parkinson's disease: preliminary analysis from the French COPARK cohort. Eur J Neurol 2012; **19**: 28–37.

20 Rana AQ, Khondker S, Kabir A, Owalia A, Khnodker S, Emre M. Impact of cognitive dysfunction on drooling in Parkinson's disease. Eur Neurol 2013; **70**: 42–5.

21 Evatt M, Chaudhuri KR, Chou KL, et al. Dysautonomia rating scales in Parkinson's disease: sialorrhea, dysphagia, and constipation. Critique and recommendations to Movement Disorders Task Force on Rating Scales for Parkinson's disease. Mov Disord 2009; **24**: 635–46.

22 Volonté MA, Porta M, Comi G. Clinical assessment of dysphagia in early phases of Parkinson's disease, Neurol Sci 2002; **23**: 121–2.

23 Thomas-Stonell N, Greenberg J. Three treatment approaches and clinical factors in the reduction of drooling. Dysphagia 1988; **3**: 73–8.

24 Perez Lloret S, Piran Arce G, Rossi M, et al. Validation of a new scale for the evaluation of sialorrhea in patients with Parkinson's disease. Mov Disord 2007; **22**: 107–11.

25 Ondo WG, Hunter C, Moore W. A double-blind placebo-controlled trial of botulinum toxin B for sialorrhea in Parkinson's disease. Neurology 2004; **62**: 37–40.

26 Chaudhuri KR, Martinez-Martin P, Schapira AHV, et al. An international multicentre pilot study of the first comprehensive self-completed non motor symptoms questionnaire for Parkinson's disease: the NMSQuest study. Mov Disord 2006; **21**: 916–23.

27 Chaudhuri KR, P Martinez-Martin, RG Brown, et al. The metric properties of a novel non-motor symptoms scale for Parkinson's disease: results from an international pilot study. Mov Disord 2007; **22**: 1901–11.

28 South AR, Somers SM, Jog MS. Gum chewing improves swallow frequency and latency in Parkinson patients: a preliminary study. Neurology 2010; **74**: 1198–202.

29 Marks L, Turner K, O'Sullivan J, et al. Drooling in Parkinson's disease: a novel speech and language therapy intervention. Int J Lang Commun Disord 2001; **36**(Suppl): 282–7.

30 Hockstein NG, Samadi DS, Gendron K, et al. Sialorrhoea; a management challenge. Am Fam Physician 2004; **69**: 2628–34.

31 **Hyson HC, Johnson A, Jog MS**. Survey of sialorrhea in parkinsonian patients in southwestern Ontario. Can J Neurol Sci 2001; **28**: S46–S47.

32 **Thomsen TR, Galpern WR, Asante A**. Ipratropium bromide spray as treatment for sialorrhoea in Parkinson's disease. Mov Disord 2007; **22**: 2268–73.

33 **Seppi K, Weintraub D, Coelho M, et al**. The Movement Disorder Society evidence-based medicine review update: treatments for the non-motor symptoms of Parkinson's disease. Mov Disord 2011; 26(Suppl 3): S42–S80.

34 **Dogu O, Apaydin D, Sevim S, et al**. Ultrasound-guided versus 'blind' intraparotid injections of botulinum toxin-A for the treatment of sialorrhoea in patients with Parkinson's disease. Clin Neurol Neurosurg 2004; **106**: 93–6.

35 **Contarino MF, Pompili M, Tittoto P, et al**. Botulinum toxin B ultrasound-guided injections for sialorrhea in amyotrophic lateral sclerosis and Parkinson's disease. Parkinsonism Relat Disord 2007; **13**: 299–303.

36 **Su CS, Lan MY, Liu JS, et al**. Botulinum toxin type A treatment for Parkinsonian patients with moderate to severe sialorrhea. Acta Neurol Taiwan 2006; **15**: 151–3.

37 **Nobrega AC, Rodrigues B, Torres AC, et al**. Does botulinum toxin decrease frequency and severity of sialorrhea in Parkinson's disease? J Neurol Sci 2007; **253**: 85–7.

38 **Lagalla G, Millevolte M, Capecci M, et al**. Botulinum toxin type A for drooling in Parkinson's disease: a double-blind, randomized, placebo-controlled study. Mov Disord 2006; **21**: 704–7.

39 **Chinnapongse R, Gullo K, Nemeth P, Zhang Y, Griggs L**. Safety and efficacy of botulinum toxin type B for treatment of sialorrhea in Parkinson's disease: a prospective double-blind trial. Mov Disord 2012; **27**: 219–26.

40 **Neppelberg E, Haugen DF, Thorsen L, et al**. Radiotherapy reduces sialorrhea in amyotrophic lateral sclerosis. Euro J Neurol 2007; **14**: 1373–7.

41 **Kasarskis EJ, Hodskins J, St Clair WH**. Unilateral parotid electron beam radiotherapy as palliative treatment for sialorrhea in amyotrophic lateral sclerosis J Neurol Sci 2011; **308**: 155–7.

42 **Postma AG, Heesters M, van Laar T**. Radiotherapy to the salivary glands as treatment of sialorrhea in patients with parkinsonism. Mov Disord 2007; **22**: 2430–5.

43 **Manrique D, do Brasil Ode O, Ramos H**. Drooling: analysis and evaluation of 31 children who underwent bilateral submandibular gland excision and parotid duct ligation. Rev Bras Otorhinolaringol (Engl Ed) 2007; **73**: 40–4.

44 **Stern Y, Feinmesser R, Collins M, et al**. Bilateral submandibular gland excision with parotid duct ligation for treatment of sialorrhea in children: long-term results. Arch Otolaryngol Head Neck Surg 2002; **128**: 801–3.

Chapter 22

Olfaction in Parkinson's disease

Heinz Reichmann and Birgit Herting

Background

As more than 95% of Parkinson's disease (PD) patients present with hyposmia [1,2], it could be argued that hyposmia should be considered as the fifth general feature of PD in addition to tremor, rigidity, bradykinesia and postural instability. In contrast to these symptoms, however, hyposmia occurs earlier and may indeed turn out to be one of the most sensitive features for the early and differential diagnosis of PD.

Hyposmia as a cardinal feature of Parkinson's disease

According to a recent study by Politis et al. [3], olfactory loss is one of the top five most prevalent motor and non-motor symptoms in early stage PD patients. Some patients do not realize they have hyposmia because olfactory deficits in general start subtly and progress slowly. Others, however, feel that this symptom affects their quality of life. A first clue that hyposmia is associated with PD was given by Ansari and Johnson [4] who described this phenomenon in 22 patients. In the 1990s, several groups published convincing data on olfactory dysfunction in PD patients [5–7]. These studies employed the University of Pennsylvania Smell Identification Test (UPSIT). This test uses cards with encapsulated smelly substances which are liberated by scratching. Subjects have to name 40 smelly substances which are presented at high concentrations following the forced-choice method (the correct answer must be selected from a choice of four options). Doty et al. [2] reported that the ability to identify smells was diminished in 90% of 81 PD patients studied. In addition, the odour threshold was analysed in 38 PD patients and was found to be significantly more impaired than in an age- and sex-matched control group. This was independent of age, gender, duration and state of the disease. Clinical symptoms, cognitive impairment and medication did not have any influence either. These data were supported by a paper by Hawkes et al. [6] who found that 70% of 96 patients tested with the UPSIT presented with hyposmia. In our recent multicentre study [1] using Sniffin' Sticks (Fig 22.1) in 400 PD patients from three independent populations, 96.7% of PD patients presented with significant olfactory loss when compared with young normosmic subjects. This number, however, decreased to 74.5%, when adjusted to age-related norms.

In their paper Hawkes et al. [6] stated that PD patients have problems with distinct smelly substances. In our work using Sniffin' Sticks [8–10] we found that, in accordance

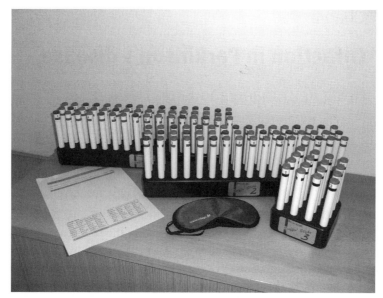

Fig. 22.1 A set of Sniffin' Sticks.

with Hawkes et al.'s study, PD patients indeed have more difficulties in identifying some odours than others—interestingly, however, people with other forms of hyposmia (e.g. post-infectious or post-traumatic hyposmia) had the same preferences [11].

The Sniffin' Sticks test can be performed with 12 common smelly substances and forced-choice answers. For scientific assessments, the more comprehensive test battery which consists of 48 individual tests should be used. In general, we use three subtests: determination of odour threshold, discrimination and identification. The results are summarized in the form of a differentiation and identification threshold value. The threshold is analysed with different concentrations of smelly substances, while differentiation is assessed with a triplet of sticks, where one stick contains a smelly substance that is different from the other two. Identification is tested by offering a choice of four smells to the patient. We analysed which of the three tests may be the most discriminatory and found that the combined testing of these components of olfaction provides the most significant approach to the diagnosis of smell loss [12].

Doty et al. [13] were the first to show that hyposmia is present to the same degree no matter which of the two nostrils is tested and that there is no correlation between disease stage and olfactory dysfunction. Similar to the situation in controls, olfaction in PD is more impaired in men than in women [1,5].

Barz et al. [14] further demonstrated that olfactory-evoked potentials are significantly delayed in PD compared with age- and sex-matched controls. Stimulation of the trigeminal system did not show any deficits, confirming selective impairment of the olfactory system in PD. Olfactory-evoked potentials deteriorated as the disease progressed further [15]. Thus, in 12 patients it could be demonstrated that hyposmia worsened during the course of the disease. Using this method it could be shown that olfaction itself is impaired in PD and not sniffing alone (i.e. not just an impairment in the nose but in the brain itself).

As already mentioned, other authors have described a missing correlation between olfactory loss and both disease duration and the clinical severity of PD [2,5,6]. To further investigate these contradictory results, we analysed 27 consecutive patients (22 male and 5 female) with PD using Sniffin' Sticks. The patients were aged from 27 to 64 years and their disease duration ranged from 0 to 19 years. All patients were examined at least twice during a 3–6-year period. We investigated the patients again after 4.4 years [16]. The average score at baseline was 17.5 points (with scores below 30 indicating hyposmia and below 15 indicating functional anosmia). Again there was no correlation between age, gender, duration and severity of PD and hyposmia. The second analysis after 4.4 years yielded an average score of 17.5 points. Interestingly, we found a conversion from hyposmia to functional anosmia in five patients and a conversion from anosmia to hyposmia in three patients. The use of quantitative methods such as Sniffin' Sticks confirms that olfaction changes in PD, only a limited number of PD patients develop anosmia and that no patient was normosmic. This work raises the question of why some patients deteriorate and some even improve. A possible answer can be found in the paper by Huisman et al. [17], who showed that the number of dopaminergic cells in the olfactory bulb is twice as high in PD patients as in controls when stained for tyrosine hydroxylase. This finding contrasts with the fact that PD patients show a loss of dopaminergic neurons in the substantia nigra. In the glomeruli of the olfactory bulb, dopamine inhibits signal transduction between the olfactory receptor neurons and the mitral cells, which control the first and most important step in odour perception. The authors stress that the increased number of dopaminergic neurons in the olfactory bulb could explain the loss of olfaction [18]. This hypothesis also explains why dopaminergic medication is unlikely to improve olfaction in PD patients [2,19].

In post-mortem analyses, other investigators [20] demonstrated a loss of neurons in the olfactory bulb in seven PD patients which correlated well with disease duration. Lewy bodies were found in all patients in both the olfactory bulb and tract.

More recent studies were performed by Braak et al. [21] and will be discussed in detail later (see the section Loss of olfaction as an early marker of Parkinson's disease). This group showed typical α-synuclein deposits in neurons but not in the glomeruli.

In the near future, immunohistochemical, volumetric and functional neuroimaging studies of the olfactory system might become relevant for PD diagnosis [22]. Witt and Hummel compared biopsy material from PD patients for histological/histochemical changes with that from patients with olfactory dysfunction due to other causes [23]. However, they found no specific changes in the nasal mucosa of PD patients. A non-significant decrease in the volume of the olfactory bulb was found using magnetic resonance imaging volumetry [24]. This study included 11 PD patients (six with functional anosmia and five hyposmic patients) and nine healthy normosmic controls. It is difficult to speculate why olfactory neurons are so vulnerable, but this could reflect damage or the uptake of a pathogen early in life with consecutive neurodegeneration. Selective vulnerability could originate from the fact that the ciliary surface is not protected by the blood–brain barrier.

Finally, neuropathological studies indicate a progressive loss of neurons in the amygdala which contribute to the secondary olfactory system [25].

Functional magnetic resonance imaging has been used in an effort to identify the brain structures responsible for smell loss in PD. Overall, the results of these studies [26,27] show that neuronal activity in the amygdala and hippocampus is reduced in PD patients which may have a specific impact on olfactory sensitivity. In addition, neuronal activity in components of the corticostriatal loops appears to be upregulated, indicating compensatory processes involving the dopaminergic system.

Cognitive impairment hampers studies on olfaction because these patients have problems in validating and recognizing smelly substances [28]. We have no evidence that medication improves olfaction, and this contrasts with our observation that deep brain stimulation (DBS) improves olfaction in PD [29]. This could be due to cognitive improvement or improvement of alertness following DBS.

Impairment of olfaction as a differential diagnostic tool

Wenning et al. [30] were the first to demonstrate different degrees of olfactory impairment in patients with idiopathic PD (IPD), multisystem atrophy (MSA), progressive supranuclear palsy (PSP) and corticobasal degeneration (CBD). Using the UPSIT they found in their cohorts that IPD patients showed the well-known impairment of olfaction, but this was less pronounced in MSA and did not occur in PSP and CBD. This is in agreement with the lack of tau pathology in the olfactory bulbs of patients who died from PSP or CBD [31].

This finding was confirmed using Sniffin' Sticks. MSA patients showed less hyposmia and PSP patients no olfactory impairment at all, while PD patients demonstrated hyposmia or functional anosmia in 86% of cases [32,33]. We have also reported that hyposmia/anosmia was equally present in the various iPD subtypes, including the tremor-dominant type, the rigid–akinetic type and the equivalence type [5]. However, subsequent data from Ondo and Lai [34] have shown that patients with a tremor-dominant type of PD have a less marked reduction of olfaction. In contrast to patients with iPD, who have a loss of olfaction in more than 95% of cases at the time of diagnosis, MSA patients show normal values for quite some time and only deteriorate later in the course of the disease [13,16,35]. In PSP patients olfaction also deteriorates as the disease progresses, and although the reason for this is not yet clear a contribution from cognitive impairment has been discussed [16]. A recent American Academy practice parameter on the diagnosis and prognosis of PD concluded that olfactory testing 'should be considered' to differentiate PD from PSP and CBD but not from MSA [36].

Patients with Alzheimer's dementia are also hyposmic, which again confirms the link between cognitive impairment and impaired olfaction [35]. In addition, the use of Sniffin' Sticks should permit reliable differential diagnosis between essential tremor and tremor-dominant types of PD in most patients and also of vascular Parkinsonism or PD or parkin-induced parkinsonism (Table 22.1) [37–39] (for review see Haehner et al. [22] and Doty [40]).

Table 22.1 Olfactory dysfunction in neurodegenerative disorders—its role in differential diagnosis [37,40]

Neurodegenerative disorder	Olfactory dysfunction
Idiopathic Parkinson`s disease, Alzheimer's disease, Lewy body disease, *PARK8* locus mutations	+ + +
Multiple system atrophy, Huntington's disease	+ +
Progressive supranuclear palsy, amyotrophic lateral sclerosis, *PARK1* locus mutations	+
Corticobasal degeneration, *PARK2* locus mutations, vascular parkinsonism, essential tremor	+/0

+ + +, marked olfactory dysfunction; + +, moderate olfactory dysfunction; +, mild olfactory dysfunction; 0, intact olfaction.

Loss of olfaction as an early marker of Parkinson's disease

There is good evidence that most PD patients develop impairment of olfaction some 4–6 years before they start to present with motor symptoms [41]. This is supported by work from Braak's group [21]. They claim that abnormalities first occur in the Meissner and Auerbach plexus, then in the olfactory bulb and the dorsal vagal nucleus before they ascend to other parts of the brain including the substantia nigra. They demonstrated the presence of Lewy bodies and Lewy neuritis in the olfactory bulb even in individuals who were suspected of being in the pre-motor phase of PD. Based upon these findings, idiopathic hyposmia may be a very early sign of PD. However, hyposmia is unspecific in the elderly population. Thus, the identification of further pre-motor signs of imminent PD would be essential for any future application of neuroprotective agents. Apart from hyposmia, rapid eye movement sleep behaviour disorder [42,43], depression and constipation might also be considered as potential candidate signs [44–47].

Several studies have been performed to test the hypothesis that hyposmia may be a valuable tool for the detection of early pre-motor PD. Our group investigated 30 patients with idiopathic hyposmia (19 male, 11 female; average age 59 years; average duration of hyposmia 5.8 years) [48]. None of these patients had pre-existing neurological disease. A careful neurological examination including the Unified Parkinson Disease Rating Scale (UPDRS) Parts II and III and substantia nigra sonography was performed in all patients. Sonography of the substantia nigra was abnormal in many cases of PD [49]. These patients show hyperechogenicity of the substantia nigra, probably due to the incorporation of iron ions and activated microglia [50]. A ^{123}I-FP-CIT (dopamine transporter scan) was performed in all patients with abnormalities in the UPDRS or in the substantia nigra sonography. One patient showed typical clinical features of PD and two patients had suspected PD. Parenchymal sonography was abnormal in 11 patients. A dopamine transporter scan was performed in 10 of these 11 patients and was abnormal in five and equivocal in two, while only three patients showed normal activities. A further two patients developed motor symptoms of PD 2 years later [51].

Berendse and colleagues [52,53] used another approach. In a prospective study they examined 361 asymptomatic first-degree relatives of PD patients (parents, children and siblings) aged 50–75 years. Using olfactory tests they identified 40 people with impaired olfactory function and compared them with 38 with normal olfaction. Both groups received a dopamine transporter scan at baseline and after 2 years. The other 283 relatives were followed up with a validated questionnaire which was aimed at the specific features of IPD. Two years after the baseline examination, 10 of the relatives with initial hyposmia showed motor symptoms indicative of PD, and another 12% presented with abnormalities of dopamine transporter single-photon emission computed tomography (SPECT). None of the 38 normosmic relatives had developed PD symptoms. These results suggest that idiopathic hyposmia may lead to PD in 10% of cases. However, if abnormal SPECT data are also considered, the proportion may rise to 22%. In a follow-up study, 5 years after baseline testing [54] five relatives had developed clinical PD, with initial clinical (motor) symptoms appearing 9 to 52 months (median 15 months) after baseline testing.

In summary, the occurrence of specific symptoms that allow the clinical diagnosis of PD is preceded by a long prodromal phase in which the neurodegenerative process leads to substantial neuronal loss. To enable earlier disease-modulating or even neuroprotective therapy it is essential to identify individuals in this early phase. There are a number of ongoing studies (e.g. <http://www.trend-studie.de> and <http://www.parsinfosource.com>) investigating the pre-motor diagnosis of PD.

References

1 Haehner A, Bosveldt S, Berendse HW, et al. Prevalence of smell loss in Parkinson's disease—a multicenter study. Parkinsonism Relat Disord 2009; **15**: 490–4.

2 Doty RL, Deems DA, Stellar S. Olfactory dysfunction in parkinsonism: a general deficit unrelated to neurologic signs, disease stage, or disease duration. Neurology 1988; **38**: 1237–44.

3 Politis M, Wu K, Molloy S et al. Parkinson's disease symptoms: the patient's perspective. Mov Disord 2010; **25**: 1646–51.

4 Ansari KA, Johnson A. Olfactory function in patients with Parkinson's disease. J Chron Dis 1975; **28**: 493–7.

5 Stern MB, Doty RL, Dotti M, et al. Olfactory function in Parkinson's disease subtypes. Neurology 1994; **44**: 266–8.

6 Hawkes CH, Shephard BC, Daniel SE. Olfactory dysfunction in Parkinson's disease. J Neurol Neurosurg Psych 1997; **62**: 436–46.

7 Daum RF, Sekinger B, Kobal G, Lang C. Riechprüfung mit 'Sniffin' Sticks' zur klinischen Diagnostik des Morbus Parkinson [Olfactory testing with 'sniffin' sticks' for clinical diagnosis of Parkinson disease]. Nervenarzt 2000; **71**: 643–50.

8 Hummel T, Sekinger B, Wolf SR, et al. 'Sniffin' sticks': olfactory performance assessed by the combined testing of odor identification, odor discrimination and olfactory threshold. Chem Senses 1997; **22**: 39–52.

9 Kobal G, Klimek L, Wolfensberger M, et al. Multicenter investigation of 1,036 subjects using a standardized method for the assessment of olfactory function combining tests of odor identification, odor discrimination, and olfactory thresholds. Eur Arch Otorhinolaryngol 2000; **257**: 205–11.

10 Hummel T, Kobal G, Gudziol H, Mackay-Sim A. Normative data for the 'Sniffin' Sticks' including tests of odor identification, odor discrimination, and olfactory thresholds: an upgrade based on a group of more than 3,000 subjects. Eur Arch Otorhinolaryngol 2007; **264**: 237–43.

11 Herting B, Bietenbeck S, Scholz K, et al. Olfactory dysfunction in Parkinson's disease: its role as a new cardinal sign in early and differential diagnosis. Nervenarzt 2008; **79**: 175–84.

12 Loetsch J, Reichmann H, Hummel T. Different odor tests contribute differently to the evaluation of olfactory loss. Chem Senses 2008; **33**: 17–21.

13 Doty RL, Stern MB, Pfeiffer C, et al. Bilateral olfactory dysfunction in early stage treated and untreated idiopathic Parkinson's disease. J Neurol Neurosurg Psychiatry 1992; **55**: 138–42.

14 Barz S, Hummel T, Pauli E, et al. Chemosensory event-related potentials in response to trigeminal and olfactory stimulation in idiopathic Parkinson's disease. Neurology 1997; **49**: 1424–31.

15 Hummel T. Olfactory evoked potentials as a tool to measure progression of Parkinson's disease. In: T Chase, P Bedard (eds) Focus on medicine, Vol. **14**: New developments in the drug therapy of Parkinson's disease, pp. 47–53. Oxford: Blackwell Science, 1999.

16 Herting B, Schulze S, Reichmann H, Haehner A, Hummel T. A longitudinal study of olfactory function in patients with idiopathic Parkinson's disease. J Neurol 2008; **255**: 367–70.

17 Huisman E, Uylings HB, Hoogland PV. A 100% increase of dopaminergic cells in the olfactory bulb may explain hyposmia in Parkinson's disease. Mov Disord 2004; **19**: 687–92.

18 Winner B, Geyer M, Couillard-Despres S, et al. Striatal deafferentation increases dopaminergic neurogenesis in the adult olfactory bulb. Exp Neurol 2006; **197**: 113–21.

19 Roth J, Radil T, Ruzickas E, et al. Apomorphine does not influence olfactory thresholds in Parkinson's disease. Funct Neurol 1998; **13**: 99–103.

20 Pearce RKB, Hawkes CH, Daniel SE. The anterior olfactory nucleus in Parkinson's disease. Mov Disord 1995; **10**: 283–7.

21 Braak H, Ghebremedhin E, Rub U, et al. Stages in the development of Parkinson's disease-related pathology. Cell Tissue Res 2004; **318**: 121–34.

22 Haehner A, Hummel T, Reichmann H. Olfactory loss in Parkinson's disease. Parkinson's Dis. 2011; 2011: article ID 450939.

23 Witt M, Hummel T. Vomeronasal versus olfactory epithelium: is there a cellular basis for human vomeronasal perception? Int Rev Cytol 2006; **248**: 209–59.

24 Müller A, Abolmaali N, Hakimi AR, et al. Olfactory bulb volumes in patients with idiopathic Parkinson's disease—a pilot study. J Neural Transm 2005; **112**: 1363–70.

25 Harding AJ, Stimson E, Henderson JM, Halliday GM. Clinical correlates of selective pathology in the amygdala of patients with Parkinson's disease. Brain 2002; **125**: 2431–45.

26 Westermann B, Wattendorf E, Schwerdtfeger U, et al. Functional modulation of cortical olfactory pathways in Parkinson's disease: an fMRI study J Neurol Neurosurg Psychiatry 2008; **79**: 19–24.

27 Hummel T, Fliessbach K, Abele M, et al. Olfactory fMRI in patients with Parkinson's disease. Front Integr Neurosci. 2010; **4**: 125.

28 Hudry J, Thobois S, Broussolle E, et al. Evidence for deficiencies in perceptual and semantic olfactory processes in Parkinson's disease. Chem Senses 2003; **28**: 537–43.

29 Hummel T, Jahnke U, Sommer U, et al. Olfactory function in patients with idiopathic Parkinson's disease: effects of deep brain stimulation in the subthalamic nucleus. J Neural Transm 2005; **112**: 669–76.

30 Wenning GK, Shephard B, Hawkes C, et al. Olfactory function in atypical parkinsonian syndromes. Acta Neurol Scand 1995; **91**: 274–50.

31 Tsuboi Y, Wszolek ZK, Graff-Radford NR, et al. Tau pathology in the olfactory bulb correlates with Braak stage, Lewy body pathology and apolipoprotein epsilon4. Neuropathol Appl Neurobiol 2003; **29**: 503–10.

32 **Müller A, Reichmann H, Livermore A, Hummel T**. Olfactory function in idiopathic Parkinson's disease (IPD): results from cross-sectional studies in IPD patients and long-term follow-up of de-novo IPD patients. J Neural Transm 2002; **109**: 805–11.

33 **Müller A, Müngersdorf M, Reichmann H, et al.** Olfactory function in parkinsonian syndromes. J Clin Neurosci 2002; **9**: 521–4.

34 **Ondo WG, Lai D**. Olfaction testing in patients with tremor-dominant Parkinson's disease: is this a distinct condition? Mov Disord 2005; **20**: 471–5.

35 **Doty RL, Perl DP, Steele JC, et al.** Odor identification deficit of the parkinsonism-dementia complex of Guam: equivalence to that of Alzheimer's an idiopathic Parkinson's disease. Neurology 1991; **41**(Suppl 2): 77–80.

36 **McKinnon JH, Demaerschalk BM, Caviness JN, et al.** Sniffing out Parkinson disease: can olfactory testing differentiate parkinsonian disorders? Neurologist 2007; **13**: 382–5.

37 **Katzenschlager R, Lees AJ.** Olfaction and Parkinson's syndromes: its role in differential diagnosis. Curr Opin Neurol 2004; **17**: 417–23.

38 **Katzenschlager R, Zijlmans J, Evans A, et al.** Olfactory function distinguishes vascular parkinsonism from Parkinson's disease. J Neurol Neurosurg Psychiatry 2004; **75**: 1749–52.

39 **Khan NL, Katzenschlager R, Watt H, et al.** Olfaction differentiates parkin disease from early-onset parkinsonism and Parkinson disease. Neurology 2004; **62**: 1224–6.

40 **Doty RL.** Olfaction in Parkinson's disease and related disorders. Neurobiol Dis 2012; **46**: 527–52.

41 **Müller A, Abolmaali N, Hummel T, Reichmann H.** Riechstörungen—ein frühes Kardinalsymptom des idiopathischen Parkinson-Syndroms [Cardinal symptoms of idiopathic Parkinson disease]. Akt Neurol 2003; **30**: 239–43.

42 **Stiasny-Kolster K, Doerr Y, Moller JC, et al.** Combination of 'idiopathic' REM sleep behaviour disorder and olfactory dysfunction as possible indicator for alpha-synucleinopathy demonstrated by dopamine transporter FP-CIT-SPECT. Brain 2005; **128**: 126–37.

43 **Postuma RB, Lang AE, Massicotte-Marquez J, Montplaisir J.** Potential early markers of Parkinson disease in idiopathic REM sleep behavior disorder. Neurology 2006; **66**: 845–51.

44 **Leentjens AF, Van den Acker M, Metsemakers JF, et al.** Higher incidence of depression preceding the onset of Parkinson's disease: a register study. Mov Disord 2003; **18**: 414–18.

45 **Ishihara-Paul L, Wainwright NW, Khaw KT, et al.** Prospective association between emotional health and clinical evidence of Parkinson's disease. Eur J Neurol 2008; **15**: 1148–54.

46 **Hawkes CH, Del Tredici K, Braak H.** A timeline for Parkinson's disease. Parkinsonism Relat Disord 2010; **16**: 79–84.

47 **Postuma RB, Aarsland D, Barone P, et al.** Identifying prodromal Parkinson's disease: pre-motor disorders in Parkinson's disease. Mov Disord 2012; **27**: 617–26.

48 **Sommer U, Hummel T, Cormann K, et al.** Detection of presymptomatic Parkinson's disease: combination of olfactory tests, transcranial sonography, and 123-I-FP-CIT-SPECT. Mov Disord 2004; **19**: 1196–202.

49 **Becker G, Seufert J, Bogdahn U, et al.** Degeneration of substantia nigra in chronic Parkinson's disease visualized by transcranial color-coded real-time sonography. Neurology 1995; **45**: 182–4.

50 **Berg D, Roggendorf W, Schröder U, et al.** Echogenicity of the substantia nigra: association with increased iron content and marker for susceptibility to nigrostriatal injury. Arch Neurol 2002; **59**: 999–1005.

51 **Haehner A, Hummel T, Hummel C, et al.** Olfactory loss may be a first sign of idiopathic Parkinson's disease. Mov Disord 2007; **22**: 839–42.

52 **Berendse HW, Booij J, Francot CM, et al**. Subclinical dopaminergic dysfunction in asymptomatic Parkinson's disease patients' relatives with decreased sense of smell. Ann Neurol 2001; **50**: 34–41.

53 **Ponsen MM, Stoffers D, Booji J, et al**. Idiopathic hyposmia as a preclinical sign of Parkinson's disease. Ann Neurol 2004; **56**: 173–81.

54 **Ponsen MM, Stoffers D, Twisk JW et al**. Hyposmia and executive dysfunction as predictors of future Parkinson's disease: a prospective study. Mov Disord 2009; **24**: 1060–5.

Chapter 23

Chronic pain and Parkinson's disease

Santiago Perez-Lloret, Estelle Dellapina,
Jean Pelleprat, María Verónica Rey, Christine
Brefel-Courbon and Olivier Rascol

Introduction

Despite increasing interest in the non-motor signs of Parkinson's disease (PD) [1,2], pain remains one of the symptoms that is most rarely considered in patients suffering from this disorder. For example, a bibliographic search of the PubMed database using the key words 'pain' and 'Parkinson' will identify less than a few hundred references over the last 10 years on the topic. The same search done over the same time period using the term 'dementia' leads to several thousand articles. Nevertheless, pain is a common and relevant problem in PD, although its exact prevalence, its main causes and pathophysiological mechanisms, its consequences for patients' quality of life and its therapeutic management remain incompletely known and poorly understood.

The prevalence of chronic pain in Parkinson's disease

The limited data available in the literature make it possible to conclude that sensory disorders are common in PD; indeed, it is estimated that 30–85% of PD patients suffer from such problems [3–12]. The exact prevalence of pain, however, remains difficult to define because most epidemiological surveys in the literature fail to provide a clear definition of the term 'pain'. In addition, these studies have tended to select their patients from tertiary specialized referral centres which are not representative of the general population. Furthermore, only a few studies include a group of non-PD subjects for comparison.

Two recent large prospective epidemiological surveys, however, have helped to clarify this issue [6,11]. The first one, known as the DoPaMiP survey, was conducted in southwest France in collaboration with 25 neurologists from the public and private sectors in both rural and urban areas [11]. The main purpose of this study was to define the prevalence of 'chronic pain' in 450 patients suffering from idiopathic PD and compare this with age- and sex-matched subjects suffering from chronic disorders other than PD. The results of this survey showed that 278/450 patients (61.8%) suffered from at least one form of chronic pain as defined by the International Association for the Study of Pain ('an unpleasant sensory and emotional experience linked to an existing or potential lesion in the tissue or described in terms evoking such a lesion; occurring for more than 3–6 months and/or likely to negatively affect the patient's behaviour or well-being, attributable to any non-malignant cause'). The proportion of PD patients suffering from chronic pain was twice that observed using the same criteria in the group of patients suffering from chronic disorders other than PD, after adjusting for the main co-morbidity factors, particularly that of degenerative osteoarthritis, which is common in the people aged over 50 years. This type of pain had an average intensity of 60 mm on a visual analogue scale of 1–100 mm.

Interestingly, the DoPaMiP results are consistent with those of another large case–control survey conducted by a group of Italian neurologists who reported an overall frequency of pain of 69.9% (281/402 patients with PD) in their population [6]. In line with the DoPaMiP survey, this proportion was significantly greater than that observed in age- and sex-matched healthy control subjects.

Recently, pain prevalence was explored by a systematic review of the literature [4]. The modified Quality Assessment of Diagnostic Accuracy Studies tool was used, which is specially designed for judging the methodological quality of prevalence studies. Only eight articles out of 18 met the predefined criteria for use in the review. Pain prevalence frequency ranged from 40 to 85% with a mean of 67.6%. Pain was most frequently located in the lower limbs, with almost half of all PD patients complaining of musculoskeletal pain (46.4%). In a recent review, differences in the prevalence between pain subtypes were noted: dystonic pain affected 4–35% of patients, musculoskeletal pain 19–58%, radicular pain 3–38% and central pain 2–8% [13].

A difference in the location of pain between men and women has also been observed [14]. While women reported that pain more frequently affected their left arm, men reported more frequent leg pain. Regarding duration, more than 70% of patients manifesting pain suffered it for more than 6 months [15]. Finally, pain can precede the diagnosis of PD; this has been show to be the case in 25% of PD patients in a recent study [16].

Clinical presentation of chronic pain in Parkinson's disease

The broad spectrum of pain felt by patients suffering from PD is highlighted by empirical clinical experience. In a population of PD patients older than 50 years not all forms of chronic pain are necessarily due to PD. Accidental associations are not uncommon and it is not always easy to define what is causing pain: PD or co-morbidity. Unfortunately, there are no validated scales or questionnaires for assessing this question. PD-related pain can be defined as the pain that starts after diagnosis of PD, responds to antiparkinsonian treatment, is more prominent on the side maximally affected and/or that does not have any other clear cause [6,10]. Based on this method, it was concluded that among the 278 PD patients in the DoPaMiP survey who suffered from chronic pain, the majority (167 patients) had pain that was directly or indirectly attributable to PD. In other words, PD was either a direct cause of pain on its own or PD indirectly aggravated pain of another origin (mainly osteoarthritis) [11]. This group represents 37.1% of the DoPaMiP survey population. In the 111 remaining patients (24.6% of the total), chronic pain was considered by the neurologists to be unrelated to PD; in these cases osteoarthritis was the most frequent aetiology, which is in line with what would be expected in elderly subjects [17].

Once pain unrelated to PD has been excluded there is still great clinical heterogeneity when focusing on chronic pain directly caused by PD. A synthesis is difficult to establish due to the ambiguity of reported clinical pictures and without consensus or a precise framework for the classification of syndromes. In some instances, classifications referring, for example, to 'musculoskeletal', 'dystonic' and 'joint' pains [18] or 'dystonic' and 'non-dystonic' pains [19] have been proposed according to empirical non-validated experience. In practice, in some patients it is relatively easy to identify and describe the pain and even associate it with a specific mechanism. For example, one of the most easily identified types is cramp-like pain related to the muscular contraction of painful parkinsonian dystonia, a syndrome commonly reported in many studies [6,11,19]. In other instances, however, the painful symptoms prove more difficult to characterize. Many patients report rather vague (although sometimes intense) painful sensations such as ill-defined muscular or articular pain. Some cases of PD are diagnosed in the initial stages by a rheumatologist without there necessarily being any sign of the classic, but rare, inaugural algo-dystrophic syndrome of the disease [20]. Indeed, in up to a quarter of PD patients with chronic pain, pain precedes the occurrence of motor symptoms or the initiation of antiparkinsonian medications [16]. Shoulder pain represents a frequent presenting symptom [21]. A proportion of patients also report painful, sometimes superficial and cutaneous, paraesthesias like burning or painful pins and needles, electrical charge-like sensations or sometimes deep pain like grinding and oppression of one or several limbs, the thorax or the abdomen, which recall 'neuropathic' pain [22], despite the absence of any objective clinical signs of a neurological lesion other than parkinsonism. More rarely, 'visceral' pain has been described in the abdomen, mouth and even genitals of PD patients [23,24]. In general, PD patients who suffer from neuropathic or visceral pain report that 'off' episodes worsen such painful sensations. A few PD patients also have painful sensations which could be likened to akathisia or restless legs syndrome. Recently an integrative classification of pain in PD has been proposed [25]. The authors propose a taxonomy of pain in PD that combines various elements of previous studies and allows a global vision of pain in this disease. This pain classification integrates the relationship to PD (related or unrelated), the broad pain system (nociceptive, neuropathic or miscellaneous), the broad type (musculoskeletal, central, peripheral, etc.) and finally the specific structures and pathology (back pain, radicular pain, central parkinsonian pain, etc.). This is a promising approach, but more research is needed.

The subjective limits of these clinical definitions sometimes prove to be puzzling and difficult to delimit, and often make comparisons difficult. One patient is rarely like another. It is a common observation that patients can actually suffer simultaneously from more than one type of pain. A few clinical pictures have become apparent (e.g. painful forms of dystonia, 'pseudo-neuropathic' pain), but in most cases there is much fundamental work that still needs to be done to specify the complex pain symptomatology of PD patients. Only this will allow us to establish the foundations that practitioners and researchers can use as a basis for caring for patients and furthering knowledge.

The pathophysiological mechanisms responsible for chronic pain in Parkinson's disease

The heterogeneity of the multiple painful syndromes encountered by the PD patient makes it difficult to attempt any universal or specific explanation of the causal mechanism. It would seem reasonable to suggest two main aetiological frameworks for pain in PD: a domain of pain apparently due to a peripheral 'mechanical' cause and pain which seems more legitimately due to 'central' neurological dysfunction, possibly related to the dopaminergic deficit.

Certain forms of PD pain are intuitively associated with a peripheral cause. This is the case for pain associated with the muscle cramps caused by dystonia or for pain related to specific deformities caused by PD, like camptocormia [26] or the parkinsonian 'hand'. Sometimes, however, it is more difficult to be certain about the contribution due to the disease. Thus, for osteoarthritic or established radicular conflicts, for example, the extent to which PD makes these different forms of pain worse by postural disturbances, rigidity or abnormal movements, or even by the changes it can induce in the pain perception threshold, is often unclear [27,28].

Conversely, in some cases observations strongly suggest a primary central neurological mechanism with a probable contribution of the dopaminergic deficit to nociceptive symptoms. Many arguments in favour of such a mechanism exist. Some patients describe their pain in terms reminiscent of the criteria for the diagnosis of neuropathic pain [22]. In these cases, no 'peripheral' mechanical or muscular cause for the pain can be found. Pain can be predominant in the limb(s) most severely affected by parkinsonian motor signs. Sometimes, pain becomes worse or returns during the 'off' episodes in fluctuating patients [29] and is reported to be improved by levodopa and other dopaminergic medications [30]. Favourable effects of deep brain stimulation of the subthalamic nucleus have also been reported in patients who have had this procedure [31].

In the light of these clinical arguments, other factors that support the hypothesis of the involvement of basal ganglia and the central dopaminergic deficit in the genesis of parkinsonian pain should be noted. Anatomically, several nuclei of the basal ganglia have connections with cerebral structures involved in nociception, both as inputs to the thalamus, cortex or amygdala and as outputs of the thalamus or medulla (see Chudler and Dong [32] for review). Electrophysiologically, neurons in the substantia nigra and the striatum which have an electrical activity that varies in response to painful stimulation have been described in animals [33]. Nociceptive stimulation evokes the expression of Fos in the subthalamus of hemiparkinsonian rats [34]. Moreover, rats depleted of dopamine by intrastriatal 6-hydroxydopamine (6-OHDA) displayed increased nociceptive responses to chemical stimulation of the face and hyperalgesic responses to thermal stimulation of the hind paw [35]. In another experiment, rats with lesions induced by 6-OHDA displayed a significantly reduced response latency for nociceptive thermal stimuli [36]. Moreover, parkinsonian rats exhibited a lower nociceptive threshold (i.e. hypersensitivity) to the stimulus on the lesioned side of the body compared with the contralateral side, and with both sides of the sham-operated group. These results suggest the involvement of basal ganglia in pain processing and their alteration in PD.

Pharmacologically, the administration of levodopa has an analgesic effect at certain doses in rats [37]. In functional imaging, bilateral activation of the putamen has been reported in healthy men and women in response to peripheral nociceptive stimulations [38]. Certain painful syndromes like 'burning mouth syndrome' have been associated with anomalies of cerebral dopaminergic markers observed using positron emission tomography (PET) [39] and have been reported to be improved by dopaminergic agents [39,40]. At the other extreme, hyposensitivity to pain is common in patients with schizophrenia, which has been linked to excessive dopamine neurotransmission [41].

The release of dopamine in the striatum may modulate different aspects of pain processing [42]. Indeed, release of dopamine to the ventral striatum may be related to anticipatory responses and to the emotional aspects of the processing of pain in humans, whereas release to the dorsal part has been correlated with the subjective perception of the intensity of the pain.

In patients with PD, the analysis of pain perception thresholds also corroborates the dopaminergic hypothesis. The pain perception threshold for heat was significantly lowered in a group of PD patients with pain compared with patients not complaining of pain, and this abnormality was more pronounced on the most affected side [28]. The pain perception threshold and the RIII reflex were also reported to be abnormal in PD patients compared with age- and sex-matched controls, such abnormalities being improved by levodopa [27,43,44]. Other neurophysiological techniques support the concept of abnormal processing of nociceptive inputs in patients with PD [45,46]. Finally, PET functional imaging revealed abnormal overactivation of several nociceptive cerebral areas in response to nociceptive stimulation in PD patients; levodopa reduced such abnormalities [28].

Nevertheless, central mechanisms other than the dopaminergic deficit cannot be excluded from the pathophysiology of parkinsonian pain. For example, pathological lesions in lamina I of the spinal cord have been reported at autopsy of PD patients [47]. Moreover, more severe levodopa-unresponsive axial sign scores have been observed in patients with chronic pain caused by PD compared with pain-free PD patients [11]. Finally, descending inhibitory influences on pain beginning in the nucleus gigantocellularis, the bulbar raphe nuclei and the periaqueductal grey and parabrachial nuclei might be compromised in PD [48].

Impact of chronic pain in patients with Parkinson's disease

There is little information available about the impact of chronic pain in PD patients. The DoPaMiP survey revealed that pain in PD was associated with higher scores for depression as measured with the Hospital Anxiety and Depression Scale [11]. The same was true for health-related quality of life as measured with the Parkinson's Disease Questionnaire (PDQ-39) [11]. After adjustments for other factors (including disease severity), possible/probable depressive signs were found to be significantly correlated with the presence of parkinsonian pain compared with a group of PD patients who did not suffer from chronic pain. Whether pain is a factor contributing to depression or vice versa remains to be explored. In other surveys, depression has also been reported to be more severe in PD patients with pain, although the overall prevalence of depression in these patients was no higher than that in patients without pain [19,49]. Conversely, while sleep problems are commonly reported in PD patients with or without pain, no clear correlation has been reported between these two symptoms [11,49].

Caring for patients with Parkinson's disease suffering from chronic pain

The medical literature contains very few data on this topic. To illustrate this we can quote the Movement Disorder Society's Evidence-Based Medicine Review which offers an exhaustive up-to-date analysis of the level of proof of all treatments used in PD. However, it does not once mention the question of caring for patients suffering from pain due to PD [50,51].

In the DoPaMiP survey, analysis of analgesic consumption showed that about 50% of patients who presented with chronic pain caused by PD took at least one analgesic during the previous month [11]. Level I analgesics (according to the World Health Organization definition) were the most frequently consumed, in particular paracetamol. Overall, the consumption of analgesics was significantly lower in this group than in PD patients who suffered from chronic pain caused by a disorder other than PD (68%) and in patients suffering from a chronic disorder other than PD who also had chronic pain (70%). This difference was observed despite greater indices of pain intensity and impact on health-related quality of life in the PD patients with PD pain. About 20% of the patients in the DoPaMiP survey with chronic pain caused or aggravated by their disease also took level II–III analgesics or co-analgesics (opiates, antidepressants, antiepileptics or benzodiazepines). These results are in agreement with other studies [52]. Most notably, analgesic drug prescription was compared between PD patients ($n = 11\,466$), diabetes patients ($n = 11\,459$), osteoarthritis patients ($n = 11\,329$) and the general population ($n = 11\,200$) in the database of the French health insurance system [53]. Analgesic drugs were prescribed more frequently to PD patients than to the general population (82% versus 77%, $P < 0.0001$) but less frequently than that to patients with osteoarthritis (90%, $P < 0.0001$).

This lower level of analgesic consumption in cases of chronic pain caused by PD compared with pain of other origin deserves further exploration. Several possibilities may explain this observation. It may reflect the low frequency with which PD patients report such pain to their physicians, as opposed to other types of pain. It may also reflect the poor knowledge that doctors have of painful parkinsonian symptoms. It is also possible that a poor understanding of the mechanisms underlying parkinsonian pain has raised doubts about the efficacy of analgesics in this situation, or that other types of management, such as dopaminergic drug adjustment, are preferred. Indeed, analgesics have never proven their efficacy for this type of pain and the level of evidence for their use in this condition is low.

Therefore it would appear legitimate to question the prescription and consumption of analgesics in this population in the future because their efficacy and safety have not been evaluated specifically for the treatment of PD pain. On the other hand, preliminary evidence from double-blind controlled clinical trials suggests that transdermal rotigotine or cranial electrotherapy stimulation might be effective for pain control in PD [52]. Furthermore, results from open-label studies warrant further research on duloxetine, a norepinephrine and serotonin reuptake blocker, stimulation or lesion of subthalamic or pallidum nuclei or levodopa. Finally, some case reports indicate that repetitive transcranial magnetic stimulation or apomorphine could be effective for relieving painful 'off'-period dystonia.

In practice, without objective data and a high level of evidence, empiricism and clinical common sense are still necessary [25,54,55]. It is essential to question and examine patients thoroughly to identify the presence or absence of pain and define the type of pain and its possible mechanism(s). Indeed, in certain cases patients do not spontaneously report their pain, maybe due to cultural acceptance of illness, resignation or fatalism, and instead focus their complaints on other symptoms. Likewise, doctors commonly do not ask the patient about the possible presence of pain or do not hear them complain about it, perhaps for the same reasons.

Whenever a link is suspected between pain, motor symptoms, fluctuations and dopamine response, efforts must be made to optimize the antiparkinsonian treatment, for example by adjusting the levodopa dose, adding a dopamine agonist, a monoamine oxidase B or catechol-O-methyltransferase inhibitor, or the use of injectable subcutaneous apomorphine, enteral levodopa/caridopa infusion or even functional surgery (stimulation of subthalamic nuclei) [52]. Pain dues to such apparently different causes as painful dystonias—whether from 'early morning' or 'off' periods—and painful pseudo-neuropathic syndromes observed during 'off' periods can benefit from this strategy. Of course, if the pain appears to be related to 'on' episodes, as can be the case in radicular pain due to osteoarticular conditions made worse by peak-dose dyskinesias, the antiparkinsonian treatment should be adapted accordingly, adjusting the dose and prescribing amantadine to treat dyskinesia or, again, considering functional surgery.

In some cases, it is impossible to establish a convincing link between the evolution of pain and the effect of antiparkinsonian medication. It is not always possible to adjust antiparkinsonian medications sufficiently to obtain the desired analgesic effect. In such a situation, one may well turn to non-specific, symptomatic treatments for pain, starting with level I analgesics and then co-analgesics, despite any convincing placebo-controlled studies [52], with the hope of achieving at least a placebo effect [56]. Whether it is a medical prescription or self-medication, polymedication and extended prescriptions renewed without re-evaluation should be strongly discouraged. This is particularly true in the case of level II (opiate) analgesics and co-analgesics (antidepressants and antiepileptics) due to the risk of adverse drug reactions and drug interactions to which such practice exposes patients. On the other hand, behavioural therapies and a global approach to pain, as are usually offered by specialized centres in this field, might be more effective than isolated drug strategies.

In summary, chronic pain constitutes a common, yet still too often neglected, symptom of PD that is likely to have a significant impact on the everyday lives of many PD patients. The broad spectrum of clinical pictures of pain; its complexity and our ignorance of underlying mechanisms, whether or not they are dopamine-responsive; and the absence of an evaluation of the benefit/risk relationship of any specific therapeutic strategy often leaves the doctor helpless and the patient frustrated. We must fill the gaps in symptomatology, physiology and pathology, pharmacology and therapy to improve this situation.

References

1 **Chaudhuri KR, Healy DG, Schapira AH**. Non-motor symptoms of Parkinson's disease: diagnosis and management. Lancet Neurol 2006; **5**: 235–45.

2 **Witjas T, Kaphan E, Azulay JP, et al**. Nonmotor fluctuations in Parkinson's disease: frequent and disabling. Neurology 2002; **59**: 408–13.

3 **Beiske AG, Loge JH, Ronningen A, Svensson E**. Pain in Parkinson's disease: prevalence and characteristics. Pain 2009; **141**: 173–7.

4 **Broen MP, Braaksma MM, Patijn J, Weber WE**. Prevalence of pain in Parkinson's disease: a systematic review using the modified QUADAS tool. Mov Disord 2012; **27**: 480–4.

5 **Broetz D, Eichner M, Gasser T, et al**. Radicular and nonradicular back pain in Parkinson's disease: a controlled study. Mov Disord 2007; **22**: 853–6.

6 **Defazio G, Berardelli A, Fabbrini G, et al**. Pain as a nonmotor symptom of Parkinson disease: evidence from a case-control study. Arch Neurol 2008; **65**: 1191–4.

7 **Etchepare F, Rozenberg S, Mirault T, et al**. Back problems in Parkinson's disease: an underestimated problem. Joint Bone Spine 2006; **73**: 298–302.

8 **Giuffrida R, Vingerhoets FJ, Bogousslavsky J, Ghika J**. [Pain in Parkinson's disease]. Rev Neurol (Paris) 2005; **161**: 407–18.

9 **Hanagasi HA, Akat S, Gurvit H, et al**. Pain is common in Parkinson's disease. Clin Neurol Neurosurg 2011; **113**: 11–13.

10 **Lee MA, Walker RW, Hildreth TJ, Prentice WM**. A survey of pain in idiopathic Parkinson's disease. J Pain Symptom Manage 2006; **32**: 462–9.

11 **Negre-Pages L, Regragui W, Bouhassira D, et al**. Chronic pain in Parkinson's disease: the cross-sectional French DoPaMiP survey. Mov Disord 2008; **23**: 1361–9.

12 **Quittenbaum BH, Grahn B**. Quality of life and pain in Parkinson's disease: a controlled cross-sectional study. Parkinsonism Relat Disord 2004; **10**: 129–36.

13 **Defazio G, Gigante A, Mancino P, Tinazzi M**. The epidemiology of pain in Parkinson's disease. J Neural Transm 2013; **120**: 583–6.

14 **Skogar O, Fall PA, Hallgren G, et al**. Parkinson's disease patients' subjective descriptions of characteristics of chronic pain, sleeping patterns and health-related quality of life. Neuropsychiatr Dis Treat 2012; **8**: 435–42.

15 **Ford B**. Pain in Parkinson's disease. Mov Disord 2010; **25**(Suppl 1): S98–S103.

16 **Farnikova K, Krobot A, Kanovsky P**. Musculoskeletal problems as an initial manifestation of Parkinson's disease: a retrospective study. J Neurol Sci 2012; **319**: 102–4.

17 **Breivik H, Collett B, Ventafridda V, et al**. Survey of chronic pain in Europe: prevalence, impact on daily life, and treatment. Eur J Pain 2006; **10**: 287–333.

18 **Goetz CG, Tanner CM, Levy M, et al**. Pain in Parkinson's disease. Mov Disord 1986; **1**: 45–9.

19 **Tinazzi M, Del VC, Fincati E, et al**. Pain and motor complications in Parkinson's disease. J Neurol Neurosurg Psychiatry 2006; **77**: 822–5.

20 **Vaserman-Lehuede N, Verin M**. Shoulder pain in patients with Parkinson's disease. Rev Rhum Engl Ed 1999; **66**: 220–3.

21 **Stamey W, Davidson A, Jankovic J**. Shoulder pain: a presenting symptom of Parkinson disease. J Clin Rheumatol 2008; **14**: 253–4.

22 **Bouhassira D, Attal N, Fermanian J, et al**. Development and validation of the Neuropathic Pain Symptom Inventory. Pain 2004; **108**: 248–57.

23 **Ford B, Louis ED, Greene P, Fahn S**. Oral and genital pain syndromes in Parkinson's disease. Mov Disord 1996; **11**: 421–6.

24 **Quinn NP, Koller WC, Lang AE, Marsden CD**. Painful Parkinson's disease. Lancet 1986; **1**: 1366–9.

25 **Wasner G, Deuschl G**. Pains in Parkinson disease—many syndromes under one umbrella. Nat Rev Neurol 2012; **8**: 284–94.

26 **Melamed E, Djaldetti R**. Camptocormia in Parkinson's disease. J Neurol 2006; 253(Suppl 7): VII14–VII16.

27 **Brefel-Courbon C, Payoux P, Thalamas C, et al**. Effect of levodopa on pain threshold in Parkinson's disease: a clinical and positron emission tomography study. Mov Disord 2005; **20**: 1557–63.

28 **Djaldetti R, Shifrin A, Rogowski Z, et al**. Quantitative measurement of pain sensation in patients with Parkinson disease. Neurology 2004; **62**: 2171–5.

29 **Storch A, Schneider CB, Wolz M, et al**. Nonmotor fluctuations in Parkinson disease: Severity and correlation with motor complications. Neurology 2013; **80**: 800–9.

30 **Nebe A, Ebersbach G**. Pain intensity on and off levodopa in patients with Parkinson's disease. Mov Disord 2009; **24**: 1233–7.

31 **Dellapina E, Ory-Magne F, Regragui W, et al**. Effect of subthalamic deep brain stimulation on pain in Parkinson's disease. Pain 2012; **153**: 2267–73.

32 **Chudler EH, Dong WK**. The role of the basal ganglia in nociception and pain. Pain 1995; **60**: 3–38.

33 **Pay S, Barasi S**. A study of the connections of nociceptive substantia nigra neurones. Pain 1982; **12**: 75–89.

34 **Heise CE, Reyes S, Mitrofanis J**. Sensory (nociceptive) stimulation evokes Fos expression in the subthalamus of hemiparkinsonian rats. Neurol Res 2008; **30**: 277–84.

35 **Chudler EH, Lu Y**. Nociceptive behavioral responses to chemical, thermal and mechanical stimulation after unilateral, intrastriatal administration of 6-hydroxydopamine. Brain Res 2008; **1213**: 41–7.

36 **Chen CC, Shih YY, Chang C**. Dopaminergic imaging of nonmotor manifestations in a rat model of Parkinson's disease by fMRI. Neurobiol Dis 2012; **49C**: 99–106.

37 **Paalzow GH**. L-dopa induces opposing effects on pain in intact rats: (-)-sulpiride, SCH 23390 or alpha-methyl-DL-p-tyrosine methylester hydrochloride reveals profound hyperalgesia in large antinociceptive doses. J Pharmacol Exp Ther 1992; **263**: 470–9.

38 **Tracey I, Becerra L, Chang I, et al**. Noxious hot and cold stimulation produce common patterns of brain activation in humans: a functional magnetic resonance imaging study. Neurosci Lett 2000; **288**: 159–62.

39 **Jaaskelainen SK, Rinne JO, Forssell H, et al**. Role of the dopaminergic system in chronic pain—a fluorodopa-PET study. Pain 2001; **90**: 257–60.

40 **Stuginski-Barbosa J, Rodrigues GG, Bigal ME, Speciali JG**. Burning mouth syndrome responsive to pramipexol. J Headache Pain 2008; **9**: 43–5.

41 **Jarcho JM, Mayer EA, Jiang ZK, et al**. Pain, affective symptoms, and cognitive deficits in patients with cerebral dopamine dysfunction. Pain 2012; **153**: 744–54.

42 **Juri C, Rodriguez-Oroz M, Obeso JA**. The pathophysiological basis of sensory disturbances in Parkinson's disease. J Neurol Sci 2010; **289**: 60–5.

43 **Gerdelat-Mas A, Simonetta-Moreau M, Thalamas C, et al.** Levodopa raises objective pain threshold in Parkinson's disease: a RIII reflex study. J Neurol Neurosurg Psychiatry 2007; **78**: 1140–2.

44 **Slaoui T, Mas-Gerdelat A, Ory-Magne F, et al.** Levodopa modifies pain thresholds in Parkinson's disease patients. Rev Neurol (Paris) 2007; **163**: 66–71.

45 **Schestatsky P, Kumru H, Valls-Sole J, et al.** Neurophysiologic study of central pain in patients with Parkinson disease. Neurology 2007; **69**: 2162–9.

46 **Tinazzi M, Del VC, Defazio G, et al.** Abnormal processing of the nociceptive input in Parkinson's disease: a study with CO_2 laser evoked potentials. Pain 2008; **136**: 117–24.

47 **Braak H, Sastre M, Bohl JR, et al.** Parkinson's disease: lesions in dorsal horn layer I, involvement of parasympathetic and sympathetic pre- and postganglionic neurons. Acta Neuropathol 2007; **113**: 421–9.

48 **Scherder E, Wolters E, Polman C, et al.** Pain in Parkinson's disease and multiple sclerosis: its relation to the medial and lateral pain systems. Neurosci Biobehav Rev 2005; **29**: 1047–56.

49 **Goetz CG, Wilson RS, Tanner CM, Garron DC.** Relationships among pain, depression, and sleep alterations in Parkinson's disease. Adv Neurol 1987; **45**: 345–7.

50 **Goetz CG, Poewe W, Rascol O, Sampaio C.** Evidence-based medical review update: pharmacological and surgical treatments of Parkinson's disease: 2001 to 2004. Mov Disord 2005; **20**: 523–39.

51 **Seppi K, Weintraub D, Coelho M, et al.** The Movement Disorder Society Evidence-Based Medicine Review Update: treatments for the non-motor symptoms of Parkinson's disease. Mov Disord 2011; **26**(Suppl 3): S42–S80.

52 **Perez-Lloret S, Rey MV, Dellapina E, et al.** Emerging analgesic drugs for Parkinson's disease. Expert Opin Emerg Drugs 2012; **17**: 157–71.

53 **Brefel-Courbon C, Grolleau S, Thalamas C, et al.** Comparison of chronic analgesic drugs prevalence in Parkinson's disease, other chronic diseases and the general population. Pain 2009; **141**: 14–18.

54 **Ha AD, Jankovic J.** Pain in Parkinson's disease. Mov Disord 2012; **27**: 485–91.

55 **Sophie M, Ford B.** Management of pain in Parkinson's disease. CNS Drugs 2012; **26**: 937–48.

56 **Colloca L, Lopiano L, Lanotte M, Benedetti F.** Overt versus covert treatment for pain, anxiety, and Parkinson's disease. Lancet Neurol 2004; **3**: 679–84.

Chapter 24

Visual function in Parkinson's disease

T. Baba, I. Estrada-Bellmann, E. Mori and A. Takeda

Introduction

Visual problems are common in Parkinson's disease (PD). A wide variety of visual symptoms have been described in PD, including blurred vision, diplopia, impaired colour vision, contrast insensitivity and visuospatial deficits [1]. Additionally, about a third of PD patients undergoing long-term dopaminergic treatment can present with visual hallucinations [2], although they may occur independently of dopaminergic medication. These symptoms affect the daily life of PD patients to varying degrees, and visual hallucinations in particular may be followed by cognitive decline and nursing home placement [3].

The neural basis of visual dysfunction in PD is not completely understood, but a combination of impairments in both bottom-up and top-down visual processing (i.e. the afferent flow of visual information and higher-order cognitive influences, respectively) may play a fundamental role [4–6]. Emerging evidence suggests that several levels of the visual pathway, from the retina to the primary visual cortex (the geniculostriate pathway), are preferentially affected in PD, causing impaired bottom-up visual processing [4]. Moreover, several functional imaging studies have reported alterations in top-down modulation of visual processing in PD, especially in association with visual hallucinations [7–9]. It seems to be plausible that many of the visual symptoms in PD can be explained by the interplay between these two mechanisms. This view may be somewhat oversimplified because it neglects the contribution of attentional deficits, brainstem dysregulation and the effects of administered drugs on visual function in PD [1,10,11]. However, such a systematic perspective will be helpful for a better understanding of the complexity of the visual symptoms in PD.

Overview of visual processing

It is generally thought that visual information is analysed at three levels—low, intermediate and high [12]. Particular sets of brain structures in the visual pathway are involved in each of these levels, with some overlap (Fig. 24.1).

Initially, elementary features of a visual scene, such as local contrast, orientation, colour and motion, are discriminated by low-level visual processing [13]. This first stage of visual processing starts at the retina [4]. The photoreceptor cells located in the outermost layer of the retina absorb light, and from there visual transduction starts. Then, retinal bipolar

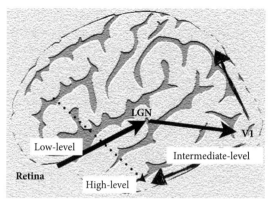

Fig. 24.1 Overview of visual processing. Visual information is analysed at three levels—low, intermediate and high. Solid lines suggest the bottom-up flow of visual information and the dotted line indicates the top-down modulation of visual information. Low-level visual information is processed in the geniculostriate pathway from the retina through the lateral geniculate nucleus (LGN) into the primary visual cortex. Low-level visual information is integrated into intermediate-level visual processing and delivered to the inferior temporal cortex, which is considered as the centre of high-level visual processing and the target of top-down modulation from various regions such as the prefrontal cortex and medial temporal lobe.

cells transfer the light signal to the retinal ganglion cells located in the inner retina. After leaving the retina, visual information is relayed via thalamic nuclei, including the lateral geniculate nucleus (LGN) and pulvinar, to the primary visual cortex (area V1). In this way, the retinal circuitry decomposes the retinal image into signals representing contrast, colour and movement.

Next, low-level visual information is assembled into contours and surfaces, and then those combined features are assigned to the representations of specific objects or background in intermediate-level visual processing. Many cortical areas are involved in these processes. Area V1 plays a role in contour integration and surface segmentation, in addition to the low-level perception of orientation and colour [13,14]. From area V1, visual information flows into the parietal lobe (dorsal stream) and the temporal lobe (ventral stream) [15]. The dorsal stream is involved in the analysis of movement and spatial localization. In contrast, the ventral stream, which contributes to object recognition, runs from areas V1 and V2 to area V4 and then into the high-level processing stage. In this way, elementary visual features are assembled into unified representations of objects and background, and the information is utilized as bottom-up signals in the next step.

Finally, object recognition is accomplished in high-level visual processing by the interplay between bottom-up inputs derived from the preceding stages and top-down signals converging from a variety of sources. The inferior temporal cortex plays a central role in high-level visual processing [16]. This area is known as the end stage of the ventral stream. Beyond the primary and secondary visual cortices, the ventral stream goes through the temporo-occipital (TPO) junction and culminates in the inferior temporal cortex [17,18].

In addition, it receives inputs from various cortical areas, including the prefrontal cortex and medial temporal lobe, and serves as a target of top-down modulation [18,19]. It is clinically well known that a lesion in the inferior temporal cortex causes impaired object recognition, known as visual agnosia [20]. Thus, the inferior temporal cortex, where bottom-up and top-down signals meet, is thought of as the primary centre for object recognition.

We will now discuss patterns of visual dysfunctions in PD, emphasizing their association with these visual processing stages.

Impairment in low-level visual processing in Parkinson's disease

As already mentioned, low-level visual processing starts at the retina and resolves the retinal image into minimal units of information concerned with contrast, colour and movement [4]. The retina comprises three layers of cell bodies and two interposed layers of fibres and synapses. It is known that dopaminergic cell bodies are located within the layer of amacrine cells at the border of the inner nuclear and inner plexiform layers. Dopamine exerts multiple effects on retinal cells, and helps to switch the active visual pathway from being rod-mediated to cone-mediated during periods of light—the process known as light adaptation [12].

Contrast sensitivity

In PD, marked dopaminergic deficiency is evident in the retina, in addition to the degeneration of nigrostriatal dopaminergic neurons [21,22]. Various visual impairments in PD are attributed to dopamine depletion within the retinal circuitry; one of the most well-known visual impairments is abnormal contrast sensitivity [23]. Contrast sensitivity is the visual ability to distinguish differences in luminance. Contrast sensitivity is predominantly regulated by the mechanisms of light adaptation, leading to perceptual constancy of contrast under varying conditions of illumination. Thus, dopamine depletion, either due to PD itself or during relatively unmedicated periods such as overnight, may cause altered light adaptation and result in contrast insensitivity, especially in the medium spectral frequencies at which human contrast perception is most sensitive [13]. Supporting this notion, the restoration of a normal spatial tuning function was noted upon the administration of levodopa [24,25]. Furthermore, it has been suggested that drug-induced parkinsonism exhibits deficits in contrast sensitivity in a pattern similar to that of PD [26]. Conversely, during levodopa-induced dyskinesias, a period of dopaminergic overstimulation, patients may experience pathologically increased inhibition of the 'surround' input for short periods of time, causing contrast sensitivity to fluctuate rapidly, leading to complaints of blurred vision [13,27].

Overall, dopamine is a vital neuromodulator for light adaptation. It seems likely that contrast insensitivity in PD may stem from the lack of retinal dopamine. However, orientation-specific loss of contrast sensitivity is observed in some PD patients which cannot be explained just by the retinal dysfunction, and the cortical influence on contrast insensitivity remains controversial [24,28].

Colour vision

Colour vision also begins in the retina [12]. In general, primates have three types of cone photoreceptors, distinguished on the basis of their wavelength preferences, specifically red, green and blue cones. Light stimuli absorbed in these photoreceptors are transformed into active potentials in the retinal bipolar cells and transmitted to the retinal ganglion cells. From the retinal ganglion cells, visual information is carried into the LGN and the primary visual cortex via segregated parallel visual pathways: parvocellular, magnocellular and koniocellular pathways. Among them, the parvocellular (red–green) and koniocellular (blue–yellow) pathways are involved in colour vision, whereas the magnocellular pathway has a major role in contrast vision. After the primary visual cortex, colour information is analysed as object surface information at subsequent processing stages.

Reduced colour vision is often an early feature of PD, and the most prominent deficits have been shown to be in the tritan (blue–yellow) axis [29,30]. Abnormality in the tritan axis in PD may be due to the simple fact that blue cones are more sparsely distributed in the retina and also lack surround inhibition, thus leaving the tritan axis particularly vulnerable. The Lanthony D-15 test and the Farnsworth–Munsell 100-hue test are the most widely used in the clinic for testing colour discrimination, but these tests have limited quantitative power. Thus, it may be somewhat difficult to detect impairments in colour vision in the early stages of PD, leading to inconsistent results [29,31]. Using more sophisticated colour discrimination tasks, a recent study suggested that the impairment in the tritan axis is due to normal ageing, and impaired protan (red–green)/deutan (luminance) axes are specific to PD [32]. It is also known that colour discrimination becomes worse with the progression of PD. Retinal dopaminergic deficiency may play a role in the colour discrimination deficits in PD, but many regions along the visual pathway participate in colour vision, and it is difficult to attribute impaired colour vision to retinal dysfunction alone. In addition, a recent study suggested that impaired colour vision is accompanied by a pre-motor parkinsonian state characterized by several non-motor symptoms including rapid eye movement sleep behaviour disorder [33].

Motion perception

Retinal ganglion cells and neurons in the LGN have concentric centre-surround receptive fields. These types of receptive fields are sensitive to moving objects. In low-level visual processing, information about an object's movement is transferred mainly by the magnocellular pathway. It has been thought that a dysfunction in the magnocellular pathway may cause a deficit in motion perception in PD, but a recent study described dorsal stream impairment as more important [34,35].

Impairment in intermediate-level visual processing in Parkinson's disease

In intermediate-level visual processing, low-level visual information is assembled into contours and surfaces through a hierarchy of cortical areas (Fig. 24.2 and Plate 5). It is

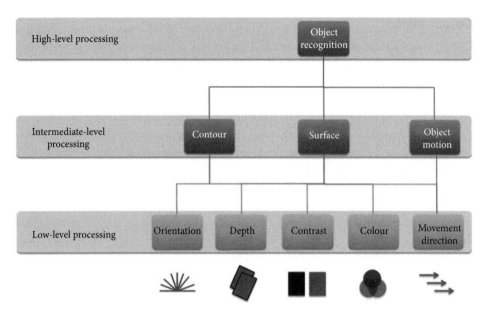

Fig. 24.2 The visual system is organized in both a hierarchical and a parallel manner. Low-level visual information is integrated at the intermediate-level processing stage. (See also Plate 5)

widely accepted that intermediate-level visual areas fall into two distinct streams, ventral and dorsal streams. The ventral stream is involved in object recognition, and the dorsal stream is engaged in the analysis of movement and spatial localization [12].

The following paragraphs describe how visual information is processed in each visual area (V1–V5) in the intermediate-level processing stage.

Area V1 is located on the surface of the occipital cortex, which receives inputs from the LGN and sends their projections into the ventral and dorsal streams. This area has orientation columns and blobs (clusters of colour-selective neurons). Orientation specificity, surface texture information and the integration of inputs from both eyes are developed in this area, leading to contour integration and surface segmentation.

Area V2 analyses information about an object's surface and depth (binocular disparity). It is also reported that this area responds to illusory contour stimuli. In addition, information from the magnocellular pathway enters the dorsal stream through areas V1 and V2. Area V4 is included in the ventral stream, and this area integrates information about colour and object shape, whereas area V5/MT is involved in the dorsal stream, integrates motion signals across space and is involved in the control of ocular movement.

There is evidence that intermediate-level visual processing is also impaired in PD. Imaging studies have demonstrated reduced metabolism and hypoperfusion in the occipital cortex as early characteristics of PD [36,37]. Furthermore, recent studies suggested that cortical cholinergic dysfunction occurs in the occipital cortex in early PD. The distribution of these radiographic abnormalities extends to higher-order visual areas along with disease progression in PD. Moreover, a pathological study demonstrated that the visual association cortex is among the most vulnerable cortical regions in PD [38]. Based on these findings, it is little wonder that damage to intermediate-level visual areas causes various visual symptoms in PD. In fact, impairments in orientation and motion perception are frequently described. Furthermore, pre-attentive 'pop-out' of complex shapes, a phenomenon that is attributed to early visual cortical processing, is also impaired in PD [39].

There is insufficient evidence at present about impairments in contour integration and surface segmentation in PD. However, a recent study using the overlapping figure identification test seems to have provided an important clue. This test consists of overlapping line drawings of objects, for all of which the subjects are instructed to provide names (Fig. 24.3). In order to succeed at this task, it is necessary to detect the edges of objects and to correctly identify which edge belongs to which object. Thus proper contour integration and surface segmentation abilities are required to accomplish this test. Mori and colleagues [40] used this test for dementia with Lewy bodies (DLB), and reported significant impairments in DLB patients. Recently, the overlapping figure identification test was used for the assessment of PD, and the results suggested that ventral pathway dysfunction is associated with incorrect responses in this task [41], although the most prominent correlation was observed at the TPO junction (which participates in high-level visual processing).

Impairment in intermediate-level visual processing may lead to various visuoperceptual dysfunctions in PD, although we still do not have the full picture.

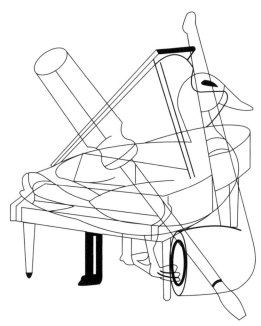

Fig. 24.3 The overlapping figure identification test. In this example, achromatic line drawings of a duck, a grand piano, a pipe and a flathead screwdriver overlap one another. Subjects are instructed to name all the objects.

Reproduced with permission from Ishioka T, Hirayama K, Hosokai Y, Takeda A, Suzuki K, Nishio Y, et al. Illusory misidentifications and cortical hypometabolism in Parkinson's disease. Mov Disord 2011; 26(5): 837–43.

Impairment in high-level visual processing in Parkinson's disease

Neurons in the inferior temporal cortex respond to complex visual stimuli, and dysfunction in this area causes impaired object recognition. A lesion in this area is known to cause impaired object recognition (visual agnosia) [20]. Indeed, impairments in object shape recognition were demonstrated in PD, and this finding may reflect a dysfunction in high-level visual processing. Impairment of high-level visual processing may also be involved in the pathogenesis of visual hallucinations in PD.

Visual hallucination occurs in about a third of PD patients during long-term dopaminergic therapy [11]. Visual hallucinations may also occur independently of dopaminergic therapy, based on reports from the pre-levodopa era, which suggests that dopaminergic medication is not the direct cause but seems to serve as a precipitating factor. In general, visual hallucinations are categorized into complex visual hallucinations and other minor hallucinations. Complex visual hallucinations have specific forms and are often animate, while other minor hallucinations include passage and presence hallucinations. These hallucinations affect activities of daily life in PD, and they are also known as a risk factor for nursing home placement and the development of dementia [3]. Thus, we need to understand the characteristics of these symptoms. Many factors are assumed to be involved in the pathogenesis of visual hallucinations in PD [10], such as dopaminergic overactivation, cholinergic deficits [42], retinal dysfunction, alteration in the sleep–wake cycle and impaired attention. However, an imbalance between bottom-up visual processing and top-down modulation may play an important role in the development of visual hallucinations in PD [5]. In the context of impairment of bottom-up visual processing, the occurrence of visual hallucinations has been thought of as a type of Charles Bonnet syndrome [43]. Furthermore, it has been shown that PD patients whose performance in the Lanthony D-15 colour test is one standard deviation below the mean have more than a four-fold increased risk of experiencing visual hallucinations [44]. In imaging studies, both hypoperfusion in the inferior temporal cortex and hyperperfusion/hypermetabolism in the frontal cortex were shown to be associated with visual hallucinations [7–9]. Pathological extension to the temporal lobe and amygdala was also reported to be associated with visual hallucinations in PD [45]. It has been suggested that visual hallucinations in PD might occur due to a dysregulation of gating and filtering of external perception and internal image production, but the pathogenesis of visual hallucinations in PD remains uncertain [43].

Despite its importance, there is no gold standard for testing and rating visual hallucinations in PD. The Unified Parkinson's Disease Rating Scale and the Neuropsychiatric Inventory have been used, but they have limitations in their detection sensitivity for visual hallucinations. Recently, the pareidolia test was invented as a tool to elicit visual hallucinations in the clinical setting [46], and the utility of this test for assessing visual hallucinations in DLB has been demonstrated (Fig. 24.4 and Plate 6). Considering the symptomatic similarities in the visual hallucinations of DLB and PD, it is expected that this test will also be useful for the evaluation of PD patients.

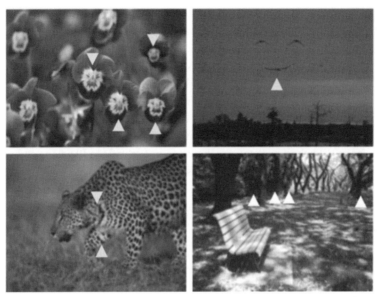

Fig. 24.4 Examples of the pareidolia test. Patients with dementia with Lewy bodies often misidentify objects or patterns in a picture as human faces (top left, top right and bottom left) or as people and animals (bottom right). (See also Plate 6)

Reproduced with permission from Uchiyama M, Nishio Y, Yokoi K, Hirayama K, Imamura T, Shimomura T, et al. Pareidolias: complex visual illusions in dementia with Lewy bodies. Brain: a Journal of Neurology 2012; 135(8): 2458–69.

Other visual symptoms in Parkinson's disease

Up to this point, we have discussed visual dysfunctions in PD and their relationship to the stages of visual processing. However, there are visual symptoms in PD patients that originate from outside the visual pathways, and these include abnormal ocular or eyelid movements (including diplopia). Ocular signs in PD are usually subtle, and studies have reported a high frequency of oculomotor signs and symptoms in PD patients with early, untreated disease, as well as those with moderate to late-stage PD. Deficits include disordered dynamic eye movements such as saccades and pursuit, convergence insufficiency, decreased blink rate, square wave jerks, blepharospasm, apraxia of eyelid opening and ocular micro-tremor [47].

Symptoms associated with oculomotor abnormalities include diplopia and difficulty reading, although the exact interplay between oculomotor abnormalities and the actual symptoms reported by patients has yet to be definitively elucidated.

Ocular movements

In PD, saccadic eye movements are often slow and hypometric, especially during vertical movements. The saccades most commonly affected are those conducted towards the remembered location of a previous visual target after its stimulus has been lost (so-called remembered saccades) [47]. In addition to impaired saccadic movements, abnormalities in smooth pursuit eye movements are also impaired when following moving targets. The pursuit gain is reduced, and thus the eyes cannot keep up with the target, necessitating the aid of catch-up saccades to compensate. This results in a characteristic effect known as cogwheel pursuit, although despite the name, the underlying pathogenesis is different from cogwheel rigidity [48]. Fixation of the gaze on a specific visual target is often interrupted in PD via a phenomenon known as square wave jerks, which are back-to-back involuntary saccades of tiny amplitude that result in eye movement away from the fixed target and then rapidly back onto it again. Such movements are, however, not specific to PD alone and may occur in normal individuals. Following the administration of levodopa, an improvement is seen in saccadic accuracy and smooth pursuit gain, thus implicating dopamine or a downstream neurotransmitter system modulated by dopamine in controlling aspects of ocular movement.

Diplopia

Diplopia is a relatively common complaint in PD patients with normal visual acuity. One study described that more than a third of patients with PD reported symptoms consistent with diplopia. The recently reported NMSQuest study has suggested that diplopia may be under-reported and therefore an under-diagnosed problem in PD [49]. Bye and Chaudhuri [50], comparing a subset of 11 treated PD patients with and without symptomatic diplopia, reported that those with diplopia suffered a longer duration of PD (mean 9.5 years) than those without diplopia (mean 3.0 years). This suggests that diplopia may be more prevalent in PD sufferers with moderate-advanced stage disease than in patients with early-stage disease [47]. The mechanism of diplopia in PD is still unclear, although Bye and Chaudhuri [50] found that 64% of a diplopia group versus just 33% of a control group had demonstrable convergence insufficiency, supporting the previous study.

Nebe and Ebersach [51] reported a 'selective diplopia', in which double vision was limited to the duplication of single objects. All but one subject in this study reported that the double vision effect was extinguished when one eye was covered, thus indicating a binocular cause, correlating with the work of Bye and Chaudhuri. They also reported that more than half of the patients were suffering from current or previous visual hallucinations and three more patients developed hallucinations within 3 years of the onset of diplopia. These results raise the possibility that, in addition to distorted higher-level visual processing, selective diplopia is also related to the pathogenesis of visual hallucinations in PD. Furthermore, a link between dopaminergic medication and the onset of symptoms was reported in some cases.

Taken together, these studies on diplopia indicate a multifactorial aetiology, including subtle oculomotor abnormalities and convergence insufficiency, as well as a possible effect of medication.

Conclusions

A range of visual problems occurs in PD with varying frequency. Although the whole picture has not yet been elucidated, the underlying pathophysiology of visual dysfunction in PD has become clearer with recent advances in neuroscience. Emerging evidence suggests that impairments in both bottom-up and top-down visual processing are related to the visual deficits in PD. Additionally, oculomotor abnormalities may also influence visual function in PD. Further study is needed to untangle the complexity of visual symptoms in PD.

References

1 **Chaudhuri KR, Schapira AH**. Non-motor symptoms of Parkinson's disease: dopaminergic pathophysiology and treatment. Lancet Neurol 2009; **8**: 464–74.

2 **Barnes J, David AS**. Visual hallucinations in Parkinson's disease: a review and phenomenological survey. J Neurol Neurosurg Psychiatry 2001; **70**: 727–33.

3 **Goetz CG, Stebbins GT**. Risk factors for nursing home placement in advanced Parkinson's disease. Neurology 1993; **43**: 2227–9.

4 **Archibald NK, Clarke MP, Mosimann UP, Burn DJ**. The retina in Parkinson's disease. Brain 2009; **132**: 1128–45.

5 **Shine JM, Halliday GM, Naismith SL, Lewis SJ**. Visual misperceptions and hallucinations in Parkinson's disease: dysfunction of attentional control networks? Mov Disord 2011; **26**: 2154–9.

6 **Diederich NJ, Goetz CG, Stebbins GT**. Repeated visual hallucinations in Parkinson's disease as disturbed external/internal perceptions: focused review and a new integrative model. Mov Disord 2005; **20**: 130–40.

7 **Nagano-Saito A, Washimi Y, Arahata Y, et al**. Visual hallucination in Parkinson's disease with FDG PET. Mov Disord 2004; **19**: 801–6.

8 **Stebbins GT, Goetz CG, Carrillo MC, et al**. Altered cortical visual processing in PD with hallucinations: an fMRI study. Neurology 2004; **63**: 1409–16.

9 **Oishi N, Udaka F, Kameyama M, Sawamoto N, Hashikawa K, Fukuyama H**. Regional cerebral blood flow in Parkinson disease with nonpsychotic visual hallucinations. Neurology 2005; **65**: 1708–15.

10 **Gallagher DA, Parkkinen L, O'Sullivan SS, et al**. Testing an aetiological model of visual hallucinations in Parkinson's disease. Brain 2011; **134**: 3299–309.

11 **Diederich NJ, Fenelon G, Stebbins G, Goetz CG**. Hallucinations in Parkinson disease. Nat Rev Neurol 2009; **5**: 331–42.

12 **Kandel E, Schwartz J, Jessell T, Siegelbaum S, Hudspeth AJ**. Principles of neural science, 5th edn. New York: McGraw-Hill Education, 2012.

13 **Bodis-Wollner I, Marx MS, Mitra S, Bobak P, Mylin L, Yahr M**. Visual dysfunction in Parkinson's disease. Loss in spatiotemporal contrast sensitivity. Brain 1987; **110**: 1675–98.

14 **Tebartz van Elst L, Greenlee MW, Foley JM, Lucking CH**. Contrast detection, discrimination and adaptation in patients with Parkinson's disease and multiple system atrophy. Brain 1997; **120**: 2219–28.

15 **Van Essen DC, Gallant JL**. Neural mechanisms of form and motion processing in the primate visual system. Neuron 1994; **13**: 1–10.

16 **Sary G, Vogels R, Orban GA**. Cue-invariant shape selectivity of macaque inferior temporal neurons. Science 1993; **260**: 995–7.

17 **Malach R, Levy I, Hasson U**. The topography of high-order human object areas. Trends Cogn Sci 2002; **6**: 176–84.

18 **Miyashita Y**. Inferior temporal cortex: where visual perception meets memory. Ann Rev Neurosci 1993; **16**: 245–63.

19 **Webster MJ, Bachevalier J, Ungerleider LG.** Connections of inferior temporal areas TEO and TE with parietal and frontal cortex in macaque monkeys. Cereb Cortex 1994; **4**: 470–83.

20 **Ffytche DH, Blom JD, Catani M.** Disorders of visual perception. J Neurol Neurosurg Psychiatry 2010; **81**: 1280–7.

21 **Nguyen-Legros J.** Functional neuroarchitecture of the retina: hypothesis on the dysfunction of retinal dopaminergic circuitry in Parkinson's disease. Surg Radiol Anat 1988; **10**: 137–44.

22 **Harnois C, Di Paolo T.** Decreased dopamine in the retinas of patients with Parkinson's disease. Invest Ophthalmol Vis Sci 1990; **31**: 2473–5.

23 **Bulens C, Meerwaldt JD, van der Wildt GJ, Keemink CJ.** Contrast sensitivity in Parkinson's disease. Neurology 1986; **36**: 1121–5.

24 **Bulens C, Meerwaldt JD, Van der Wildt GJ.** Effect of stimulus orientation on contrast sensitivity in Parkinson's disease. Neurology 1988; **38**: 76–81.

25 **Hutton JT, Morris JL, Elias JW.** Levodopa improves spatial contrast sensitivity in Parkinson's disease. Arch Neurol 1993; **50**: 721–4.

26 **Bulens C, Meerwaldt JD, van der Wildt GJ, Keemink CJ.** Visual contrast sensitivity in drug-induced Parkinsonism. J Neurol Neurosurg Psychiatry 1989; **52**: 341–5.

27 **Bodis-Wollner I, Onofrj M.** The visual system in Parkinson's disease. Adv Neurol 1987; **45**: 323–7.

28 **Regan D, Maxner C.** Orientation-selective visual loss in patients with Parkinson's disease. Brain 1987; **110**: 415–32.

29 **Pieri V, Diederich NJ, Raman R, Goetz CG.** Decreased color discrimination and contrast sensitivity in Parkinson's disease. J Neurol Sci 2000; **172**: 7–11.

30 **Haug BA, Trenkwalder C, Arden GB, Oertel WH, Paulus W.** Visual thresholds to low-contrast pattern displacement, color contrast, and luminance contrast stimuli in Parkinson's disease. Mov Disord 1994; **9**: 563–70.

31 **Birch J, Kolle RU, Kunkel M, Paulus W, Upadhyay P.** Acquired colour deficiency in patients with Parkinson's disease. Vision Res 1998; **38**: 3421–6.

32 **Silva MF, Faria P, Regateiro FS, et al.** Independent patterns of damage within magno-, parvo- and koniocellular pathways in Parkinson's disease. Brain 2005; **128**: 2260–71.

33 **Postuma RB, Gagnon JF, Vendette M, Desjardins C, Montplaisir JY.** Olfaction and color vision identify impending neurodegeneration in rapid eye movement sleep behavior disorder. Ann Neurol 2011; **69**: 811–18.

34 **Uc EY, Rizzo M, Anderson SW, Qian S, Rodnitzky RL, Dawson JD.** Visual dysfunction in Parkinson disease without dementia. Neurology 2005; **65**: 1907–13.

35 **Castelo-Branco M, Mendes M, Silva F, et al.** Motion integration deficits are independent of magnocellular impairment in Parkinson's disease. Neuropsychologia 2009; **47**: 314–20.

36 **Bohnen NI, Minoshima S, Giordani B, Frey KA, Kuhl DE.** Motor correlates of occipital glucose hypometabolism in Parkinson's disease without dementia. Neurology 1999; **52**: 541–6.

37 **Hu MT, Taylor-Robinson SD, Chaudhuri KR, et al.** Cortical dysfunction in non-demented Parkinson's disease patients: a combined (31)P-MRS and (18)FDG-PET study. Brain 2000; **123**: 340–52.

38 **Braak H, Del Tredici K, Rub U, de Vos RA, Jansen Steur EN, Braak E.** Staging of brain pathology related to sporadic Parkinson's disease. Neurobiol Aging 2003; **24**: 197–211.

39 **Lieb K, Brucker S, Bach M, Els T, Lucking CH, Greenlee MW.** Impairment in preattentive visual processing in patients with Parkinson's disease. Brain 1999; **122**: 303–13.

40 **Mori E, Shimomura T, Fujimori M, et al.** Visuoperceptual impairment in dementia with Lewy bodies. Arch Neurol 2000; **57**: 489–93.

41 **Ishioka T, Hirayama K, Hosokai Y, et al.** Illusory misidentifications and cortical hypometabolism in Parkinson's disease. Mov Disord 2011; **26**: 837–43.

42 Manganelli F, Vitale C, Santangelo G, et al. Functional involvement of central cholinergic circuits and visual hallucinations in Parkinson's disease. Brain 2009; **132**: 2350–5.

43 Diederich NJ, Goetz CG, Raman R, Pappert EJ, Leurgans S, Piery V. Poor visual discrimination and visual hallucinations in Parkinson's disease. Clin Neuropharmacol 1998; **21**: 289–95.

44 Trick GL, Kaskie B, Steinman SB. Visual impairment in Parkinson's disease: deficits in orientation and motion discrimination. Optom Vis Sci 1994; **71**: 242–5.

45 Harding AJ, Stimson E, Henderson JM, Halliday GM. Clinical correlates of selective pathology in the amygdala of patients with Parkinson's disease. Brain 2002; **125**: 2431–45.

46 Uchiyama M, Nishio Y, Yokoi K, et al. Pareidolias: complex visual illusions in dementia with Lewy bodies. Brain 2012; **135**: 2458–69.

47 Biousse V, Skibell BC, Watts RL, Loupe DN, Drews-Botsch C, Newman NJ. Ophthalmologic features of Parkinson's disease. Neurology 2004; **62**: 177–80.

48 Waterston JA, Barnes GR, Grealy MA, Collins S. Abnormalities of smooth eye and head movement control in Parkinson's disease. Ann Neurol 1996; **39**: 749–60.

49 Chaudhuri KR, Martinez-Martin P, Schapira AH, et al. International multicenter pilot study of the first comprehensive self-completed nonmotor symptoms questionnaire for Parkinson's disease: the NMSQuest study. Mov Disord 2006; **21**: 916–23.

50 Bye L, Chaudhuri KR. Diplopia in Parkinson's disease: a clinical and optometric study. Mov Disord 2007; **22**: S182–S183.

51 Nebe A, Ebersbach G. Selective diplopia in Parkinson's disease: a special subtype of visual hallucination? Mov Disord 2007; **22**: 1175–8.

Section 3

Quality of life, co-morbidity, drug effects and surgery

Chapter 25

Non-motor symptoms and health-related quality of life: an overview

Pablo Martinez-Martin, Francisco J. Carod Artal and Jesus de Pedro Cuesta

Background

Quality of life and health-related quality of life

The term 'quality of life' (QoL) first surfaced in the public debate sparked by the deterioration of the environment and urban living conditions in western countries in the 1950s. It has since become a widely used expression, accorded different meanings and—more often than not—philosophical connotations linked to well-being and satisfaction in diverse aspects of life, as seen through the perspective of personal judgment and social standards. QoL has been defined by the World Health Organization (WHO) as an individual's 'perception of their position in life in the context of the culture and value systems in which they live and in relation to their goals, expectations, standards and concerns' [1]. However, there is no universally accepted definition of the QoL construct, as it lacks a gold standard and may be interpreted in a multitude of ways.

The QoL concept is multidimensional and is made up of many possible components connected with the individual, social networks, environment and society (e.g. vocational satisfaction, familial relationships, social status, spirituality and financial status). One such component is health, and the aspects related to it are collectively termed 'health-related QoL' (HRQoL). HRQoL may, in turn, be construed and defined in different ways. Schipper et al. [2] stated that 'QoL in clinical medicine represents the functional effect of an illness and its consequent therapy upon a patient, as perceived by the patient'. Following this definition, what HRQoL means in practical terms is the 'perception and evaluation, by patients themselves, of the impact that the disease and its consequences have on their life' [3]. Essentially, the components of the HRQoL concept are those contained in the WHO definition of health [4], namely symptoms and physical functioning, mental status and social well-being. Other aspects, such as role activities and global judgments of health and bodily appearance, are included in some measures of HRQoL.

Controversies concerning the conceptual framework, meaning and interpretation of HRQoL are frequent, yet the diversity of important applications based on the HRQoL measure has nevertheless promoted its use in clinical research and health policy. Indeed, beyond the debate, pragmatic application of HRQoL measures and growing interest in HRQoL outcomes have become the order of the day and, at present, these measures are commonly applied in areas such as clinical trials, evaluation of clinical practice and cost–benefit studies.

Assessment of health-related quality of life

HRQoL is assessed by means of questionnaires and other instruments which are diversely defined as addressing QoL, health status, functional well-being, subjective health, etc., a terminology intended to highlight the main purpose of a given tool. However, the terms 'health status' and 'HRQoL' are loosely used to embrace any type of tool designed to obtain information directly from individuals on their health and on the impact of their health status upon aspects of their lives, such as role functioning and social activities. The term 'patient-based outcome measure' is more comprehensive still [5].

This chapter focuses on HRQoL, and, while this will therefore be the preferred term, 'QoL' will at times be used interchangeably in line with normal usage in the clinical environment.

Depending upon the target population and concept to be assessed, HRQoL measures are classified as generic or specific. Generic instruments seek to evaluate the most important health domains (health profiles) or determine a value that is representative of health status in relation to perfect health (value = 1.0) and death (value = 0.0) (utility measures). These instruments are more appropriate for health programmes, general population health surveys and comparisons between groups or illnesses. Their disadvantage resides in their potential inability to address areas of specific interest and their lack of sensitivity for detecting change. Some of the most frequently used generic instruments applied to studies on Parkinson's disease (PD) are the Sickness Impact Profile, the Nottingham Health Profile (NHP), the Medical Outcomes Study Short Form (SF-36) health survey and the EuroQoL.

Specific instruments, in contrast, are aimed at assessing particular areas of interest for certain illnesses, populations or symptoms. Their advantage lies in their capacity to evaluate health problems that are highly prevalent in the specific setting of their application, and to detect change. Owing to their specificity, they are only useful for the concrete condition or population for which they have been designed. While specific instruments are more appropriate for clinical trials, their generic counterparts can also provide important data. Some of the most frequently used PD-specific HRQoL measures are: the Parkinson's Disease Questionnaire (PDQ-39), the Parkinson's Disease Quality of Life Questionnaire (PDQL), the Parkinson's Impact Scale (PIMS), the Parkinson's Disease Quality of Life Instrument (PDQUALIF) and Scales for Outcomes in PD–Psychosocial (SCOPA-PS).

Although clinical aspects, psychological factors, personal attitudes, social support and perception of health are unquestionably interrelated [6], some factors linked to the emotional and psychosocial impact of PD on patients continue to lie outside the scope of routine medical assessment. Measurement of HRQoL helps to identify and evaluate such factors and thereby enables interventions aimed at neutralizing their effect to be implemented. Furthermore, the side effects of therapy can have a strong impact on patients' HRQoL, so that assessment of HRQoL can also help when it comes to making decisions about treatment.

Health-related quality of life in Parkinson's disease

PD is a chronic, progressive disorder, characterized by typical motor manifestations which progress over time and give rise to growing physical disability. In advanced phases of the disease, with loss of mobility and inability to communicate, even the basic activities of daily living such as dressing and feeding oneself and maintaining personal hygiene become almost impossible to perform unaided.

Non-motor symptoms (NMS) are also present in PD and are currently receiving growing attention from researchers and clinicians [7]. Various NMS appear among the predominant sources of PD patient stress. These include constipation, dribbling, dysphagia, fatigue, pain, sexual dysfunction, sleep disturbances, a sensation of breathlessness and mental symptoms (e.g. depression, anxiety, problems with memory, difficulty in concentrating, episodes of confusion, hallucinations and delusions) [8–10] (Table 25.1).

In a survey of PD patients, 265 consecutive people were asked to rank their five most troublesome symptoms in the last 6 months. In the early PD group, the five most prevalent complaints (ranked in descending order) were slowness, tremor, stiffness, pain and loss of smell and/or taste. In the advanced PD group, fluctuating response to their medication, mood changes, drooling, sleep problems and tremor were the top five [11]. In a multicentre, international, cross-sectional study on 411 PD patients assessed by means of the Non-Motor Symptoms Scale (NMSS), nocturia (68.4%), fatigue (65.9%) and dribbling saliva (56.7%), were the most frequent complaints [12]. In the PRIAMO study, a multicentre survey using a semi-structured interview in 1072 consecutive PD patients, the most common NMS were fatigue (58%), anxiety (56%), leg pain (38%), insomnia (37%), nocturia (35%) and drooling (31%) [13].

Non-motor symptoms may have a greater impact on HRQoL than motor symptoms [12]. In the absence of a cure, preservation of patients' QoL is a primary goal of health care. NMS contribute to the impairment of HRQoL in PD, both directly (e.g. depression is a determinant of HRQoL) and indirectly through their contribution to disability [7,14,15]. Indeed, scores from a unified NMS Scale were strongly associated with those from PD-specific HRQoL measures (PDQ-8 and PDQ-39) [12]. Values of the correlation coefficient for the NMS Scale and PDQ-8 were higher by far than those observed for the HRQoL instrument and motor state or mental complications [16], suggesting that, as a whole, NMS may be more important than other aspects in determining HRQoL.

Table 25.1 Non-motor symptoms and health-related quality of life (HRQoL) assessment status in Parkinson's disease

No empirical data found	Ageusia
	Olfactory dysfunction
	Choking
	Reflux
	Seborrhoea
	Dry eye
	Xerostomia
	Blurred vision
	Diplopia
	Dysphonia
	Vivid dreaming
	Rapid eye movement (REM) sleep behaviour disorder
	Non-REM-sleep-related movement disorder
	Periodic limb movement
	Attention deficit
	Delusions
	Confusion
	Delirium
	Anhedonia
	Panic attack
	Pathological gambling
	Obsessive and repetitive behaviour
	Paraesthesias
	Taste/smell disturbances
	Weight loss/weight gain
Poorly assessed (fewer than five published papers)	Dysphagia
	Drooling
	Orthostatic hypotension
	Falls
	Sweating
	Insomnia
	Daytime somnolence
	Fatigue
	Hallucinations
	Psychosis
	Impulse control disorder
	Bladder dysfunction
	Constipation
	Faecal incontinence
Assessed, with more than four HRQoL studies	Sexual dysfunction
	Sleep disorders
	Mood disorders (depression/anxiety)
	Dementia
	Pain

Dyskinesias and (motor and non-motor) fluctuations exacerbate functional limitations and have a harmful effect on mood status, social activities, communication, sleep and the like, thus contributing to the deterioration in QoL. Non-motor fluctuations, manifested as anxiety, sweating, bradyphrenia or fatigue, may be experienced by some patients as being more disabling than motor fluctuations [17,18].

PD has an increasing impact on HRQoL as the disease progresses [19], although few longitudinal studies have assessed NMS and HRQoL in PD. A 2-year prospective study that included 336 PD patients from the SCOPA-PROPARK study showed that patients who have autonomic dysfunction, nighttime sleep problems and cognitive dysfunction were at risk of deterioration in HRQoL, as assessed with the EQ-5D [20].

At present, the treatment available for PD provides symptomatic relief and prolonga-tion of functional capacity—two components of HRQoL. Nevertheless, the side effects of treatment, frequently manifested as NMS (nausea and vomiting, gastric upset, orthostatic hypotension, sensation of sickness, etc.), may be present at any stage of the disease, for example nausea during the initial phases and psychotic symptoms during the advanced phases. As the illness progresses, dosages of medications will have to be increased and drugs combined, something that inevitably tends to accentuate both side effects and de-terioration in HRQoL [21].

This chapter takes the form of a narrative review of studies that furnish empirical data on the relationship between NMS and HRQoL in PD.

Methods

Two of the authors made independent searches of the medical literature in PubMed, using the following search terms for automatic selection purposes: (1) 'PD' plus 'quality of life'; and (2) 'PD' plus 'quality of life' plus the corresponding NMS, namely urinary dysfunction, bladder dysfunction, nocturia, urgency, polyuria, sexual dysfunction, constipation, faecal incontinence, dysphagia, choking, ageusia, drooling, orthostatic hypotension, sweating, seborrhoea, dry eye, xerostomia, dysphonia, sleep disorders, insomnia, vivid dreaming, daytime somnolence, rapid eye movement sleep behavioural disorder, periodic limb movement, fatigue, depression, anxiety, panic attacks, anhedonia, attention, hallucin-ations, delusions, psychosis, dementia, delirium, confusion, obsessive–compulsive behav-iour, impulse control, pain, paraesthesias, olfactory dysfunction, diplopia, weight loss and weight gain. For both searches, selection criteria were: (1) an established HRQoL measure was applied in the study; and (2) the effect of NMS on HRQoL was analysed. A manual search of the authors' own records was also carried out.

Each author independently reviewed the abstracts of around 1200 articles retrieved until 4 February 2013, and selected 107 for review.

Review articles were considered only if they were systematic reviews conducted in ac-cordance with the criteria for evidence-based medicine. The full text of selected papers was reviewed to extract the most informative and concise aspects relevant to the main topic.

To display the results of this narrative review, the same headings are used as in Panel 1 of Chaudhuri et al. [7].

Results

Neuropsychiatric symptoms

A number of different neuropsychiatric symptoms are prevalent among PD patients. Their presence poses a serious problem for both patients and caregivers. Moreover, the therapeutic approach to such symptoms complicates patient management, sometimes inducing more disability and adverse drug reactions.

Depression

Depression is frequently present in PD patients and was found to be the single most featured NMS in HRQoL studies. When properly measured and analysed, it has been consistently observed to have a negative effect on patients' HRQoL. A series of studies analysing multiple aspects of the disease have shown that depression is the most constant and influential factor underlying the deterioration of HRQoL in PD [22]. Indeed, the impact of depression surpasses that of other factors, such as motor function, motor complications, disease duration or sleep disorders [23–28]. This finding is shared by studies conducted in a diversity of cultural scenarios, using different designs and measures [29–39]. Some studies highlight the combined effect of and interrelationship between depression and disability [40,41]—another determinant of HRQoL—thus indicating a potentially indirect way in which depression can act on HRQoL. HRQoL seems to be significantly lower in PD patients with subthreshold depression than in non-depressed patients [42]. The combined effect of anxiety and depression on HRQoL has also been reported, though the connection between these two affective disorders renders interpretation of this finding complex [43].

High-level evidence confirming that HRQoL is improved by a beneficial response to antidepressant treatment has yet to be produced [44].

Anxiety

Despite being a highly prevalent symptom in PD, anxiety has received less attention from researchers than has depression, probably due to the close link between both disorders and the more severe consequences of the latter. In some studies that analysed self-perceived anxiety and depression separately, anxiety displayed an independent effect, equivalent to that of depression [33,43,45]. Additional studies, designed specifically to demonstrate the influence of anxiety and the effects of antianxiety treatment on HRQoL, are thus called for.

Apathy

Usually defined in pragmatic terms as lack of interest, apathy is frequent among PD patients. It has not been extensively studied, however, perhaps due to the difficulty of delimiting it conceptually and linking it to depression [46]. Apathy induces an increase in disability and would therefore be expected to have a negative effect on HRQoL [47]; however, one study did not observe it to have an independent effect on HRQoL in PD [45].

The ANIMO study recruited 557 PD patients who were assessed with the Lille Apathy Rating Scale and the EQ-5D index. Apathy was diagnosed in 52% of PD patients, and apathetic PD patients had mean EQ-5D scores that were significantly lower than those without apathy [48]. In the PRIAMO study, apathy was the NMS associated with worst PDQ-39 score, although the presence of fatigue, attention/memory and psychiatric symptoms had also a negative impact on HRQoL [13].

Hallucinations

The prevalence of psychotic symptoms in a community-based sample of 250 PD patients was reported to be 26%, with 47.7% of those having isolated minor symptoms and 52.3% having hallucinations and/or delusions [49].

The presence of hallucinations is usually disruptive for patients and caregivers alike, and may well induce fear and anxiety. In addition, the therapeutic measures required to neutralize this symptom may have side effects or limit the dosage of dopaminergic drugs, thereby bringing about subsequent impairment of the patient's motor condition. Hallucinations should thus be associated with deterioration of HRQoL, a fact that has been demonstrated by some studies [50]. After motor symptoms had been controlled for, hallucinations proved—along with depression and anxiety—to be a predictor of poor HRQoL (PDQ-39) [45].

Dementia

The association between dementia and poor HRQoL has been established. The presence of dementia significantly increases caregiver burden and diminishes HRQoL in PD patients [51]. In an Italian cohort of 70 PD patients, motor fluctuations, depression and dementia were independent predictors of HRQoL as evaluated by means of the EQ-5D [28]. In a cross-sectional study that included 100 Russian PD patients and 100 controls, dementia, depression and social support were also clinical determinants of lower HRQoL as measured by the EQ-5D and the Visual Analog Scale [36].

The relationship between cognitive performance and HRQoL in PD patients without dementia has been recently assessed in 124 PD patients. A better cognitive performance was associated with better HRQoL as measured by the PD-39 [52].

Impulse control disorder

A study of 99 PD patients, including 35 with impulse control disorders, showed that impulsivity had a negative impact on disability and HRQoL as measured with the PDQ-8 [47].

Sleep disorders

Sleep disorders are very frequent in PD, with a number of factors giving rise to poor-quality nighttime sleep and so decreasing physical and mental well-being [35]. Excessive daytime sleepiness, on the other hand, may limit daily activities. Sudden sleep attacks are less prevalent, but can be dangerous in certain circumstances. Several studies have highlighted the association between mood disturbances and sleep disorders [53–55]. This relationship is relevant because anxiety and depression, respectively, impair HRQoL and are treatable conditions [56].

Nocturnal hypokinesia has been reported to negatively affect the quality of sleep in PD in a sample of 240 PD patients who were assessed using question 35 of the PDQ-39 and the Pittsburgh Sleep Quality Index Questionnaire. In this study, there was a linear relationship between frequency of nocturnal hypokinesia and sleep quality [57].

Nocturnal sleep

Karlsen et al. [29] found a close correlation between self-reported nocturnal sleep disturbances and the sleep dimension of the NHP. Patients with insomnia have shown impaired HRQoL, with an impact on all SF-36 scales, but insomnia has also been closely linked to depressive symptoms [58]. A significant reduction in health state values as measured by the EQ-5D has been attributed to insomnia (–0.11) [59].

Poor nighttime sleep and anxiety are significant contributors to a worse HRQoL. Nighttime sleep disorders such as urinary incontinence, nighttime restlessness, morning fatigue and somnolence have been associated with poor scores on the PDQ-39 SI [60]. Havlikova et al. [61] studied 93 PD patients using the Epworth Sleepiness Scale (ESS), the Pittsburgh Sleep Quality Index (PSQI), the PDQ-39 and the Hospital Anxiety and Depression Scale. In a linear regression analysis the PSQI remained significant, accounting for 82% of the variance in PDQ-39.

However, low correlation values between nocturnal sleep (SCOPA–Nocturnal Sleep subscale) and HRQoL (EuroQoL) were reported by another study [62]. Using specific sleep measures (Parkinson's Disease Sleep Scale) and HRQoL (PDQ-39), Scaravilli et al. [63] observed a moderate correlation between both constructs. Such variability in results may be related to different study designs and the use of different sleep and HRQoL measures by the respective studies.

In Japanese study of 93 patients with PD and 93 age- and sex-matched control subjects, the stepwise linear regression analyses revealed the PDQ-39 SI and the PSQI global score were significant predictors for the total score on the Parkinson's disease sleep scale (PDSS)-2 [64].

Daytime sleepiness

Low correlation values have been reported between daytime sleepiness (SCOPA–Sleep, daytime sleepiness) and HRQoL (EuroQoL) [62].

In a population study of 426 PD patients, excessive daytime sleepiness [odds ratio (OR) 3.84, 95% confidence interval (CI) 2.56–5.75] and depression (OR 2.99, 95% CI 1.93–4.65) was elevated in patients with PD compared with controls, with similar findings seen in both early- and late-onset groups [65].

To ascertain the impact of each sleep type of disturbance and determine the differential effect of mood and sleep disorders on HRQoL, additional studies using the same sleep and HRQoL measures are called for.

Autonomic symptoms

A high prevalence of autonomic disorders, such as erectile dysfunction, sensation of incomplete bladder or bowel emptying, urgency, constipation, dysphagia and orthostatic dizziness, has been described in PD, suggesting a potential impact on patients' QoL [66,67]. Autonomic symptoms, mainly urinary, as well as constipation and postural dizziness, were more prevalent and severe among PD patients with dementia than among controls or sufferers from Alzheimer's disease. Furthermore, in patients with dementia associated with PD, the total autonomic symptom score was an independent predictor of HRQoL when measured by the SF-36 [68].

Bladder dysfunction

Lower urinary tract symptoms are prevalent in PD and may be present during the early stages of the disease. To improve the patient's condition, prompt evaluation and treatment of these symptoms is advisable at a time when they are more readily treatable. Decreased urinary QoL and overall subjective satisfaction with bladder functioning, measured by means of an ad hoc questionnaire, have been observed in clinical samples of PD patients, with a greater degree of impairment at more advanced Hoehn and Yahr stages [69]. Bowel dysfunction (incontinence) was not only associated with urinary incontinence but also increased with disease severity. Both disorders were found to cause deterioration in HRQoL by four studies addressing these symptoms [70–73]. Urinary, gastrointestinal, sleep and mood symptoms were the NMS domains that influenced the HRQoL, as measured with the PDQ-39, in a sample of Chinese PD patients [74]. Nocturia (observed in 68.4% of a sample of 411 PD patients) was significantly associated with the PDQ-39 index [12]. In the study by Gallagher et al. [15] the most common NMS were autonomic dysfunction, particularly urinary, and the HRQoL scores correlated strongly with urinary symptoms ($r = 0.84$).

Sexual dysfunction

Sexual dysfunction has been reported as having no effect on subjective satisfaction with sexual functioning [71] or on QoL [75]. A positive response (improvement in erectile dysfunction) to treatment with sildenafil, however, was accompanied by an improvement in the quality of sex life [75]. A specific Quality of Sexual Life Questionnaire (QoSL-Q), proposed as a complement to the PDQ-39, showed that satisfaction with sexual performance decreased with ageing and disease progression. No significant correlation was observed between PDQ-39 and QoSL-Q [76].

Sexual function was assessed in a case–control study of 45 PD patients and 45 age- and sex-matched healthy controls by means of the Arizona Sexual Experience Scale (ASEX), and showed that female PD patients had reduced sexual drive and less satisfaction with orgasm while male PD patients had easier orgasm that the controls [77].

Insofar as interventions are concerned, a small though positive effect on satisfaction with sexual functioning has been reported in male PD patients who underwent deep brain stimulation of the subthalamic nucleus [78]. Improvement in HRQoL associated with rasagiline treatment has been attributed to differential benefit in the self-image/sexuality domain [79].

Sweating disturbances

In a study by Swinn et al. [80], sweating disturbances were found to be present in approximately two-thirds of PD patients: they correlated with other symptoms of autonomic dysfunction and were linked to fluctuations (in 'off' and in 'on' with dyskinesia). Despite the fact that sweating disturbances were reported by many patients as having a physical, social and emotional impact, they showed no correlation with global HRQoL beyond a correlation with the visual analogue scale of the EuroQoL. However, an association was observed between sweating disturbances and the bodily pain domain of the PDQ-39.

Orthostatic hypotension

Orthostatic hypotension can lead to falls in some PD patients. Falls, in turn, have a negative influence on HRQoL [15]. One study reported that falls, including a small proportion caused by orthostatism, negatively affected all domains evaluated by the PDQ-39. This effect was more pronounced for mobility and activities of daily living [81]. In another small study that included 36 PD patients, only the PDQ-39 pain domain correlated with the risk of falls [82].

Gastrointestinal symptoms

Although the gastrointestinal symptoms present in PD could be considered autonomic disorders, they are nevertheless reviewed separately, due to the diversity of clinical manifestations affecting this area (and in order to maintain the topic classification as shown in Panel 1 of [7]).

Drooling

The dribbling of saliva is regarded as an important problem in PD; in the PRIAMO study 31% of PD patients reported drooling of saliva [13], whereas in another international collaborative study the prevalence of drooling was 56.7% [12]. It has physical, emotional and social consequences, dimensions that coincide with the basic components of HRQoL. QoL impairment tends to be more severe among patients with more severe drooling [83].

A seven-question survey on drooling was administered to 58 PD patients and 51 age-matched controls in a recent study [84]. The age, disease duration, motor scores, PDQ-39 and levodopa equivalent daily dosage (LEDD) were compared between PD patients who drooled and those who did not. The patients who drooled had significant difficulty in speaking, eating and social interaction compared with the non-droolers.

The Sialorrhoea Clinical Scale for PD (SCS-PD) has been designed to assess discomfort and social problems relating to drooling [85], although additional validation studies are needed.

Dysphagia

The prevalence of dysphagia in 106 PD patients was reported to be 32%. The impact of swallowing problems was significantly correlated with cognitive function, anxiety, depression, quality of life and postural instability [86].

A cross-sectional study evaluated the impact of dysphagia on HRQoL in 16 healthy subjects and 32 PD patients using the Swallowing Quality of Life (SWAL-QOL) questionnaire. Significant differences were found in all but one subsection of the SWAL-QOL. Disease progression had a detrimental impact on HRQoL, and subjects in later-stage PD experienced further reduction in their desire to eat, difficulty with food selection and prolonged duration of eating [87]. In another study, 36 PD patients with and without dysphagia filled out self-report assessments of the SWAL-QOL, PDQ-39 and Beck Depression Inventory. Significant relationships were detected between swallow-specific quality of life and general HRQoL ($r_s = -0.56$, $P = 0.000$) and depression [88].

Using a semi-structured interview, Miller et al. [89] addressed the in-depth impact of swallowing impairment on the physical and psychosocial aspects of patients' lives. Dysphagia was associated with motor status and complications (dyskinesias) and with dribbling of saliva. Patients reported perceived stigma, fear of choking, problems in taking their medication and abnormal throat sensation. Dysphagia contributed to the social isolation of patients and generated additional distress and burden for caregivers.

Bowel dysfunction

Bowel dysfunction, including constipation as its most frequent manifestation, was found to have a negative influence on HRQoL based on satisfaction with bowel functioning. Bowel dysfunction increased with Hoehn and Yahr stage [71].

In a clinical trial with macrogol, treated patients registered a significant improvement in constipation-related parameters, such as bowel movement frequency, straining and stool consistency, but HRQoL (PDQ-39) evinced no differences *vis-à-vis* the placebo group [90].

Pain

A systematic review using the modified Quality Assessment of Diagnostic Accuracy Studies (QUADAS) tool showed that prevalence of pain in PD ranges from 40 to 85%, with a mean of 67.7%, and with almost half of all PD patients complaining of musculoskeletal problems [91].

Pain negatively influences HRQoL in any situation, with a worse HRQoL being generally perceived by PD patients for all domains, including pain.

An impairment of health status, as measured with the EQ-5D, has been reported in relation to the increase in pain syndromes in a survey performed in 4086 PD patients. Female PD patients reported pain more often and more frequently received drug treatment for pain than did male patients [92].

Data from 162 PD patients enrolled in a community-based incidence study showed that significant reductions in health status values (EQ-5D) were also attributable to pain, motor fluctuations, depression and insomnia [59]. In fact, pain was associated with depression in PD patients in some studies [34], and predicted a worst HRQoL, as measured with the SF-36 and the Brief Pain Inventory in a sample of 159 PD patients [93].

However, no significant differences in the association between pain and HRQoL impairment were evident on comparison with matched controls from the general population [94,95]. Using a generic measure (the Nottingham Health Profile) over a 4-year follow-up, Karlsen et al. [96] observed a significant decrease in HRQoL in terms of the impairment of physical mobility, emotional reaction, pain and social-isolation dimensions. Deterioration of HRQoL in these dimensions was associated with disease progression, measured by the Unified Parkinson's Disease Rating Scale (UPDRS) and Hoehn and Yahr staging. In PD, significant correlations have also been observed between pain and sweating disturbances [80].

Certain interventions (pallidotomy, unilateral thalamotomy and conversion from standard to controlled-release levodopa) have been shown to improve the pain-related HRQoL domain significantly [97].

Fatigue

Fatigue is a highly prevalent non-motor symptom in PD, with a reported frequency of around 50–60% of cases [13,98]. Some studies did not identify fatigue as a determinant of HRQoL in PD, but in a community-based study Larsen et al. [99] observed more fatigue and poorer HRQoL in non-fluctuating PD patients than in patients with diabetes mellitus and healthy elderly individuals. Subsequent studies demonstrated that fatigue was associated with impaired HRQoL in non-depressed PD patients without dementia. Furthermore, the SF-36 and PDQ-39 emotional well-being, mobility, physical functioning, role physical and social functioning dimensions displayed significant deterioration in fatigued versus non-fatigued patients [100]. Fatigue, depression and disability have all been shown to exert an independent effect on HRQoL, as measured by the PDQ-8 [27].

The multidimensional Fatigue Inventory, the PDQ-39 and the UPDRS were used to evaluate fatigue in a sample of 175 PD patients from eastern Slovakia. Fatigue combined with worse functional status was a significant contributor to poor HRQoL [101]. In another study, the occurrence of fatigue correlated closely with more advanced PD, as well as with depression, anxiety and sleep disorders, hinting at a common underlying basis [102].

In a Japanese study of 361 PD patients without dementia, multiple logistic regression analysis indicated that the significant independent variables related to the presence of fatigue were the PDSS and PDQ-39 scores [103].

Conclusions and future developments

More than 45 NMS are listed in the panel used as a guide to display the results of this review [7]. An international study that included all disease stages and applied the NMS Questionnaire reported a mean of over 10 NMS per patient [67]. This figure suggests the considerable extent to which the lives of PD patients may be affected by any potential combination of several NMS [16], to which motor symptoms and complications should be added.

The respective negative effects on HRQoL of depression, anxiety, hallucinations, pain and fatigue have been sufficiently described by studies that applied appropriate statistical methodology and included adequate assessment tools designed to measure NMS and HRQoL. Furthermore, in some of these cases HRQoL may well be subject to an additional indirect influence. This is because disability, which is a determinant of HRQoL and is often due to other causes, can be rendered more severe by these NMS.

Other NMS (bladder and bowel dysfunction, sleep disorders, sweating disturbances, dribbling of saliva and dysphagia) have been found to be associated with impairment of HRQoL, with a correlation between the concrete symptom and the observed deterioration in QoL. Nevertheless, more studies targeting these symptoms and using appropriate measures and statistical methods should be undertaken so that the question of their influence on HRQoL can be definitively laid to rest. It is highly likely that most of these NMS will be confirmed as HRQoL predictors, but evidence is still wanting.

Finally, there is a lack of empirical data on the potential relationship between certain NMS (confusion, restless legs, vivid dreaming, orthostatism, xerostomia, ageusia, olfactory disturbance, etc.) and HRQoL. This field must therefore be further explored in order to complete our knowledge of factors with the potential capacity to impoverish the QoL of PD patients.

Several clinical trials have used measures of HRQoL to assess the effect of some drugs on NMS in PD. The RECOVER clinical trial assessed the impact of rotigotine on NMS using the PDQ-8, and showed that this drug may benefit patients with sleep, pain and mood problems [104]. In a prospective open-label observational study, the effects of intrajejunal levodopa/carbidopa gel infusion on NMS in 22 PD patients based on standard assessments utilizing the NMSS and PDQ-8 were investigated. Significant improvement was found in the PDQ-8 mean scores, which correlated significantly with the changes in NMSS mean scores [105].

The limitations of the review in this chapter mainly lie in: (1) its restricted ability to capture all the information available in the literature on the topic, as only one database (Pub-Med) was used for the identification of papers; (2) the methodology used to select such papers; and (3) a possibly erroneous interpretation of the results. However, the relevance of the database targeted and the independent search undertaken by the authors using a different approach together ensure the pertinence of the information retrieved. A potential supplementary approach using meta-analysis would require the selection of specific NMS that had been repeatedly studied in patient series fulfilling certain quality criteria.

To summarize, there are many NMS associated with PD and they affect patients' HRQoL to an important degree. Depression, autonomic dysfunction, psychiatric complications, pain, fatigue and sleep problems are major correlates of poor HRQoL. There is an urgent need for further studies to address the role of NMS and the effect of their treatment on HRQoL.

References

1 **The WHOQOL Group**. The World Health Organization Quality of Life assessment (WHOQOL): position paper from the World Health Organization. Soc Sci Med 1995; **41**: 1403–9.

2 Schipper H, Clinch JJ, Olweny CLM. Quality of life studies: definitions and conceptual issues. In: B Spilker (ed.) Quality of life and pharmacoeconomics in clinical trials, 2nd edn, pp. 11–23. Philadelphia, PA: Lippincott-Raven, 1996.

3 Martinez-Martin P. An introduction to the concept of 'quality of life in Parkinson's disease'. J Neurol 1998; **245**(Suppl 1): 2–6.

4 World Health Organization. Handbook of basic documents, 5th edn, pp. 3–20. Geneva: WHO, 1952.

5 Fitzpatrick R, Davey C, Buxton M, Jones D. Evaluating patient-based outcomes measures for use in clinical trials. Health Technol Assess 1998; **2**: 1–74.

6 World Health Organization. International classification of functioning, disability and health. Geneva: WHO, 2001.

7 Chaudhuri KR, Healy DG, Schapira AHV. Non-motor symptoms in Parkinson's disease: diagnosis and management. Lancet Neurol 2006; **5**: 235–45.

8 Fitzsimmons B, Bunting LK. Parkinson's disease. Quality of life issues. Nursing Clin N Am 1993, **28**: 807–18.

9 Shindler JS, Brown R, Welburn P, Parkes JD. Measuring the quality of life of patients with Parkinson's disease. In: SR Walker, RM Rosser (eds) Quality of life assessment: key issues in the 1990s, pp. 289–300. Dordrecht: Kluwer, 1993.

10 Gulati A, Forbes A, Stegie F, et al. A clinical observational study of pattern and occurrence of non-motor symptoms in Parkinson's disease. Mov Disord 2004; **19**(Suppl 9): 406.

11 Politis M, Wu K, Molloy S, et al. Parkinson's disease symptoms: the patient's perspective. Mov Disord 2010; **25**: 1646–51.

12 Martinez-Martin P, Rodriguez-Blazquez C, Kurtis MM, et al.; NMSS Validation Group. The impact of non-motor symptoms on health-related quality of life of patients with Parkinson's disease. Mov Disord 2011; **26**: 399–406.

13 Barone P, Antonini A, Colosimo C, et al.; PRIAMO study group. The PRIAMO study: a multicenter assessment of nonmotor symptoms and their impact on quality of life in Parkinson's disease. Mov Disord 2009; **24**: 1641–9.

14 Hely MA, Morris JGL, Reid WGJ, Trafficante R. Sydney multicenter study of Parkinson's disease: non-L-dopa-responsive problems dominate at 15 years. Mov Disord 2005; **20**: 190–9.

15 Gallagher DA, Lees AJ, Schrag A. What are the most important nonmotor symptoms in patients with Parkinson's disease and are we missing them? Mov Disord 2010; **25**: 2493–500.

16 Chaudhuri KR, Martinez-Martin P, Brown RG, et al. The metric properties of a novel non-motor symptoms scale for Parkinson's disease: results from an international pilot study. Mov Disord 2007; **22**: 1901–11.

17 Witjas T, Kaphan E, Azulay JP, et al. Nonmotor fluctuations in Parkinson's disease: frequent and disabling. Neurology 2002; **59**: 408–13.

18 Chapuis S, Ouchchane L, Metz O, et al. Impact of the motor complications of Parkinson's disease on the quality of life. Mov Disord 2005; **20**: 224–30.

19 Forsaa EB, Larsen JP, Wentzel-Larsen T, et al. Predictors and course of health-related quality of life in Parkinson's disease. Mov Disord 2008; **23**: 1420–7.

20 Visser M, Verbaan D, van Rooden S, et al. A longitudinal evaluation of health-related quality of life of patients with Parkinson's disease. Value Health 2009; **12**: 392–6.

21 Koller WC. Drug treatment for Parkinson's disease: impact on the patient's quality of life. In: P Martinez-Martin, WC Koller (eds) Quality of life in Parkinson's disease, pp. 79–91. Barcelona: Masson, 1999.

22 Visser M, van Rooden SM, Verbaan D, et al. A comprehensive model of health-related quality of life in Parkinson's disease. J Neurol 2008; **255**: 1580–7.

23 **Kuopio AM, Marttila RJ, Helenius H, et al.** The quality of life in Parkinson's disease. Mov Disord 2000; **15**: 216–23.

24 **Schrag A, Jahanshahi M, Quinn N.** What contributes to quality of life in patients with Parkinson's disease? J Neurol Neurosurg Psychiatry 2000; **69**: 308–12.

25 **Global Parkinson's Disease Survey Steering Committee.** Factors impacting on quality of life in Parkinson's disease: results from an international survey. Mov Disord 2002; **17**: 60–7.

26 **Slawek J, Derejko M, Lass P.** Factors affecting the quality of life of patients with idiopathic Parkinson's disease: a cross-sectional study in an outpatient clinic attendees. Parkinsonism Relat Disord 2005; **11**: 465–8.

27 **Martinez-Martin P, Catalan MJ, Benito-Leon J, et al.** Impact of fatigue in Parkinson's disease: the Fatigue Impact Scale for Daily Use (D-FIS). Qual Life Res 2006; **15**: 597–606.

28 **Winter Y, von Campenhausen S, Arend M, et al.** Health-related quality of life and its determinants in Parkinson's disease: results of an Italian cohort study. Parkinsonism Relat Disord 2011; **17**: 265–9.

29 **Karlsen KH, Larsen JP, Tandberg E, Maeland JG.** Influence of clinical and demographic variables on quality of life in patients with Parkinson's disease. J Neurol Neurosurg Psychiatry 1999; **66**: 431–5.

30 **Cubo E, Rojo A, Ramos S, et al.** The importance of educational and psychological factors in Parkinson's disease quality of life. Eur J Neurol 2002; **9**: 589–93.

31 **Zach M, Friedman A, Sławek J, Derejko M.** Quality of life in Polish patients with long-lasting Parkinson's disease. Mov Disord 2004; **19**: 667–72.

32 **Behari M, Srivastava AK, Pandey RM.** Quality of life in patients with Parkinson's disease. Parkinsonism Relat Disord 2005; **11**: 221–6.

33 **Carod-Artal FJ, Vargas AP, Martinez-Martin P.** Determinants of quality of life in Brazilian patients with Parkinson's disease. Mov Disord 2007; **22**: 1408–15.

34 **Roh JH, Kim BJ, Jang JH, et al.** The relationship of pain and health-related quality of life in Korean patients with Parkinson's disease. Acta Neurol Scand 2009; **119**: 397–403.

35 **Andreadou E, Anagnostouli M, Vasdekis V, et al.** The impact of comorbidity and other clinical and sociodemographic factors on health-related quality of life in Greek patients with Parkinson's disease. Aging Ment Health 2011; **15**: 913–21.

36 **Winter Y, von Campenhausen S, Popov G, et al.** Social and clinical determinants of quality of life in Parkinson's disease in a Russian cohort study. Parkinsonism Relat Disord 2010; **16**: 243–8.

37 **Winter Y, von Campenhausen S, Gasser J, et al.** Social and clinical determinants of quality of life in Parkinson's disease in Austria: a cohort study. J Neurol 2010; **257**: 638–45.

38 **Rahman S, Griffin HJ, Quinn NP, et al.** Quality of life in Parkinson's disease: the relative importance of the symptoms. Mov Disord 2008; **23**: 1428–34.

39 **Arun MP, Bharath S, Pal PK, et al.** Relationship of depression, disability, and quality of life in Parkinson's disease: a hospital-based case-control study. Neurol India 2011; **59**: 185–9.

40 **Weintraub D, Moberg PJ, Duda JE, et al.** Effect of psychiatric and other nonmotor symptoms on disability in Parkinson's disease. J Am Geriatr Soc 2004; **52**: 784–8.

41 **Ravina B, Camicioli R, Como PG, et al.** The impact of depressive symptoms in early Parkinson disease. Neurology 2007; **69**: 342–7.

42 **Reiff J, Schmidt N, Riebe B, et al.** Subthreshold depression in Parkinson's disease. Mov Disord 2011; **26**: 1741–4.

43 **Carod-Artal FJ, Ziomkowski S, Mourao Mesquita H, Martinez-Martin P.** Anxiety and depression: main determinants of health-related quality of life in Brazilian patients with Parkinson's disease. Parkinsonism Relat Disord 2008; **14**: 102–8.

44 **Schrag A.** Quality of life and depression in Parkinson's disease. J Neurol Sci 2006; **248**: 151–7.

45 McKinlay A, Grace RC, Dalrymple-Alford JC, et al. A profile of neuropsychiatric problems and their relationship to quality of life for Parkinson's disease patients without dementia. Parkinsonism Relat Disord 2008; **14**: 37–42.

46 Oguru M, Tachibana H, Toda K, et al. Apathy and depression in Parkinson disease. J Geriatr Psychiatry Neurol 2010; **23**: 35–41.

47 Leroi I, Ahearn DJ, Andrews M, et al. Behavioural disorders, disability and quality of life in Parkinson's disease. Age Ageing 2011; **40**: 614–21.

48 Benito-León J, Cubo E, Coronell C; ANIMO Study Group. Impact of apathy on health-related quality of life in recently diagnosed Parkinson's disease: the ANIMO study. Mov Disord 2012; **27**: 211–18.

49 Mack J, Rabins P, Anderson K, et al. Prevalence of psychotic symptoms in a community-based Parkinson disease sample. Am J Geriatr Psychiatry 2012; **20**: 123–32.

50 Schrag A, Selai C, Jahanshahi M, Quinn NP. The EQ-5D—a generic quality of life measure is a useful instrument to measure quality of life in patients with Parkinson's disease. J Neurol Neurosurg Psychiatry 2000; **69**: 67–73.

51 Leroi I, McDonald K, Pantula H, Harbishettar V. Cognitive impairment in Parkinson disease: impact on quality of life, disability, and caregiver burden. J Geriatr Psychiatry Neurol 2012; **25**: 208–14.

52 Klepac N, Trkulja V, Relja M, et al. Is quality of life in non-demented Parkinson's disease patients related to cognitive performance? A clinic-based cross-sectional study. Eur J Neurol 2008; **15**: 128–33.

53 Happe S, Ludemann P, Berger K; for the FAQT study investigators. The association between disease severity and sleep-related problems in patients with Parkinson's disease. Neuropsychobiology 2002; **46**: 90–6.

54 Pal PK, Thennarasu K, Fleming J, et al. Nocturnal sleep disturbances and daytime dysfunction in patients with Parkinson's disease and in their caregivers. Parkinsonism Relat Disord 2004; **10**: 157–68.

55 Qin Z, Zhang L, Sun F, et al; Chinese Parkinson Study Group. Health related quality of life in early Parkinson's disease: impact of motor and non-motor symptoms, results from Chinese levodopa exposed cohort. Parkinsonism Relat Disord 2009; **15**: 767–71.

56 Borek LL, Kohn R, Friedman JH. Mood and sleep in Parkinson's disease. J Clin Psychiatry 2006; **67**: 958–63.

57 Louter M, Munneke M, Bloem BR, et al. Nocturnal hypokinesia and sleep quality in Parkinson's disease. J Am Geriatr Soc 2012; **60**: 1104–8.

58 Caap-Ahlgren M, Dehlin O. Insomnia and depressive symptoms in patients with Parkinson's disease. Relationship to health-related quality of life. An interview study of patients living at home. Arch Gerontol Geriatr 2001; **32**: 23–33.

59 Shearer J, Green C, Counsell CE, et al. The impact of motor and non motor symptoms on health state values in newly diagnosed idiopathic Parkinson's disease. J Neurol 2012; **259**: 462–8.

60 Gómez-Esteban JC, Tijero B, Somme J, et al. Impact of psychiatric symptoms and sleep disorders on the quality of life of patients with Parkinson's disease. J Neurol 2011; **258**: 494–9.

61 Havlikova E, van Dijk JP, Nagyova I, et al. The impact of sleep and mood disorders on quality of life in Parkinson's disease patients. J Neurol 2011; **258**: 2222–9.

62 Martinez-Martin P, Cubo-Delgado E, Aguilar-Barbera M, et al. A pilot study on a specific measure for sleep disorders in Parkinson's disease: SCOPA-Sleep. Rev Neurol 2006; **43**: 577–83.

63 Scaravilli T, Gasparoli E, Rinaldi F, et al. Health-related quality of life and sleep disorders in Parkinson's disease. Neurol Sci 2003; **24**: 209–10.

64 Suzuki K, Miyamoto M, Miyamoto T, et al. Nocturnal disturbances and restlessness in Parkinson's disease: using the Japanese version of the Parkinson's disease sleep scale-2. J Neurol Sci 2012; **318**: 76–81.

65 Knipe MD, Wickremaratchi MM, Wyatt-Haines E, et al. Quality of life in young- compared with late-onset Parkinson's disease. Mov Disord 2011; **26**: 2011–18.

66 Singer C, Weiner WJ, Sanchez-Ramos JR. Autonomic dysfunction in men with Parkinson's disease. Eur Neurol 1992; **32**: 134–40.

67 Martinez-Martin P, Schapira AH, Stocchi F, et al. Prevalence of nonmotor symptoms in Parkinson's disease in an international setting: study using nonmotor symptoms questionnaire in 545 patients. Mov Disord 2007; **22**: 1623–9.

68 Allan L, McKeith I, Ballard C, Kenny RA. The prevalence of autonomic symptoms in dementia and their association with physical activity, activities of daily living and quality of life. Dement Geriatr Cogn Disord 2006; **22**: 230–7.

69 Ragab MM, Mohammed ES. Idiopathic Parkinson's disease patients at the urologic clinic. Neurourol Urodyn 2011; **30**: 1258–61.

70 Lemack GE, Dewey RB Jr, Roehrborn CG, et al. Questionnaire-based assessment of bladder dysfunction in patients with mild to moderate Parkinson's disease. Urology 2000; **56**: 250–4.

71 Sakakibara R, Shinotoh H, Uchiyama T, et al. Questionnaire-based assessment of pelvic organ dysfunction in Parkinson's disease. Auton Neurosci 2001; **92**: 76–85.

72 Iacovelli E, Gilio F, Meco G, et al. Bladder symptoms assessed with overactive bladder questionnaire in Parkinson's disease. Mov Disord 2010; **25**: 1203–9.

73 Sammour ZM, Gomes CM, Barbosa ER, et al. Voiding dysfunction in patients with Parkinson's disease: impact of neurological impairment and clinical parameters. Neurourol Urodyn 2009; **28**: 510–15.

74 Li H, Zhang M, Chen L, et al. Nonmotor symptoms are independently associated with impaired health-related quality of life in Chinese patients with Parkinson's disease. Mov Disord 2010; **25**: 2740–6.

75 Hussain IF, Brady CM, Swinn MJ, et al. Treatment of erectile dysfunction with sildenafil citrate (Viagra) in parkinsonism due to Parkinson's disease or multiple system atrophy with observations on orthostatic hypotension. J Neurol Neurosurg Psychiatry 2001; **71**: 371–4.

76 Moore O, Gurevich T, Korczyn AD, et al. Quality of sexual life in Parkinson's disease. Parkinsonism Relat Disord 2002; **8**: 243–6.

77 Celikel E, Ozel-Kizil ET, Akbostanci MC, et al. Assessment of sexual dysfunction in patients with Parkinson's disease: a case–control study. Eur J Neurol 2008; **15**: 1168–72.

78 Castelli L, Perozzo P, Genesia ML, et al. Sexual well being in parkinsonian patients after deep brain stimulation of the subthalamic nucleus. J Neurol Neurosurg Psychiatry 2004; **75**: 1260–4.

79 Biglan KM, Schwid S, Eberly S, et al. Rasagiline improves quality of life in patients with early Parkinson's disease. Mov Disord 2006; **21**: 616–23.

80 Swinn L, Schrag A, Viswanathan R, et al. Sweating dysfunction in Parkinson's disease. Mov Disord 2003; **18**: 1459–63.

81 Michalowska M, Fiszer U, Krygowska-Wajs A, Owczarek K. Falls in Parkinson's disease. Causes and impact on patients' quality of life. Funct Neurol 2005; **20**: 163–8.

82 Cano-de la Cuerda R, Vela-Desojo L, Miangolarra-Page JC, et al. [Health-related quality of life in Parkinson's disease]. Medicina (B Aires) 2010; **70**: 503–7.

83 Kalf JG, Smit AM, Bloem BR, et al. Impact of drooling in Parkinson's disease. J Neurol 2007; **254**: 1227–32.

84 Leibner J, Ramjit A, Sedig L, et al. The impact of and the factors associated with drooling in Parkinson's disease. Parkinsonism Relat Disord 2010; **16**: 475–7.

85 Perez Lloret S, Pirán Arce G, Rossi M, et al. Validation of a new scale for the evaluation of sialorrhea in patients with Parkinson's disease. Mov Disord 2007; **22**: 107–11.

86 Walker RW, Dunn JR, Gray WK. Self-reported dysphagia and its correlates within a prevalent population of people with Parkinson's disease. Dysphagia 2011; **26**: 92–6.

87 **Leow LP, Huckabee ML, Anderson T, et al**. The impact of dysphagia on quality of life in ageing and Parkinson's disease as measured by the swallowing quality of life (SWAL-QOL) questionnaire. Dysphagia 2010; **25**: 216–20.

88 **Plowman-Prine EK, Sapienza CM, Okun MS, et al**. The relationship between quality of life and swallowing in Parkinson's disease. Mov Disord 2009; **24**: 1352–8.

89 **Miller N, Noble E, Jones D, Burn D**. Hard to swallow: dysphagia in Parkinson's disease. Age Ageing 2006; **35**: 614–18.

90 **Zangaglia R, Martignoni E, Glorioso M, et al**. Macrogol for the treatment of constipation in Parkinson's disease. A randomized placebo-controlled study. Mov Disord 2007; **22**: 1239–44.

91 **Broen MP, Braaksma MM, Patijn J, et al**. Prevalence of pain in Parkinson's disease: a systematic review using the modified QUADAS tool. Mov Disord 2012; **27**: 480–4.

92 **Müller T, Muhlack S, Woitalla D**. Pain perception, pain drug therapy and health status in patients with Parkinson's disease. Neuroepidemiology 2011; **37**: 183–7.

93 **Santos-García D, Abella-Corral J, Aneiros-Díaz Á, et al**. [Pain in Parkinson's disease: prevalence, characteristics, associated factors, and relation with other non motor symptoms, quality of life, autonomy, and caregiver burden]. Rev Neurol 2011; **52**: 385–93.

94 **Schrag A, Jahanshahi M, Quinn N**. How does Parkinson's disease affect quality of life? A comparison with quality of life in the general population. Mov Disord 2000; **15**: 1112–18.

95 **Quittenbaum BH, Grahn B**. Quality of life and pain in Parkinson's disease: a controlled cross-sectional study. Parkinsonism Relat Disord 2004; **10**: 129–36.

96 **Karlsen KH, Tandberg E, Arsland D, Larsen JP**. Health related quality of life in Parkinson's disease: a prospective longitudinal study. J Neurol Neurosurg Psychiatry 2000; **69**: 584–9.

97 **Martinez-Martin P, Deuschl G**. Effect of medical and surgical interventions on health-related quality of life in Parkinson's disease. Mov Disord 2007; **22**: 757–65.

98 **Miwa H, Miwa T**. Fatigue in patients with Parkinson's disease: impact on quality of life. Intern Med 2011; **50**: 1553–8.

99 **Larsen JP, Karlsen K, Tandberg E**. Clinical problems in non-fluctuating patients with Parkinson's disease: a community based study. Mov Disord 2000; **15**: 826–9.

100 **Herlofson K, Larsen JP**. The influence of fatigue on health-related quality of life in patients with Parkinson's disease. Acta Neurol Scand 2003; **107**: 1–6.

101 **Havlikova E, Rosenberger J, Nagyova I, et al**. Impact of fatigue on quality of life in patients with Parkinson's disease. Eur J Neurol 2008; **15**: 475–80.

102 **Metta V, Logishetty K, Martinez-Martin P, et al**. The possible clinical predictors of fatigue in Parkinson's disease: a study of 135 patients as part of international nonmotor scale validation project. Parkinsons Dis 2011; **2011**: 125271.

103 **Okuma Y, Kamei S, Morita A, et al**. Fatigue in Japanese patients with Parkinson's disease: a study using Parkinson fatigue scale. Mov Disord 2009; **24**: 1977–83.

104 **Ghys L, Surmann E, Whitesides J, et al**. Effect of rotigotine on sleep and quality of life in Parkinson's disease patients: post hoc analysis of RECOVER patients who were symptomatic at baseline. Expert Opin Pharmacother 2011; **12**: 1985–98.

105 **Honig H, Antonini A, Martinez-Martin P, et al**. Intrajejunal levodopa infusion in Parkinson's disease: a pilot multicenter study of effects on nonmotor symptoms and quality of life. Mov Disord 2009; **24**: 1468–74.

Chapter 26

Non-motor symptoms and co-morbidity in Parkinson's disease

Graeme J. A. Macphee and Douglas G. MacMahon

Background

The importance of the non-motor symptoms of Parkinson's disease (PD) is now increasingly recognized, and the monitoring of such symptoms is becoming incorporated into best practice. However, non-motor symptoms declared by individual PD patients may reflect clinical manifestations of other unrelated co-morbid conditions as well as the underlying pathology of PD—the primary focus of this book. As both PD and common co-morbidities become more prevalent with advancing age, co-morbidities have an increasing impact as the disease progresses. As the patient ages, they almost become the norm.

In one of the first studies in the world literature, Diedrich et al. [1] reported in 2003 that patients with onset of PD in old age were more likely to have co-morbid conditions than patients with onset in middle age. The specific co-morbidities that were more common in older patients in this select population of 47 patients were cerebrovascular disease, auditory deficits, especially presbycusis, and visual impairment (cataracts, glaucoma and macular degeneration). The Movement Disorders Section of the British Geriatrics Society undertook a prospective multicentre cohort study of the effects of age on the features of PD at diagnosis [2]. One hundred patients with a mean age of 75.6 years were studied. There was a high rate of co-morbidity, with a prevalence of cardiac disease of 32%, hypertension 32% (with 4% having suffered a previous stroke), arthritis 32%, cataracts 13%, respiratory disease 8% and depression 11%.

Consequently, clinicians responsible for the care of patients with PD should familiarize themselves with the diagnosis, management and sequelae of common co-morbidities in PD.

This chapter will review co-morbidity unrelated to the primary pathology of PD. Recognition and appropriate management of co-morbidity should be part of the remit of clinicians primarily responsible for PD patients. We will also consider the implications for resource use, expenditure and opportunities for improvement in holistic management of PD for patients who may receive unscheduled episodes of care under non-specialist clinical teams.

Assessment of co-morbidity: clinical and trial issues

The detection, assessment and measurement of co-morbidity is important in PD as coexisting but unrelated conditions may influence diagnosis, prognosis and therapy. Furthermore, comprehensive assessment of co-morbidity is crucial to the appropriate interpretation of randomized control trials, and several tools are available for this purpose. Principally, the detection and measurement of co-morbidity permits correction for confounding factors and improvement of the internal validity of studies, and improves statistical efficiency [3]. Secondly, co-morbidity may predict study outcome or the natural disease trajectory. The review by De Groot and colleagues [3] reported that the Charlson Index, the Cumulative Illness Rating Scale (CIRS), the Index of Coexisting Diseases (ICED) and the Kaplan Index (developed for diabetes research) are valid and reliable methods that can be used in clinical research to measure co-morbidity generically.

Visser et al. [4] assessed the accuracy of an interview-based assessment using the Cumulative Illness Rating Scale—Geriatric (CIRS-G) in an interview with 31 PD patients and their caregivers, as well as reviewing the patients' medical charts from general practice. They found that all patients had some co-morbidity, with 84% having one or more moderate co-morbid diseases. The most frequently affected systems were the lower gastrointestinal and genitourinary. The agreement between interview-based and chart-based assessment for the six summary scores ranged from 0.69 to 0.81. Fifteen per cent of patients had severe co-morbidity. Chart-based scores were higher than the interview-based summary scores. Agreement between interview and chart was higher for the more severe disorders. Patients with more cognitive impairment tended to demonstrate more difference between interview-based and chart-based CIRS-G scores, and so the use of chart review CIRS-G is preferable to interview in patients with significant cognitive impairment.

The frequency and length of hospital admission in patients with Parkinson's disease and co-morbidities

A study from the United States [5] investigated the impact of co-morbid disease and injuries on resource use and expenditure in patients with parkinsonism, utilizing the National Long Term Care Survey. This study included patients over the age of 65 years and followed 790 patients with parkinsonism and over 24 000 without parkinsonism using Medicare administrative records. They determined that patients with parkinsonism were 1.5 times more likely to be hospitalized than those without. Woodford and Walker [6] surveyed emergency hospital admissions in patients with idiopathic PD in the UK and found a significantly longer mean length of stay—21.3 days compared with 17.8 days for non-PD patients.

Pressley et al. [5] demonstrated significant differences in patterns of delivery of care and resource use in elderly patients with and without parkinsonism (assessed by a non-specialist) across a variety of co-morbid conditions. They measured co-morbid disease risk using age-adjusted odds ratios and developed co-morbidity cost ratios (i.e. the ratio of average annual charges per person for parkinsonism alone versus that for those who also had co-morbid conditions). Patients with parkinsonism were older and had more injuries resulting in fractures (including hip fractures), and these were more prevalent among both genders with parkinsonism and were reflected in cost ratios two- to three-fold higher in those with parkinsonism—particularly for dementia, fractures and diabetes.

Woodford and Walker [6] described the profile of emergency hospital admissions in a geographically defined population where the accuracy of diagnosis was likely to be high. The population admitted was representative of the PD population generally in terms of age and sex distribution. During the 4-year period of the study, there were 246 emergency admissions with a mean length of stay of 17.3 days. The core study population was made up of 129 PD patients with a mean age of 78 years, of whom 48% were male. The most common reason for admission was intercurrent infections, accounting for 21% of admissions (pneumonia 11%, urinary tract infection 9%, cellulitis 1%). Cardiovascular causes including angina and heart failure accounted for 20%. Stroke and transient ischaemic attack accounted for around 2% of admissions. Falls were common, accounting for 13% of admissions, with a further 8% accounted for by decreased mobility or dyskinesia. Fractures accounted for 4% and orthostatic hypotension accounted for 4% of admissions. Other co-morbidities included surgical causes, upper gastrointestinal bleeds and myocardial infarction. Increased dependency was evidenced by 16 of 179 patients previously living in their own home who were unable to return, and an increase in patients requiring nursing home care from previous residential care environments following hospital admission. Psychiatric manifestations such as delirium and hallucinations accounted for only 8% of admissions and did not appear to be the major determinant of nursing home placement in contrast to previous observations. The relatively low rate of admissions with neuropsychiatric symptoms may be explained by the intense screening and management of complications that this service offers in the community setting.

Guttman et al. [7] reported a large study of parkinsonism (rather than PD) in over 15 000 patients in Ontario and showed higher rates of hospitalization among patients compared with controls for aspiration pneumonia [6.34, confidence interval (CI) 5.23–7.93], affective psychosis (2.71, CI 2.13–3.32), hip fracture (2.56, CI 2.35–2.76), other urinary tract disorders including infections (2.50, CI 2.17–2.86), septicaemia (2.39, CI 2.02–2.85) and fluid and electrolyte disorders (2.27, CI 1.93–2.66). Rates for cardiac, cerebrovascular and peripheral vascular disease were not significantly different.

A retrospective cross-sectional study from Italy [8] examined a well-defined population of patients with PD using a standard interview with patients and caregivers. Only ambulant patients were considered and patients with advanced PD were excluded. Consultations and admissions for reasons related to PD were excluded from the survey. Specialist visits accounted for 41.5% of resource use, followed by visits to the general practitioner (27%), emergency room consultations (22.3%) and hospital admissions (19.2%). This study highlighted the lower rate of consultations with general practitioners and non-neurological specialists, which may reflect preferential consultation with the specialist PD and movement disorder centre. Interestingly, new drug treatments for co-morbidity (unrelated to PD) were issued to 66% of patients, and over 80% of these were prescribed in general practice or the emergency room. This highlights the need for generalists to be aware of treatment updates and potential drug interactions (see Drug interactions). This study suggests that the patients using emergency facilities or those admitted to hospital tended to be older and have longer disease duration. The most frequent causes of emergency room consultations were injuries and fractures. Martignoni et al. [9] reported a 1-year prospective study of co-morbid events leading to hospitalization in an unselected group of 180 PD patients. The most frequent acute co-morbid events were trauma secondary to falls in 30%, vascular disorders in 29% and diverse medical causes such as hepatitis, cancer and anaemia, and yet more than half did not require specific treatment for the acute co-morbid event

The high rates of utilization of emergency care and hospital facilities emphasize the need for a holistic, coordinated view of specific and non-specific co-morbidities in PD. Within the UK, PD nurse specialists are often the key workers who will help to coordinate management and changes in medication. Patients and family should be encouraged to inform their specialist nurse regarding elective and emergency hospital admissions and report changes in medication to their specialist PD team [10]. Reconciliation of medicines should be undertaken during every clinical encounter.

Practical guidelines on emergency treatment for patients with Parkinson's disease

It is clear that patients with PD will experience episodes of unscheduled care. During these periods they may be cared for by a variety of non-PD specialists. Dissemination of good practice by in-house education and written guidelines may be helpful [11]. Two recent papers highlight the importance of guidelines and education for teams undertaking care of PD patients [12,13].

For many patients, timing of medication is vital, and accordingly inpatient facilities should ensure that drug doses and timings are accurate and wherever possible patients are able to self-administer medication. Factors contributing to non-conformity include inflexible timing of drug rounds and a lack of understanding on the part of ward staff regarding the importance of accurate treatment regimens in maintaining control and preventing hypostatic complications such as pneumonia and peripheral and pulmonary thromboembolism. Parkinson-hyperpyrexia syndrome (PHS) may be a serious consequence of admission. Most commonly this syndrome occurs in association with a delay in implementing dopaminergic therapy or where a patient is unable to swallow medication. A simple five-step guideline for non-specialists with key points is shown in Box 26.1. A comprehensive review is provided by MacMahon and MacMahon [14].

Neuroleptic malignant syndrome and Parkinson-hyperpyrexia syndrome in Parkinson's disease

Neuroleptic malignant syndrome is a potentially fatal drug-induced movement disorder characterized by hyperthermia, muscle rigidity, dysautonomia and changes in mental status. It was first described in psychiatric patients, particularly those treated with neuroleptic drugs. In the 1980s, a similar disorder was described in patients with PD precipitated by

Box. 26.1 Five-step guidelines on supportive therapy for patients with Parkinson's disease admitted to hospital

1. Ensure the received treatment schedule is accurate including use of as-required medications

Drug formulations Madopar (co-beneldopa) and Sinemet (co-careldopa) are interchangeable if only one is available and equivalent doses of levodopa are used. Levodopa is the active constituent. Benserazide (Madopar) and carbidopa (Sinemet) are peripheral DOPA decarboxylase inhibitors which prevent breakdown of levodopa to dopamine in the peripheral circulation and reduce dopaminergic side effects.

2. Ensure an appropriate route of administration of dopaminergic drugs

Most PD drugs are only available in oral preparations. If the patient is unable to take the drug by mouth then a nasogastric tube is likely to be required. Madopar dispersible tablets in solution (in levodopa-equivalent doses) can be used, although adjustments in dosage may be necessary because of shorter action than standard release levodopa. Apomorphine is the only non-oral drug that is licensed but rotigotine (transdermal) could also be used. These are dopamine agonists. Both should generally be used under the guidance of a PD specialist or with specialist pharmacy input. Apomorphine is not suitable generally for emergency administration in a drug naïve patient, but patients admitted on apomorphine should have this continued.

3. Ensure emergency supplies of common antiparkinsonian drugs are available and treatment is not delayed

Make drugs available at a defined setting in emergency care facilities. It is crucial that PD drugs are not stopped for any length of time as there is a significant risk of parkinsonism-hyperpyrexia syndrome (neuroleptic malignant-like syndrome) (see 4e). Patients with acute illness may have an increased requirement for dopaminergic medications on a temporary basis and it is important not to reduce total dopaminergic treatment unnecessarily unless there are clear signs of toxicity.

4. Ensure regular review for common complications and serious sequelae

(a) Neuropsychiatric features, such as confusion, hallucinations

Review the patient's mental status history. Neuropsychiatric features may reflect intrinsic PD pathology but first exclude underlying causes of confusion and delirium, e.g. infection, constipation, dehydration, metabolic upset, any recently prescribed medications. Only if necessary treat with low-dose benzodiazepines, e.g. 0.5 mg of lorazepam,

> **Box 26.1 Five-step guidelines on supportive therapy for patients with Parkinson's disease admitted to hospital** *(continued)*
>
> or very low dose atypical antipsychotic, e.g. quetiapine. Note that benzodiazepines such as lorazepam may prolong or worsen delirium. Do not use typical antipsychotics, e.g. haloperidol or chlorpromazine.
>
> ### (b) Nausea and vomiting
>
> Use domperidone (Motilium) or ondansetron (may be constipating). Avoid metoclopramide (Maxolon) and prochlorperazine (Stemetil).
>
> ### (c) Constipation
>
> Severe faecal impaction can impair absorption of antiparkinsonian drugs. Clear the bowel if necessary.
>
> ### (d) Dizziness and falls
>
> Check for postural hypotension. Consider stopping or deintensifying drugs which may lower blood pressure, e.g. antihypertensives, antianginals, antiheart failure drugs. Alpha-blockers may be prescribed for urinary obstructive symptoms. Check timings of medications if the time of dizziness appears fixed and review standing blood pressure. In patients with falls, consider sequelae such as fractures, subdural haematoma (particularly if receiving anticoagulants or antiplatelet agents) and pneumothorax.
>
> ### (e) Parkinson hyperpyrexia syndrome
>
> [Pyrexia, altered mental status (agitation confusion and stupor), autonomic dysfunction including labile blood pressure.] Laboratory findings may show leucocytosis and elevated creatinine kinase. Monitor temperature, pulse, blood pressure, mental status regularly.
>
> ## 5. Ensure that the specialist team (e.g. PD nurse specialist) is aware of admission as soon as possible

sudden withdrawal of dopaminergic medications, notably levodopa and amantadine. This syndrome has been reported under a number of different and somewhat similar sounding names. PHS may be the most specific and overarching term [15].

 The true prevalence of PHS is unknown as there is probably a spectrum from mild to life-threatening and several scenarios may trigger the condition. Classically, it occurred following a well-intentioned, but totally inadvisable, 'drug holiday', which should no longer be used. However, patients may stop medications themselves or on the advice of a clinician, believing that confusion is due to dopaminergic medication. Substitution of controlled-release formulations for immediate-release levodopa at equivalent doses may precipitate the syndrome due to lower bioavailability. Patients admitted with acute delirium may inadvisably be treated with typical neuroleptics such as haloperidol. Other reported triggers of

PHS include menstruation and metabolic upsets, particularly hypernatraemia, and abrupt reduction of dopaminergic medication following deep brain stimulation (DBS) [16]. These treatment-related effects are discussed in more detail in Chapter 29.

The clinical features of PHS appear very similar to those of neuroleptic malignant syndrome [17]. Increasing rigidity, tremor and progression to immobility may occur over hours to days. Patients can develop pyrexia and altered mental status ranging from agitation and confusion to stupor and coma. Autonomic signs such as tachycardia, tachypnoea, labile blood pressure, urinary incontinence, pallor and sweating are often also present. Temperatures as high as 41.7°C have been reported. Acute worsening of parkinsonian features may occur in the context of transient unresponsiveness to the patient's regular medication or to an increase in dopaminergic therapy [18]. Laboratory findings usually reveal a leucocytosis and elevated creatinine kinase. Mutism may occur, and other less common neurological features include seizures and myoclonus. Serrano-Duenas [17] performed a comparison of 11 patients with PHS and 21 with neuroleptic malignant syndrome. He reported that latency to onset of symptoms appeared longer (93 versus 49 hours for PHS and neuroleptic malignant syndrome, respectively). In addition, in PHS elevation of creatinine phosphokinase and the white blood cell count was significantly less marked and may be less helpful in diagnosis. PHS may have serious sequelae including increased disability or death. Medical complications include deep-vein thrombosis, pulmonary embolus, disseminated intravascular coagulation (DIC), aspiration pneumonia and acute renal failure secondary to myoglobinuria [16,17].

Management

PHS is a medical emergency. Early recognition of the syndrome is crucial to the outcome and its importance in emergency care facilities should be emphasized. The medication regimen and compliance should be reviewed, as should the covert use of neuroleptic drugs, including 'hidden neuroleptics' such as tricyclic/neuroleptic combinations. Poor absorption of levodopa secondary to faecal impaction should be considered. Other management is similar to that for neuroleptic malignant syndrome, and is essentially supportive, including rehydration with intravenous fluids and treatment of hyperpyrexia with antipyretics and cooling blankets. Cardiovascular monitoring, intravenous access, nasogastric suction, feeding and prevention of thrombotic complications, exclusion of infection and review of possible aspiration are all required. Although there are no controlled trials, the literature supports the use of a dopamine agonist. Bromocriptine is the most studied, but it is presumed that a non-ergot would be more sensible, and may need to be given by a non-oral route, perhaps in the form of apomorphine (subcutaneous) or rotigotine (transdermal) [14] from which the authors have had favourable results (unpublished) and recent reports corroborate these anecdotal findings [19]. Dantrolene has been used in severe cases despite significant adverse effects, but may only be beneficial in fully expressed cases with significant rigidity and hyperthermia. One double-blind study randomized patients to receive placebo or 1000 mg of methylprednisolone [20]. This study showed marked variability in patient response but suggested that steroid pulse therapy might shorten the duration of the illness.

The prognosis is variable, and the condition may prove fatal. With appropriate, timely intervention the symptoms should reverse but may take up to 7–14 days and most patients endure a prolonged hospital stay. Patients with acute renal failure and DIC have a particularly poor outcome.

Serotonin syndrome

A similar but unrelated syndrome, so-called serotonin syndrome, may also occur [21]. This comprises three symptom domains—cognitive behavioural features (confusion, agitation, coma, anxiety and hallucinations), autonomic features and neuromuscular features (myoclonus and hyperreflexia, muscle rigidity, restlessness, tremor, ataxia and extensor plantar responses). It is an iatrogenic disorder related to drugs that augment serotonin transmission. PD patients are significantly at risk because increased dopaminergic transmission in the central nervous system (CNS) can promote the release of serotonin. Further, PD patients are often treated with antidepressant agents, commonly a selective serotonin reuptake inhibitor (SSRI), along with dopaminergics. While rare, the specific interaction of the monoamine oxidase inhibitor (MAOI) selegiline and SSRIs is highlighted as a potential cause of serotonin syndrome. Patients on fluoxetine appear to be at specific risk as this drug has an active metabolite with a half-life of 7–14 days.

Narcotic analgesics such as meperidine, dextromethorphan and tramadol increase CNS serotonin. Following discontinuation, patients need a wash-out period of at least 5 weeks before starting another serotonergic agent. Herbal remedies including St John's Wort, ginseng and brewer's yeast may also increase the activity of serotonin [22]. Alterations in hepatic or renal function may contribute to elevated SSRI levels in patients receiving serotoninergic agents. Patients with PD may inadvertently receive more than one serotoninergic agent. Tricyclic antidepressants inhibit serotonin uptake to some extent, particularly clomipramine and trazodone. Apart from dopaminergic agents, other drugs that may cause elevation in serotonin levels include opioid drugs (oxycodone, buprenorphine), moclobemide, amphetamines, lithium and sumatriptan. Management of serotonin syndrome is beyond the scope of this chapter, but serotonin syndrome is an important differential diagnosis of PHS in parkinsonian patients. Gordon and Leder [22] give a comprehensive review and a list of other potentiating serotoninergic drugs.

Prescribing for co-morbidity in Parkinson's disease

Because PD becomes increasingly prevalent with advancing age, the general principles of prescribing for the elderly apply in many PD patients [23,24]. Drug therapy should be introduced at low doses with slow titration. Specific problems of mobility and dexterity should be considered in PD patients [25]. Elderly patients will receive multiple drugs and blanket implementation of disease management protocols in primary care (e.g. secondary prophylaxis of vascular disease), meaning that polypharmacy is the norm. Commonly, elderly patients may receive anticoagulant or antiplatelet drugs for atrial fibrillation, antihypertensives, statins and drugs for osteoporosis. The risk of adverse drug reactions is greatly increased in such patients and the benefit–risk ratio should be regularly reviewed. Swallowing difficulties are common, and suitable formulations and pharmacy review should be considered good practice because residual tablets in the mouth or oesophagus may be associated with ulceration.

Age-associated changes in physiology frequently lead to non-specific complaints such as dizziness, and patients and carers should be warned to avoid drug therapies such as metoclopramide, prochlorperazine or other labyrinthine sedatives which may worsen PD.

Patients with PD are particularly susceptible to orthostatic hypotension, which may be exacerbated by drugs used to treat co-morbid conditions, commonly antihypertensive agents. Regular routine review of medication with lying/standing blood pressure measurement is mandatory and reduction of antihypertensive therapy may be necessary, particularly with up-titration of dopaminergic drugs and with advancing disease. In patients who have had a fall the possibility of a subdural haematoma should be considered, particularly in those who are also receiving anticoagulants or antiplatelet agents.

Adverse drug reactions as a mimic of non-motor symptoms

Adverse drug reactions may present in a non-specific fashion in older patients mimicking non-motor symptoms such as confusion or delirium, depression, sleep disturbance or urinary incontinence [24]. Hypnotics and sedatives should be avoided as far as possible to reduce the risk of drowsiness, unsteadiness, falls and confusion. Non-steroidal anti-inflammatory drugs are commonly used in musculoskeletal disorders but present a particular hazard in older patients because of the risks of bleeding and acute renal impairment. Simple analgesics and non-pharmacological inputs should be considered as first steps in patients requiring analgesia.

Practical therapeutics in the older PD patient

The most pertinent effect of age on pharmacokinetics is a reduction in renal clearance [23]. Reduced renal excretion of a drug or its metabolites may cause toxicity. Infection or dehydration during acute illness in patients with PD may lead to rapid decompensation in renal clearance and increased sensitivity to drug effects.

Pramipexole and amantadine are both renally eliminated [23]. Accordingly, dose reduction or adjustment may be necessary in patients whose renal function is compromised. Domperidone, which is commonly used to treat co-morbid nausea and vomiting, carries a manufacturer's recommendation to reduce the dose in renal impairment. Tolcapone should be used with caution if creatinine clearance is less than 30 pmol min^{-1}. Cholinesterase inhibitors used in the treatment of dementia, such as rivastigmine, may require a dose reduction in renal impairment. Commonly used antibiotics such as amoxicillin and clarithromycin require adjustment in moderate to severe renal impairment. It should be remembered that many older patients with PD will have renal impairment, but because of reduced muscle mass, serum creatinine may appear 'normal'. Mild impairment in renal function should be assumed in all older patients, and use of estimated glomerular filtration rates or calculations of creatinine clearance based on the Cockroft and Gault formula will improve recognition of the severity of renal impairment.

The commonly used non-ergot dopamine agonist drugs ropinirole and rotigotine predominantly undergo hepatic metabolism and should be used with caution in patients with concurrent liver disease. Ergot dopamine agonists such as bromocriptine, cabergoline and pergolide have been associated with serosal fibrosis of the pleura, pericardium and retroperitoneum [26]. Non-motor symptoms intrinsic to PD, such as breathlessness, chest and abdominal pain and peripheral oedema, may be mimicked by the side effects of such ergot agonists. The acute respiratory side effects of dopamine agonists usually regress after ergot withdrawal but established fibrosis may not.

Cardiac valvulopathy with multiple valve involvement and features similar to fenfluramine/carcinoid syndrome has been described with ergot-based drugs and is probably related to 5-HT_{2B} agonism effects [27]; this has led to the restrictions on the use of these drugs and a need for monitoring, such that they have now been generally downgraded to second-line treatment options in many countries. Where they are used, patients should be appropriately monitored with haematological, biochemical and imaging investigations such as chest X-ray and echocardiography. As yet there is no evidence to link non-ergot dopamine agonists to fibrotic effects but it would seem prudent to keep these under consideration during clinical review.

A drug safety alert in 2012 from the Medicines and Healthcare Products Regulatory Agency (MHRA) in the UK [28] focused on the small risk of serious ventricular arrhythmia and sudden cardiac death with domperidone. This is considered to be associated with QT prolongation on electrocardiogram (ECG) and the risk of *torsade de pointes*. Where necessary, domperidone should be used in the lowest possible dose and the benefit–risk ratio regularly reassessed. *Recent MHRA guidance (2014) suggests domperidone should be used at the lowest effective dose (no more than three 10 mg tablets per day) *for the shortest possible duration*. Clinicians should also be aware of other drugs commonly used in PD that may be implicated in QTc prolongation (see Table 26.1).

Table 26.1 Drugs commonly used in PD patients that may prolong QTc

Substantial evidence as prescribed	Amiodarone
	Antifungals
	Antihistamines
	Citalopram
	Erythromycin/clarithromycin
Substantial evidence	Alfusozin
	Amantadine
	Clozapine/quetiapine
	Venlafaxine
	Ondansetron
Conditional	Amitriptyline
	Ciprofloxacin
	Galantamine
	Solifenacin

Derived from CredibleMeds® (http://crediblemeds.org/).

Drug interactions

Patients with PD are frequently treated with other medications for co-morbid disorders and vigilance for drug interactions is necessary. There are a large number of potential interactions with PD drugs [29].

Dopamine agonists such as ropinirole, rotigotine, cabergoline, pergolide and bromocriptine (but not pramipexole) have the potential for drug–drug interactions mediated by the cytochrome P450 enzyme system. Information about cytochrome P450 and drug interactions is readily available [30].

The most important drug interaction occurring with antiparkinsonian drugs is the risk of hypotension. This may occur when antihypertensive drugs are given with either levodopa, dopamine agonists or MAOI B drugs alone or in combination. Common culprits are angiotensin-converting enzyme (ACE) inhibitor drugs, alpha-blocker drugs (also used in the treatment of obstructive urinary symptoms in men), other antihypertensives such as beta-blockers, calcium-channel blocking agents, diuretics and moxonodine and antianginal drugs such as nitrates and nicorandil.

Other important interactions are the risk of hypertensive crisis and hyperexcitability if levodopa is given with MAOIs (e.g phenelzine, isocarboxacid, tranylcypromine and moclobemide). Some of the more important interactions with antiparkinsonian drugs are shown in Table 26.2.

Co-morbidity and the need for anaesthesia

Patients with PD commonly require surgical interventions such as orthopaedic procedures for arthritis or following fractures and urological and cataract operations. Careful pre-operative assessment of patients with PD is mandatory and should include careful assessment of the respiratory system because obstructive and restrictive respiratory dysfunction are common non-motor symptoms in PD. Unrelated co-morbidities which are common in an ageing population, such as chronic obstructive pulmonary disease or kyphosis secondary to osteoporosis, may impair ventilatory capacity.

It is important that the usual PD treatment schedule is adhered to as closely as possible. Anaesthetic considerations in PD patients have been reviewed by Nicholson et al. [31] and Kalenka and Schwarz [32]. Halothane and fluothane should be avoided in patients receiving levodopa because these agents sensitize the heart to catecholamines. Data regarding the safety of various anaesthetic agents is often based on small case series. Patients should have oral medication continued as near to anaesthesia and surgery as feasible and their treatment regimen recommenced as soon as possible after intervention, either with sips of water or via a nasogastric tube. Where this is not possible, consideration can be given to using apomorphine with domperidone suppositories or transdermal rotigotine. All potential drug interactions should be considered (especially when MAOIs are used). Brennan and Genever [33] have recently published a comprehensive review on the management of PD during surgery.

Following surgery, early mobilization and rehabilitation efforts are crucial for favourable outcomes and to avoid hypostatic complications.

Table 26.2 Important drug interactions with antiparkinsonian drugs (this list is not exhaustive—see main text).

Drug	Interaction
Levodopa	Synergism with antihypertensive drugs Reduced blood pressure with antianginal, ACE inhibitor, calcium antagonist drugs, beta-blockers, dipyridamole Reduced blood pressure with alpha-blockers for urinary obstruction Reduced absorption with oral iron and possibly with antimuscarinic agents Risk of hypertensive crisis when levodopa given with MAO inhibitors Reduced therapeutic effect with neuroleptic drugs, opioids, reserpine and alpha-methyldopa
Dopamine agonists	Synergism with antihypertensive and cardioactive drugs Elevation of macrolide antibiotics with bromocriptine and cabergoline Pramipexole renal excretion may be reduced by amantadine, cimetidine and other renally excreted drugs Reduced therapeutic effect with neuroleptic drugs, opioids and reserpine and alpha-methyldopa
Selegiline/ rasagiline MAO-B inhibitors	SSRI antidepressant drugs—risk of serotonin syndrome MAO inhibitors/tricyclic drugs—risk of serotonin syndrome Caution in combination with COMT inhibitors if selegiline dose >10 mg Linezolid contraindicated Ciprofloxacin increases AUC of rasagiline—other inhibitors of cytochrome P450 isoenzyme CYP1A2 may also do so Pethidine and opioid analgesics—may precipitate serotonin syndrome
COMT inhibitors	Do not use with non-selective MAO inhibitors or combination of RIMA and MAO-B inhibitor Caution with selegiline doses >10 mg May enhance effect of apomorphine Potential warfarin interaction (enhanced effect) through inhibition of cytochrome P450 Chelates ferrous sulphate—give medications 2–3 hours apart
Amantadine	Memantine contraindicated in combination – memantine may possibly enhance effects of dopaminergic therapy generally Toxicity with drugs that reduce renal clearance (e.g. diuretics, NSAIDs, ACE inhibitors) Accentuates adverse effects of anticholinergic drugs, for example, confusion, hallucinations Decreases tolerance of alcohol

ACE, angiotensin converting enzyme; SSRI, selective serotonin reuptake inhibitor; MAO, monoamine oxidase; COMT, catechol-O-methyltransferase; AUC, area under the plasma concentration curve; NSAID, non-steroidal anti inflammatory drug; RIMA, reversible inhibitor of monoamine oxidase Type A.

Source: British Medical Association, 2013 [23] and Jost and Bruck, 2002 [29].

Co-morbid cerebrovascular disease

The presence of cerebrovascular disease as an age-associated co-morbidity is common in elderly patients with neurodegenerative conditions such as PD and Alzheimer's disease [34] and may contribute to the early appearance or worsening of non-motor features such as depression, cognitive decline, orthostatic hypotension, urinary incontinence and gait disorder. Neuroimaging should be considered in such circumstances [35]. However, the relationship between cerebrovascular disease and PD is controversial [36]. Some studies have suggested a reduced frequency of stroke possibly related to smoking history or the protective effects of dopamine depletion [37]. Haugervoll et al. [38] suggested that cerebrovascular risk factors do not contribute to the risk of dementia in PD. In contrast, Beyer et al. [39] have reported significantly high levels of white-matter hyperintensities (WMH) in patients with PD dementia compared with a group without dementia. These findings suggest that WMH in the deep white matter may contribute to dementia in PD, along with other factors such as Alzheimer and Lewy body pathology. Several factors may cause WMH, including altered cerebral blood flow autoregulation, amyloid angiopathy and haemodynamic changes. Guerini et al. [40] reported that increasing subcortical cerebrovascular load was associated with a poorer functional recovery after rehabilitation in patients with gait disturbance and levodopa-refractory parkinsonism. Secondary prophylaxis of cerebrovascular disease in PD patients is therefore worthy of further attention. Co-morbid cerebrovascular disease in PD was comprehensively reviewed by Nanhoe-Mahabier et al. [41].

Co-morbid cardiovascular disease

Ischaemic heart disease, angina pectoris and atrial fibrillation are common co-morbidities in older patients with PD. A study in the United States [42] has suggested an increased incidence of heart failure in patients with PD; however, the study was cross-sectional in nature with potential surveillance bias. One study has suggested increased cardiovascular and ECG abnormalities in patients receiving combination dopaminergic therapy compared with levodopa [43]. In practice, routine ECGs should be carried out in older patients, particularly if drugs which may affect atrioventricular function (e.g. acetylcholinesterase inhibitors) or prolong the QT interval (e.g. quetiapine), as discussed in 'Practical therapeutics in the older PD patient', are used for neuropsychiatric symptoms. Any patients remaining on ergot-based agonists should be screened for pleuro-pericardial, retroperitoneal and cardiac fibrotic reactions as already noted. Oedema is a common side effect of dopamine agonist drugs. A history of coronary artery disease may increase the risk [44].

Co-morbidity and the endocrine system

Surveillance for thyroid disorders should be considered because non-specific symptoms may be similar to those of PD. Hypothyroidism may mimic or exacerbate symptoms of apathy and slowness while thyrotoxicosis may worsen tremor and weight loss. Screening for hypothyroidism may be most appropriately done before the first morning dose of levodopa as thyroid-stimulating hormone (TSH) may be suppressed for a few hours after levodopa treatment [45]. Apathy and other non-motor symptoms are associated with testosterone deficiency in male PD patients [46], although the benefits of supplementation have not been clearly demonstrated [47].

Co-morbid diabetes

Diabetes is a common co-morbidity in PD patients. Hu et al. [48] reported an increased risk of PD in Type 2 diabetes, although surveillance bias may be responsible for the findings. Another recent study [49] found no increased risk of PD in people with diabetes, hypertension or elevated cholesterol. Hyperuricaemia and gout appear to be inversely related to the risk of PD [50]. A recent systematic review has concluded that there is no conclusive evidence for diabetes being a risk factor for PD [51].

Diabetes is frequently associated with autonomic dysfunctions, such as gastroparesis, orthostatic hypotension, urinary dysfunction, diarrhoea or constipation and erectile dysfunction, which may augment or be confused with classical non-motor features in PD. Diabetic neuropathy may be occasionally confused with PD pain syndromes because radicular, burning or dysaesthetic pain syndromes may be common to both. Objective sensory testing may help to detect diabetic neuropathy.

Statins (HMG-CoA reductase inhibitors) may cause myopathy with elevation of creatinine phosphokinase and worsen mobility in PD patients. Managing hypertension in PD patients with diabetes is challenging because of the need to treat mildly elevated blood pressure to reduce cardiovascular risk while avoiding orthostatic hypotension.

Co-morbidity, weight loss and disorders of the digestive system

Weight loss is a common non-motor feature in PD [52] but the possibility of alternative pathology such as thyrotoxicosis, depression, tuberculosis or other cryptic infection and neoplasia should always be borne in mind. Antiparkinsonian and other co-morbid drugs may impair appetite and contribute to weight loss. Cancer is a relatively common co-morbidity in people with PD although there remains controversy as to whether there is an increased incidence of cancer in PD populations [53]. Acute environmental exposures to pesticides and oxidative stress mechanisms may be linked to both PD and cancer, although reduced rates of smoking may be protective.

Acute onset or worsening of dysphagia or constipation in the context of weight loss, iron-deficiency anaemia or rectal bleeding in a PD patient should prompt consideration of an investigation of the gastrointestinal tract. Constipation, once considered a coincidental co-morbidity, is now recognized as part of the non-motor disease complex and shares the same pathological hallmark of Lewy bodies in the myenteric plexus; it may pre-date the diagnosis of PD by many years [54]. Antiparkinsonian drug doses may need to be revised when weight loss is dramatic as dyskinesia may relate to mean body weight [55].

Co-morbid osteoporosis

Using bone densitometry, Wood and Walker [56] reported a high prevalence of osteoporosis in a population of PD patients with a median age of 75 years. There were associations between osteoporosis and age, depression and disease duration, but not disease severity. Although the prevalence did not exceed that of other people of a similar age, osteoporosis or osteopenia was present in all women in the study. Detection and management of osteoporosis (both primary and secondary) should be actively considered in all PD patients. Sato et al. [57] reported that treatment with risedronate and vitamin D_2 (1000 IU) for 2 years produced a reduced risk of hip fracture in elderly men with PD when compared with a PD group receiving a placebo and vitamin D_2. The relative risk of a hip fracture in the risedronate versus placebo group was 0.33 (95% CI 0.09–1.20). Because of the high prevalence of falls and risk of skeletal damage in PD, empirical treatment with vitamin D in all PD patients has been suggested [58]. That literature review highlighted the lack of prospective studies in this relatively neglected area.

Co-morbid urinary disorders

Symptoms of urinary dysfunction such as urgency, frequency, incontinence and nocturia are common in old age and also in PD [59]. After exclusion of infection, benign prostatic hypertrophy is a common co-morbidity in men and may complicate the intrinsic bladder dysfunction of PD. Both obstructive and irritable symptoms may occur. The conventional view that PD patients have a poor outcome after prostatic surgery has been challenged [59] as some earlier studies may have included patients with multiple system atrophy. However, it may be reasonable to give a cautious trial of anticholinergic drug therapy in patients with irritable symptoms after exclusion of obstruction and considering the potential for side effects such as constipation, confusion, dry mouth or blurred vision. If surgery is contemplated, formal urodynamic studies are mandatory [59]. Outflow obstruction due to PD may be reversible with subcutaneous apomorphine, and this has been proposed as a diagnostic test to distinguish symptoms from those of prostatic hypertrophy before surgery is contemplated. Stenosis of the bladder neck may contribute to obstructive uropathies in women. If there is reason to suspect a prostatic malignancy in men then a prostate-specific antigen test and digital rectal examination should be performed. A recent study [60] has reported a novel association between PD and prostate cancer, which extended to first-degree, second-degree and third-degree relatives as well as confirming the reported risk association for melanoma in patients with PD (see 'Co-morbidity and the skin').

Co-morbidity and the skin

Seborrhoea, common disorders of sweating and other skin abnormalities are common non-motor manifestations in PD. Clinicians should be aware of other important co-morbidities such as a possible increased risk of melanoma and other malignant skin tumours in patients with PD [61]. There is speculation that levodopa therapy increases the risk of cutaneous malignant melanoma; however, a recent study suggested that there is no epidemiological or experimental evidence of a causal role of levodopa increasing the risk of incidence or progression of melanoma [62,63] and that it is PD per se that carries the higher risk of melanoma rather than its treatment.

Skin rashes have been reported as side effects of levodopa preparations, and amantadine has been associated with livedo reticularis (Fig. 26.1). Chou and Stacy [64] have highlighted

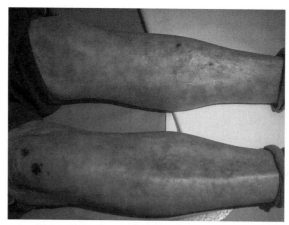

Fig. 26.1 Livedo reticularis in a patient receiving amantidine.

the association of a rash with allergic reaction to the yellow dye in some Sinemet® preparations of co-careldopa.

Conclusions

Co-morbidities are common particularly with advancing age and duration of PD. Clinicians who attend PD patients should have a working knowledge of the diagnosis and management of PD related and unrelated co-morbidities and how they may impact and interact with the treatment of PD. The appearance of serious or multiple co-morbidities may merit management in an intensive care unit setting [65].

All PD practitioners have an important role to play in spreading and sharing knowledge with other teams who may find themselves managing co-morbidities in patients with PD. A multidisciplinary and multiprofessional approach, particularly around pharmaceutical care, is necessary to optimize outcomes [66]. Further studies are needed to determine the impact of co-morbidities on the clinical expression and course of PD.

References

1 Diederich NJ, Moore CG, Leurgans SE, et al. Parkinson's disease with old-age onset. A comparative study with subjects with middle-age onset. Arch Neurol 2003; **60**: 529–33.

2 Playfer JR. The therapeutic challenges in the older Parkinson's disease patient. Eur J Neurol 2002; **9**(Suppl 3): 55–8.

3 De Groot V, Beckerman H, Lankhorst GJ, Bouter LM. How to measure comorbidity: a critical review of available methods. J Clin Epidemiol 2003; **56**: 221–9.

4 Visser M, Marinus J, van Hilten JJ, et al. Assessing comorbidity in patients with Parkinson's disease. Mov Disord 2004; **19**: 824–8.

5 Pressley JC, Louis ED, Tang M-X, et al. The impact of comorbid disease and injuries on resource use and expenditures in Parkinsonism. Neurology 2003; **60**: 87–93.

6 Woodford H, Walker R. Emergency hospital admissions in idiopathic Parkinson's disease. Mov Dis 2005; **20**: 1104–8.

7 Guttman M, Slaughter PM, Theriault M-E, et al. Parkinsonism in Ontario: comorbidity associated with hospitalization in a large cohort. Mov Dis 2004; **19**: 49–53.

8 Cosentino M, Martignoni E, Michielotto D, et al. Medical healthcare use in Parkinson's disease: survey in a cohort of ambulatory patients in Italy. BMC Health Serv Res 2005; **5**: 26.

9 Martignoni E, Godi L, Cittorio, A, et al. Comorbid disorders and hospitalisation in Parkinson disease: a prospective study. Neurol Sci 2004; **25**: 66–71.

10 MacMahon DG. PD nurse specialists-an important role in disease management. Neurology 1999; **52**(Suppl 3): S21–S25.

11 Magdalinou KN, Martin A, Kessel B. Prescribing medications in Parkinson's disease patients during acute admissions to a district general hospital. Parkinsonism Relat Disord 2007; **13**: 539–40.

12 Aminoff MJ, Christine CW, Friedman JH, et al. Management of the hospitalized patient with Parkinson's disease: current state of the field and need for guidelines. Parkinsonism Relat Disord 2011; **17**: 139–45.

13 Gerlach OHH, Winogrodzka A, Weber WEJ. Clinical problems in the hospitalised Parkinson's disease patient: systematic review. Mov Disord 2011; **26**: 197–208.

14 MacMahon M, MacMahon DG. Management of Parkinson's disease in the acute hospital environment. J R Coll Physicians Edinburgh 2012; **42**: 157–62.

15 Factor SA, Santiago A. Parkinsonism-hyperpyrexia syndrome in Parkinson's disease. In: SJ Frucht, S Fahn (eds) Current clinical neurology: movement disorders emergencies: diagnosis and treatment, pp. 29–40. Totowa, NJ: Humana Press, 2005.

16 Mizuno Y, Takubo H, Mizuta E, Kuno S. Malignant syndrome in Parkinson's disease: concept and review of the literature. Parkinsonism Relat Disord 2003; **9**: S3–S9.

17 Serrano-Dueñas M. Neuroleptic malignant syndrome-like, or dopaminergic malignant syndrome due to levodopa therapy withdrawal. Clinical features in 11 patients. Parkinsonism Relat Disord 2003; **9**: 175–8.

18 Onofrj M Thomas A. Acute akinesia in Parkinson's disease. Neurology 2005; **64**: 1162–9.

19 Wüllner U, Kassubek J, Odin P, et al.; NEUPOS Study Group. Transdermal rotigotine for the perioperative management of Parkinson's disease. J Neural Transm 2010; **117**: 855–9.

20 Sato Y, Asoh T, Metoki N, Satoh K. Efficacy of methylprednisolone pulse therapy on neuroleptic malignant syndrome in Parkinson's disease J Neurol Neurosurg Psychiatry 2001; **71**: 111–13.

21 Mason PJ, Morris VA, Balcezak TJ. Serotonin syndrome: presentation of 2 cases and review of the literature. Medicine 2000; **79**: 201–9.

22 Gordon MF, Leder A. Serotonin syndrome. In: SJ Frucht, S Fahn (eds) Current clinical neurology: movement disorders emergencies: diagnosis and treatment, pp. 175–85. Totowa, NJ: Humana Press, 2005.

23 British Medical Association. Prescribing for the elderly. In: British national formulary. London: British Medical Association, Royal Pharmaceutical Society, 2013

24 Simonson W, Feinberg JL. Medication-related problems in the elderly. Defining the issues and identifying solutions. Drugs Aging 2005; **22**: 559–69.

25 Thwaites JH. Practical aspects of drug treatment in elderly patients with mobility problems. Drugs Aging 1999; **14**: 105–14.

26 Titner R, Manian P, Gauthier P, Jancovic J. Pleuropulmonary fibrosis after long term treatment with the dopamine agonist pergolide for Parkinson's disease. Arch Neurol 2005; **62**: 1290–5.

27 Roth BL. Drugs and valvular heart disease. N Engl J Med 2007; **356**: 6–8.

28 MHRA. Domperidone: small risk of serious ventricular arrhythmia and sudden cardiac death. Drug Safety Update 2012; 5(issue 10): A2. Available at: <http://www.mhra.gov.uk/Safetyinformation/DrugSafetyUpdate/CON152725> (last accessed March 2014).

29 **Jost WH, Brück C**. Drug interactions in the treatment of Parkinson's disease. J Neurol 2002; 249: III/24–III/29.

30 **Flockhart DA**. Drug interactions: cytochrome P450. Indiana University School of Medicine Drug Interaction Table (last updated 12 July 2013). Available at: <http://medicine.iupui.edu/clinpharm/ddis/table.aspx> (last accessed March 2014).

31 **Nicholson G, Pereira AC, Hall GM**. Parkinson's disease and anaesthesia. Br J Anaesthesia 2002; **89**: 904–16.

32 **Kalenka A, Schwarz A**. Anaesthesia and Parkinson's disease: how to manage with new therapies. Curr Opin Anaesthesiol 2009; **22**: 419–24.

33 **Brennan KA, Genever RW**. Managing Parkinson's disease during surgery. Br Med J 2010; **341**: c5718.

34 **Jellinger KA, Attems J**. Prevalence and impact of cerebrovascular pathology in Alzheimer's disease and parkinsonism. Acta Neurol Scand 2006; **114**: 38–46.

35 **Grosset DG, Macphee GJA, Nairn M**. Diagnosis and management of Parkinson's disease: summary of SIGN guidelines. Br Med J 2010; **340**: b5614.

36 **Nataraj A, Rajput AH**. Parkinson's disease, stroke, and related epidemiology. Mov Dis 2005; **20**: 1476–80.

37 **Korten A, Lodder J, Vreeling F, et al**. Stroke and IPD: does a shortage of dopamine offer protection against stroke? Mov Disord 2002; **16**: 119–23.

38 **Haugarvoll K, Aarsland D, Wentzel-Larsen T, Larsen JP**. The influence of cerebrovascular risk factors on incident dementia in patients with Parkinson's disease. Acta Neurol Scand 2005; **112**: 386–90.

39 **Beyer MK, Aarsland D, Greve OJ, Larsen JP**. Visual rating of white matter hyperintensities in Parkinson's disease. Mov Dis 2006; **21**: 223–9.

40 **Guerini F, Frisoni GB, Bellwald C, et al**. Subcortical vascular lesions predict functional recovery after rehabilitation in patients with L-dopa refractory parkinsonism. J Am Geriatr Soc 2004; **52**: 252–6.

41 **Nanhoe-Mahabier W, Karlijn F, de Laat JE, et al**. Parkinson disease and comorbid cerebrovascular disease. Nat Rev Neurol 2009; **5**: 533–41.

42 **Zesiewicz TA, Strom JA, Borenstein AR, et al**. Heart failure in Parkinson's disease: analysis of the United States Medicare current beneficiary survey. Parkinsonism Relat Disord 2004; **10**: 417–20.

43 **Korchounov A, Kessler KR, Schipper HI**. Differential effects of various treatment combinations on cardiovascular dysfunction in patients with Parkinson's disease. Acta Neurol Scand 2004; **109**: 45–51.

44 **Kleiner-Fisman G, Fisman DN**. Risk factors for development of pedal oedema in patients using pramipexole. Arch Neurol 2007; **64**: 820–4.

45 **Munhoz RP, Teivea HAG, Troianoa AR, et al**. Parkinson's disease and thyroid dysfunction. Parkinsonism Relat Dis 2004; **10**: 381–3.

46 **Okun MS, McDonald WM, De Long MR**. Refractory non-motor symptoms in male patients with Parkinson's disease due to testosterone deficiency. Arch Neurol 2002; **59**: 807–11.

47 **Okun MS, Fernandez HH, Rodriguez RL**. Testosterone therapy in men with Parkinson's disease: results of the TEST PD study. Arch Neurol 2006; **63**: 729–35.

48 **Hu G, Jousilahti P, Bidel S, et al**. Type 2 diabetes and the risk of Parkinson's disease. Diabetes Care 2007; **30**: 842–7.

49 **Simon KC, Chen H, Schwarzchild M, Ascherio A**. Hypertension hypercholesterolaemia diabetes and risk of Parkinson's disease. Neurology 2007; **69**: 1688–95.

50 **Alonso A, Garda Rodriguez LA, Lagroscino G, Hernan MA**. Gout and risk of Parkinson disease: a prospective study. Neurology 2007; **69**: 1698–700.

51 **Cereda E, Barichelli M, Pedrolli C, et al.** Diabetes and risk of Parkinson's disease: a systematic review and meta analysis. Diabetes Care 2011; **34**: 2614–23.

52 **Kashihara K.** Weight loss in Parkinson's disease. J Neurol 2006; 253: VII/38–VII/41.

53 **Elbaz A, Peterson BJ, Bower JH.** Risk of cancer after the diagnosis of Parkinson's disease: a historical cohort study. Mov Disord 2005; **20**: 720–5.

54 **Abbot Ross GW, Abbott RD, Petrovitch H, Tanner CM, White LR.** Pre-motor features of Parkinson's disease: the Honolulu-Asia Aging Study experience. Parkinsonism Relat Disord 2012; **18**(Suppl 1): S199–S202.

55 **Sharma JC, Ross IN, Rascol O, Brooks D.** Relationship between weight, levodopa and dyskinesia: the significance of levodopa dose per kilogram body weight. Eur J Neurol 2008; **15**: 493–6.

56 **Wood B, Walker R.** Osteoporosis in Parkinson's disease. Mov Disord 2005; **20**: 1636–7.

57 **Sato Y, Honda Y, Iwamoto J.** Risedronate and ergocalciferol prevent hip fracture in elderly men with Parkinson disease. Neurology 2007; **68**: 911–15.

58 **Gnädingera M, Mellinghoff H-U, Kaelin-Lang A.** Parkinson's disease and the bones. Swiss Med Wkly 2011; **141**: w13154.

59 **Winge K, Fowler CJ.** Bladder dysfunction in parkinsonism: mechanisms prevalence symptoms and management. Mov Disord 2006; **21**: 737–45.

60 **Kareus SA, Figueroa KP, Cannon-Albright LA, Pulst SM.** Shared predispositions of parkinsonism and cancer: a population-based pedigree-linked study. Arch Neurol 2012; **69**: 1572–7.

61 **Olsen JH, Friis S, Frederiksen K.** Malignant melanoma and other types of cancer preceding Parkinson disease. Epidemiology 2006; **17**: 582–7.

62 **Olsen JH, Tangerud K, Wermuth L, et al.** Treatment with levodopa and malignant melanoma. Mov Disord 2007; **22**: 1252–7.

63 **Liu R, Gao X, Lu Y, Chen H.** Meta-analysis of the relationship between Parkinson disease and melanoma. Neurology 2011; **76**: 2002–9.

64 **Chou KL, Stacy MA.** Skin rash associated with Sinemet does not equal levodopa allergy. Neurology 2007; **68**: 1078–9.

65 **Freeman WD, Tan KM, Glass GA, et al.** ICU management of patients with Parkinson's disease or parkinsonism. Curr Anaesth Crit Care 2007; **18**: 227–36.

66 **Thomson FC, Muir A, Stirton J, et al.** Pharmaceutical care: Parkinson's disease. Pharm J 2001; **267**: 600–12.

Chapter 27

Non-motor symptoms of Parkinson's disease and the effects of deep brain stimulation surgery

Shen-Yang Lim, Elena Moro, Ai Huey Tan
and Anthony E. Lang

Introduction

Deep brain stimulation (DBS) of the subthalamic nucleus (STN) and globus pallidus internus (GPi) dramatically improves motor symptoms, daily functioning and quality of life (QoL) in well-selected patients with Parkinson's disease (PD) [1]. Since their introduction into clinical practice in the late 1990s, these procedures have become established, evidence-based treatment options for patients with severe motor response complications [1–3]. More recently, DBS has also been shown to provide superior outcomes compared with medical therapy alone in relatively early-stage PD [4]. Indeed, after levodopa, DBS is widely considered to be the most important advance in therapy for PD [5]. However, DBS is a complex procedure and successful treatment depends on the careful selection of appropriate candidates, optimal placement of the stimulating electrodes and post-operative adjustment of stimulation parameters and antiparkinsonian medications. Factors that may influence patient outcomes are listed in Table 27.1 [6].

Most studies have focused on the motor outcomes of treatment, but important changes in non-motor symptoms (NMS) are also seen post-operatively. It is important to consider NMS when selecting patients for surgery [6,7]. Some changes in NMS after DBS [e.g. in non-motor fluctuations (NMFs), pain or sleep disturbances] are very beneficial, but development or worsening of other NMS (mostly in the cognitive-behavioural domains) can also occur and potentially offset the benefits of DBS. It is now recognized that NMS have a significant impact on the QoL of PD patients, sometimes exceeding that of motor symptoms [8]. Thus, patient perceptions of outcome after DBS surgery may sometimes be more associated with non-motor domains of QoL than with motor or physical factors [9].

Table 27.1 Factors that may influence outcome after deep brain stimulation surgery for Parkinson's disease (PD)

Patient factors including levodopa response, age, gender, duration of PD, nature of patient's PD (e.g. cognitive impairment, extent of mesolimbic dopaminergic denervation), co-morbidities (e.g. psychiatric or personality disorder, substance abuse), adherence to treatment, coping skills, brain imaging factors

Surgical factors (e.g. electrode passes, surgical trajectory, electrode placement)

Target selection

Post-operative management (e.g. medication changes, fine-tuning of electrical parameters, attention to cognitive-behavioural issues)

Psychosocial adaptation to a life-changing event (e.g. loss of the 'sick role', unrealistic expectations), social environment (including adequacy of social supports) and culture

Natural progression of the underlying disease

Target selection—subthalamic nucleus or globus pallidus internus?

Bilateral DBS is performed much more frequently than unilateral DBS, although unilateral or staged implants can be considered in individual cases (e.g. where parkinsonian features are highly asymmetric) [3,10,11].

Whether the STN or the GPi is the better target continues to be debated [12,13]. Earlier studies suggested that STN DBS may be superior in improving the motor features of PD, and this became the procedure of choice in most centres [3,14,15]. To date, there are five randomized controlled trials that have compared STN DBS with GPi DBS (one pilot study included only nine patients and will not be discussed further) [16]. These studies demonstrate that, overall, both procedures have comparable efficacy in terms of motor outcomes [17–21].

It has been suggested that GPi DBS may be associated with less non-motor morbidity than STN DBS [3,14,22–25]. For example, in a 4-year multicentre study, cognitive-behavioural dysfunction occurred in a greater proportion of patients undergoing bilateral STN DBS ($n = 49$) versus GPi DBS ($n = 20$), in whom adverse events were relatively few (note, however, that subjects were not randomized to DBS target, and thus the study was not designed to enable direct comparisons between the two targets) [22,26]. Even so, similar improvements in QoL were seen at 6 months and 3–4 years post-surgery [27]. The perception of higher rates of adverse events after STN DBS may also be due in part to reporting bias, because of the preponderance of STN procedures being performed [28]. A meta-analysis of publications from 1996 to 2007 found that cognitive-behavioural events were more common in STN than GPi DBS patients, but the authors noted that the lack of consistent reporting was a major obstacle preventing accurate estimation; for example, the category of cognitive-behavioural adverse events was not reported in 22% and 33% of STN DBS and GPi DBS studies, respectively [14].

An early study randomizing patients to bilateral STN versus GPi DBS reported that cognitive-behavioural complications only occurred with STN DBS [19]. However, this study included a very small number of patients (10 in each group with 12 months of follow-up) and, as acknowledged by the authors, cognitive-behavioural changes were not examined in a rigorous way.

Indeed, of the five randomized controlled studies comparing STN DBS with GPi DBS, only two were relatively large and involved *bilateral* DBS [17,18]. Patients and evaluators were blinded to target site and both studies received 'high-quality' designations from the Movement Disorder Society [1]. In the study by Odekerken et al. [18] (the NSTAPS study; 65 GPi, 63 STN), a co-primary outcome was a composite score for cognitive, mood and behavioural effects 1 year after surgery. Patients fulfilling one or more of the following were given a negative composite score: clinically significant worsening on neuropsychological tests; psychosis, depression or anxiety lasting for 3 months or more; the loss of a professional activity; or the loss of an important relationship (e.g. marriage). The authors included the latter item because this may reflect subtle cognitive-behavioural problems that affect daily life but that may not be detected by standard questionnaires. There was no between-group difference in the number of patients with a negative composite score (56% for STN DBS versus 58% for GPi DBS, $P = 0.94$). The authors thus concluded that GPi DBS was *not* superior to STN DBS with respect to cognitive-behavioural outcomes. In the study by Follett et al. [17] (the Veterans Affairs Co-operative Studies Program 468 study; 147 STN, 152 GPi), non-motor variables were evaluated as secondary outcomes. At 24 months, both groups had similarly slight decrements in all measures of neurocognitive function, except for a greater decline in the STN patients for visuomotor processing speed (a mean between-group difference of 2.5 points on the Wechsler Adult Intelligence Scales III, range of scale 54–150 points). Verbal fluency scores worsened similarly in both groups ($P = 0.33$ and $P = 0.99$ for between-group differences in phonemic and semantic fluency, respectively). The communication subscale of the PD Questionnaire-39 (PDQ-39) worsened slightly for both groups post-DBS ($P = 0.54$ for between-group difference). Beck Depression Inventory (BDI) scores worsened slightly in the STN group, but improved slightly for GPi patients (mean between-group difference of 1.9 points, range of scale 0–63). It is unclear if the differences were clinically significant [29]. At 36 months (70 STN, 89 GPi), small differences were seen in favour of the GPi group with respect to the Mattis Dementia Rating Scale and the Hopkins Verbal Learning Test, whilst many other measures of cognitive functioning declined similarly in both groups, probably reflecting disease progression [30]. The authors suggested that these differences should be interpreted cautiously because STN patients were also slightly worse on baseline cognitive tests.

In the COMPARE trial, Okun et al. [21] assessed mood and cognition as co-primary outcomes 7 months after *unilateral* DBS (22 STN, 23 GPi), using the Visual Analogue Mood Scale (VAMS) and tests of verbal fluency. The study revealed no significant between-group differences in pre- to post-DBS change scores. A trend for a worsening in letter verbal fluency with STN versus GPi DBS did not reach the pre-defined $P < 0.025$ significance level ($P = 0.03$). Interestingly, the authors demonstrated that adverse mood effects (less 'happy', less 'energetic' and more 'confused') occurred when patients were stimulated ventrally at either target. The authors later reported smaller improvements in QoL in the STN group and postulated that changes in verbal fluency may have contributed to this [31]. The study by Rothlind et al. [20] comparing the neuropsychological performance of patients randomized to *unilateral* STN DBS (n = 19) and *unilateral* GPi DBS (n = 23) found mostly comparable outcomes. BDI scores improved after GPi DBS, but not after STN DBS.

Therefore, taken together, the more recent and relatively large randomized trials point to only small differences in cognitive and neuropsychiatric outcomes after STN and GPi DBS.

Nevertheless, some differences between the two procedures are still likely to be relevant, and they may potentially be associated with a different profile of cognitive-behavioural effects. Medications are reduced more after STN DBS [17,18,32]; this may ameliorate not only dyskinesia but also medication-related NMS [33] such as impulsive–compulsive behaviours (ICBs), psychosis or hypersomnolence [34]. However, in other patients a reduction of medication has been linked to the development of apathy, depression or anxiety ('hypodopaminergic' symptoms) [28,35]. The STN has broader influences than the GPi physiologically due to its extensive projections (serving as a nexus that integrates motor, cognitive and emotional processes). Moreover, the STN has a volume of only 200 mm³, its subdivisions being separated by functional gradients rather than by sharp boundaries [28,36–38]. Thus, it is unlikely that STN DBS selectively influences the motor part of this nucleus without impinging on domains (within the STN itself or in neighbouring structures) that are associated with cognitive and emotional functions.

Most of the rest of this chapter deals with STN DBS. A summary of the (much more limited) literature on the non-motor effects of GPi DBS will be presented towards the end.

Less commonly used targets

DBS of the ventral intermediate nucleus of the thalamus

This procedure improves tremor but not other parkinsonian features or dyskinesia and has largely been replaced by STN or GPi DBS [6,39]. Unilateral or bilateral ventral intermediate (Vim) DBS does not appear to have a significant effect on cognitive abilities, and to our knowledge there are no reports of adverse psychiatric outcomes in PD patients after this procedure [7,39].

DBS of the pedunculopontine nucleus

The pedunculopontine nucleus (PPN) is a new target currently being studied for the management of axial signs that fail to respond to levodopa and conventional DBS targets. However, small blinded trials showed only a subjective reduction in falls with no impact on other manifestations of PD [40,41]. Therefore, the data do not support the use of PPN DBS in routine clinical practice at this time.

Neurocognitive and neuropsychiatric sequelae of STN DBS

Cognitive-behavioural symptoms account for the majority of non-motor adverse effects that occur following STN DBS [28].

Post-operative delirium

This complication typically occurs during the first few post-operative days and is usually self-limiting. It is the most frequent reason for delayed discharge from hospital following DBS surgery [42]. Older age, pre-operative cognitive impairment or depression and multiple frontal lobe tracts during surgery may be risk factors [42–45]. Several studies have reported very similar rates of this complication (22–24%) [17,18,46], but this was only 3% (5/183 patients) and 4% (5/136 patients) in the studies by Williams et al. [15] and Okun et al. [47], respectively.

Cognitive symptoms

STN DBS in carefully selected patients is relatively safe and does not lead to global cognitive deterioration [4,7,48–50]. In a recent large randomized controlled multicentre trial, there was no difference in overall cognitive functioning at 6 months in operated versus medically managed patients [48]. A low incidence of dementia at longer-term follow-up in some studies (0–10% after 5–8 years) is likely to reflect a selection bias, since patients undergoing DBS are generally younger and healthier and those with pronounced cognitive deficits or severe brain atrophy on imaging are excluded [6,46,51,52].

Older patients and those with cognitive impairment or poorer executive functions may be at risk of sustaining global cognitive deterioration after STN DBS, perhaps reflecting lower levels of cognitive reserve [43,44,53–56]. The presence of hallucinations or a low levodopa response at baseline may also be risk factors [54,55]. There appears to be a small incremental neuropsychological burden associated with bilateral DBS compared with unilateral treatment [20,57].

The most consistent cognitive side effect is a decline in verbal fluency, typically of a mild to moderate degree [7,48,49,58]. Microlesions produced by the surgical procedure may be responsible, as this complication is typically observed immediately after surgery [50,51,53,59,60]. Consistent with this, Okun et al. [47] demonstrated that verbal fluency deteriorated similarly after STN implantation regardless of whether the stimulator was turned on. Some authors suggested that declines in verbal fluency may result from apathy, commonly seen after STN DBS [59,61], but one study specifically evaluating this relationship found no correlation between these two features [62]. One study found that left-sided treatment was more associated with reductions in verbal fluency [20], but no laterality effect was observed by Okun et al. [21]. A degree of recovery may be seen with longer-term follow-up [58,60,63,64].

In addition, DBS may have a small adverse effect on other neuropsychological domains sensitive to frontal-subcortical dysfunction [48,49,55]. In their meta-analysis, Parsons et al. [49] found significant but small declines in executive functions and verbal learning and memory. It is currently uncertain if, or to what extent, these changes in neuropsychological test performance impact on the performance of activities of daily living, QoL or caregiver burden [31,48,51,63]. Some authors reported that the worsening in executive functions after DBS can be transient, returning to baseline by 12 months post-surgery [58,64].

There are only a few reported cases of severe cognitive decline due to misplaced electrodes; these patients recovered after repositioning of the contacts or electrodes [65,66].

Apathy

The majority of studies that have quantified apathy after STN DBS found increased apathy after surgery [67]. Apathy is the most frequent long-term adverse psychiatric effect of STN DBS [28]. Some authors have proposed that STN stimulation itself could contribute to the development of apathy [68], but this seems unlikely since acute STN DBS has psycho-stimulant effects (albeit to a lesser degree than acute levodopa challenge) [35,59,69,70]. In the study by Thobois et al. [35], 54% of patients developed apathy post-operatively. This higher than usual incidence was probably due to the drastic reduction in dopaminergic medication (immediate discontinuation of dopamine agonists and a mean 82% reduction of levodopa over 2 weeks). Apathy had resolved by 12 months in half the cases; at this time, 37% of patients had resumed dopamine agonist therapy. Using ^{11}C-raclopride positron emission tomography (PET), the authors found that individual variation in mesolimbic dopaminergic denervation (due to the neurodegenerative process) plus post-operative dopamine reduction leads to apathy [35]. The presence of neuropsychiatric fluctuations at baseline emerged as a major risk factor for the development of post-operative apathy (a 2.5-fold increased risk). Notably, the appearance of apathy may be delayed by many months after the reduction of dopaminergic medications.

Post-operative apathy often responds to an increase in dopaminergic medications [35,46], especially dopamine agonist therapy [35,71]. Apathy that does not respond to dopaminergic treatment also occurs, typically much later and often in parallel with worsening of frontal cognitive functions related to disease progression [46].

Depression

The effects of STN DBS on depressive symptoms are highly variable. A systematic review including 1398 patients from 82 studies reported a frequency of post-operative depression of 8% [72], but it was as high as 25% (moderate to severe depression) in a small prospective study of 24 patients (remarkably, half of these patients were also transiently suicidal, despite clear motor improvement) [73]. Other prospective studies reported that depressive symptoms improved post-operatively, although the effect size may be small [4,47,48,59,62,74,75]. Risk factors for post-operative depression include excessive withdrawal of dopaminergic medications and a previous history of depression [28,35,70]. Psychosocial factors are also likely to play a role, and similar adverse responses (including suicide) have been reported after dramatically life-changing surgery for other chronic disabling diseases. Reports of depressive states with an onset time-locked to stimulation are rare and are probably due to the effects of stimulation outside the STN [76–78]. Resuming or increasing dopaminergic medication may be appropriate, even if this treatment is not required to control parkinsonian motor symptoms [7,35,46,59]. In severe and refractory cases, electroconvulsive therapy may be a safe and effective option [79].

Anxiety

Anxiety worsened after surgery in one retrospective study, with 63% of operated patients experiencing a fear that the stimulator would suddenly fail; the duration of this specific phobic symptom is not known [70]. In the study by Weaver et al. [80], anxiety occurred more frequently in patients randomized to DBS (STN or GPi) versus medically treated patients, but no further details were provided. However, subsequent prospective studies found either no change [4,81] or an improvement [48,74,75,82] in anxiety levels 3–24 months after surgery.

Emotional hyperactivity/lability

Excessive mood-congruent emotional responses to minor triggers were reported in 75% of operated patients in one retrospective study [70]. Odekerken et al. [18] reported an 84% incidence of emotional lability after STN DBS. In a study by Smeding et al. [83], family members reported an increase in irritability/lability on the Neuropsychiatric Inventory (NPI) compared with a non-operated control group. In the COMPARE trial, an exploratory analysis suggested that that there was increased anger in patients randomized to unilateral STN DBS, but not GPi DBS [21]. Analysis of a larger dataset of patients (STN 195, GPi 56) revealed that both groups of patients were significantly angrier at 1–3 months post-surgery, with no significant difference between the two groups [84]. Changes in anger scores were associated with the number of microelectrode passes, suggesting that this may be a lesional effect. In contrast, Lhommee et al. [34] reported (non-significant) reductions in the prevalence of patients scoring ≥2 on the Ardouin scale for 'irritability/aggressiveness' and 'hyper-emotivity' (from 14.5 to 6.5% and 35.5 to 24.2%, respectively) 1 year post-surgery.

Hypomania/mania

A systematic review found a 4% frequency of post-operative hypomania or mania [72]. However, no cases of this complication were reported in more recent series involving relatively large cohorts of patients [15,17,48]. This complication typically occurs within the first 3–6 months after surgery and is usually transient [28,46,59,85–87]. Implicated factors include pre-morbid vulnerability (e.g. a history of medication-induced mania), brain microlesions from the surgical procedure and a synergistic psychotropic effect of stimulation and dopaminergic medication (the latter is likely to be the predominant factor) [7,46,69,86,87]. Acute STN stimulation induces feelings of well-being and euphoria, increases motivation and decreases fatigue, anxiety and tension [69]. In one study, uncontrollable laughter was induced in two patients by an acute increase in stimulation; chronic stimulation at therapeutic parameters led to hypomania in one of these patients [88].

Electrode contacts within the anteromedial STN [28,38,89] or caudal to the STN at the midbrain level (e.g. the substantia nigra) [85,90] were implicated in several cases. One small study suggested that men may be more prone to developing transient manic psychosis post-operatively [91]. Management strategies include: a decrease in stimulation or a change in stimulation contacts (e.g. to more dorsal contacts), a decrease in dopaminergic medication and/or treatment with an atypical antipsychotic or mood stabilizer [86,87,92–94].

Impulsive–compulsive behaviours: impulse control disorders, compulsive medication use/dopamine dysregulation syndrome and punding

In three studies the overall frequency of these behaviours in patients presenting for DBS was 7% [34], 16% [95] and 48% [96]. The largest prospective study to date, by Eusebio et al. [97] ($n = 110$ consecutive patients undergoing bilateral STN DBS), reported pre-operative prevalence rates of 16% for CMU (11% DDS) and 32% for one or more ICDs. Risk factors for ICBs include dopamine agonist therapy, higher doses of dopaminergic medications, male gender, younger age of onset of PD, a history of ICBs or substance misuse, depression and single status [96,98,99]. Treatment is often difficult, with reduction of antiparkinsonian drugs being the most important management approach; however, this is often limited by the deterioration of parkinsonian symptoms. Some patients improved dramatically after STN DBS coupled with medication reduction [34,35,96,100–102], but in other patients these behaviours can decompensate or even develop for the first time post-operatively [70,95,99,102,103].

Lhommee et al. [34] reported that 1 year after surgery, ICBs had disappeared in all 30 patients (17 with behavioural addictions, 4 DDS, 9 isolated CMU). The authors used a strategy of immediate post-operative discontinuation of dopamine agonists and a marked reduction of levodopa over 2 weeks (mean 69% reduction in levodopa equivalent units at 1 year). In their series of 63 patients undergoing bilateral STN DBS there was only one case of new-onset CMU (a patient with misplaced electrodes) [34]. Eusebio et al. [97] also reported dramatic improvement in CMU/DDS (resolving in at least 83% of cases, and with no new occurrences) and ICDs (with the exception of binge eating, which increased) 1 year after DBS. In this study, post-operative adjustment of PD medications and stimulation settings followed the centre's 'routine' procedure, but this was not explained further. Levodopa equivalent daily dose (LEDD) reduced by 48% in the dopamine misuse group versus 32% in the group without dopamine misuse (P not significant). Similarly, in the series by Shotbolt et al. [96], no new cases of ICBs were observed in 29 patients undergoing DBS surgery, although it is not clear if the STN was the surgical target in all of these patients.

In some studies, poor behavioural outcomes were associated with a lack of reduction of dopaminergic medication after surgery, either because the motor outcome would be suboptimal or because patients resisted drug withdrawal (e.g. to avoid anxiety, dysphoria or other NMS) [95,97,102,103]. In some patients, STN DBS seems to induce impulsive behaviours/premature responding, proposed to be due to functional inactivation of the normal subthalamic 'no-go/hold your horses' signal (i.e. the normal ability to slow down when faced with decision conflicts), while on DBS, PD patients actually sped up [28,104,105]. In the addiction literature, a reduced ability to inhibit impulses is a vulnerability factor for developing substance and behavioural addictions [106]. Recognition of the presence of these behaviours by the DBS team is important [35,70,96,102], and a strategy of relatively rapid post-operative drug withdrawal may be important in some patients [35,101]. Compliance and motivation to wean medication should be considered when selecting these patients for surgery [101,102,107]. The need to reduce or withdraw medication to improve these behaviours should be balanced with careful assessments of consequent apathy or the features of the dopamine agonist withdrawal syndrome [35,108]. Adjustment of stimulation settings was reported to be useful in managing a few cases of ICBs [109,110].

Psychosis

Studies have reported a 35–72% prevalence of hallucinations or delusions in patients presenting for DBS [111,112]. STN DBS may be associated with a lower risk of psychosis due to significant reductions in antiparkinsonian medications. In randomized controlled studies, psychosis occurred in 0–5% of DBS versus 5–9% of medically treated patients [4,48]. Retrospective surveys also reported improvement of psychotic symptoms after bilateral STN DBS and reduction of dopaminergic medications [111,113]. Umemura et al. [113] reported complete disappearance of psychotic symptoms in all 10 patients with severe pre-operative hallucinations or delusions (although in two patients these features initially worsened, before gradually disappearing over a few months). There is only one case report of a patient developing new-onset of visual hallucinations time-locked to STN stimulation [114].

Psychosocial maladjustment

Despite marked improvement in parkinsonism, an absence of significant changes in cognitive status and improvement in activities of daily living and QoL, STN DBS can result in poor adjustment of the patient to socioprofessional aspects of life [70,115]. Currently, patients undergoing DBS typically have advanced PD, with disease duration of 10–15 years [3,6]. The sudden breakdown in patterns of dependency built up over years can have a marked impact on interpersonal relationships. Therefore, there may be a role for DBS earlier, rather than being solely a treatment of 'last resort' when QoL, psychosocial competence and professional activities are already severely impaired [4,27,82]. In the recent study by Schupbach et al. [4], which demonstrated that STN DBS provided superior outcomes compared with medical therapy alone, patients had a mean disease duration of 7.5 years and levodopa-induced motor complications were present for only 1.7 years.

Suicide

Patients can become suicidal despite a dramatic improvement in motor function [70,73,116,117]. An international survey involving 55 centres and 5311 patients undergoing STN DBS reported a 0.5% rate of completed suicide and 0.9% rate of attempted suicide [118]. This was considerably lower than the 4.3% completed suicide rate reported in an earlier single-centre study (140 patients with various movement disorders treated with bilateral DBS) [116]. Another single-centre study reported rates of 1% completed suicide and 2% attempted suicide [117]. In the study by Voon et al. [118], the highest risk was during the first two post-operative years. Single status, post-operative depression and a history of ICDs accounted for 51% of the variance for attempted suicide risk. Other potential risk factors include male gender, young-onset PD, impulsiveness, a previous suicide attempt, substance abuse, multiple DBS surgeries and post-operative apathy [116–118]. It has been suggested that patients presenting for DBS may represent a select group with a higher risk for suicidal behaviour—and indeed a higher burden of psychiatric disorders overall—compared with the general PD population [4,112].

Non-motor fluctuations

NMS commonly occur in association with the 'off' medication state [119,120]. Some NMFs (e.g. fluctuating pain, or rebound worsening of affect during 'off' periods) may also reflect, at least in part, a process of pharmacological sensitization and aberrant plasticity in limbic and cognitive brain regions (e.g. the ventral striatum) induced by chronic levodopa treatment [121–123].

Witjas et al. [124] reported striking improvements in a range of NMF (sensory, cognitive, dysautonomic, e.g. drenching sweats, and, to a lesser extent, psychic fluctuations) 1 year after STN DBS ($n = 40$). Lhommee et al. [34] reported that psychic fluctuations were markedly diminished 12 months post-surgery. The proportion of patients with significant (Ardouin scale score ≥ 2) off-period dysphoria in everyday life was reduced from 42% to 14%, and on-period 'artificial' euphoria from 35% to 6% [34]. Likewise, another study involving 20 patients reported a reduction in the frequency and severity of NMF in the 'off'-medication state 2 years after STN DBS [125]. The improvement in off-period symptoms may be due to diffusion of DBS current to the non-motor territories of the STN, whilst the reduction in the acute psychostimulant effects of levodopa after chronic STN DBS may be due to desensitization of the ventral striatum (as pulsatile dopaminergic treatment is replaced with continuous stimulation) [123].

Studies focusing on pain outcomes are discussed further later (Sensory symptoms; Pain).

Sleep disorders

Nocturnal sleep disturbance

STN DBS improves sleep time and quality, probably due to improvement of overnight akinesia or dystonia and reductions in antiparkinsonian medication [123–131]. In some studies, restless legs syndrome (RLS) and periodic leg movements in sleep (PLMS) emerged after DBS, presumably as a result of reductions in dopaminergic medication [127,132], although others reported marked improvement despite reductions in levodopa equivalents of 50% or more [131,133]. Rapid eye movement sleep behaviour disorder is not improved by DBS [126,127].

Excessive daytime sleepiness

The combination of reduction of medication and improvement in sleep may be associated with reduced daytime somnolence [134], but this was not found in other studies [128,130,131].

Autonomic symptoms

Bladder dysfunction

This issue has only been investigated in small studies (n = 5–16) [135–137]. Normalization of urodynamic parameters (delaying the first desire to void and increasing bladder capacity) was demonstrated using 'on' versus 'off' STN stimulation protocols [136,137]. In contrast, Winge et al. [135] reported that, compared with pre-operative status, urodynamic parameters were unchanged after 6 months of chronic STN DBS. Although scores for total lower urinary tract symptoms (LUTS) did not change and the International Prostate Symptom Score for symptoms of overactive bladder improved, the Danish Prostate Symptom Score (5–8) questionnaire score for *troublesome* symptoms of overactive bladder was slightly worse at 6 months compared with pre-DBS, and more patients experienced *severe troublesome* LUTS 3–6 months post-DBS [135].

Sexual dysfunction

In one study evaluating changes in sexual function following bilateral STN DBS (n = 31), Castelli et al. [138] found no changes in female patients, whereas male patients reported slightly (but significantly) more satisfaction with their sexual life 9–12 months post-operatively. The authors reported that improvements were more evident in male patients under 60 years of age (but n = 7 only in this subgroup). The changes in total Sexual Functioning Inventory (SFI) scores were not statistically significant in either males or females. No correlation was found between sexual functioning and variables such as depression, severity of motoric function or dopaminergic treatment.

Gastrointestinal dysfunction

In one study of 18 patients without dysphagia pre-operatively, STN DBS (evaluated 20 months post-surgery) had no clinically relevant influence on deglutition; videofluoroscopic images were evaluated blindly [139]. However, and in accord with the results of another study (n = 14) [140], improvements were seen in quantitative parameters of the pharyngeal phase of deglutition in the DBS 'on'-stimulation state compared with the 'off' state and the pre-operative condition. Arai et al. [141] evaluated gastric emptying using the ^{13}C-acetate breath test (n = 16) and found that bilateral STN DBS significantly improved gastric emptying time (30.0 min in the 'on'-stimulation state versus 44.0 min 'off'-stimulation, $P < 0.001$); gastric emptying was not improved by levodopa administration before surgery. However, upper gastrointestinal symptoms were not assessed. A retrospective chart review (n = 36) reported that the prevalence of constipation was lower 24 months after bilateral STN DBS compared with the pre-surgical baseline (41 versus 67%) [142]. In the PD SURG trial, constipation classified as a 'serious' adverse event was reported for three patients randomized to DBS versus two patients receiving medical therapy alone [15].

Cardiovascular dysfunction

Using 'on' versus 'off' STN stimulation protocols, one study (n = 14) showed that STN stimulation had no influence on cardiovascular autonomic function [143] whereas another study ($n = 14$) reported stabilization of blood pressure during tilt table testing with DBS 'on' [144]. In a controlled study of patients with advanced PD (84% of whom had subclinical dysautonomia as assessed by heart rate variability and orthostatic tests), no difference in cardiovascular autonomic dysfunction was seen 1 year after STN DBS despite significant reduction in pharmacotherapy, compared with control (pharmacologically managed) patients [145].

Weight gain

The majority of patients gain weight after STN DBS, on average 3–10 kg [46,146–152]. Two studies documented an increased proportion of overweight patients [body mass index (BMI) ≥ 25 kg m^{-2}] from 13% and 16% pre-operatively to 47% and 37%, respectively, one year after surgery, although obesity (BMI ≥ 30 kg m^{-2}) was uncommon [147,148]. This mostly occurs in the first three post-operative months and may be rapid, although slower gain beyond the first post-operative year has also been documented [46,147,148,152]. One study reported that body weight may return towards pre-operative baseline in the ensuing years, possibly related to disease progression [153].

This phenomenon remains largely unexplained; possible factors include decreased energy expenditure due to amelioration of dyskinesia or parkinsonism, spread of current into hypothalamic-associated homeostatic control centres or fibre bundles, or abnormal eating behaviour/food craving [147,148,154,155]. One study found that medial contacts were associated with greater weight gain than those located laterally [152]. Overweight and obesity are risk factors for other health problems (diabetes, cardiovascular disease, etc.) and may exacerbate the impairment of motor function; therefore, patients should be given nutritional advice before or very soon after DBS to prevent excessive weight gain [156,157]. However, in other patients with unintended weight loss, the weight gain after surgery may be beneficial.

Sensory symptoms

Pain

In one early study selecting PD patients with disabling 'off'-period dystonia ($n = 8$), STN DBS reduced 'off'-period dystonia and 'off'-period pain by 90 and 66%, respectively [158]. Witjas et al. [124] reported striking improvements in a range of non-motor fluctuations 1 year post-STN DBS ($n = 40$), with the greatest reductions observed for pain and sensory fluctuations (the score for pain/sensory symptoms improving by 84%; note that the analysis excluded dystonic pain). Kim et al. [159] reported that pain (experienced by 79% of 29 patients at baseline) disappeared or improved at 3 months after STN DBS in 87% of patients; fluctuating 'off'-period pain improved in 94% of patients. Further improvement was seen at 24 months, although 43% reported new pain (mostly musculoskeletal) that was not present at baseline; despite this, the mean pain score at follow-up was lower than at baseline (4.1 versus 6.8; range of scale 0–10) [160]. One small study selecting patients with PD-related central neuropathic pain ($n = 8$) found a significant reduction in mean pain Visual Analog Scale score 3 months or more after STN DBS (5.4 versus 7.5) [161]. Another study of 12 patients with primarily nociceptive pain reported reduction in pain intensity 1–40 weeks post-STN DBS (1.9 versus 4.3); fewer patients also experienced sensory symptoms other than pain post-DBS (33 versus 75%) [162]. The study by Ciampi de Andrade et al. [163], involving 25 patients a mean of 2.4 years after bilateral STN DBS, aimed primarily to evaluate sensory thresholds but the authors also reported a significantly lower prevalence of chronic pain (36 versus 72%) post-surgery. Postulated mechanisms underlying a reduction of pain with STN DBS include reduction of dystonia or muscle rigidity, modulation of the cerebral processing of pain and improvement in mood [161,164,165].

Hyposmia

Some studies reported that odour identification improved significantly in the ON-stimulation condition [166,167]. Improved cortical integration of olfactory information mediated by STN DBS was proposed to underlie these changes.

Overall improvement in NMS after STN DBS

A few studies used recently validated scales encompassing a broad range of NMS—the PD NMS Questionnaire (NMSQuest; which evaluates the presence or absence of symptoms) and/or the PD Non-motor Scale (NMSS; which measures the severity and frequency of individual symptoms)—before and after STN DBS. Nazzaro et al. [168] reported that 1 year after bilateral STN DBS (*n* = 24), the mean number of NMS decreased from 12 to 7, and 27 of the 30 items in the NMSQuest (i.e. 90% of items) were reported less frequently. The improvement in NMS was associated with improvement in QoL as measured by the PDQ-39. Other small studies of bilateral and unilateral STN DBS reported broadly similar outcomes (reduction in overall NMS burden) [169,170].

GPi DBS and non-motor effects

Cognitive-behavioural outcomes

Many studies reported minimal cognitive-behavioural changes after GPi DBS. The most consistent decline is in verbal fluency, probably comparable to that seen after STN DBS (reviewed by Rothlind et al. [20]; see also the section 'Target selection—subthalamic nucleus or globus pallidus internus?'). However, in one open-label study of 17 patients undergoing bilateral GPi DBS (nine with baseline cognitive dysfunction considered by the authors to contraindicate treatment with STN DBS), neuropsychological performance (including tests of verbal fluency) remained stable at 6 months post-surgery [23].

There are isolated case reports of cognitive deterioration (severe executive dysfunction) and psychiatric complications including mania and hypersexuality after GPi DBS [171–173]. There are a few reported cases of pre-operative DDS and/or ICDs persisting after GPi DBS [95,102]. In one series, of the 17 patients (out of 159, or 11%) developing new-onset

ICDs after DBS of the GPi or STN, nine cases were after GPi DBS (seven unilateral, two bilateral) [95]. In the study by Odekerken et al. [18] emotional lability was reported in 72% of GPi patients (versus 84% of STN patients, $P = 0.29$). The rate of post-operative delirium (20–22%) in randomized controlled studies was similar to that seen with STN DBS [17,18], but in one series involving 'high-risk' patients this complication was observed in only 1/17 (6%) patients [23].

Weight gain

Sauleau et al. [149] reported less weight gain after bilateral GPi DBS (1.7 kg; $n = 14$) than bilateral STN DBS (mean 5.7 kg; $n = 32$) 6 months post-operation. Volkmann et al. [174] reported similar results, with weight gain of over 10 kg in 27% of bilateral GPi DBS patients ($n = 11$) versus 37% of STN patients ($n = 16$). However, target selection in these studies was non-randomized. In the study by Mills et al. [175], patients randomized to bilateral STN DBS had slightly greater weight gain than those undergoing bilateral GPi DBS, but this difference (3 kg) was not statistically significant. Locke et al. [150] reported that patients randomized to undergo unilateral GPi DBS ($n = 23$) gained a similar amount of weight at 6 months post-surgery (2.4 kg; $n = 23$) as patients undergoing unilateral STN DBS (1.9 kg; $n = 21$).

Management of patients undergoing DBS

The complexity of the management required for DBS stresses the need for an expert multidisciplinary team approach, consisting of a movement disorders neurologist, neurosurgeon, neuropsychologist and psychiatrist [9,176]. Specially trained nurses or nurse practitioners are often important members of this team. Allied health therapists such as occupational therapists, speech therapists, dieticians, physiotherapists and social workers should also be involved.

Pre-operative management

A careful evaluation of the patient's cognitive and psychiatric function, coping skills, adequacy of social support, adherence to treatment and expectations of surgery is mandatory [6,28,176]. Patients should be educated about the *broad* potential impact of DBS [177]. Unrealistic expectations need to be addressed.

DBS is not appropriate for patients with moderate or severe cognitive impairment who risk sustaining further loss of cognition that may, despite motor improvement, increase dependency [43,54]. However, there is currently no consensus on the type of testing for establishing cognitive impairment or on the cut-off level of performance that should be respected for eligibility for DBS [3].

Psychiatric areas to be assessed include mood, anxiety, apathy, psychotic symptoms, ICBs, impulsivity and suicidal tendencies. Attention needs to be given to prior (lifetime) as well as to current issues. Patients should be instructed to be as frank as possible; even so, some patients may not volunteer such histories readily, perhaps for fear of not qualifying for surgery [28,70,102,112]. Surgery should generally be deferred in patients with unstable psychiatric conditions until treatments have been optimized and symptoms adequately controlled. Surgery is contraindicated in patients with active and severe treatment-refractory psychiatric disorders or a non-modifiable high suicide risk. In some patients, it may be advisable to delay the decision to operate and to monitor the patient over time.

Selection criteria for DBS continue to evolve; in one study based on the Core Assessment Program for Surgical Interventional Therapies in Parkinson's Disease (CAPSIT-PD) criteria, only 1.6% of 641 consecutive PD patients attending movement disorders centres were considered eligible for STN DBS [107,178]. A common reason for exclusion was drug-induced psychosis; however, as discussed in the subsections above on Psychosis and Cognitive symptoms, whilst the presence of hallucinations may be a risk factor for post-operative cognitive decline, even patients with severe psychosis may derive significant benefit from STN DBS.

Nutritional counselling by a dietician should be given before, or very soon after, DBS to prevent excessive weight gain [157].

Target selection should be individualized taking into consideration the potential differences in motor as well as non-motor outcomes, as discussed throughout this chapter.

Post-operative management

Close post-operative follow-up is important to help patients and caregivers cope with the sudden changes that can occur following successful surgery and to facilitate early intervention if required. The patient's usual psychotropic medications (antidepressants, benzodiazepines, atypical neuroleptics, mood stabilizers, etc.) should typically be continued in the post-operative period. Judicious management of medications and stimulation parameters may reduce the risk of complications (see Table 27.2). A strategy of relatively rapid

Table 27.2 Post-operative management of neuropsychiatric symptoms following deep brain stimulation (DBS) surgery for Parkinson's disease (PD)

Non-motor symptom	Management
Cognitive impairment	In cases of acute or subacute post-operative cognitive decline, verify electrode placement and/or try different stimulation contacts Less potent PD medications (e.g. anticholinergics) should be eliminated Multidisciplinary management; compensatory strategies (e.g. cueing, simplifying complex tasks) Cholinesterase inhibitors (e.g. rivastigmine) Memantine has conflicting data for efficacy in PD dementia
Apathy	Education of patients and caregivers that this is a common symptom in PD and after subthalamic nucleus DBS, different from 'laziness' Increase dopaminergic medication (dopamine agonists may be particularly helpful) Exclude/treat cognitive impairment, depression, daytime somnolence, anaemia and hypothyroidism Implementation of a structured daily routine and increased psychological stimulation by caregivers Consider methylphenidate

Table 27.2 (continued) Post-operative management of neuropsychiatric symptoms following deep brain stimulation (DBS) surgery for Parkinson's disease (PD)

Non-motor symptom	Management
Depression, suicidal ideation	Involvement of a neuropsychiatrist; cognitive behavioural therapy Verify electrode placement and/or try different (e.g. more dorsal) stimulation contacts Increase dopaminergic medication; dopamine agonists (e.g. pramipexole, ropinirole or piribedil) may have antidepressant effects Antidepressant medication Assess for suicidal ideation; standard psychiatric management of suicidal ideation Electroconvulsive therapy may be a safe and effective option in refractory cases
Anxiety	Involvement of a neuropsychiatrist; cognitive behavioural therapy Depression is highly co-morbid with anxiety; both symptoms may improve with antidepressant treatment Benzodiazepines (e.g. lorazepam)—there are no clinical trial data concerning treatment choice for anxiety in PD
Hypomania/ mania	Involvement of a neuropsychiatrist Assess for suicidal ideation and risk-taking behaviours (e.g. reckless driving, excessive spending, hypersexuality) Verify electrode placement and/or try different (e.g. more dorsal) stimulation contacts Decrease dopaminergic medication and/or stimulation Consider discontinuation of antidepressant medication Mild cases may not require pharmacological treatment Atypical antipsychotic (quetiapine or clozapine) and/or mood stabilizer (carbamazapine, valproic acid)
Impulsive-ompulsive behaviours	Rule out hypomania/mania Dopaminergic medication (especially dopamine agonists) should be used at the lowest possible dose (may need to withdraw dopamine agonist therapy completely, as this is an 'all-or-none' phenomenon in some patients) Non-pharmacological measures (e.g. family involvement, financial guardianship, addiction counselling) Trial of decreasing stimulation? Consider atypical antipsychotics (quetiapine or clozapine) Treatment with amantadine is controversial
Psychosis	Decrease PD medication(s)—less potent ones (e.g. anticholinergics) should be eliminated first Atypical antipsychotic (quetiapine or clozapine) Cholinesterase inhibitor if dementia present (may have antipsychotic effects)
Psychosocial maladjustment	Multidisciplinary management

Adapted with permission from Voon V, Kubu C, Krack P, Houeto J-L, Troster AI. Deep brain stimulation: neuropsychological and neuropsychiatric issues. Mov Disord 2006; 21(Suppl 14): S305–S326.

post-operative drug withdrawal may be important in selected patients, for example those with severe ICBs or psychosis [35,101,102,113]. However (and especially in potentially predisposed individuals), medication reduction should generally be undertaken gradually to reduce the risk of hypodopaminergic withdrawal syndromes [3,34,35]. Complete elimination of medication post-STN DBS is not necessary for alleviation of dyskinesia or fluctuations (motor and non-motor) and should not be considered the final goal of DBS surgery, nor necessarily a measure of good outcome. If a strategy of rapid medication reduction is undertaken, patients should undergo repeated psychological follow-up, especially during the first post-operative year [34]. Some centres have used a protocol for systematic monitoring of suicidal ideation (including evaluations at least every 2 months and mandatory immediate psychiatric assessment if there is a suspicion of suicide risk) [4].

References

1 Fox SH, Katzenschlager R, Lim SY, et al. The Movement Disorder Society evidence-based medicine review update: treatments for the motor symptoms of Parkinson's disease. Mov Disord 2011; **26**(Suppl. 3): S2–S41.

2 Limousin P, Krack P, Pollak P, et al. Electrical stimulation of the subthalamic nucleus in advanced Parkinson's disease. N Engl J Med 1998; **339**: 1105–11.

3 Bronstein JM, Tagliati M, Alterman RL, et al. Deep brain stimulation for Parkinson disease: an expert consensus and review of key issues. Arch Neurol 2011; **68**: 165–71.

4 Schupbach WMM, Rau J, Knudsen K, et al. Neurostimulation for Parkinson's disease with early motor complications. N Engl J Med 2013; **368**: 610–22.

5 Rascol O, Lozano A, Stern M, Poewe W. Milestones in Parkinson's disease therapeutics. Mov Disord 2011; **26**: 1072–82.

6 Lang AE, Houeto J-L, Krack P, et al. Deep brain stimulation: preoperative issues. Mov Disord 2006; 21(Suppl. **14**): S171–S196.

7 Voon V, Kubu C, Krack P, Houeto J-L, Troster AI. Deep brain stimulation: neuropsychological and neuropsychiatric issues. Mov Disord 2006; **21**(Suppl. 14): S305–S326.

8 Martinez-Martin P, Rodriguez-Blazquez C, Kurtis MM, Chaudhuri KR; NMSS Validation Group. The impact of non-motor symptoms on health-related quality of life of patients with Parkinson's disease. Mov Disord 2011; **26**: 399–406.

9 Okun MS, Foote KD. Parkinson's disease DBS: what, when, who and why? The time has come to tailor DBS targets. Expert Rev Neurother 2010; **10**: 1847–57.

10 Alberts JL, Hass CJ, Vitek JL, Okun MS. Are two leads always better than one: an emerging case for unilateral subthalamic deep brain stimulation in Parkinson's disease. Exp Neurol 2008; **214**: 1–5.

11 Taba HA, Wu SS, Foote KD, et al. A closer look at unilateral versus bilateral deep brain stimulation: results of the National Institutes of Health COMPARE cohort. J Neurosurg 2010; **113**: 1224–9.

12 Krack P, Hariz MI. Deep brain stimulation in Parkinson's disease: reconciliation of evidence-based medicine with clinical practice. Lancet Neurol 2013; **12**: 25–6.

13 Okun MS, Foote KD. Subthalamic nucleus vs globus pallidus interna deep brain stimulation, the rematch: Will pallidal deep brain stimulation make a triumphant return? Arch Neurol 2005; **62**: 533–6.

14 Videnovic A, Metman LV. Deep brain stimulation for Parkinson's disease: prevalence of adverse events and need for standardized reporting. Mov Disord 2008; **23**: 343–9.

15 **Williams A, Gill S, Varma T, et al**. Deep brain stimulation plus best medical therapy versus best medical therapy alone for advanced Parkinson's disease (PD SURG trial): a randomised, open-label trial. Lancet Neurol 2010; **9**: 581–91.

16 **Burchiel KJ, Anderson VC, Favre J, Hammerstad JP**. Comparison of pallidal and subthalamic nucleus deep brain stimulation for advanced Parkinson's disease: results of a randomized, blinded pilot study. Neurosurgery 1999; **45**: 1375–82.

17 **Follett KA, Weaver FM, Stern M, et al**. Pallidal versus subthalamic deep-brain stimulation for Parkinson's disease. N Engl J Med 2010; **362**: 2077–91.

18 **Odekerken VJJ, van Laar T, Staal MJ, et al**. Subthalamic nucleus versus globus pallidus bilateral deep brain stimulation for advanced Parkinson's disease (NSTAPS study): a randomised controlled trial. Lancet Neurol 2013; **12**: 37–44.

19 **Anderson VC, Burchiel KJ, Hogarth P, Favre J, Hammerstad JP**. Pallidal vs subthalamic nucleus deep brain stimulation in Parkinson disease. Arch Neurol 2005; **62**: 554–60.

20 **Rothlind JC, Cockshott RW, Starr PA, Marks WJ Jr**. Neuropsychological performance following staged bilateral pallidal or subthalamic nucleus deep brain stimulation for Parkinson's disease. J Int Neuropsychol Soc 2007; **13**: 68–79.

21 **Okun MS, Fernandez HH, Wu SS, et al**. Cognition and mood in Parkinson's disease in subthalamic nucleus versus globus pallidus interna deep brain stimulation: the COMPARE trial. Ann Neurol 2009; **65**: 586–95.

22 **Hariz MI, Rehncrona S, Quinn NP, Speelman JD, Wensing C; Multicentre Advanced Parkinson's Disease Deep Brain Stimulation Group**. Multicenter study on deep brain stimulation in Parkinson's disease: an independent assessment of reported adverse events at 4 years. Mov Disord 2008; **23**: 416–21.

23 **Rouaud T, Dondaine T, Drapier S, et al**. Pallidal stimulation in advanced Parkinson's patients with contraindications for subthalamic stimulation. Mov Disord 2010; **25**: 1839–46.

24 **Fasano A, Daniele A, Albanese A**. Treatment of motor and non-motor features of Parkinson's disease with deep brain stimulation. Lancet Neurol 2012; **11**: 429–42.

25 **Borgohain R, Kandadai RM, Jabeen A, Kannikannan MA**. Nonmotor outcomes in Parkinson's disease: Is deep brain stimulation better than dopamine replacement therapy? Ther Adv Neurol Disord 2012; **5**: 23–41.

26 **Moro E, Lozano AM, Pollak P, et al**. Long-term results of a multicenter study on subthalamic and pallidal stimulation in Parkinson's disease. Mov Disord 2010; **25**: 578–86.

27 **Volkmann J, Albanese A, Kulisevsky J, et al**. Long-term effects of pallidal or subthalamic deep brain stimulation on quality of life in Parkinson's disease. Mov Disord 2009; **24**: 1154–61.

28 **Volkmann J, Daniels C, Witt K**. Neuropsychiatric effects of subthalamic neurostimulation in Parkinson disease. Nat Rev Neurol 2010; **6**: 487–98.

29 **Follett KA, Torres-Russotto D**. Deep brain stimulation of globus pallidus interna, subthalamic nucleus, and pedunculopontine nucleus for Parkinson's disease: which target? Parkinsonism Relat Disord 2012; **18**(Suppl 1): S165–S167.

30 **Weaver FM, Follett KA, Stern M, et al**. Randomized trial of deep brain stimulation for Parkinson disease: thirty-six-month outcomes. Neurology 2012; **79**: 55–65.

31 **Zahodne LB, Okun MS, Foote KD, et al**. Greater improvement in quality of life following unilateral deep brain stimulation surgery in the globus pallidus as compared to the subthalamic nucleus. J Neurol 2009; **256**: 1321–9.

32 **Rodriguez-Oroz MC, Obeso JA, Lang AE, et al**. Bilateral deep brain stimulation in Parkinson's disease: a multicentre study with 4 years follow-up. Brain 2005; **128**: 2240–9.

33 **Lim SY, Lang AE**. The nonmotor symptoms of Parkinson's disease: an overview. Mov Disord 2010; **25**(Suppl. 1): S123–S130.

34 Lhommee E, Klinger H, Thobois S, et al. Subthalamic stimulation in Parkinson's disease: restoring the balance of motivated behaviours. Brain 2012; **135**: 1463–77.

35 Thobois S, Ardouin C, Lhommee E, et al. Non-motor dopamine withdrawal syndrome after surgery for Parkinson's disease: predictors and underlying mesolimbic denervation. Brain 2010; **133**: 1111–27.

36 Hamani C, Saint-Cyr JA, Fraser J, Kaplitt M, Lozano AM. The subthalamic nucleus in the context of movement disorders. Brain 2004; **127**: 4–20.

37 Temel Y, Blokland A, Steinbusch HW, Visser-Vandewalle V. The functional role of the subthalamic nucleus in cognitive and limbic circuits. Prog Neurobiol 2005; **76**: 393–413.

38 Mallet L, Schupbach M, N'Diaye K, et al. Stimulation of subterritories of the subthalamic nucleus reveals its role in the integration of the emotional and motor aspects of behavior. Proc Natl Acad Sci USA 2007; **104**: 10661–6.

39 Hariz MI, Krack P, Alesch F, et al. Multicentre European study of thalamic stimulation for parkinsonian tremor: a 6 year follow-up. J Neurol Neurosurg Psychiatry 2008; **79**: 694–9.

40 Moro E, Hamani C, Poon YY, et al. Unilateral pedunculopontine stimulation improves falls in Parkinson's disease. Brain 2010: **133**; 215–24.

41 Ferraye MU, Debu B, Fraix V, et al. Effects of pedunculopontine nucleus area stimulation on gait disorders in Parkinson's disease. Brain 2010: **133**; 205–14.

42 Mikos A, Pavon J, Bowers D, et al. Factors related to extended hospital stays following deep brain stimulation for Parkinson's disease. Parkinsonism Relat Disord 2010; **16**: 324–8.

43 Hariz MI, Johansson F, Shamsgovara P, Johansson E, Hariz GM, Fagerlund M. Bilateral subthalamic nucleus stimulation in a parkinsonian patient with preoperative deficits in speech and cognition: persistent improvement in mobility but increased dependency: A case study. Mov Disord 2000; **15**: 136–9.

44 Saint-Cyr JA, Trepanier LL, Kumar R, et al. Lozano AM, Lang AE. Neuropsychological consequences of chronic bilateral stimulation of the subthalamic nucleus in Parkinson's disease. Brain 2000; **123**: 2091–108.

45 Pilitsis JG, Rezai AR, Boulis NM, et al. A preliminary study of transient confusional states following bilateral subthalamic stimulation for Parkinson's disease. Stereotact Funct Neurosurg 2005; **83**: 67–70.

46 Krack P, Batir A, Van Blercom N, et al. Five-year follow-up of bilateral stimulation of the subthalamic nucleus in advanced Parkinson's disease. N Engl J Med 2003; **349**: 1925–34.

47 Okun MS, Gallo BV, Mandybur G, et al. Subthalamic deep brain stimulation with a constant-current device in Parkinson's disease: an open-label randomised controlled trial. Lancet Neurol 2012; **11**: 140–9.

48 Witt K, Daniels C, Reiff J, et al. Neuropsychological and psychiatric changes after deep brain stimulation for Parkinson's disease: a randomised, multicentre study. Lancet Neurol 2008; **7**: 605–14.

49 Parsons TD, Rogers SA, Braaten AJ, Woods SP, Tröster AI. Cognitive sequelae of subthalamic nucleus deep brain stimulation in Parkinson's disease: a meta-analysis. Lancet Neurol 2006; **5**: 578–88.

50 Zangaglia R, Pasotti C, Mancini F, Servello D, Sinforiani E, Pacchetti C. Deep brain stimulation and cognition in Parkinson's disease: an eight-year follow-up study. Mov Disord 2012; **27**: 1192–4.

51 Contarino MF, Daniele A, Sibilia AH, et al. Cognitive outcome 5 years after bilateral chronic stimulation of subthalamic nucleus in patients with Parkinson's disease. J Neurol Neurosurg Psychiatry 2007; **78**: 248–52.

52 Fasano A, Romito LM, Daniele A, et al. Motor and cognitive outcome in patients with Parkinson's disease 8 years after subthalamic implants. Brain 2010; **133**: 2664–76.

53 Morrison CE, Borod JC, Perrine K, et al. Neuropsychological functioning following bilateral subthalamic nucleus stimulation in Parkinson's disease. Arch Clin Neuropsychol 2004; **19**: 165–81.

54 Aybek S, Gronchi-Perrin A, Berney A, et al. Long-term cognitive profile and incidence of dementia after STN-DBS in Parkinson's disease. Mov Disord 2007; **22**: 974–81.

55 Smeding HMM, Speelman JD, Huizenga HM, Schuurman PR, Schmand B. Predictors of cognitive and psychosocial outcome after STN DBS in Parkinson's disease. J Neurol Neurosurg Psychiatry 2011; **82**: 754–60.

56 Rektorova I, Hummelova Z, Balaz M. Dementia after DBS Surgery: a case report and literature review. Parkinson's Dis 2011; **2011**: 679283.

57 Sjoberg RL, Lidman E, Häggström B, et al. Verbal fluency in patients receiving bilateral versus left-sided deep brain stimulation of the subthalamic nucleus for Parkinson's disease. J Int Neuropsychol Soc 2012; **18**: 606–11.

58 Zangaglia R, Pacchetti C, Pasotti C, et al. Deep brain stimulation and cognitive functions in Parkinson's disease: a three-year controlled study. Mov Disord 2009; **24**: 1621–8.

59 Funkiewiez A, Ardouin C, Caputo E, et al. Long term effects of bilateral subthalamic nucleus stimulation on cognitive function, mood, and behaviour in Parkinson's disease. J Neurol Neurosurg Psychiatry 2004; **75**: 834–9.

60 Lefaucheur R, Derrey S, Martinaud O, et al. Early verbal fluency decline after STN implantation: is it a cognitive microlesion effect? J Neurol Sci 2012; **321**: 96–9.

61 Pillon B, Ardouin C, Damier P, et al. Neuropsychological changes between 'off' and 'on' STN or GPi stimulation in Parkinson's disease. Neurology 2000; **55**: 411–18.

62 Castelli L, Lanotte M, Zibetti M, et al. Apathy and verbal fluency in STN-stimulated PD patients: an observational follow-up study. J Neurol 2007; **254**: 1238–43.

63 Alegret M, Valldeoriola F, Martı M, et al. Comparative cognitive effects of bilateral subthalamic stimulation and subcutaneous continuous infusion of apomorphine in Parkinson's disease. Mov Disord 2004; **19**: 1463–9.

64 Yamanaka T, Ishii F, Umemura A, et al. Temporary deterioration of executive function after subthalamic deep brain stimulation in Parkinson's disease. Clin Neurol Neurosurg 2012; **114**: 347–51.

65 Smeding HMM, van den Munckhof P, Esselink RAJ, Schmand B, Schuurman PR, Speelman JD. Reversible cognitive decline after DBS STN in PD and displacement of electrodes. Neurology 2007; **68**: 1235–6.

66 Cakmakli GY, Oruckaptan H, Saka E, Elibol B. Reversible acute cognitive dysfunction induced by bilateral STN stimulation. J Neurol 2009; **256**: 1360–2.

67 Kirsch-Darrow L, Zahodne LB, Marsiske M, Okun MS, Foote KD, Bowers D. The trajectory of apathy after deep brain stimulation: from pre-surgery to 6 months post-surgery in Parkinson's disease. Parkinsonism Relat Disord 2011; **17**: 182–8.

68 Le Jeune F, Drapier D, Bourguignon A, et al. Subthalamic nucleus stimulation in Parkinson disease induces apathy: a PET study. Neurology 2009; **73**: 1746–51.

69 Funkiewiez A, Ardouin C, Krack P, et al. Acute psychotropic effects of bilateral subthalamic nucleus stimulation and levodopa in Parkinson's disease. Mov Disord 2003; **18**: 524–30.

70 Houeto JL, Mesnage V, Mallet L, et al. Behavioural disorders, Parkinson's disease and subthalamic stimulation. J Neurol Neurosurg Psychiatry 2002; **72**: 701–7.

71 Czernecki V, Schupbach M, Yaici S, et al. Apathy following subthalamic stimulation in Parkinson disease: a dopamine responsive symptom. Mov Disord 2008; **23**: 964–9.

72 Temel Y, Kessels A, Tan S, Topdag A, Boon P, Visser-Vandewalle V. Behavioural changes after bilateral subthalamic stimulation in advanced Parkinson disease: a systematic review. Parkinsonism Relat Disord 2006; **12**: 265–72.

73 Berney A, Vingerhoets F, Perrin A, et al. Effect on mood of chronic subthalamic DBS for Parkinson's disease: a consecutive series of 24 patients. Neurology 2002; **59**: 1427–9.

74 Daniele A, Albanese A, Contarino MF, et al. Cognitive and behavioural effects of chronic stimulation of the subthalamic nucleus in patients with Parkinson's disease. J Neurol Neurosurg Psychiatry 2003; **74**: 175–82.

75 Houeto J-L, Mallet L, Mesnage V, et al. Subthalamic stimulation in Parkinson disease: behavior and social adaptation. Arch Neurol 2006; **63**: 1090–5.

76 Bejjani BP, Damier P, Arnulf I, et al. Transient acute depression induced by high-frequency deep-brain stimulation. New Engl J Med 1999; **340**: 1476–80.

77 Stefurak T, Mikulis D, Mayberg H, et al. Deep brain stimulation for Parkinson's disease dissociates mood and motor circuits: a functional MRI case study. Mov Disord 2003; **18**: 1508–16.

78 Tommasi G, Lanotte M, Albert U, et al. Transient acute depressive state induced by subthalamic region stimulation. J Neurol Sci 2008; **273**: 135–8.

79 Chou KL, Hurtig HI, Jaggi JL, Baltuch GH, Pelchat RJ, Weintraub D. Electroconvulsive therapy for depression in a Parkinson's disease patient with bilateral subthalamic nucleus deep brain stimulators. Parkinsonism Rel Disord 2005; **11**: 403–6.

80 Weaver FM, Follett K, Stern M, et al. Bilateral deep brain stimulation vs best medical therapy for patients with advanced Parkinson disease: a randomized controlled trial. J Am Med Assoc 2009; **301**: 63–73.

81 Drapier D, Drapier S, Sauleau P, et al. Does subthalamic nucleus stimulation induce apathy in Parkinson's disease? J Neurol 2006; **253**: 1083–91.

82 Schupbach WMM, Maltete D, Houeto JL, et al. Neurosurgery at an earlier stage of Parkinson disease: a randomized, controlled trial. Neurology 2007; **68**: 1–5.

83 Smeding HMM, Speelman JD, Koning-Haanstra M, et al. Neuropsychological effects of bilateral STN stimulation in Parkinson disease: a controlled study. Neurology 2006; **66**: 1830–6.

84 Burdick AP, Foote KD, Wu S, et al. Do patients get angrier following STN, GPi, and thalamic deep brain stimulation. NeuroImage 2011; **54**(Suppl 1): S227–S232.

85 Kulisevsky J, Berthier ML, Gironell A, Pascual-Sedano B, Molet J, Parés P. Mania following deep brain stimulation for Parkinson's disease. Neurology 2002; **59**: 1421–4.

86 Romito LM, Raja M, Daniele A, et al. Transient mania with hypersexuality after surgery for high-frequency stimulation of the subthalamic nucleus in Parkinson's disease. Mov Disord 2002; **17**: 1371–4.

87 Herzog J, Reiff J, Krack P, et al. Manic episode with psychotic symptoms induced by subthalamic nucleus stimulation in a patient with Parkinson's disease. Mov Disord 2003; **18**: 1382–4.

88 Krack P, Kumar R, Ardouin C, et al. Mirthful laughter induced by subthalamic nucleus stimulation. Mov Disord 2001; **16**: 867–75.

89 Coenen VA, Honey CR, Hurwitz T, et al. Medial forebrain bundle stimulation as a pathophysiological mechanism for hypomania in subthalamic nucleus deep brain stimulation for Parkinson's disease. Neurosurgery 2009; **64**: 1106–15.

90 Ulla M, Thobois S, Llorca PM, et al. Contact dependent reproducible hypomania induced by deep brain stimulation in Parkinson's disease: clinical, anatomical and functional imaging study. J Neurol Neurosurg Psychiatry 2011; **82**: 607–14.

91 Romito LM, Contarino FM, Albanese A. Transient gender-related effects in Parkinson's disease patients with subthalamic stimulation. J Neurol 2010; **257**: 603–8.

92 Voon V, Moro E, Saint-Cyr J, Lozano A, Lang A. Psychiatric symptoms following surgery for Parkinson's disease with an emphasis on subthalamic stimulation. Adv Neurol 2005; **96**: 130–47.

93 Raucher-Chene D, Charrel CL, de Maindreville AD, Limosin F. Manic episode with psychotic symptoms in a patient with Parkinson's disease treated by subthalamic nucleus stimulation: Improvement on switching the target. J Neurol Sci 2008; **273**: 116–17.

94 Chopra A, Tye SJ, Lee KH, et al. Underlying neurobiology and clinical correlates of mania status after subthalamic nucleus deep brain stimulation in Parkinson's disease: a review of the literature. J Neuropsychiatry Clin Neurosci 2012; **24**: 102–10.

95 Moum SJ, Price CC, Limotai N, et al. Effects of STN and GPi deep brain stimulation on impulse control disorders and dopamine dysregulation syndrome. PLoS One 2012; **7**: e29768.

96 Shotbolt P, Moriarty J, Costello A, et al. Relationships between deep brain stimulation and impulse control disorders in Parkinson's disease, with a literature review. Parkinsonism Relat Disord 2012; **18**: 10–16.

97 Eusebio A, Witjas T, Cohen J, et al. Subthalamic nucleus stimulation and compulsive use of dopaminergic medication in Parkinson's disease. J Neurol Neurosurg Psychiatry 2013; **84**: 868–74.

98 Lim SY, Evans AH, Miyasaki JM. Impulse control and related disorders in Parkinson's disease: review. Ann NY Acad Sci 2008; **1142**: 85–107.

99 Lim SY, Zuroswski M, Moro E. Impulsive-compulsive behaviors and subthalamic nucleus deep brain stimulation in Parkinson's disease: review of the literature. Eur Neurol J 2010: 2; 61.

100 Ardouin C, Voon V, Worbe Y, et al. Pathological gambling in Parkinson's disease improves on chronic subthalamic nucleus stimulation. Mov Disord 2006; **21**: 1941–6.

101 Witjas T, Baunez C, Henry JM, et al. Addiction in Parkinson's disease: impact of subthalamic nucleus deep brain stimulation. Mov Disord 2005; **20**: 1052–5.

102 Lim SY, O'Sullivan SS, Kotschet K, et al. DDS, ICDs and punding after DBS surgery for Parkinson's disease. J Clin Neurosci 2009; **16**: 1148–52.

103 De la Casa-Fages B, Grandas F. Dopamine dysregulation syndrome after deep brain stimulation of the subthalamic nucleus in Parkinson's disease. J Neurol Sci 2012; **312**: 191–3.

104 Frank MJ, Samanta J, Moustafa AA, Sherman SJ. Hold your horses: impulsivity, deep brain stimulation, and medication in Parkinsonism. Science 2007; **318**: 1309–12.

105 Ballanger B, van Eimeren T, Moro E, et al. Stimulation of the subthalamic nucleus and impulsivity: release your horses. Ann Neurol 2009; **66**: 817–24.

106 Bechara A. Decision making, impulse control and loss of willpower to resist drugs: a neurocognitive perspective. Nat Neurosci 2005; **8**: 1458–63.

107 Morgante L, Morgante F, Moro E, et al. How many parkinsonian patients are suitable candidates for deep brain stimulation of subthalamic nucleus? Results of a questionnaire. Parkinsonism Relat Disord 2007; **13**: 528–31.

108 Rabinak CA, Nirenberg MJ. Dopamine agonist withdrawal syndrome in Parkinson disease. Arch Neurol 2010; **67**: 58–63.

109 Sensi M, Eleopra R, Cavallo MA, et al. Explosive-aggressive behaviour related to bilateral subthalamic stimulation. Parkinsonism Relat Disord 2004; **10**: 247–51.

110 Smeding HMM, Goudriaan AE, Foncke EMJ, Schuurman PR, Speelman JD, Schmand B. Pathological gambling after bilateral subthalamic nucleus stimulation in Parkinson disease. J Neurol Neurosurg Psychiatry 2007; **78**: 517–19.

111 Yoshida F, Miyagi Y, Kishimoto J. Subthalamic nucleus stimulation does not cause deterioration of preexisting hallucinations in Parkinson's disease patients. Stereotact Funct Neurosurg 2009; **87**: 45–9.

112 Voon V, Saint-Cyr JA, Lozano AM, Moro E, Poon YY, Lang AE: Psychiatric symptoms in patients with Parkinson disease presenting for deep brain stimulation surgery. J Neurosurg 2005; **103**: 246–51.

113 Umemura A, Oka Y, Okita K, Matsukawa N, Yamada K. Subthalamic nucleus stimulation for Parkinson disease with severe medication-induced hallucinations or delusions. J Neurosurg 2011; **114**: 1701–5.

114 Diederich NJ, Alesch F, Goetz CG. Visual hallucinations induced by deep brain stimulation in Parkinson's disease. Clin Neuropharmacol 2000; **23**: 287–9.

115 Schupbach M, Gargiulo M, Welter ML, et al. Neurosurgery in Parkinson disease: a distressed mind in a repaired body? Neurology 2006; **66**: 1811–16.

116 Burkhard PR, Vingerhoets FJ, Berney A, Bogousslavsky J, Villemure JG, Ghika J. Suicide after successful deep brain stimulation for movement disorders. Neurology 2004; **63**: 2170–2.

117 Soulas T, Gurruchaga JM, Palfi S, Cesaro P, Nguyen JP, Fenelon G. Attempted and completed suicides after subthalamic nucleus stimulation for Parkinson's disease. J Neurol Neurosurg Psychiatry 2008; **79**; 952–4.

118 Voon V, Krack P, Lang AE, et al. A multicentre study on suicide outcomes following subthalamic stimulation for Parkinson's disease. Brain 2008; **131**: 2720–8.

119 Riley DE, Lang AE. The spectrum of levodopa-related fluctuations in Parkinson's disease. Neurology 1993; **43**: 1459–64.

120 Witjas T, Kaphan E, Azulay JP, et al. Nonmotor fluctuations in Parkinson's disease: frequent and disabling. Neurology 2002; **59**: 408–13.

121 Lim SY, Farrell MJ, Gibson SJ, Helme RD, Lang AE, Evans AH. Do dyskinesia and pain share common pathophysiological mechanisms in Parkinson disease? Mov Disord 2008; **23**: 1689–95.

122 Evans AH, Farrell MJ, Gibson SJ, Helme RD, Lim SY. Dyskinetic patients show rebound worsening of affect after an acute L-dopa challenge. Parkinsonism Relat Disord 2012; **18**: 514–19.

123 Castrioto A, Kistner A, Klinger H, et al. Psychostimulant effect of levodopa: reversing sensitisation is possible. J Neurol Neurosurg Psychiatry 2013; **84**: 18–22.

124 Witjas T, Kaphan E, Régis J, et al. Effects of chronic subthalamic stimulation on nonmotor fluctuations in Parkinson's disease. Mov Disord 2007; **22**: 1729–34.

125 Ortega-Cubero S, Clavero P, Irurzun C, et al. Effect of deep brain stimulation of the subthalamic nucleus on non-motor fluctuations in Parkinson's disease: two-year follow-up. Parkinsonism Relat Disord 2013; **19**: 543–7.

126 Arnulf I, Bejjani BP, Garma L, et al. Improvement of sleep architecture in PD with subthalamic nucleus stimulation. Neurology 2000; **55**: 1732–4.

127 Iranzo A, Valldeoriola F, Santamaria J, Tolosa E, Rumia J. Sleep symptoms and polysomnographic architecture in advanced Parkinson's disease after chronic bilateral subthalamic stimulation. J Neurol Neurosurg Psychiatry 2002; **72**: 661–4.

128 Hjort N, Ostergaard K, Dupont E. Improvement of sleep quality in patients with advanced Parkinson's disease treated with deep brain stimulation of the subthalamic nucleus. Mov Disord 2004; **19**: 196–9.

129 Monaca C, Ozsancak C, Jacquesson JM, et al. Effects of bilateral subthalamic stimulation on sleep in Parkinson's disease. J Neurol 2004; **251**: 214–18.

130 Lyons KE, Pahwa R. Effects of bilateral subthalamic nucleus stimulation on sleep, daytime sleepiness, and early morning dystonia in patients with Parkinson disease. J Neurosurg 2006; **104**: 502–5.

131 Chahine LM, Ahmed A, Sun Z. Effects of STN DBS for Parkinson's disease on restless legs syndrome and other sleep-related measures. Parkinsonism Relat Disord 2011; **17**: 208–11.

132 Kedia S, Moro E, Tagliati M, Lang AE, Kumar R. Emergence of restless legs syndrome during subthalamic stimulation for Parkinson disease. Neurology 2004; **63**: 2410–12.

133 **Driver-Dunckley E, Evidente VGH, Adler CH, et al**. Restless legs syndrome in Parkinson's disease patients may improve with subthalamic stimulation. Mov Disord 2006; **21**: 1287–9.

134 **Lopiano L, Rizzone M, Bergamasco B, et al**. Daytime sleepiness improvement following bilateral chronic electrical stimulation of the subthalamic nucleus in Parkinson's disease. Eur Neurol 2001; **46**: 49–50.

135 **Winge K, Nielsen KK, Stimpel H, Lokkegaard A, Jensen SR, Werdelin L**. Lower urinary tract symptoms and bladder control in advanced Parkinson's disease: effects of deep brain stimulation in the subthalamic nucleus. Mov Disord 2007; **22**: 220–5.

136 **Finazzi-Agro E, Peppe A, d'Amico A, et al**. Effects of subthalamic nucleus stimulation on urodynamic findings in patients with Parkinson's disease. J Urol 2003; **169**: 1388–91.

137 **Seif C, Herzog J, van der Horst C, et al**. Effect of subthalamic deep brain stimulation on the function of the urinary bladder. Ann Neurol 2004; **55**: 118–20.

138 **Castelli L, Perozzo P, Genesia ML, et al**. Sexual well being in parkinsonian patients after deep brain stimulation of the subthalamic nucleus. J Neurol Neurosurg Psychiatry 2004; **75**: 1260–4.

139 **Lengerer S, Kipping J, Rommel N, et al**. Deep-brain-stimulation does not impair deglutition in Parkinson's disease. Parkinsonism Relat Disord 2012; **18**: 847–53.

140 **Ciucci MR, Barkmeier-Kraemer JM, Sherman SJ**. Subthalamic nucleus deep brain stimulation improves deglutition in Parkinson's disease. Mov Disord 2008; **23**: 676–83.

141 **Arai E, Arai M, Uchiyama T, et al**. Subthalamic deep brain stimulation can improve gastric emptying in Parkinson's disease. Brain 2012; **135**: 1478–85.

142 **Zibetti M, Torre E, Cinquepalmi A, et al**. Motor and nonmotor symptom follow-up in Parkinsonian patients after deep brain stimulation of the subthalamic nucleus. Eur Neurol 2007; **58**: 218–23.

143 **Ludwig J, Remien P, Guballa C, et al**. Effects of subthalamic nucleus stimulation and levodopa on the autonomic nervous system in Parkinson's disease. J Neurol Neurosurg Psychiatry 2007; **78**: 742–5.

144 **Stemper B, Beric A, Welsch G, Haendl T, Sterio D, Hilz MJ**. Deep brain stimulation improves orthostatic regulation of patients with Parkinson disease. Neurology 2006; **67**: 1781–5.

145 **Holmberg B, Corneliusson O, Elam M**. Bilateral stimulation of nucleus subthalamicus in advanced Parkinson's disease: no effects on, and of, autonomic dysfunction. Mov Disord 2005; **20**: 976–81.

146 **Romito LMA, Scerrati M, Contarino MF, Bentivoglio AR, Tonali P, Albanese A**. Long-term follow up of subthalamic nucleus stimulation in Parkinson's disease. Neurology 2002; **58**: 1546–50.

147 **Barichella M, Marczewska AM, Mariani C, Landi A, Vairo A, Pezzoli G**. Body weight gain rate in patients with Parkinson's disease and deep brain stimulation. Mov Disord 2003; **18**: 1337–40.

148 **Macia F, Perlemoine C, Coman I, et al**. Parkinson's disease patients with bilateral subthalamic deep brain stimulation gain weight. Mov Disord 2004; **19**: 206–12.

149 **Sauleau P, Leray E, Rouaud T, et al**. Comparison of weight gain and energy intake after subthalamic versus pallidal stimulation in Parkinson's disease. Mov Disord 2009; **24**: 2149–55.

150 **Locke M, Wu S, Foote K, et al**. Weight changes in STN versus GPi DBS: results from the COMPARE Parkinson's disease DBS cohort. Neurosurgery 2011; **68**: 1233–8.

151 **Bannier S, Montaurier C, Derost PP**. Overweight after deep brain stimulation of the subthalamic nucleus in Parkinson's disease: long-term follow-up. J Neurol Neurosurg Psychiatry 2009; **80**: 484–8.

152 **Ruzicka F, Jech R, Novakova L, Urgosik D, Vymazal J, Ruzicka E**. Weight gain is associated with medial contact site of subthalamic stimulation in Parkinson's disease. PLoS One 2012; **7**: e38020.

153 **Castrioto A, Lozano AM, Poon YY, Lang AE, Fallis M, Moro E**. Ten-year outcome of subthalamic stimulation in Parkinson disease: a blinded evaluation. Arch Neurol 2011; **68**: 1550–6.

154 **Montaurier C, Morio B, Bannier S, et al**. Mechanisms of body weight gain in patients with Parkinson's disease after subthalamic stimulation. Brain 2007; **130**: 1808–18.

155 **Zahodne LB, Susatia F, Bowers D, et al**. Binge eating in Parkinson's disease: prevalence, correlates and the contribution of deep brain stimulation. J Neuropsychiatry Clin Neurosci 2011; **23**: 56–62.

156 **Rieu I, Derost P, Ulla M, et al**. Body weight gain and deep brain stimulation. J Neurol Sci 2011; **310**: 267–70.

157 **Guimaraes J, Matos E, Rosas MJ, et al**. Modulation of nutritional state in Parkinsonian patients with bilateral subthalamic nucleus stimulation. J Neurol 2009; **256**: 2072–8.

158 **Krack P, Pollak P, Limousin P, et al**. From off-period dystonia to peak-dose chorea: the clinical spectrum of varying subthalamic nucleus activity. Brain 1999; **122**: 1133–46.

159 **Kim HJ, Paek SH, Kim JY, et al**. Chronic subthalamic deep brain stimulation improves pain in Parkinson disease. J Neurol 2008; **255**: 1889–94.

160 **Kim HJ, Jeon BS, Lee JY, Paek SH, Kim DG**. The benefit of subthalamic deep brain stimulation for pain in Parkinson disease: a 2-year follow-up study. Neurosurgery 2012; **70**: 18–24.

161 **Dellapina E, Ory-Magne F, Regragui W, et al**. Effect of subthalamic deep brain stimulation on pain in Parkinson's disease. Pain 2012; **153**: 2267–73.

162 **Gierthmuhlen J, Arning P, Binder A, et al**. Influence of deep brain stimulation and levodopa on sensory signs in Parkinson's disease. Mov Disord 2010; **25**: 1195–202.

163 **Ciampi de Andrade D, Lefaucheur JP, Galhardoni R, et al**. Subthalamic deep brain stimulation modulates small fiber-dependent sensory thresholds in Parkinson's disease. Pain 2012; **153**: 1107–13.

164 **Kim HJ, Jeon BS, Paek SH**. Effect of deep brain stimulation on pain in Parkinson disease. Effect of deep brain stimulation on pain in Parkinson disease. J Neurol Sci 2011; **310**: 251–5.

165 **Juri C, Rodriguez-Oroz MC, Burguera JA, Guridi J, Obeso JA**. Pain and dyskinesia in Parkinson's disease. Mov Disord 2010; **25**: 130–2.

166 **Guo X, Gao G, Wang X, et al**. Effects of bilateral deep brain stimulation of the subthalamic nucleus on olfactory function in Parkinson's disease patients. Stereotact Funct Neurosurg 2008; **86**: 237–44.

167 **Hummel T, Jahnke U, Sommer U, Reichmann H, Muller A**. Olfactory function in patients with idiopathic Parkinson's disease: effects of deep brain stimulation in the subthalamic nucleus. J Neural Transm 2005; **112**: 669–76.

168 **Nazzaro JM, Pahwa R, Lyons KE**. The impact of bilateral subthalamic stimulation on non-motor symptoms of Parkinson's disease. Parkinsonism Relat Disord 2011; **17**: 606–9.

169 **Reich MM, Chaudhuri KR, Ashkan K, et al**. Changes in the non-motor symptom scale in Parkinson's disease after deep brain stimulation. Basal Ganglia 2011; **1**: 131–3.

170 **Hwynn N, Ul Haq I, Malaty IA, et al**. Effect of deep brain stimulation on Parkinson's nonmotor symptoms following unilateral DBS: a pilot study. Parkinson's Dis 2011; **2011**: 507416.

171 **Dujardin K, Krystkowiak P, Defebvre L, Blond S, Destee A**. A case of severe dysexecutive syndrome consecutive to chronic bilateral pallidal stimulation. Neuropsychologia 2000; **38**: 1305–15.

172 **Miyawaki E, Perlmutter JS, Troster AI, Videen TO, Koller WC**. The behavioral complications of pallidal stimulation: a case report. Brain Cogn 2000; **42**: 417–34.

173 **Roane DM, Yu M, Feinberg TE, Rogers JD**. Hypersexuality after pallidal surgery in Parkinson disease. Neuropsychiatry Neuropsychol Behav Neurol 2002; **15**: 247–51.

174 **Volkmann J, Allert N, Voges J, Weiss PH, Freund HJ, Sturm V**. Safety and efficacy of pallidal or subthalamic nucleus stimulation in advanced PD. Neurology 2001; **56**: 548–51.

175 **Mills KA, Scherzer R, Starr PA, Ostrem JL**. Weight change after globus pallidus internus or subthalamic nucleus deep brain stimulation in Parkinson's disease and dystonia. Stereotact Funct Neurosurg 2012; **90**: 386–93.

176 **Moro E, Lang AE**. Criteria for deep-brain stimulation in Parkinson's disease: review and analysis. Expert Rev Neurother 2006; **6**: 1695–705.

177 **Woopen C, Pauls KA, Koy A, Moro E, Timmermann L**. Early application of deep brain stimulation: clinical and ethical aspects. Prog Neurobiol. 2013; **110**: 74–88.

178 **Defer G-L, Widner H, Marie R-M, Remy P, Levivier M; conference participants**. Core assessment program for surgical interventional therapies in Parkinson's disease (CAPSIT-PD). Mov Disord 1999; **14**: 572–84.

Chapter 28

Impulse dyscontrol and dopamine dysregulation syndrome

Regina Katzenschlager and Andrew Evans

Background

Dopaminergic medications used to treat Parkinson's disease (PD) improve symptoms, reduce motor handicap and may prolong survival. However, in some individuals they may induce a range of disabling symptoms beyond those attributable to the disease process. These include a variety of compulsive and addictive behaviours.

The term 'dopamine dysregulation syndrome' (DDS) refers to the compulsive use of dopaminergic medications well beyond the dose needed to optimally control motor disability and in the face of a mounting number of harmful physical, psychiatric and social sequelae.

Impulse control disorders are characterized as the failure to resist an impulse, drive or temptation to perform an act that is harmful to the person or to others. These may be induced by dopaminergic therapy, particularly dopamine agonists. Moreover, ICDs are frequently seen in patients with DDS, indicating a global sensitizing effect of dopaminergic drugs on motivational systems.

Some PD patients display repetitive and aimless behaviours, called punding, which tend to reflect pre-morbid interests and may be socially disabling. Punding is currently not well described by any DSM criteria. It is important to note that while many patients with DDS also have ICDs as part of the clinical syndrome and many ICD patients overuse medication, these behavioural disorders may occur in isolation. Similarly, punding may be associated with DDS, ICDs or both, but may also occur without associated other disorders (Table 28.1).

Nearly all patients with PD receive dopaminergic medications for the management of motor symptoms, but only a small percentage develop medication-related compulsive behaviours. Therefore, individual vulnerability factors are critical in the expression of these disorders. Important clinical risk factors are summarized in Table 28.2. Their identification may help the clinician with prevention or early identification of these disorders.

Dopamine dysregulation syndrome, punding and impulse control disorders: phenomenology and prevalence

Dopamine dysregulation syndrome

In PD, dopaminergic dosage requirements increase over time as disability increases and neurodegeneration progresses. In many patients this is associated with a shortened

Table 28.1 Diagnostic criteria for dopamine dysregulation syndrome

Parkinson's disease with documented levodopa responsiveness
Need for increased doses of dopamine replacement therapy (DRT) in excess of those normally required to relieve parkinsonian symptoms and signs
Pattern of pathological use: expressed need for increased DRT in the presence of excessive and significant dyskinesias despite being 'on', drug hoarding or drug-seeking behaviour, unwillingness to reduce DRT
Impairment of social or occupational functioning: fights, violent behaviour, loss of friends, absence from work, loss of job, legal difficulties, arguments or family difficulties
Development of hypomanic, manic or cyclothymic affective syndrome in relation to DRT
Development of a withdrawal state characterized by dysphoria, depression, irritability and anxiety with reduction of DRT
Duration of disturbance is of at least 6 months

duration of drug response, dose failures and unpredictable 'off' states. In patients who develop DDS, doses increase beyond the level required to treat motor disability, resulting in a pattern of compulsive medication overuse associated with cognitive and behavioural disturbances. These patients often also develop ICDs or punding behaviour, but each of these disorders may occur in isolation [1–4].

Patients report craving their drugs and usually experience a range of unpleasant sensations, particularly dysphoria, during 'off' states. Conversely, euphoric effects following

Table 28.2 Vulnerability factors for impulse control and related disorders

Vulnerability factor	Dopamine dysregulation syndrome	Punding	Impulse control disorders
Young age at onset	Yes	Yes	Yes
Gender	No	No (but modifies phenomenology)	Male: pathological, gambling, hypersexuality Female: impulsive eating, shopping
Impulsive sensation seeking	Yes	Yes	Yes
Levodopa equivalent dose	Yes	Yes	Yes
Dopamine agonist treatment	No (but may modify expression of impulse control disorders)	Possibly	Yes
Depression	Yes	Unknown	Yes
Alcohol consumption	Yes	Unknown	Hypersexuality: no Pathological gambling: yes
Dyskinesias	Yes	Yes	Possibly
Rescue doses	Yes	Yes	No

drug intake are uncommonly reported. The doses required to satisfy the craving tend to increase over time. This may develop out of prescribed 'as required' medication or as a result of demands for increasing doses for reported 'off' periods. Alternative drug sources may be sought, such as 'doctor shopping' or internet purchases, and drug hoarding and hiding are typical behaviours. Most patients develop 'on' period dyskinesias as a result of increased dopaminergic drug load. They use frequent rescue doses despite an external impression of good mobility and often disabling dyskinesias.

One recent proposal [5] to expand the spectrum of DDS behaviours emphasizes the central role of an anticipatory anxiety or panic about being off, culminating in a phobic avoidance that impacts on social/occupational function. However, this construct remains untested in clinical practice.

The phenomenology of the fully developed syndrome is characterized by cognitive and behavioural changes in addition to drug-seeking strategies. These include impulsivity, compulsivity and impatience. Dishonesty, manipulation and addictive denial systems are frequently coupled with a lack of insight into the harm caused. Heightened aggression is common and includes irritability, low tolerance of frustration, angry outbursts and occasional violence. Hypomania is usually short-lived or cyclical, with euphoria or exaggerated feelings of power and dominance. Patients often devote a great deal of time to complex dosing schedules and may take medications throughout the night. Excessive doses may lead to delirium, agitation or psychosis. Enforced drug withdrawal may cause worsened parkinsonism but typically involves dysphoric or aggressive responses and enhanced efforts to obtain further drugs. The syndrome frequently results in marked social disruption.

The prevalence of DDS has not been fully studied. Observations from movement disorder referral centres suggest an occurrence in up to 3.4–4% of PD patients [2,6].

Individual differences in impulsive sensation-seeking traits reflect partly heritable variations in the activity of brain dopamine systems [7]. Individuals scoring highly on impulsive sensation-seeking inventories exhibit risky, sensation-seeking behaviours and are predisposed to various kinds of disinhibited behaviours, criminality, sexuality and substance use and abuse. As a group, PD patients are generally described as anancastic and show reduced scores on impulsive sensation-seeking inventories [8]. In contrast, DDS patients score higher on such ratings, have greater past experimental drug use and tend to have higher current alcohol intake [1].

DDS is associated with high doses of levodopa and total levodopa equivalent dose, but not with any class of dopaminergic drugs, such as dopamine agonists, in particular. Predisposing factors also include young age at onset and depression, whereas gender does not appear to strongly influence susceptibility to DDS [1] but is relevant to its behavioural manifestations and the degree of social disruption that may result. Moreover, PD-related factors have a role. The neuroplastic changes that accompany behavioural sensitization in animal models are more prominent when nigrostriatal dopamine denervation is more profound [9]. Consistent with this, DDS patients have a longer disease duration than those with isolated pathological gambling [10].

Punding

Punding refers to the prolonged performance of repetitive tasks, often involving a degree of fascination with the activities. These complex repetitive behaviours were first described in psychostimulant addicts [11] and the term was coined by affected addicts. The phenomenon is believed to be homologous to the behaviours seen in animals with amphetamine-induced stereotypies. The behaviours are idiosyncratic, develop from preexisting habits and depend on an individual's previous occupation, interests and pastimes. Examples include spending excessive time on a computer (without a need to do so), hoarding, handling and sorting objects, writing or drawing, and aimless walkabouts. Men typically manipulate or dismantle machines and tools including the lead connector following DBS or apomorphine pumps [12]. Examples in women include a retired seamstress continuously sorting her button collection, or housewives who excessively tidy their homes, often creating an increasing mess. Punding usually becomes disabling when it occurs at night and tends to take up a longer and longer time, in some cases becoming the patient's predominant activity, causing them to miss meals or to neglect personal hygiene and social interaction. External attempts to interrupt these behaviours are typically met with acute dysphoria. These cognitive and behavioural disturbances lead to significant impairment in social, occupational or recreational functioning.

On questioning, patients often realize that their behaviours are not productive, although many try to rationalize them. They rarely report them spontaneously and it is usually the carers who bring up problems caused by punding. These patients have a significantly shorter overall sleep duration [12].

Misinterpretation as obsessive–compulsive disorder (OCD) may occur. The two disorders share some features: Both involve complex, stereotyped and meaningless behaviours which have a soothing effect and which are phenomenologically influenced by gender and personal history. In both, there may be a dissociation of insight into the uselessness of the behaviours. However differences exist which allow a clear distinction: Punding is often experienced as pleasurable and is not performed to relieve inner tensions or fear, as in OCD. Typical OCD contents are lacking, such as counting, checking, desire for symmetry or fear of contamination. Unlike OCDs, punding is unresponsive to serotonin reuptake inhibitors (SSRIs).

Limited data on prevalence are available at this stage. One group reported 14% of 123 PD patients on higher dopaminergic doses (800 mg levodopa equivalent per day) to be affected [12], while another reported a frequency of 1.4% in 373 unselected PD outpatients [13]. Another estimation of 8.2% in North American patients would seem to be more realistic [14]. Both reports are from specialized referral clinics, potentially limiting the generalizability of the findings to the PD population at large.

The phenomenology of punding behaviours (but not necessarily their incidence) is strongly influenced by gender. The mean age of disease onset was 47.8 years [12]. A strong association between drug dose and punding was found, with a mean daily levodopa equivalent dose of 1580 mg [12]. An association with agonist use was found in one study [15], but not in another [16]. Punding patients use a significantly higher number of rescue doses, including during the night [12]. One study found an association of excessive 'punding-like' involvement with hobbies/activities in PD patients with higher impulsive sensation-seeking traits [15].

An association of punding with DDS and with ICDs may occur. In one study of 17 DDS patients, 10 were also punders [12], and other small studies also found this association [6,17]. Hypersexuality and pathological gambling are significantly more prevalent in punders [12]. Moreover, patients classified with punding are significantly more likely to show hoarding behaviours [18].

Although the motor stereotypies observed in many dementia patients resemble the motor pattern in punding, dementia is relatively rare in cohorts of punders. In a small case series, one out of eight patients was mildly cognitively impaired and three had dementia [15,19]. However, a series of 17 patients [12] found no differences in Mini Mental Scores between the punding and non-punding groups which were matched for disease duration. Psychosis and hallucinations have occasionally been reported in the context of punding [19].

Many patients are only able to pund when in an 'on' state. Daily levodopa equivalent doses have been found to be higher in punding patients [12] and many punders also report dyskinesias [16]. Dyskinesias and punding are both thought to relate to drug-induced sensitization of neural systems mediating motor and behavioural functions that seem to be favoured by a more pulsatile (self-) administration of levodopa. Dyskinesias are correlated with punding severity, even when correcting for levodopa equivalent dose, which suggests that a sensitizing mechanism similar to that inducing behavioural changes might be involved in the development of dyskinesias [16]. The finding also suggests that punding should be screened for in dyskinetic patients.

Impulse control disorders

ICDs are characterized by the failure to resist an impulse, drive or temptation to perform an act that is harmful to the person or to others. ICDs in PD encompass a broad range of disorders including pathological gambling, compulsive sexual behaviours, compulsive buying or shopping, binge eating, intermittent explosive disorder, kleptomania and pyromania. However, the concept of pathologizing excessive behaviours such as sexual behavior has been an ongoing source of significant controversy. In general, the phenomenology is characterized by impulsivity, compulsivity and preoccupation with a behaviour or mood state. ICDs commonly have a detrimental impact on social and occupational functioning and may lead to breakdowns in interpersonal relationships and to financial and legal difficulties.

Lifetime prevalence in patients seen in specialized clinics has been found to be 3–8% [20–22], but this figure increased to 13.7% when only patients on dopamine agonists were considered [20]. A large North American multicentre survey conducted in 3090 PD patients found at least one ICD in 13.6% of them [24]. The four variants of ICDs included in the assessment tool used (QUIP) were pathological gambling, hypersexuality and compulsive eating and shopping, which occurred at similar frequencies. However, gender determined the type of ICD, with gambling and hypersexuality being more common in men and the other two disorders more common in women. More than one ICD was present in 3.9% of patients.

There is a strong association between dopamine agonist therapy and ICDs, but not with any one dopamine agonist in particular [20,23,24]. In the large survey of 3090 PD patients [24], ICDs were found in 17.1% of patients on dopamine agonists compared with 6.9% of those not taking an agonist. There is some dose relationship with dopamine agonists, but it is important to note that these abnormal behaviours may occur on regular doses, including on agonist monotherapy as initial treatment of early PD. This is highlighted by the observation of ICDs brought on by the small doses used in the treatment of restless legs syndrome: 7.1% of patients with restless legs syndrome treated with dopamine agonists were found to have an ICD [25,26]. Other risk factors identified in the large survey [24] included age, single status, smoking and a family history of gambling. In a case–control analysis of the same cohort, patients with ICDs were significantly more likely to report greater depressive, state and trait anxiety, more obsessive–compulsive symptoms and greater novelty-seeking and impulsivity, including choice impulsivity [27]. Frequent use of short-acting rescue therapy with apomorphine injections for 'off' periods was linked to hypersexuality (associated with dysregulation) in one small series [28].

Hypersexuality

Hypersexuality in PD is characterized by excessive preoccupation with sexual thoughts, a desire for frequent stimulation, compulsive masturbation, promiscuity, use of telephone sex lines, (internet) pornography, contact with sex workers or paraphilias. Cross-dressing exhibitionism and transvestic fetishism may occur. More extreme expressions have been described, including paraphilic disorders that may result in forensic consequences, such as paedophilia, sadomasochism or zoophilia. A few cases of serious sexual assault have been reported [1].

The prevalence of hypersexuality was found to be 3.5% in a large cross-sectional survey [24]. An association with the use of dopamine agonists has been demonstrated, without significant association with any particular agonist. The combination of levodopa and an agonist also increases the risk, albeit to a smaller extent than agonist monotherapy [21]. Sexual function often 'normalizes' after initiation of drug therapy in newly diagnosed PD, and there were reports on sexual excess following levodopa treatment even in the early years after its introduction [30]. Other reports have related hypersexuality to selegiline, pallidotomy and subthalamic stimulation [31–33].

Patients affected by this problem are overwhelmingly male [21,28]. They tend to have developed PD at an earlier age than average: the mean age at onset reported was between 42.9 and 51.4 (range 20–71) years [3,21,28].

Pathological gambling

All varieties of gambling occur in PD patients and internet use for this purpose has an increasing role. For current definitions of pathological gambling see <http://www.ncdhhs.gov/mhddsas/providers/problemgambling/pg-dsm10-11.pdf>. DDS may be associated, but this is by no means always the case and isolated pathological gambling is considerably more common than co-occurrence with DDS [10].

In the general population, pathological gambling has a prevalence of 0.25–1.7% [21,22]. This has been found to be considerably higher (2.3–8%) in PD patients [24,29].

There is considerable overlap between individual vulnerability factors for DDS and ICDs in PD and similarities to susceptibility factors for pathological gambling in the general population. Pathological gambling in PD is linked to male gender, having co-morbid psychiatric [10] or alcohol use disorders and having higher impulsive sensation-seeking traits. Patients tend to have a relatively young age of onset [27].

Other impulse control disorders

Compulsive eating The phenomenology of compulsive eating in PD may bear little resemblance to eating disorders affecting adolescents. In general, PD patients have a tendency to lose weight. In contrast, new-onset food cravings (e.g. for sweets) and compulsive and binge eating (including in the middle of the night) have been found in PD patients and often result in undesired weight gain. Pre-morbid obesity, female gender and young-onset PD appear to be risk factors [23]. The prevalence of this ICD in PD has been reported to be 4.3% [24].

Compulsive buying Although not officially recognized as a mental disorder, compulsive buying is seen as a serious condition characterized by excessively or poorly controlled preoccupations, urges, or behaviours with regard to shopping or buying, which can lead to negative consequences such as remorse, excessive debt and marital and family conflict [34]. The prevalence has been found to be 0.4–5.7% [21,24]. This disorder may include buying for others ('reckless generosity') [18] and occurs more commonly in women.

Explosive aggressive behaviour This has been considered to be one of the ICDs. It is rarely reported in PD, although it has been recognized as one of the behavioural changes in DDS and may occur transiently following deep brain stimulation (DBS) [31].

Hoarding Hoarding disorder has recently been recognized by DSM-5 as persistent difficulty in discarding or parting with possessions, regardless of the value others may attribute to these possessions. The behaviour usually has harmful effects. In PD, compulsive hoarding has been linked to the presence of ICDs, with hoarders showing a higher impulsive buying tendency score, punding, compulsive buying, binge eating and compulsive medication use. In PD patients, measures of clutter correlated with measures of obsessive–compulsion symptoms. Excessive acquisition was correlated with measures of impulse buying tendencies [35].

Pathophysiology

The impulse control-related behavioural disorders observed in PD patients on dopaminergic therapy are likely to be linked by overlaps in their pathophysiology. The neuroanatomical regions implicated in all behaviours include the ventral striatum where repetitive stimulation by long-term dopaminergic medication is believed to induce sensitization processes. The disorders share many, but not all, individual susceptibility factors, which are likely to shape the type of phenotypical expression.

Dopamine dysregulation syndrome

Negative reinforcement—avoiding aversive 'offs'

End-of-dose effects in isolation seem insufficient to explain DDS, as the majority of PD patients will experience some wearing-off effects if the course of the illness is long enough. Patients with early dyskinesia experience rebound worsening in affect [36] that is likely to progressively worsen with time, but the majority of patients do not compulsively self-medicate. Conversely, DDS patients commonly report self-medicating to avoid an unpleasant experience resembling the withdrawal state in abusers of psychostimulants. Their medication withdrawal state is characterized by reduced positive affect, a broader range of negative affective symptoms and worse motor function [37]. Negative reinforcement models of addiction propose that addicts are motivated to take drugs not for the initial pleasure but by the desire to avoid withdrawal symptoms that result from drug-induced plastic changes as the body seeks to restore its 'hedonic equilibrium'.

Negative reinforcement also includes self-medication of an existing aversive state. Consistent with this, higher depression scores have been found in DDS patients than in patients without DDS and with comparable motor disability [27,37].

Incentive-motivational accounts—'hunger' for medication

Incentive-motivational models of addiction equate the withdrawal state to natural motivational states such as hunger where repeated experiences with withdrawal enhance the incentive value of the drug [38]. In PD, repeated experience with end-of-dose wearing-off and coexistence of a chronic depressive state may further enhance the incentive value of the drug. However, this is unlikely to be the only explanation for DDS, as a negative affective state during 'off' periods is experienced by many more PD patients than those who develop DDS, and not all patients with DDS experience 'off' period withdrawal symptoms.

Conditioned reinforcement—medication taking 'habit'

A habit is an automatic action in a given situation, without direct reference to the goal of that action. Despite beginning as a goal-directed action, in which individuals seek drugs based on the knowledge of the pleasure they produce, in patients susceptible to the development DDS there is a progression to an automatic behaviour in which voluntary control is lost. In addition, stimuli consistently present in the environment gain motivational power through association.

Habit theory also provides an explanation for the development of punding. These stereotyped behaviours include pleasurable habitual routines which are homologous to the complex stereotyped responses in rats seen during hyperdopaminergic states. Dopaminergic drugs may enhance conditioned reinforcement (such as responding to financial incentives), and this effect is particularly striking in punders [37].

Incentive sensitization theory—enhanced drug 'wanting'

According to incentive sensitization theory, compulsive drug use results from neuroadaptations induced in dopamine projections to the accumbens-related circuitry, which can include long-lasting changes in dopaminergic and GABA-ergic neurotransmission and in intracellular signalling pathways, and to persistent changes in the physical structure of neurons [39–41]. Critical neuroadaptations make these systems hypersensitive to the rewarding effects of repeatedly administered drugs. According to this theory, the sensitized systems mediate a subcomponent of reward: incentive salience. Incentive salience is neither a hunger nor a withdrawal state, but one component of normal appetite which, if attributed to stimuli, causes them to become attractive and 'wanted' [39]. This 'wanting' is separate from 'liking', or sensory pleasure, and may result in pathological craving [38].

PD patients with DDS exhibit enhanced levodopa-induced ventral striatal dopamine release compared with PD patients without DDS [42]. This sensitized ventral striatal dopamine neurotransmission correlates with self-reported compulsive drug 'wanting' but not 'liking' [42] and DDS patients report increased drug 'wanting' during 'on' periods compared with non-dysregulating patients, despite having similar motor disability and more disabling dyskinesias [37].

Cortical inhibition of behaviour

The descending influences on striatal mechanisms from the prefrontal cortex may have a role in progressive loss of control over compulsive behaviours [43]. Dopamine mediates many cognitive functions of the frontal cortex [44]. Unmedicated PD patients in the early stage of the disease have reduced activation of the orbitofrontal cortex, the amygdala and the striatum [45] and medicated PD patients show reduced activity in the mesial–frontal areas during gambling tasks [46]. Decreased activity of the orbitofrontal cortex has been consistently reported in imaging studies of drug addicts [47] and frontal–striatal disconnection has been described in PD patients with isolated gambling [48].

Punding

Many of the mechanisms already outlined are likely to also have in role in the emergence of disabling punding behaviour in susceptible individuals, and overlaps are more likely in patients who additionally overuse their medication. The pathophysiology of punding is currently less well understood than that of DDS, but a sensitization process induced by repeated dopaminergic striatal stimulation is believed to be involved.

Dysfunction in orbitofrontal cortical systems is likely to have an important role [13,49]. Consistent with this, patients display an inability to control automatic stimulus-response selection mechanisms and to discontinue initiated habitual routines.

Impulse control disorders

Dopamine has long been known to have a central role in natural reward systems and reward-related disorders in people without PD. There is evidence from animal studies showing that unpredicted rewards induce phasic activity in the ventral tegmentum, whereas maximum reward uncertainty was associated with tonic increase in activity. Dopamine has a role in conditioned learning. Its physiological role in reward processing may be affected by dopaminergic treatment [50].

In keeping with this, it has been found that PD patients taking dopamine agonist medication make choices more rapidly and that learning from rewards is enhanced. In contrast, learning from negative outcomes is impaired, which may be due to the continuous presence of dopaminergic stimulation, precluding the physiological drop in dopaminergic release following unexpected punishment [51].

Similarly to DDS, a sensitization process with increasing incentive salience of behaviours has been implicated in the formation of ICDs. The release of dopamine following a reward may shift to cues of the reward, triggering a reward response [52]. This has been demonstrated in imaging studies in subjects without PD with substance and gambling addiction and in PD patients with pathological gambling [52,53].

Through imaging studies, dysfunction of the orbitofrontal cortex has been implicated in ICDs in individuals without PD. PD patients on dopaminergic medication have shown reduced orbitofrontal activity on positron emission tomography studies [54]. In keeping with this, a controlled brain perfusion single-photon emission computed tomography (SPECT) study in PD patients with pathological gambling found dysfunction in the brain network implicated in decision making, risk processing and response inhibition, which included the ventrolateral prefrontal, anterior and posterior cingulate and medial prefrontal cortex, the insula and the striatum. PD gamblers showed a disconnection between the anterior cingulate cortex and the striatum [48]. Clinically, impaired cognitive function has been found in PD patients with ICDs and prefrontal and memory functions were predominantly affected [55].

Genetic factors are very likely to play a role in the emergence of all impulsive behavioural disorders in PD. Polymorphisms linked to ICDs that have been identified so far are related to dopamine and glutamate receptor and serotonin transporter genes [56].

Management

Prevention and early detection

In assessing a patient with PD, potential factors that may influence individual susceptibility to compulsive behavioural disturbances should be taken into account. Gender, past drug and alcohol history, personal and family psychiatric disorders, gambling behaviours, evidence of a risk-taking personality in professional and recreational choices and attitudes to medications and social support systems are all relevant.

In individuals at risk, the minimum effective dose of dopaminergic drug therapy should be prescribed and non-medication-based therapies emphasized for the treatment of exacerbations, or during times of stress. The reinforcing effects of dopaminergic drugs may be more potent with short-acting pulses of therapy and there is evidence to suggest that rescue drugs such as apomorphine injections or soluble levodopa preparations may increase the risk in susceptible persons [16]. Adherence to regular dosing intervals should be encouraged rather than use of medications on an as-required basis.

When initiating dopamine agonist treatment, patients and relevant others should be informed of the small but existing risk of developing ICDs.

To detect possible punding behaviour early, it is essential to consider unreported punding when discussing insomnia, and to enquire whether patients engage in activities or use additional dopaminergic drug doses during those hours when they report being unable to sleep.

Treatment

Dopamine dysregulation syndrome

Once DDS has been identified, those patients who are able to significantly decrease dopaminergic doses can be expected to achieve remission or improvement, often without worsening of motor symptoms [40]. However, in many cases all attempts to reduce doses are met with resistance and management is often difficult because of a typical lack of insight into the nature of the problem, withdrawal symptoms or overwhelming drug craving. Treatment options focus on dose reductions as well as monitoring and supervision of medications, which requires the involvement of informed others. Attempts to restrict supplies may lead to medication hoarding or seeking alternative drug sources. Moreover, even when medication reductions are achieved, there is an enduring tendency for the individual to relapse.

A few cases of response to atypical neuroleptics such as clozapine [57] and quetiapine [13] have been observed. If associated with hypersexuality, antiandrogens have been used in selected severe cases [13]. DBS may provide another treatment option that allows drug reduction. Seven PD patients with active pathological gambling—four with DDS—were reported to improve following subthalamic DBS [58]. However, pre-operative DDS or ICDs may be a risk factor for post-operative suicide attempts [20].

Co-morbid disorders including depression, anxiety, psychosis, mania and dementia should be specifically screened for and treated in individuals with impulse-related disorders.

Involving informed others in the assessment and management has a central role in limiting harm.

Punding

No randomized controlled treatment studies or even observational long-term follow-up data exist for punding. Improvement with reduction of dopamine agonists (or, possibly, levodopa equivalent dose) has been reported, at least in some patients [13,40,59], but achieving dose reductions is often difficult due to a lack of insight. Improvement following amantadine or quetiapine has been observed [59]. Despite the repetitive behaviours sharing superficial similarity with OCD, SSRIs are ineffective [13].

Informing the patient's caregivers is important to involve them in the management of the problem and to avoid accusations or tensions which may arise from the behavioural changes they observe and which are hardly ever attributed to the disease or drugs by the patients or their relatives unless this is specifically addressed by the treating physician.

Impulse control disorders

One randomized cross-over study has suggested that amantadine reduces gambling behaviour in pathological gamblers with PD [60] many of whom were unable to discontinue the dopamine agonist. However, contradictory data exist with respect to amantadine as this was found to be associated with punding [13] and with impulse control disorders in two large cross-sectional studies [61,62]. Patients with ICDs usually benefit from dopamine agonist withdrawal. Reducing the dose is an alternative option, either using the same agonist or switching to a lower equivalent dose of another agonist. In many cases, this means that levodopa needs to be increased for adequate motor control. It may take weeks or months before the problematic ICD clears. Two small retrospective studies showed that full or partial response could be achieved by reducing or stopping dopamine agonists (and adding levodopa if required) [63,64].

Dopamine agonist withdrawal syndrome, which includes anxiety, dysphoria, apathy and subjective motor worsening, occurs more frequently if the agonist is discontinued because of an ICD [65].

Atypical neuroleptics such as quetiapine and clozapine [57,66] or, in cases of extreme hypersexuality, antiandrogens [13], have been reported to be helpful. Further observations of improvement have been reported with bupropione [67], topiramate, zonisamide [68], carbamazepine [69] and valproate [70]. Switching to continuous intrajejunal levodopa may be considered.

Naltrexone, a competitive opioid antagonist, has been observed to improve problem gambling in PD patients and this agent is currently under further investigation in a randomized controlled study [71].

ICDs have been reported to improve after treatment with subthalamic nucleus DBS [72], possibly due to the reduction in medication this procedure allows, although the opposite effect has also been observed [73,74].

A small randomized controlled study recently suggested a role for cognitive-behavioural therapy [6] but this approach should not be chosen without an appropriate adaptation or reduction in the medication.

Co-morbid conditions such as depression should be sought for and treated.

Additional social and legal supportive measures should always be considered and may be of particular importance in cases of pathological gambling. Involvement of the patient's close relatives or caregivers is of particular importance.

References

1 **Evans AH, Lees AJ.** Dopamine dysregulation syndrome in Parkinson's disease. Curr Opin Neurol 2004; **17**: 393–8.

2 **Evans AH, Lawrence AD, Potts J, et al.** Factors influencing susceptibility to compulsive dopaminergic drug use in Parkinson disease. Neurology 2005; **65**: 1570–4.

3 **Giovannoni G, O'Sullivan JD, Turner K, et al.** Hedonistic homeostatic dysregulation in patients with Parkinson's disease on dopamine replacement therapies. J Neurol Neurosurg Psychiatry 2000; **68**: 423–8.

4 **Katzenschlager R.** Dopamine dysregulation syndrome in Parkinson's disease. J Neurol Sci 2011; **310**: 271–5.

5 **Okai D, Askey-Jones S, Samuel M, et al.** Trial of CBT for impulse control behaviors affecting Parkinson patients and their caregivers. Neurology 2013; **80**: 792–9.

6 **Pezzella FR, Colosimo C, Vanacore N, et al.** Prevalence and clinical features of hedonistic homeostatic dysregulation in Parkinson's disease. Mov Disord 2005; **20**: 77–81.

7 **Pickering AD, Gray JA.** Dopamine, appetitive reinforcement, and the neuropsychology of human learning: an individual differences approach. In: A Eliasz, A Angleitner (eds), Advances in research on temperament, pp. 113–49. Lengerich: Pabst Science Publishers, 2001.

8 **Evans AH., Lawrence AD, Potts J, et al.** Relationship between impulsive sensation seeking traits, smoking, alcohol and caffeine intake, and Parkinson's disease. J Neurol Neurosurg Psychiatry 2006; **77**: 317–21.

9 **Oh JD, Russell DS, Vaughan CL, Chase TN.** Enhanced tyrosine phosphorylation of striatal NMDA receptor subunits: effect of dopaminergic denervation and L-DOPA administration. Brain Res 1998; **813**: 150–9.

10 **Gallagher DA, O'Sullivan SS, Evans AH, et al.** Pathological gambling in Parkinson's disease: risk factors and differences from dopamine dysregulation. An analysis of published case series. Mov Disord 2007; **22**: 1757–63.

11 **Rylander G.** Psychoses and the punding and choreiform syndromes in addiction to central stimulant drugs. Psychiatr Neurol Neurochir 1972; **75**: 203–12.

12 **Evans AH, Katzenschlager R, Paviour D, et al.** Punding in Parkinson's disease: its relation to the dopamine dysregulation syndrome. Mov Disord 2004; **19**: 397–405.

13 **Miyasaki JM, Al HK, Lang AE, Voon V.** Punding prevalence in Parkinson's disease. Mov Disord 2007; **22**: 1179–81.

14 **Nguyen FN, Chang YL, Okun MS, et al.** Prevalence and characteristics of punding and repetitive behaviors among Parkinson patients in north-central Florida. Int J Geriatr Psychiatry 2010; **25**: 540–1.

15 **Lawrence AJ, Blackwell AD, Barker RA, et al.** Predictors of punding in Parkinson's disease: results from a questionnaire survey. Mov Disord 2007; **22**: 2339–45.

16 **Silveira-Moriyama L, Evans AH, Katzenschlager R, Lees AJ.** Punding and dyskinesias. Mov Disord 2006; **21**: 2214–7.

17 **Serrano-Duenas M.** Chronic dopamimetic drug addiction and pathologic gambling in patients with Parkinson's disease—presentation of four cases. Ger J Psychiatry 2002; **5**: 62–6.

18 **O'Sullivan SS, Evans AH, Quinn NP, Lawrence AD, Lees AJ.** Reckless generosity in Parkinson's disease. Mov Disord 2010; **25**: 221–3.

19 **Kurlan R.** Disabling repetitive behaviors in Parkinson's disease. Mov Disord 2004; **19**: 433–7.

20 **Voon V, Hassan K, Zurowski MSM, et al.** Prevalence of repetitive and reward-seeking behaviors in Parkinson disease. Neurology 2006; **67**: 1254–7.

21 **Weintraub D, Siderowf AD, Potenza MN, et al.** Association of dopamine agonist use with impulse control disorders in Parkinson disease. Arch Neurol 2006; **63**: 969–3.

22 **Avanzi M, Baratti M, Cabrini S, et al.** Prevalence of pathological gambling in patients with Parkinson's disease. Mov Disord 2006; **21**: 2068–72.

23 **Grosset KA, Macphee G, Pal G, et al.** Problematic gambling on dopamine agonists: Not such a rarity. Mov Disord 2006; **21**: 2206–8.

24 **Weintraub D, Koester J, Potenza MN, et al.** Impulse control disorders in Parkinson disease: a cross-sectional study of 3090 patients. Arch Neurol 2010; **67**: 589–95.

25 **Tippmann-Peikert M, Park JG, Boeve BF, et al.** Pathologic gambling in patients with restless legs syndrome treated with dopaminergic agonists. Neurology 2007; **68**: 301–3.

26 Voon V, Schoerling A, Wenzel S, et al. Frequency of impulse control behaviours associated with dopaminergic therapy in restless legs syndrome. BMC Neurol 2011; **11**: 117.

27 Voon V, Sohr M, Lang AE, et al. Impulse control disorders in Parkinson disease: a multicentre case–control study. Ann Neurol 2011; **69**: 986–96.

28 Courty E, Durif F, Zenut M, et al. Psychiatric and sexual disorders induced by apomorphine in Parkinson's disease. Clin Neuropharmacol 1997; **20**: 140–7.

29 Djamshidian A, Cardoso F, Grosset D, Bowden-Jones H, Lees AJ. Pathological gambling in Parkinson's disease—a review of the literature. Mov Disord 2011; **26**: 1976–84.

30 Bowers MB Jr, Van Woert M, Davis L. Sexual behavior during L-dopa treatment for Parkinsonism. Am J Psychiatry 1971; **127**: 1691–3.

31 Sensi M, Eleopra R, Cavallo MA, et al. Explosive-aggressive behavior related to bilateral subthalamic stimulation. Parkinsonism Relat Disord 2004; **10**: 247–51.

32 Mendez MF, O'Connor SM, Lim GT. Hypersexuality after right pallidotomy for Parkinson's disease. J Neuropsychiatry Clin Neurosci 2004; **16**: 37–40.

33 Houeto JL, Mesnage V, Mallet L, et al. Behavioural disorders, Parkinson's disease and subthalamic stimulation. J Neurol Neurosurg Psychiatry 2002; **72**: 701–7.

34 McElroy SL, Keck PE, Pope HG Jr, Smith JMR, Strakowski SM. Compulsive buying: A report of 20 cases. J Clin Psychiatry 1994; **55**: 242–8.

35 O'Sullivan SS, Djamshidian A, Evans AH, Loane CM, Lees AJ, Lawrence AD. Excessive hoarding in Parkinson's disease. Mov Disord 2010; **25**: 1026–33.

36 Evans AH, Farrell MJ, Gibson SJ, Helme RD, Lim SY. Dyskinetic patients show rebound worsening of affect after an acute L-dopa challenge. Parkinsonism Relat Disord 2012; **18**: 514–19.

37 Evans AH, Lawrence AD, Cresswell SA, Katzenschlager R, Lees AJ. Compulsive use of dopaminergic drug therapy in Parkinson's disease: reward and anti-reward. Mov Disord 2010; **25**: 867–76.

38 Hutcheson DM, Everitt BJ, Robbins TW, Dickinson A. The role of withdrawal in heroin addiction: enhances reward or promotes avoidance? Nat Neurosci 2001; **4**: 943–7.

39 Robinson TE, Berridge KC. Addiction. Ann Rev Psychol 2000; **54**: 25–53.

40 Kimber TE, Thompson PD, Kiley MA. Resolution of dopamine dysregulation syndrome following cessation of dopamine agonist therapy in Parkinson's disease. J Clin Neurosci 2008; **15**: 205–8.

41 Berke JD, Hyman SE. Addiction, dopamine, and the molecular mechanisms of memory. Neuron 2000; **25**: 515–32.

42 Evans AH, Pavese N, Lawrence AD, et al. Compulsive drug use linked to sensitized ventral striatal dopamine transmission. Ann Neurol 2006; **59**: 852–8.

43 Cilia R, Van Eimeren T. Impulse control disorders in Parkinson's disease: seeking a roadmap to ward a better understanding. Brain Struct Funct 2011; **216**: 289–99.

44 Cohen JD, Braver TS, Brown JW. Computational perspectives on dopamine function in prefrontal cortex. Curr Opin Neurobiol 2002; **12**: 223–9.

45 Ouchi Y, Yoshikawa E, Okada H, et al. Alterations in binding site density of dopamine transporter in the striatum, orbitofrontal cortex, and amygdala in early Parkinson's disease: compartment analysis for beta-CFT binding with positron emission tomography. Ann Neurol 1999; **45**: 601–10.

46 Thiel A, Hilker R, Kessler J, et al. Activation of basal ganglia loops in idiopathic Parkinson's disease: a PET study. J Neural Transm 2003; **110**: 1289–301.

47 Volkow ND, Wang GJ, Ma Y, et al. Activation of orbital and medial prefrontal cortex by methylphenidate in cocaine-addicted subjects but not in controls: relevance to addiction. J. Neurosci 2005; **25**: 3932–9.

48 Cilia R, Cho SS, Van Eimeren T, et al. Pathological gambling in patients with Parkinson's disease is associated with fronto-striatal disconnection: a path modeling analysis. Mov Disord 2011; **26**: 225–33.

49 Spencer AH, Rickards H, Fasano A, Cavanna AE. The prevalence and clinical characteristics of punding in Parkinson's disease. Mov Disord 2011; **26**: 578–86.

50 Fiorillo CD, Tobler PN, Schultz W. Discrete coding of reward probability and uncertainty by dopamine neurons. Science 2003; **299**: 1898–902.

51 Van Eimeren, T., Ballanger B, Pellecchia G, et al. Dopamine agonists diminish value sensitivity of the orbitofrontal cortex: a trigger for pathological gambling in Parkinson's disease? Neuropsychopharmacology 2009; **34**: 2758–66.

52 Voon V, Mehta AR, Hallett M. Impulse control disorders in Parkinson's disease: recent advances. Curr Opin Neurol 2011; **24**: 324–30.

53 Frosini D, Pesaresi I, Cosottini M, et al. Parkinson's disease and pathological gambling: results from a functional MRI study. Mov Disord 2010; **25**: 2449–53.

54 Reuter J, Raedler T, Rose M, et al. Pathological gambling is linked to reduced activation of the mesolimbic reward system. Nat Neurosci 2005; **8**: 147–8.

55 Vitale C, Santangelo G, Trojano L, et al. Comparative neuropsychological profile of pathological gambling, hypersexuality and compulsive eating in Parkinson's disease. Mov Disord 2011; **26**: 830–6.

56 Cormier F, Muellner J, Corvol JC. Genetics of impulse control disorders in Parkinson's disease. J Neural Transm 2013; **120**: 665–71.

57 Fernandez HH, Durso R. Clozapine for dopaminergic-induced paraphilias in Parkinson's disease. Mov Disord 1998; **13**: 597–8.

58 Ardouin C, Voon V, Worbe Y, et al. Pathological gambling in Parkinson's disease improves on chronic subthalamic nucleus stimulation. Mov Disord 2006; **21**: 1941–6.

59 Fasano A, Ricciardi L, Pettorruso M, Bentivoglio AR. Management of punding in Parkinson's disease: an open-label prospective study. J Neurol 2011; **258**: 656–60.

60 Thomas A, Bonanni L, Gambi F, Di Iorio A, Onofrj M. Pathological gambling in Parkinson disease is reduced by amantadine. Ann Neurol 2010; **68**: 400–4.

61 Weintraub D, Sohr M, Potenza MN, et al. Amantadine use associated with impulse control disorders in Parkinson disease in cross-sectional study. Ann Neurol 2010; **68**: 963–8.

62 Lee JY, Kim HJ, Jeon BS. Is pathological gambling in Parkinson's disease reduced by amantadine? Ann Neurol 2011; **69**: 213–14.

63 Mamikonyan E, Siderowf AD, Duda JE, et al. Long-term follow-up of impulse control disorders in Parkinson's disease. Mov Disord 2008; **23**: 75–80.

64 Macphee GJ, Copeland C, Stewart D, Grosset K, Grosset DG. Clinical follow up of pathological gambling in Parkinson's disease in the West Scotland study. Mov Disord 2009; **24**: 2430–1.

65 Pondal M, Marras C, Miyasaki J, et al. Clinical features of dopamine agonist withdrawal syndrome in a movement disorders clinic. J Neurol Neurosurg Psychiatry 2013; **84**: 130–5.

66 Rotondo A, Bosco D, Plastino M, et al. Clozapine for medication-related pathological gambling in Parkinson disease. Mov Disord 2010; **25**: 1994–5.

67 Benincasa D, Pellicano C, Fanciulli A, et al. Bupropion abates dopamine agonist-mediated compulsive behaviors in Parkinson's disease. Mov Disord 2011; **26**: 355–7.

68 Bermejo PE. Topiramate in managing impulse control disorders in Parkinson's disease. Parkinsonism Relat Disord 2008; **14**: 448–9.

69 Bach JP, Oertel WH, Dodel R, et al. Treatment of hypersexuality in Parkinson's disease with carbamazepine—a case report. Mov Disord 2009; **24**: 1241–2.

70 Hicks CW, Pandya MM, Itin I, et al. Valproate for the treatment of medication-induced impulse-control disorders in three patients with Parkinson's disease. Parkinsonism Relat Disord 2011; **17**: 379–81.

71 **Eusebio A, Witjas T, Cohen J, et al**. Subthalamic nucleus stimulation and compulsive use of dopaminergic medication in Parkinson's disease. J Neurol Neurosurg Psychiatry 2013; **84**: 868–74.

72 **Bosco D, Plastino M, Colica C, et al**. Opioid antagonist naltrexone for the treatment of pathological gambling in Parkinson disease. Clin Neuropharmacol 2012; **35**: 118–20.

73 **Lu C, Bharmal A, Suchowersky O**. Gambling and Parkinson disease. Arch Neurol 2006; **63**: 298.

74 **Moum SJ, Price CC, Limotai N, et al**. Effects of STN and GPi deep brain stimulation on impulse control disorders and dopamine dysregulation syndrome. PLoS ONE 2012; **7**: e29768.

Chapter 29

Treatment-related non-motor symptoms in Parkinson's disease

Vincent Ries, J. Carsten Möller, Marcus M. Unger
and Wolfgang H. Oertel

Introduction

This chapter describes non-motor effects attributable to antiparkinsonian medication. These include rare but serious side effects such as serotonin syndrome and malignant neuroleptic syndrome, and chronic side effects such as heart-valve fibrosis. Medication-induced fluctuation of mood, cognition and perception is discussed. Lastly, the chapter describes how medication can accentuate excessive daytime sleepiness.

Serotonin-related complications

Serotonin syndrome—acute serotonergic overstimulation

Serotonin syndrome, also known as carcinoid syndrome, is not specific to Parkinson's disease (PD). It is simply induced by serotonergic overstimulation, typically due to combinations of serotonergic agents. These comprise: (1) the serotonin precursors tryptophan and 5-hydroxytryptophan; (2) serotonin liberators, namely opioids, especially tramadol, dextromethorphan and pethidine, methylenedioxymethamphetamine (MDMA), amphetamines or lithium; (3) selective and non-selective serotonin reuptake inhibitors including tricyclics; (4) selective and non-selective monoamine oxidase (MAO) inhibitors; and (5) 5-HT$_{1A}$ agonists like buspiron and 5-HT$_{1B/D}$ agonists, the triptans. In addition, some ergot dopamine (DA) agonists are also 5-HT agonists (Table 29.1) [1–3]. Special attention should be paid to ephedrine and dextromethorphan, which are present in many over-the-counter decongestants and antitussives as well as illicit drugs. Endogenous serotonin syndromes are seen in the context of carcinoid tumours. Nevertheless, due to disease-related medication and increased neurochemical susceptibility, PD patients may be at higher risk of developing serotonin syndrome.

Clinically, serotonin syndrome is marked by psychiatric, neurological and autonomic symptoms. Psychiatric symptoms are confusion, hypomania or agitation; neurological symptoms include tremor, shivering, coma, coordination problems, hyperreflexia, myoclonus and rigidity. Autonomic symptoms include flush, hypersalivation, hypersudation,

Table 29.1 Affinities of selected dopamimetics to 5-HT$_1$ receptors

Drug	5-HT$_{1A}$ (pKi)	5-HT$_{1B}$ (pKi)	5-HT$_{1D}$ (pKi)
Lisuride	8.9 (+)	7.6 (+)	8.5 (+)
Bromocriptine	7.2 (+)	6.0 (+)	7.1 (−)
Cabergoline	6.4 (+)	5.7 (+)	7.8 (+)
Pergolide	7.0 (+)	6.0 (+)	7.5 (+)
Piribedil	5.7 (+)	n.d.	n.d.
Apomorphine	5.9 (+)	<5 (−)	<5 (−)
Ropinirole	6.5	<5	5.9
Pramipexole	6.2	5.1	5.8

(+), agonist; (−), antagonist; n.d., not determined.

Adapted from [2] and [3].

diarrhoea and tensional dysregulation. The presence of at least one symptom from each of these three categories has been proposed as a diagnostic criterion.

Essentially, most reports only describe symptomatic treatment after withdrawal of the inducing drugs. The action of most symptomatic therapies is based on 5-HT$_{2A}$ receptors. The 5-HT$_{2A}$ antagonist ketanserin, licensed in the Netherlands for use in eclampsia, is the antidote of choice, starting with 10 mg for a 70-kg person, which can be increased up to 160 mg day^{-1} [4]. An alternative is cyproheptadine 4–8 mg orally repeated after 2 hours and at a maximum of 32 mg day^{-1} or, more symptomatically, beta-blockers like propranolol. Serotonin symptoms and syndrome may be largely prevented by the implementation of drug-interaction warning software.

In summary, one should avoid combinations of antidepressants and MAO-B inhibitors or tramadol, pethidine or dextromethorphan in order to prevent the precipitation of serotonin syndrome.

Fibrotic ergot-related problems

In recent years, much attention has been paid to the development of heart-valve fibrosis with different ergolinic dopamimetic drugs. A survey in a British general practice population reported a five-fold increased risk of cardiac valvular fibrosis with pergolide and cabergoline [5]. The results are summarized in Table 29.2.

In an echocardiographic prevalence study on 64 patients taking pergolide, 49 taking cabergoline, 42 taking non-ergot DA agonists and 90 controls, Zanettini et al. [6] found a six-fold increased relative risk. The tricuspid, mitral and aortic valves seem to be at comparable risk for fibrosis [6].

Based on receptor affinity profiles, several authors have assigned this effect to 5-HT$_{2B}$ agonistic action [5–9]. Fibrotic complications like retroperitoneal fibrosis and cardiac Hedinger syndrome are classical complications of chronic serotonergic overstimulation, either exogenously by ergot derivatives like ergotamine, ergometrine or dihydroergocriptine,

Table 29.2 Incidence of heart-valve fibrosis with dopamimetics and in controls

Drug	No of cases with heart-valve fibrosis	Cumulative exposure (patient-years)	Mean duration of exposure (years)	Incidence/10 000 patient-years
Bromocripine	0	1683	2.0	–
Lisuride	0	88	1.4	–
Pergolide	6	2031	2.2	30
Cabergoline	6	1812	1.5	33
Pramipexole	0	648	1.3	–
Ropinirole	0	1565	1.6	–
Controls	19	28892	3.8	6

Derived from [5].

serotonin liberators like fenfluramine or MDMA or endogenously in the context of a carcinoid syndrome. Even bleomycin lung recently proved to be indirectly induced by 5-HT$_{2A}$ and 5-HT$_{2B}$ agonism. Nevertheless, compounds like methysergide and cyproheptadine, formerly used against migraine and mostly withdrawn from the market for their well-recognized fibrotic potential, are 5-HT$_{2B}$ antagonists. The frequency of fibrosis was 2 in 10 000 in patients treated with methysergide [10]. The receptor-linked mechanism of profibrotic action is not fully understood yet, but downregulation of 5-HT$_{2B}$ receptors may be the decisive step, with the 5-HT$_{2B}$ receptor being known to be downregulated upon exposure to both agonists and antagonists [11].

The 5-HT$_2$ receptor affinities of ergot parkinsonian medications are given in Table 29.3. Only cabergoline and pergolide are 5-HT$_{2B}$ agonists; all others are 5-HT$_{2B}$ antagonists, and lisuride is the most potent blocker of 5-HT$_{2B}$ receptors [2].

Table 29.3 Affinities to 5-HT$_2$ receptors of some potentially fibrogenic drugs

Drug	5-HT$_{2A}$ (pKi)	5-HT$_{2B}$ (pKi)	5-HT$_{2C}$ (pKi)
Cabergoline	8.1 (+)	8.6 (+)	6.7 (+)
Pergolide	8.8 (+)	8.2 (+)	7.4 (+)
Piribedil	<4 (–)	6.0 (–)	<4 (–)
Apomorphine	6.4 (–)	6.2 (–)	6.1 (–)
Bromocriptine	8.2 (+)	8.9 (–)	7.0 (–)
Lisuride	8.1 (+)	9.0 (–)	8.1 (+)
Methysergide	8.6 (–)	9.1 (–)	8.6 (–)
Pizotifen	7.8 (–)	7.8 (–)	8.1 (–)
Cryproheptadine	8.5 (–)	8.0 (–)	7.9 (–)

(+), agonist; (–), antagonist.

Adapted from [2] and [10].

Table 29.4 Registered cases of fibrosis under dopamine agonists

		Fibrosis (no. of cases)		
	Available since	**Pleura**	**Pericardium**	**Peritoneum**
Pergolide	1988	104	8	19
Bromocriptine	1979	215	12	29
Cabergoline	1997	12	1	0
Lisuride	1968	6	0	1
Ropinirole	1996	4	3	0
Pramipexole	1997	0	0	0

Adapted from [12].

Cabergoline and pergolide have the highest profibrotic potential. Table 29.4 provides a summary of cases reporting fibrosis [12]. Until now, there have been almost no data on the reversibility of ergot-induced fibrosis. Current recommendations include a cardiological examination, including echocardiography, prior to the initiation of ergot derivatives. The recommendations also advise 6-monthly clinical cardiopulmonary examination and an annual echocardiogram in patients who have already been treated successfully with these compounds for a longer period. Those patients who discontinue ergot derivates should undergo cardiopulmonary examination every second year [13].

The frequency and risk of exacerbation of coronary heart disease by dopamimetics largely exceeds the incidence of heart-valve fibrosis and can be monitored clinically and by stress-electrocardiogram. Taken together, ergot-related fibrosis and valvulopathy are possibly linked to the 5-HT$_{2B}$ affinity of ergot compounds and occur with a frequency of 1 in 300 patient years. Ergot derivatives are no longer considered as first-line drugs in PD therapy and are reserved for individual cases under close monitoring.

Fluctuating non-motor symptoms

Fluctuating subjective symptoms

A large fraction of patients experience uncomfortable fluctuating subjective symptoms. The diurnal pattern of these, if carefully assessed, only partially overlaps or exceeds that of the motor symptoms and can be completely uncoupled. In a detailed characterization of 20 patients Volpe-Gillot et al. [14] categorized subjective fluctuations into: 'energetic' feelings comprising fatigue and a sensation of mental emptiness; cognitive-perceptual alterations including blurred vision, slowing of thought, loss of concentration; and emotional modifications including social withdrawal, depressive ideas and anxiety/panic. An illustrative case from their series is cited here (translated from the French, with permission):

> A woman, aged 65 years, followed up for PD since 1978, was admitted for increasingly severe blockades in 1993. The patient was sometimes forced to lie down and had the awkward sensation of shrinking or entering into a shell, with her neck regressing into her shoulders and her head into

her thorax; she felt the loss or withering of her legs, and that she was becoming self-enclosed. She was unable to move or speak. The symptoms would be accompanied by anxiety and fear of dying, attacks of panic, impulsive phobia and badly defined visual blurring. These episodes initially occurred 2.5 hours after intake of levodopa and could be relieved by 3 mg apomorphine, although this soon lost its efficiency. Later, following observation in 1995, although the patient described being completely blocked, she reported being able to move with a UPDRS [Unified Parkinson's Disease Rating Scale]-III of 15 [14].

In their wearing-off questionnaire, Stacy et al. [15,16] included six items related to fluctuating subjective symptoms: tiredness, cloudy/dull mind, slowness of thinking, anxiety, mood changes, panic attacks. Among 181 patients identified with wearing-off phenomena, tiredness and the feeling of cloudy/dull mind congruent with the 'energetic' category of Volpe-Gillot et al. [14] were the most common non-motor symptoms. There are several case reports stating complete dissociation of motor and non-motor fluctuations. An autobiographical report describes a patient who was perfectly able to walk with subthalamic nucleus deep-brain stimulation (STN DBS) 'on' but necessitated switching it 'off' for talking or thinking [17].

In summary, fluctuating subjective symptoms can be subdivided into 'energetic', cognitive-perceptual and emotional fields. Their duration can exceed that of motor fluctuations or they can be completely desynchronized from them. Fluctuating subjective symptoms can be resistant to or differentially influenced by DBS. Treatment with antidepressant medications may be possible.

Fluctuating autonomic and other symptoms

Further non-motor fluctuations that mostly present during motor 'off' phases include attacks of hypersalivation, abnormal vasomotor activity with arterial hypertension, urinary/micturition urgency, abdominal pain and inspiratory stridor. Many PD patients describe blurred vision, especially at lower luminosity during 'off' phases. The pathophysiological correlate is probably a degeneration of foveal dopaminergic neurons (A17) [18,19] which physiologically enhance visual contrast [20].

Dopamimetic withdrawal, akinetic crisis and neuroleptic malignant syndrome

The underlying mechanism of these phenomena is the abrupt stoppage of central dopaminergic neurotransmission, either by discontinuation of dopamimetic medication in PD patients or by the intake of neuroleptics, including atypical neuroleptics and the vesicular monoamine transport (VMAT) inhibitor tetrabenazine, in people with PD. Research criteria from the Diagnostic and Statistical Manual of Mental Disorders (DSM-V TR) require that both severe muscle rigidity and elevated temperature are present after recent administration of an antipsychotic as well as two associated signs, symptoms or laboratory findings [21]. The overall incidence of neuroleptic malignant syndrome is estimated to be 0.01–0.02% in people treated with neuroleptics [22]. It should be noted that cases of neuroleptic malignant syndrome have also been reported after clozapine [23,24] (the only neuroleptic approved for PD in Germany), sometimes in the context of pharmacokinetic interaction with the CYP1A2 inhibitor paroxetine [25], or quetiapine [26] (the only other neuroleptic recommended for use in PD).

Typically, neuroleptic malignant syndrome starts with a delay of 2–15 days after the onset or increase of neuroleptic medication. Cardinal symptoms are extra-pyramidal rigidity, compromised consciousness and vegetative syndromes including hyperthermia > 38.5°C, profuse sweating, unstable blood pressure and tachycardia. Rigor and dystonia can lead to contractures and a marked increase in creatine phosphokinase. Increased leucocyte counts are frequently observed, and patients may need to be admitted to an intensive care unit. Differential diagnoses include anticholinergic syndrome (warm skin without sweating, mydriasis), serotonin syndrome (flush, agitation, diarrhoea), idiopathic malignant catatonia, withdrawal from baclofen, salicylate poisoning, tetanus (hypocalcaemic or clostridial, spasms on a rigid background), stiff-man syndrome and non-convulsive status epilepticus. Knowledge of the pharmaco-toxicological context is mandatory. In the parkinsonian patient, the diagnostic workup should contain the search for dehydration, infectious pathology, mistakes in drug application, compromised drug absorption because of diarrhoea, gastroenteritis, ileus, previous use of antibiotics or exposure to heat.

Therapeutic measures recommended by various national guidelines, for example [13], include withdrawal of the neuroleptic, hydration and correction of electrolytes, cooling, sufficient calorific support and prophylaxis of thrombosis, decubitus and pneumonia. With respect to the almost obligatory aspiration pneumonia, the antibiotic dose should be adapted, after a loading dose, to the often-compromised renal function. In agitated or catatonic patients, lorazepam 1–2 mg can be tried [21]. As specific measures, levodopa or dopamimetics should be reintroduced. In severe cases, 200 mg amantadine over 3 hours can be administered up to three times a day. Apomorphine can be tried first as a bolus of 2–10 mg, later as a continuous infusion by a subcutaneous pump. Infusion rates should be 1–2 mg hour^{-1} initially, and can be increased every 12 hours in steps of 0.5–1 mg hour^{-1}. Levodopa can be administered by a nasoduodenal tube. An alternative, especially useful in a context of subileus, may be transdermal rotigotine. In case of rhabdomyolysis, 1 mg kg^{-1} dantrolene every 6 hours can be tried for up to 48 hours, but cardiovascular collapse can occur if it is used in combination with calcium channel blockers [21]. Use of dantrolene seemed to be associated with higher mortality in a review of 271 cases, especially if the prior medication consisted of more than neuroleptic monotherapy [27]. In psychiatric patients with neuroleptic malignant syndrome and prolonged catatonia, the use of electroconvulsive therapy has been reported, but there are only rare case reports for PD [21]. Woodbury and Woodbury [28] proposed five stages of neuroleptic malignant syndrome to guide the escalation of measures. Endocrinopathies like hypothyroidism or adrenal insufficiency can aggravate neuroleptic malignant syndrome. One-third or more of non-PD patients relapse with reintroduction of neuroleptic therapy.

In brief, akinetic crisis and neuroleptic malignant syndrome should be prevented through attention to drug interactions and strict avoidance of neuroleptics other than clozapine or quetiapine. Therapeutic measures include withdrawal of neuroleptics, water/

electrolyte correction and the search for intercurrent triggers. Optionally, in an akinetic crisis it may be possible to use levodopa by nasoduodenal tube, subcutaneous apomorphine, intravenous amantadine (paying attention to the potential of amantadine to induce confusion) or transdermal rotigotine.

Thermoregulatory problems

As an abortive form of neuroleptic malignant syndrome, isolated hyperthermia can occur as a phenomenon related to medication or PD, the latter being called Parkinson-hyperpyrexia syndrome (PHS). Ten to 15 days after initiation of clozapine, transitory mild hyperthermia is frequent and mostly benign, after exclusion of neuroleptic malignant syndrome, agranulocytosis and myocarditis [29]. Furthermore, hyperthermia is a stereotypic effect of any anticholinergic drug. PHS can occur after reduction of treatment and withdrawal of amantadine or anticholinergics.

Drug-induced somnolence and sudden onset of sleep

General, epidemiology

Sudden onset of sleep (SOS) in PD was highlighted by Frucht et al. in 1999 [30]; their study described eight cases of PD patients who fell asleep while driving a car and caused accidents. These patients were treated with pramipexole and ropinirole. Excessive daytime sleepiness (EDS) and SOS in PD had been known before [31]. Obviously, the disease process and dopamimetic medication contribute to sleep induction in PD.

To estimate the frequency of SOS, Paus et al. [32] screened 2952 PD patients and identified 177 as having experienced SOS during active stimulation, corresponding to a prevalence of 6%. In an even larger study, Möller [33] reported a prevalence of up to 43% in a cohort of 6620 patients recruited from the German Parkinson Association and submitted to a postal questionnaire. These were further differentiated into 10% reporting 'sleep attacks' exclusively, 40% only unintended sleep episodes with premonitory signs and the remaining 50% a mixture of both. Ferreira et al. [34] found comparable prevalences of SOS in PD patients and controls of 27 and 32%, respectively, but a significantly higher frequency and severity in PD patients in situations requiring attention (10.8 versus 1.7%). The same group reported a prevalence of 31% in a previous pharmaco-epidemiological study [35]. A Canadian survey found a prevalence of SOS of 3.8% [36], two different US surveys found 14% [37] and 20.8% [38] and a Chinese one 13.8% [39]. Younger patients seem to be at higher risk of non-ergot-induced SOS [40]. In a longitudinal study over 8 years, EDS was found in 8% of PD subjects at baseline, in 21% at 4 years and in 40.8% at 8 years. Factors associated with development of EDS included dementia and more rapid progression of parkinsonism [41,42].

Pathophysiology and phenotype

A considerable part of SOS and EDS in PD is explained by dopamimetic drug action, as levodopa can have a sedative effect in healthy volunteers [43]. A novel explanation for this phenomenon has been provided by the discovery of a dopaminergic cell group in the ventral periaqueductal grey matter (vPAG) of the rat which is selectively active during wakefulness. Expression of Fos in the vPAG underlies a precise sleep/wake cycle and its destruction led to a 20% increase in sleep in rats. This vPAG cell group projects to and receives afferent input from the most sleep-relevant structures, including the intralaminar thalamus, the medial prefrontal cortex, the basal forebrain cholinergic neurons, the ventrolateral preoptic nucleus, the lateral hypothalamic orexin/hypocretin neurons, the cholinergic pontine laterodorsal tegmental nucleus and the locus coeruleus [44]. The inhibitory effect of pre-synaptic D_2/D_3 receptors in the vPAG may promote sedation. Analogously, the A10 dopaminergic group or ventral tegmental area at the origin of the mesolimbic projections has also been assumed to be involved in dopamimetic-induced sleepiness [45].

In addition there are disease-specific mechanisms suggested by the longitudinally increasing occurrence of SOS in patients who have never taken dopamimetics [42]. These mechanisms comprise degeneration of serotonergic and noradrenergic structures promoting arousal, namely the nucleus raphe dorsalis (B7) and the locus coeruleus (A4/A6) which are already affected by Braak Stage II [46]. The precise correlation of these neurochemically defined structures with the ascending reticular activating system remains to be established. An ascending reticular activating system was postulated based on experiments in cats. Its dorsal projections from bulbo-pontal areas to the nuclei intralaminares thalami and its ventral part, projecting via subthalamic areas to the nucleus dorsomedianus thalami, may contribute to SOS [47]. Hypocretin neurons further contribute to arousal via stimulation of the vPAG and the A10 group [48]. The hypothesis of a link between the dopamine and hypocretin systems is strengthened by the association of SOS with the (–909T/C) pre-prohypocretin polymorphism and the Taq1A dopamine D2-receptor gene polymorphism [49,50]. In this context, it is of note that post-mortem studies indicate a loss of hypocretin neurons in PD [59,60]. Finally, altered sleep structure with sleep fragmentation in the second half of the night, reduced rapid eye movement (REM) and slow-wave sleep, co-morbidity with other sleep disorders such as REM sleep behaviour disorder and the presence of nocturnal motor disability [51] are likely to compromise sleep efficiency and have been proposed to aggravate EDS. However, recent epidemiological studies have shown the inverse, in other words, there is less EDS in patients who report a poorer sleep quality [42,52].

Besides the neuronal pathomechanism, the polysomnographic phenotype of SOS is of interest. An increased frequency of sleep-onset REM episodes has been reported in some PD populations. However, the majority of recorded SOS has so far been characterized by the presence of non-REM sleep [53].

Differential effect of dopamimetics

SOS is often exacerbated by dopamimetic medication. The hypnogenic potential of dopamimetics in PD patients has never been assessed systematically by prospective comparative studies. For differential information we have to rely on several retrospective surveys which are partially biased by increasing doses of dopamimetics with longer disease duration and tremor-predominant forms of PD, where the degenerative pattern differs from that of akinetic–rigid forms. Paus et al. [32] assessed 2952 PD patients and identified 177 cases of SOS. The raw prevalences of sleep attacks on all dopamimetics did not differ significantly from each other or from the total, except for patients on levodopa monotherapy, who experienced less SOS. If these prevalences are adjusted to the levodopa equivalent dose of DA agonists, lisuride is descriptively the most hypnogenic, followed by pramipexole, ropinirole and bromicriptine, cabergoline and pergolide. Similar results were obtained in the survey by Montastruc et al. [35] who assessed 64 patients taking ropinirole with the highest risk of SOS, followed by 11 patients on lisuride, 67 patients on bromocriptine and 217 patients on levodopa monotherapy, especially after adjustment for disease duration and severity. Körner et al. [40], in the largest study so far, found a significantly increased risk of SOS under a monotherapy of non-ergot derivates compared with ergot derivates and the combination of non-ergot derivates with levodopa in patients younger than 70 years; this was independent of the duration of drug intake.

It is possible that short-acting agonists and non-ergot selective D2/3 agonists tend to have a higher hypnogenic potential than long-acting ergot agonists. This seems plausible, as a short effect should be related to rapidly acting drugs rather than to slow-acting ones. In addition, the mentioned D2/3 receptor-bearing A10 and A13 groups may provide a rationale for a D2/3-dominated effect. Interestingly, disease duration was not correlated with the prevalence of SOS in some studies. However, as pergolide and cabergoline are now obsolete because of their fibrogenic potential, only the possible lower hypnogenic potential of levodopa versus any agonist is of relevance.

Predictors and tests predictive of 'sleep attacks'

Patients with and without premonitory signs should be differentiated. The latter in particular should be reminded that PD patients suffering from daytime sleepiness and/or SOS should not drive. In a pilot study using a driving simulator, the deleterious effect of SOS in PD on driving performance could be clearly shown [54]. In retrospective surveys, EDS assessed by the Epworth Sleepiness Scale (ESS; Table 29.5) [55] correlated well with the risk of SOS.

Some patients seem to be at risk for sleep attacks without appropriate warning signs and without accompanying daytime sleepiness [32]. Correspondingly, a small study comparing 10 PD patients with and 10 without sleep attacks found multiple sleep latency testing to have no predictive value, suggesting that SOS may indeed occur against a background of normal alertness [56]. The predictive value of an ESS score of 10 or more was only 40.7% in the population assessed by Ferreira et al. [34]. Notwithstanding, Möller [33] reported good sensitivity and specificity of the ESS characterized by an integral of the receiver operating characteristic (ROC) curve of 0.85 (maximum 1.0 if sensitivity = 100% and specificity = 100%). Montastruc et al. [35] proposed dysautonomia as a strong predictive factor of SOS, with an odds ratio of 25. Further risk factors identified for SOS were disease duration, age,

Table 29.5 The Epworth sleepiness scale (ESS)

Situation	Probability of falling asleep[*]
1. Sitting in a train and reading	
2. Watching television	
3. Sitting inactively in a public place (cinema, theatre, meetings . . .)	
4. Passenger in a car or a bus driving non-stop for more than one hour	
5. Lying down in the afternoon when permitted by the situation	
6. Sitting in a train and speaking with somebody	
7. Sitting in silence after a lunch without alcohol	
8. In a car standing for some minutes at a red traffic light or in a traffic jam	
Total	Out of 24

[*] 0, never; 1, weak; 2, medium; 3, strong.

Adapted from [55].

male sex and compromised quality of nighttime sleep [57]. Meindorfer et al. [58] searched for predictors of car accidents and detected previously reported SOS at the wheel as most risky, with odds ratios of 3.2 and 3.5 for involvement in and causation of car accidents, respectively.

Pharmacological prevention of 'sleep attacks'

It would be particularly interesting to find out whether SOS in PD can be relieved by analeptic drugs, including caffeine. The role of the emerging adenosine A2A receptor antagonists may provide a means to treat medication-induced SOS. Istradefylline was recently approved as an adjunct therapy in PD in Japan, but it has not yet been approved by the US Food and Drug Administration or the European Medicines Agency. Three Phase III clinical trials assessing preladenant in early and moderate to severe PD were recently halted due to lack of efficacy. To date, there is an amazing lack of data concerning caffeine. Indeed, with respect to motor symptoms it has been tested in only a few pilot trials. To our knowledge, no epidemiological studies on SOS or EDS and no marketing approval studies of A2A receptor antagonists have assessed caffeine consumption as a covariate or mentioned it as an inclusion/exclusion criterion. In 2012, however, a randomized, placebo-controlled trial studied the impact of up to 200 mg of caffeine twice daily for 6 weeks in PD-associated EDS and reported no significant benefit on EDS [61].

Modafinil failed to improve EDS in PD [62] or showed only limited benefit [63,64]. Amantadine was ineffective according to retrospective data [32]. Reboxetine, although frequently used for depression in PD [65], has not specially been tested with respect to SOS. A Phase III trial dedicated to PD-associated EDS assessing the histamine-H_3 inverse agonist pitolisant was recently completed [66].

Practical guidelines

Current guidelines recommend that patients should be given information about the sedative effect of levodopa and DA agonists and the risk of unpredictable sleep attacks prior to the initiation of a new drug and prior to each dose increase. Patients reporting somnolence or SOS should be prohibited from driving [13,67]. If SOS is reported after introduction of a new DA agonist, the drug may be switched or the dose reduced. Furthermore, discontinuation of other psychotropic drugs like benzodiazepines or antidepressants may be considered. Polysomnography may be considered for the exclusion of co-morbidity with other sleep disorders.

In conclusion, patients should be warned about unintended sleep episodes prior to initiation, change and increase of dopamimetics. Patients who have experienced unintended sleep episodes at the wheel or who suffer from daytime sleepiness should be prohibited from driving. Revision of sedative co-medication may be useful and current psychostimulants are mostly ineffective.

References

1 Sternbach H. The serotonin syndrome. Am J Psychiatry 1991; **148**: 705–13.

2 Newman-Tancredi A, Cussac D, Quentric Y, et al. Differential actions of antiparkinson agents at multiple classes of monoaminergic receptor. III. Agonist and antagonist properties at serotonin, 5-HT(1) and 5-HT(2), receptor subtypes. J Pharmacol Exp Ther 2002; **303**: 815–22.

3 Millan MJ, Maiofiss L, Cussac D, et al. Differential actions of antiparkinson agents at multiple classes of monoaminergic receptor. I. A multivariate analysis of the binding profiles of 14 drugs at 21 native and cloned human receptor subtypes. J Pharmacol Exp Ther 2002; **303**: 791–804.

4 Gustafsen J, Lendorf A, Raskov H, Boesby S. Ketanserin versus placebo in carcinoid syndrome. A clinical controlled trial. Scand J Gastroenterol 1986; **21**: 816–18.

5 Schade R, Andersohn F, Suissa S, et al. Dopamine agonists and the risk of cardiac-valve regurgitation. N Engl J Med 2007; **356**: 29–38.

6 Zanettini R, Antonini A, Gatto G, et al. Valvular heart disease and the use of dopamine agonists for Parkinson's disease. N Engl J Med 2007; **356**: 39–46.

7 Hofmann C, Penner U, Dorow R, et al. Lisuride, a dopamine receptor agonist with 5-HT$_{2B}$ receptor antagonist properties: absence of cardiac valvulopathy adverse drug reaction reports supports the concept of a crucial role for 5-HT$_{2B}$ receptor agonism in cardiac valvular fibrosis. Clin Neuropharmacol 2006; **29**: 80–6.

8 Jahnichen S, Horowski R, Pertz HH. Agonism at 5-HT$_{2B}$ receptors is not a class effect of the ergolines. Eur J Pharmacol 2005; **513**: 225–8.

9 Horowski R, Jahnichen S, Pertz HH. Fibrotic valvular heart disease is not related to chemical class but to biological function: 5-HT2B receptor activation plays crucial role. Mov Disord 2004; **19**: 1523–4.

10 Silberstein SD. Methysergide. Cephalalgia 1998; **18**: 421–35.

11 Hanley NR, Hensler JG. Mechanisms of ligand-induced desensitization of the 5-hydroxytryptamine(2A) receptor. J Pharmacol Exp Ther 2002; **300**: 468–77.

12 Chaudhuri RD. Valvular heart disease and fibrotic reactions may be related to ergot dopamine agonists, but non-ergot agonists may also not be spared. Mov Disord 2004; **19**: 1522–5.

13 Eggert K, Oertel WH, Reichmann H, et al. Parkinson-Syndrome—Diagnostik und Therapie. In: H-C Diener (ed.) Leitlinien für Diagnostik und Therapie in der Neurologie, 5th edn, pp. 124–62. Stuttgart: Thieme, 2012.

14 **Volpe-Gillot L, Creange A, Degos JD**. Subjective blockage in Parkinson's disease. Rev Neurol (Paris) 2002; **158**: 185–93.

15 **Stacy M, Bowron A, Guttman M, et al**. Identification of motor and nonmotor wearing-off in Parkinson's disease: comparison of a patient questionnaire versus a clinician assessment. Mov Disord 2005; **20**: 726–33.

16 **Stacy M, Hauser R, Oertel W, et al**. End-of-dose wearing off in Parkinson disease: a 9-question survey assessment. Clin Neuropharmacol 2006; **29**: 312–21.

17 **Dubiel A**. Deep within the brain. Munich: Kunstmann, 2006.

18 **Harnois C, Di Paolo T**. Decreased dopamine in the retinas of patients with Parkinson's disease. Invest Ophthalmol Vis Sci 1990; **31**: 2473–5.

19 **Peppe A, Stanzione P, Pierantozzi M, et al**. Does pattern electroretinogram spatial tuning alteration in Parkinson's disease depend on motor disturbances or retinal dopaminergic loss? Electroencephalogr Clin Neurophysiol 1998; **106**: 374–82.

20 **Wink B, Harris J**. A model of the Parkinsonian visual system: support for the dark adaptation hypothesis. Vision Res 2000; **40**: 1937–46.

21 **Strawn JR, Keck PE Jr, Caroff SN**. Neuroleptic malignant syndrome. Am J Psychiatry 2007; **164**: 870–6.

22 **Stubner S, Rustenbeck E, Grohmann R, et al**. Severe and uncommon involuntary movement disorders due to psychotropic drugs. Pharmacopsychiatry 2004; **37**(Suppl 1): S54–S64.

23 **Corallo CE, Ernest D**. Atypical neuroleptic malignant syndrome with long-term clozapine. Crit Care Resusc 2007; **9**: 338–40.

24 **Paparrigopoulos T, Tzavellas E, Ferentinos P, et al**. Catatonia as a risk factor for the development of neuroleptic malignant syndrome: report of a case following treatment with clozapine. World J Biol Psychiatry 2009: **10**: 70–3.

25 **Gambassi G, Capurso S, Tarsitani P, et al**. Fatal neuroleptic malignant syndrome in a previously long-term user of clozapine following its reintroduction in combination with paroxetine. Aging Clin Exp Res 2006; **18**: 266–70.

26 **Kobayashi A, Kawanishi C, Matsumura T, et al**. Quetiapine-induced neuroleptic malignant syndrome in dementia with Lewy bodies: a case report. Prog Neuropsychopharmacol Biol Psychiatry 2006; **30**: 1170–2.

27 **Reulbach U, Dutsch C, Biermann T, et al**. Managing an effective treatment for neuroleptic malignant syndrome. Crit Care 2007; **11**: R4.

28 **Woodbury MM, Woodbury MA**. Neuroleptic-induced catatonia as a stage in the progression toward neuroleptic malignant syndrome. J Am Acad Child Adolesc Psychiatry 1992; **31**: 1161–4.

29 **Lowe CM, Grube RR, Scates AC**. Characterization and clinical management of clozapine-induced fever. Ann Pharmacother 2007; **41**: 1700–4.

30 **Frucht S, Rogers JD, Greene PE, et al**. Falling asleep at the wheel: motor vehicle mishaps in persons taking pramipexole and ropinirole. Neurology 1999; **52**: 1908–10.

31 **Lesser RP, Fahn S, Snider SR, et al**. Analysis of the clinical problems in parkinsonism and the complications of long-term levodopa therapy. Neurology 1979; **29**: 1253–60.

32 **Paus S, Brecht HM, Koster J, et al**. Sleep attacks, daytime sleepiness, and dopamine agonists in Parkinson's disease. Mov Disord 2003; **18**: 659–67.

33 **Möller JC**. Tagesschläfrigkeit bei Parkinsonpatienen. Unpublished PhD thesis, Marburg University, 2005.

34 **Ferreira JJ, Desboeuf K, Galitzky M, et al**. Sleep disruption, daytime somnolence and 'sleep attacks' in Parkinson's disease: a clinical survey in PD patients and age-matched healthy volunteers. Eur J Neurol 2006; **13**: 209–14.

35 **Montastruc JL, Brefel-Courbon C, Senard JM, et al**. Sleep attacks and antiparkinsonian drugs: a pilot prospective pharmacoepidemiologic study. Clin Neuropharmacol 2001; **24**: 181–3.

36 **Hobson DE, Lang AE, Martin WR, et al.** Excessive daytime sleepiness and sudden-onset sleep in Parkinson disease: a survey by the Canadian Movement Disorders Group. J Am Med Assoc 2002; **287**: 455–63.

37 **Stover N, Okun M, Watts R.** 'Sleep attacks' and excessive daytime sleepiness in Parkinson's disease: a survey of 200 consecutive patients. Neurology 2001; **56**(Suppl 3): P03.140.

38 **Brodsky MA, Godbold J, Roth T, Olanow CW.** Sleepiness in Parkinson's disease: a controlled study. Mov Disord 2003; **18**: 668–72.

39 **Tan EK, Lum SY, Fook-Chong SM, et al.** Evaluation of somnolence in Parkinson's disease: comparison with age- and sex-matched controls. Neurology 2002; **58**: 465–8.

40 **Körner Y, Meindorfner C, Möller JC, et al.** Predictors of sudden onset of sleep in Parkinson's disease. Mov Disord 2004; **19**: 1298–305.

41 **Gjerstad MD, Aarsland D, Larsen JP.** Development of daytime somnolence over time in Parkinson's disease. Neurology 2002; **58**: 1544–6.

42 **Gjerstad MD, Alves G, Wentzel-Larsen T, et al.** Excessive daytime sleepiness in Parkinson disease: is it the drugs or the disease? Neurology 2006; **67**: 853–8.

43 **Andreu N, Chale JJ, Senard JM, et al.** L-dopa-induced sedation: a double-blind cross-over controlled study versus triazolam and placebo in healthy volunteers. Clin Neuropharmacol 1999; **22**: 15–23.

44 **Lu J, Jhou TC, Saper CB.** Identification of wake-active dopaminergic neurons in the ventral periaqueductal gray matter. J Neurosci 2006; **26**: 193–202.

45 **Monti JM, Hawkins M, Jantos H, et al.** Biphasic effects of dopamine D-2 receptor agonists on sleep and wakefulness in the rat. Psychopharmacology (Berl) 1988; **95**: 395–400.

46 **Braak H, Ghebremedhin E, Rub U, et al.** Stages in the development of Parkinson's disease-related pathology. Cell Tissue Res 2004; **318**: 121–34.

47 **Moruzzi G, Magoun HW.** Brain stem reticular formation and activation of the EEG. Electroencephalogr Clin Neurophysiol 1949; **1**: 455–73.

48 **Balcita-Pedicino JJ, Sesack SR.** Orexin axons in the rat ventral tegmental area synapse infrequently onto dopamine and gamma-aminobutyric acid neurons. J Comp Neurol 2007; **503**: 668–84.

49 **Rissling I, Körner Y, Geller F, et al.** Preprohypocretin polymorphisms in Parkinson disease patients reporting 'sleep attacks'. Sleep 2005; **28**: 871–5.

50 **Rissling I, Geller F, Bandmann O, et al.** Dopamine receptor gene polymorphisms in Parkinson's disease patients reporting 'sleep attacks'. Mov Disord 2004; **19**: 1279–84.

51 **Chaudhuri KR.** Nocturnal symptom complex in PD and its management. Neurology 2003; **61**: S17–S23.

52 **Razmy A, Lang AE, Shapiro CM.** Predictors of impaired daytime sleep and wakefulness in patients with Parkinson disease treated with older (ergot) vs newer (nonergot) dopamine agonists. Arch Neurol 2004; **61**: 97–102.

53 **Möller JC, Unger MM, Stiasny-Kolster K, et al.** Continuous sleep EEG monitoring in PD patients with and without sleep attacks. Parkinsonism Relat Disord 2009; **15**: 238–41.

54 **Möller JC, Stiasny K, Hargutt V, et al.** Evaluation of sleep and driving performance in six patients with Parkinson's disease reporting sudden onset of sleep under dopaminergic medication: a pilot study. Mov Disord 2002; **17**: 474–81.

55 **Johns MW.** A new method for measuring daytime sleepiness: the Epworth sleepiness scale. Sleep 1991; **14**: 540–5.

56 **Möller JC, Rethfeldt M, Körner Y, et al.** Daytime sleep latency in medication-matched Parkinsonian patients with and without sudden onset of sleep. Mov Disord 2005; **20**: 1620–2.

57 **Körner Y, Meindorfner C, Möller JC, et al.** Predictors of sudden onset of sleep in Parkinson's disease. Mov Disord 2004; **19**: 1298–305.

58 **Meindorfner C, Körner Y, Möller JC, et al**. Driving in Parkinson's disease: mobility, accidents, and sudden onset of sleep at the wheel. Mov Disord 2005; **20**: 832–42.

59 **Fronczek R, Overeem S, Lee SY, et al**. Hypocretin (orexin) loss in Parkinson's disease. Brain 2007; **130**:1577–85

60 **Thannickal TC, Lai YY, Siegel JM**. Hypocretin (orexin) cell loss in Parkinson's disease. Brain 2007; **130**:1586–95.

61 **Postuma RB, Lang AE, Munhoz RP, et al**. Caffeine for treatment of Parkinson disease. Neurology 2012; **79**: 651–8.

62 **Ondo WG, Fayle R, Atassi F, Jankovic J**. Modafinil for daytime somnolence in Parkinson's disease: double blind, placebo controlled parallel trial. J Neurol Neurosurg Psychiatry 2005; **76**: 1636–9.

63 **Adler CH, Caviness JN, Hentz JG, et al**. Randomized trial of modafinil for treating subjective daytime sleepiness in patients with Parkinson's disease. Mov Disord 2003; **18**: 287–93.

64 **Högl B, Saletu M, Brandauer E, et al**. Modafinil for the treatment of daytime sleepiness in Parkinson's disease: a double-blind, randomized, crossover, placebo-controlled polygraphic trial. Sleep 2002; **25**: 905–9.

65 **Pintor L, Bailles E, Valldeoriola F, et al**. Response to 4-month treatment with reboxetine in Parkinson's disease patients with a major depressive episode. Gen Hosp Psychiatry 2006; **28**: 59–64.

66 **Efficacy and safety of BF2.649** in excessive daytime sleepiness in Parkinson's disease (HARPS2). Available at: http://www.clinicaltrials.gov/ct2/show/NCT01066442 (accessed 18 March 2014).

67 **EMEA CPMP**. Position statement: dopaminergic substances and sudden sleep onset. In: CPMP578/02: evaluation of medicines for human use. London: European Agency for Evaluation of Medicinal Products, 2002.

Chapter 30

Thermoregulatory dysfunction in Parkinson's disease

Giovanni Mostile and Joseph Jankovic

Physiology of thermoregulation

An overview of the thermoregulatory system

In humans, as in all mammals, the core body temperature (T_c) is maintained within a narrow range by physiological homeostatic feedback mechanisms that are driven by the autonomic and endocrine systems [1]. After the initial vasomotor tone adjustment, sweating and shivering responses are activated at different thresholds for the determination of heat loss (HL) and heat production (HP) in response to variations in ambient temperature. Both HL and HP are reciprocally inhibited by a system involving inputs from peripheral cold sensors located in the skin and oral/urogenital mucosa as well as central warm sensors located in the preoptic anterior (regulating HL) and posterior (regulating HP) hypothalamus [2]. These responses are also modulated by non-thermal factors which principally act on system output pathways, such plasma osmolarity (dehydration reduces the sweating response and then HL) or blood glucose (hypoglycaemia reduces the shivering response and then HP) [3].

The architecture of the thermoregulatory circuitry includes peripheral thermosensors and afferent pathways that mediate signals to the central thermosensors and control mechanisms with output to the efferent pathways and effectors (see Fig. 30.1) [2]. Central thermosensors are principally warm-sensitive; in endothermic animals the central location of warm sensors may in fact prevent core overheating. Warm-sensitive neurons are principally located in the preoptic anterior hypothalamus and they are considered pacemakers as they display spontaneous membrane depolarization [2]. Peripheral thermosensory neurons, located in the skin and mucosa, are instead primarily cold-sensitive. They quickly respond to temperature changes adapting to a stable temperature. Transient receptor potential (TRP) ion channels, known as thermo-TRP channels (the heat-activated TRPV1-V4, M2, M4, and M5 and the cold-activated TRPM8 and A1), play a key role in thermosensation. Changes in T_c activate the autonomic homeostatic response by the spino-reticulo-hypothalamic pathway. Central integration of thermal signals involves the inhibitory control of the hypothalamic medial preoptic area on the dorsomedial hypothalamus projecting GABA and serotonergic output to the medullary rostral raphe pallidus [1,2].

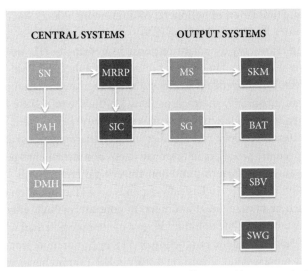

Fig. 30.1 The autonomic system regulating centres and effectors of homeostasis. Key: SN, suprachiasmatic nucleus; PAH, preoptic anterior hypothalamus; DMH, dorsomedial hypothalamus; MRRP, medullary rostral raphe pallidus; SIC, spinal cord intermediolateral column; MS, α/γ motor neuron system; SKM, skeletal muscle; SG, sympathetic ganglia; BAT, brown adipose tissue; SBV, skin blood vessel; SWG, sweat gland.

In addition, the suprachiasmatic nucleus modulates the hypothalamic preoptic area in a circadian manner, thus generating a T_c rhythm that is involved in the regulation of the circadian sleep–wake cycle. During sleep, distal vasodilatation and thus skin temperature increases whereas T_c declines [4].

The effectors of thermoregulation include blood vessels in the skin, sweat glands, skeletal muscles and brown adipose tissue (BAT). Skin vasculature, sweat glands and BAT are controlled by sympathetic thoracolumbar paravertebral ganglia. Skeletal muscles involved in shivering are modulated by the α/γ motor neurons [2,5]. The shivering phenomenon represents a remarkable thermogenic response in homeothermic animals. It is characterized by generalized, rapid, repeated skeletal muscle contractions leading to HP. Proximal muscles are principally involved during cold shivering [6,7]. Two electromyographic patterns associated with the recruitment of specific motor units have been identified during shivering: (1) a continuous, low-intensity shivering at 4–8 Hz due to slow-oxidative, fatigue-resistant type I muscle fibre recruitment and (2) bursts of high-intensity shivering at much lower frequencies (0.1–0.2 Hz) due to fast-glycolytic, fatigable type II muscle fibre recruitment [8]. Lipid and carbohydrate oxidation involved in shivering-induced HP may depend on type II muscle fibre recruitment [8]. The α/γ motor neuron circuit involved in the shivering phenomenon is centrally regulated by descending excitatory signalling through the dorsomedial hypothalamus and the rostral raphe pallidus nucleus. Warm-sensitive neurons in the preoptic anterior hypothalamus exert a tonic inhibitory control on the entire system. Stimulation of peripheral cold receptors reduces such tonic inhibition on central regulators, leading to shivering [2,9].

While sweating represents the major response in humans to HL, shivering as well as the non-shivering thermoregulatory response by BAT regulate HP. Cold-activated neural outflows are driven by independent neural pathways regulated by distinct preoptic neurons with different intrinsic T_c thermosensitivity [2,10]. The total daily HP, estimated as 'total energy expenditure', is determined by the obligatory thermogenetic processes necessary for life (the basal metabolic rate and diet-induced thermogenesis) and facultative or activated thermogenetic processes in response to environmental changes, which include physical activity as well as shivering and non-shivering thermogenesis [1]. Based on the law of conservation of energy, HP basically depends on ATP production by metabolically active tissues such as muscle, heart and liver. In contrast, in BAT, energy generated in mitochondria from oxygen consumption drives a membrane potential which is primarily dissipated via HP rather than the production of ATP by β_3-adrenoceptor stimulation.

Hormones also represent key regulating factors in HP. Thyroid hormone acts as a major regulator, increasing appetite and stimulating cardiovascular function, lipolysis and gluconeogenesis. It maximizes the autonomic adrenergic output in facultative thermogenetic processes. The responsiveness of BAT to sympathetic stimuli depends on the amount of active thyroid hormone, T_3, which is regulated by the type II iodothyronine 5'-deiodinase enzyme [11]. Thyroid hormone acts at different level in BAT, modulating the expression of β-adrenoreceptors as well as the catecholamine post-receptor signalling pathways [11]. Other regulators include insulin and leptin which increase HP and reduce food intake [1,2,11].

The goal in normal and disease states is to achieve 'thermal comfort' or *alliesthesia*, which refers to satisfaction of the entire body with the surrounding environment produced by an ambient thermic stimulus depending on internal thermal status. Discriminative temperature sensation from peripheral thermosensors involves: (1) the spinal-thalamic-cortical pathway chiefly mediated by the brainstem parabrachial nucleus and (2) extra-hypothalamic neural thermosensation centres including the insular, somatosensory and orbitofrontal cortex as well as the amygdala, which regulates the behavioural thermoregulatory responses [2,12]. At rest and during exercise, skin temperature represents the primary thermal input directing the thermobehavioural response, which is initiated by changes in the subjective indices of thermal comfort [13]. Tools like the contact heat-evoked potential, which is obtained by contact heat stimulation of the volar forearm and the dorsum of the hand at high temperature, can be helpful in evaluating central processing of sensory inputs [14].

Mechanisms of eccrine sweating

Sweating is primarily controlled by T_c and secondarily modulated by the mean skin temperature. Intermediolateral cell columns of the spinal cord receive thalamo-spinal input via axons which exit in the ventral roots and white rami to synapse in the paravertebral ganglia. Post-ganglionic non-myelinated C-fibres pass through the grey ramus communicans, combine with peripheral nerves and innervate the eccrine sweat glands. Nerve fibres synapse on eccrine sweat glands via M_3 muscarinic receptors and mediate the sudomotor response. Once muscarinic receptors are activated, intracellular Ca^{2+} concentrations increase followed by the permeability of K^+ and Cl^- channels, initiating the release of an isotonic precursor fluid from the eccrine gland cells to the duct. As the fluid travels up the duct toward the surface of the skin, Na^+ is reabsorbed depending on the sweat rate [15,16]. Sweating can also be initiated by an axon reflex by cholinergic agents that bind to the nicotinic receptors on sudomotor nerve terminals [16,17].

Sweating is influenced by various thermal factors as well as non-thermal ones. The sweat rate increases during exercise, in part by increased cortical outputs to the thalamo-spinal pathway as well as by peripheral stimulation of (1) type III mechanoreceptor fibres, that are principally sensitive to mechanical stimuli and (2) type IV metaboreceptor fibres, that are principally sensitive to ischaemic metabolites generated during exercise. Both are located within skeletal muscle [18]. In contrast, hypovolaemia due to dehydration can reduce sweating [16].

Sudomotor function may be quantified by autonomic tests. These include: thermoregulatory sweat testing (TST), the quantitative sudomotor axon reflex test (QSART), silicone impressions and quantitative direct and indirect axon reflex testing (QDIRT) [17] (a description of available tests is summarized in Table 30.1). Except for the TST, the other tests specifically explore post-ganglionic sudomotor function. A relatively specific sudomotor test is the sympathetic skin response (SSR), a direct measure of electrodermal activity which provides an indirect index of sympathetic cholinergic sudomotor function [17]. It is evoked preferably in the palm or sole using different stimuli such as inspiratory gasp, cough, a loud noise or an electric shock delivered at a peripheral nerve (usually the median nerve) opposite to the site of recording. An adequate minimal interstimulus interval should be used to avoid habituation. Once obtained, a biphasic response is often displayed with the negative component generated by the sweat gland [19]. SSR is a somato-sympathetic reflex with spinal-bulbar-suprabulbar components. Thalamo-limbic circuits involved in alertness and habituation are implicated in the control of 'emotional' or 'mental' sweating that can be quantified by the SSR. During sleep, the frequency of spontaneous SSR increases during non-rapid eye movement (REM) sleep and decreases during REM sleep [19]. Quantification of intra-epidermal and sweat gland nerve fibre density in skin biopsies provides a structural measure of small fibre cutaneous innervation complementing the investigation of small fibre neuropathies [20,21].

Clinical conditions associated with thermoregulatory dysfunction

Systemic and neurological causes of body temperature dysregulation, dysthermesthesia and dyshidrosis

Clinical conditions associated with thermoregulatory dysfunction involve pathological mechanisms which act at different levels (central or peripheral) and with different modalities (rising or decreasing T_c).

Table 30.1 Tests of sudomotor function

Test	Procedure	Evaluation targets	Quantification	Limits
Thermoregulatory sweat testing (TST)	T_c is raised and a maximal sweat response recruited by placing the subject in a heated environment. A change in colour of the indicator dye marks the site of sweat production	Pre- and post-ganglionic	Percentage of anhidrotic areas	Not routinely performed
Quantitative sudomotor axon reflex test (QSART)	Sweat glands are stimulated by iontophoresis of a cholinergic agent and sweat production is measured as an increase of humidity through a hygrometer	Post-ganglionic	Sweat output and latency	Unable to test pre-ganglionic sites
Silicone impressions	Sweat glands are stimulated by iontophoresis of acetylcholine, pilocarpine or methacholine, followed by application of a layer of moldable material on the skin	Post-ganglionic	Droplet number, size and distribution	Prone to artefacts
Quantitative direct and indirect axon reflex testing (QDIRT)	Sweat glands are stimulated by acetylcholine iontophoresis and sweat is displayed via an indicator dye followed by digital photographs over time	Post-ganglionic	Droplet number, size and distribution + response latency	High results variability
Sympathetic skin response (SSR)	Perturbation of the autonomic nervous system, through rapid inspiration or electrical stimulation, induces a change in skin potential	Pre- and post-ganglionic	Presence, amplitude and latency	High results variability

Fever is defined as an increase in T_c above the normal range of 36.5–37.5°C occurring because of an increase in the thermoregulatory set point generated by infection and inflammation. While fever is mediated by an acute phase response triggered by pyrogenic cytokines that engage physiological thermoregulation mechanisms, in *hyperthermia* the thermoregulatory control mechanisms are impaired, disabled or overwhelmed [22].

Common heat-related illnesses are the *classic slow-progressive heatstroke* (with temperatures reaching up to 44°C) due to environmental heat exposure, principally affecting the elderly, or the *exertional rapid-progressive heatstroke* affecting young active people. Tachycardia, tachypnea and normotension together with hot, dry skin and changes in mental status are key additional clinical signs. In *heat exhaustion*, which is more common and less severe than heatstroke, T_c usually ranges between 37 and 40°C. Symptoms are often non-specific and include dizziness, thirst, weakness, headache and malaise, but there is usually no change in mental status. Commonly used medications like α-adrenergics, anticholinergics, β-blockers, diuretics, laxatives or thyroid agonists may contribute to heatstroke and heat exhaustion [23]. Both *neuroleptic malignant syndrome* (NMS) and *serotonin syndrome* (SS) are manifested by changes in mental state, neurological signs, autonomic dysfunction and hyperthermia. NMS is due to exposure to antipsychotics and other D_2 receptor-blocking drugs [24]. Drug dose and potency, history of NMS and concomitant medications (such as lithium) represent potential risk factors [25]. SS is often triggered by polypharmacy which may include the combination of a selective serotonin reuptake inhibitor and a monoamine oxidase inhibitor [25]. There are clinical characteristics which may help to differentiate NMS from SS based on the available sets of diagnostic criteria for SS and the DSM-IV-TR criteria for NMS [25]. While rigidity is more frequent in NMS, myoclonus as well as tremor and ataxia are prominent in SS. Furthermore, in NMS symptoms usually begin later than in SS and the prognosis is less favourable, particularly if there is associated rhabdomyolysis with marked increase in creatine kinase and white blood cell count. Serum iron levels are typically low in NMS and gastrointestinal symptoms are more common in SS [25]. Other conditions associated with hyperthermia are *malignant hyperthermia*, another cause of rhabdomyolysis triggered by exposure to volatile anaesthetics and neuromuscular blocking agents, or specific therapeutic modalities such as hyperthermic intraperitoneal chemotherapy, hyperthermic isolated limb perfusion, pelvic and whole-body hyperthermia and radioablation [26].

The inverse of hyperthermia is hypothermia (also referred to as *anapyrexia* or *cryexia*) [27]. In hypothermia, T_c typically drops below 35°C as a complication of serious systemic disorders affecting central thermoregulation. In sepsis syndrome and septic shock, hypothermia is correlated with a high frequency of central nervous system dysfunction and even death [28]. On the other hand, hypothermia has been proposed as protective tool against ischaemia [29,30]. In different neurological conditions, hypothermia may manifest episodically and intermittently [31], leading to clinically detectable fluctuations in body temperature. Hypothermia may occur in injury, trauma, hypoxia, lipopolysaccharide-induced shock, heatstroke, ethanol intoxication, anaesthesia, starvation and other conditions [27]. Patients with multiple sclerosis may present acute relapses associated with hypothermia by direct involvement of the hypothalamus or from combined lesions affecting hypothalamic outflow to the brainstem and spinal cord [32,33]. Intermittent, episodic hypothermia has been also reported in patients with limbic encephalitis associated with N-methyl-D-aspartate receptor or voltage-gated potassium channel antibodies [34,35]. A rare hypothermic condition is Shapiro syndrome, manifested by a triad of hypothermia, hyperhidrosis and congenital agenesis of the corpus callosum [36,37]. Alcohol, which may induce hypothermia during the waking day, may increase T_c during the night, thus affecting the normal circadian temperature rhythm in alcoholic patients [38].

Discriminative temperature sensation may be altered if the spinal-thalamic-cortical pathway is affected. Excluding morphological lesions as well as neuropathy as causes of dysthermesthesia, impaired thermal perception due to altered central somatosensory processing has been reported in patients with multiple sclerosis [33], cluster headaches

[39], Parkinson's disease (PD) (see the section 'Thermoregulatory dysfunction in Parkinson's disease') [40], idiopathic restless legs syndrome [41] and motor neuron disease [42]. Although not fully investigated, dysthermesthesia may possibly occur in idiopathic focal dystonia, in which a loss of distinct sensory function of the affected hand in comparison with the contralateral hand and with matched healthy subjects has been observed [14,40]. After sympathectomy, a non-specific thermal sensation of incipient or ongoing sweating in the absence of actual sweating (so-called 'phantom sweating') may also occur [43].

Dyshidrosis can be characterzsed based on sweat production (hyper-, hypo- or anhidrosis) and localization (localized or generalized dyshidrosis). It is often related to concomitant systemic illnesses, such us generalized hyperhidrosis due to cardiological conditions, septic fever, neoplastic disease (Hodgkin's lymphoma), endocrinological disorders (diabetes mellitus, thyrotoxicosis, phaeochromocytoma) or psychiatric disorders (generalized anxiety) [44]. Dermatological conditions are instead frequent causes of localized dyshidrosis [44]. Neurological conditions may also represent specific causes of dyshidrosis, and they are summarized in Table 30.2.

Thermoregulatory dysfunction in Parkinson's disease

Pathophysiological mechanisms of thermodysregulation

Dysautonomia is frequent in patients with PD, especially in advanced stages of the disease when it may become a major therapeutic challenge [45]. Several components of the autonomic nervous system (enteric, parasympathetic cholinergic, sympathetic cholinergic, sympathetic noradrenergic and adrenomedullary hormonal) may be implicated, producing cardiovascular, sweating, bowel, urinary and sexual dysfunctions. Dysautonomia in the setting of parkinsonism should raise the possibility of not only PD but other conditions such as multiple system atrophy (MSA), dementia with Lewy bodies and other synucleinopathies, with peculiar differences in the severity of autonomic failure [46].

Patients with PD can be affected by dysregulation of body temperature, dysthermesthesia and dyshidrosis depending on differential involvement of T_c-regulating systems. Thermoregulatory dysfunction in PD gradually worsen with time as the disease progresses [47–49]. Co-morbidities, such as dehydration with hypovolaemia and infection, should be screened in patients with PD to correctly identify and treat possible secondary causes [45]. Once secondary causes are excluded primary thermoregulatory dysfunction associated with PD can be considered as a pathogenic mechanism for the abnormalities in body temperature. Dopamine, which plays a critical role in mediating PD-related motor symptoms, is also implicated in central thermoregulation. Activation of dopamine receptors in the hypothalamic preoptic area increases HL (reducing T_c), an action which is blocked by dopamine antagonists [22,50,51]. In animal models as well as in humans, dopamine agonists such as apomorphine or bromocriptine have been shown to exert a hypothermic effect which is principally mediated by activation of D_2 receptors [52,53]. Injection of sulpiride, a dopamine receptor antagonist, into the lateral hypothalamus in rats increased intracranial temperature and locally applied dopamine attenuated this sulpiride-induced

Table 30.2 Neurological causes of dyshidrosis

Hyperhidrosis	
Localized neurological causes	Processes affecting sympathetic innervation Frey's syndrome Harlequin syndrome and sign[a] Causalgia POEMS syndrome Stiff-man syndrome[b]
Generalized neurological causes	Brain lesions Spinal cord injuries Peripheral neuropathies HSAN Type III (Riley–Day syndrome)[c] Congenital autonomic dysfunction with universal pain loss Sympathectomy[d] Limbic encephalitis associated with voltage-gated potassium channel antibodies Hyperkinetic movement disorders (essential tremor, myoclonic dystonia) Hypokinetic movement disorders (Parkinson's disease, MSA, dementia with Lewy bodies)
Hypohidrosis and anhidrosis	
Localized neurological causes	Local denervation Ocular sympathetic deficit (Horner syndrome) Amyotrophic lateral sclerosis[e]
Generalized neurological causes	Fabry disease Neuropathy (diabetic, alcoholic, uremic) Guillain–Barré syndrome HSAN Type IV (congenital insensitivity to pain with anhidrosis)[c] Progressive segmental anhidrosis with Adie's tonic pupils (Ross syndrome) Pure autonomic failure Acquired idiopathic generalized anhidrosis (AIGA)[f]

POEMS, polyneuropathy, organomegaly, endocrinopathy, monoclonal gammopathy, and skin changes; HSAN, hereditary sensory and autonomic neuropathy; MSA, multisystem atrophy.

[a] Harlequin syndrome is the sudden onset of unilateral flushing and sweating in adults with apparently normal ocular sympathetic innervation. Harlequin sign is defined as excessive sweating and flushing contralateral to Horner syndrome [102].

[b] Hyperhidrosis in stiff-man syndrome has been described as multifocal [103].

[c] See [104].

[d] Sympathectomy is often associated with 'phantom sweating', a sensation of incipient or ongoing sweating in the absence of actual sweating [43].

[e] Although significant sudomotor hypofunction does not occur in amyotrophic lateral sclerosis, mild subclinical changes can be observed in weak limbs [105].

[f] Clinical features of AIGA are an acute or sudden onset of generalized anhidrosis with an onset early in life, the absence of other autonomic dysfunctions and a marked response to glucocorticoids. Concomitant sharp pain or cholinergic urticaria and elevated immunoglobulin E levels have also been described in the majority of patients. There are three subgroups of AIGA: idiopathic pure sudomotoric failure (IPSF), sudomotoric neuropathy and sweat gland failure [106].

hyperthermia [51,54]. Together with activation of central serotonin 5-HT$_{2A}$ receptors and central cholinergic M$_2$ receptor antagonism, the dopamine-mediated effect may be responsible for the increase in T_c in NMS as a complication of dopaminergic drug withdrawal in PD [22,55]. Furthermore, the endogenous opioid system may be also involved in thermal dysregulation, particularly in post-menopausal women with PD [56].

Dopaminergic striatal pathways have been shown to be implicated in the regulation of circadian rhythms in T_c [57]. Dysfunction of the central (pre-ganglionic) autonomic thermoregulatory system has been proposed in synucleinopathies [58]. For example, 48-hour monitoring of T_c revealed higher average values during both non-REM and REM sleep stages in patients with MSA compared with those with PD, thus providing evidence that the physiological nocturnal fall in T_c is blunted in MSA [59]. Besides synucleinopathies, circadian rhythmicity may also be altered in other forms of atypical parkinsonism such as progressive supranuclear palsy, in which the average value of T_c during sleep was found to be higher than in PD [60].

Involvement of the sympathetic mesencephalic–diencephalic system in the regulation of T_c in PD was suggested by observations in patients who underwent thalamotomy and developed ptosis, miosis and hemianhydrosis on the side of the body ipsilateral to the lesion [61]. Subsequently, PD patients treated with bilateral subthalamic nucleus deep brain stimulation (STN DBS) were found to have evidence of cutaneous sympathetic vasoconstriction and reduced HL [62]. Thus STN DBS may improve function of the central sympathetic autonomic system which is often impaired in PD. STN DBS has been shown to improve dyshidrosis by 66.7% [63] and to normalize thresholds for cold and warm sensation, which are typically increased in PD [64]. Rarely, hyperthermia may occur as a complication of DBS surgery for PD [65].

The caudal medial aspect of the STN and/or the caudal aspect of the ventral thalamus/ zona incerta have been implicated in the 'drenching sweats' in PD [66,67]. Drenching sweats are one of the most disabling non-motor symptoms of PD, although they do not seem to correlate with the severity of the disease. In one study, sweating dysfunction, hyperhidrosis and to a lesser extent hypohidrosis were reported by 64% of patients with PD as compared with 12.5% of controls [48]. In contrast to other non-motor symptoms, which are more frequent and more severe in the 'off' state, drenching sweats can occur in both 'on' and 'off' states in patients who experience motor fluctuations [68], although it is most frequently present during the 'off' periods and during 'on with dyskinesia' periods [49]. Because sudomotor skin response is reduced in the palms, the axial hyperhidrosis sometimes observed in patients with PD has been suggested to be compensatory phenomenon for reduced sympathetic function in the extremities [69]. The presence of α-synuclein deposits in the dermis of a patient with pure autonomic failure provides evidence that this disorder as well as other disorders associated with autonomic failure should be viewed as symptoms of synucleinopathies [70].

Dysthermesthesia could be included in the context of altered sensory processing in PD [40,71]. Pain sensitivity and spinal nociception are increased in untreated PD, as suggested by lower electrical and heat pain thresholds [72]. Chronic pain may lead to a reorganization of the somatosensory system at the thalamic level, reducing thermal sensation and enhancing pain [73]. The cortical–basal ganglia–thalamic circuit involved in motivation and emotional drive integrates motor, emotional, autonomic and cognitive responses to pain [71,74]. Studies demonstrating a decreased pain threshold in PD also provide evidence that abnormalities in thermal sensory perception reflect the involvement of spinal mechanisms [72]. Perception of heat pain in PD may be mediated by dopamine as well as other neurotransmitters. Levodopa could modulate the affective component of pain, as suggested by a cross-sectional study in which fluctuating PD patients reported a higher degree of unpleasantness in response to heat pain while on medication compared with the 'off' state [75]. Involvement of the non-dopaminergic system in the perception of pain has also been suggested by the observation that patients with progressive supra-nuclear palsy have a tendency towards higher heat pain thresholds compared with PD patients and a lower frequency of reported pain, possibly due to greater frontal lobe impairment in the former condition [76].

Clinical syndromes associated with body temperature dysregulation in PD

PD patients are at risk for developing hyperthermia as a result of heatstroke, NMS or acute akinesia. The vulnerability of PD patients to heatstroke may derive from several conditions, including motor disability or cognitive decline limiting actions normally used to avoid heat stress, concomitant use of drugs such as anticholinergic agents that affect HL or impaired sweating. PD-related heat stroke may be manifested by an altered level of consciousness, encephalopathy secondary to multiorgan failure, rhabdomyolysis and disseminated intravascular coagulopathy. The prognosis is variable because normalizing body temperature may not prevent this complication [77]. However, when diagnosed early and appropriately treated with cooling and hydration most patients recover fully.

NMS may be encountered not only in PD but also in atypical and secondary parkinsonism. NMS may be triggered by the abrupt reduction or withdrawal of antiparkinsonian drugs, particularly levodopa and dopamine agonists [55]. Elevation of T_c and an altered level of consciousness are the most common clinical features; other features include rigidity, autonomic dysfunction, elevated serum creatine kinase and leukocytosis. Although the majority of affected PD patients recover, in some cases, particularly the elderly, the course may be complicated by or associated with severe complications including pneumonia, disseminated intravascular coagulopathy and acute renal failure [51,78]. Treatment of NMS includes supportive therapy (intravenous fluid infusion and body cooling) and pharmacological therapy, including oral or intravenous levodopa, dopamine agonists and dantrolene sodium [55,78].

Acute akinesia is a rare syndrome with multiple etiologies which may include hyperthermia and NMS-like syndrome [79,80]. It is occasionally encountered as an acute motor complication of PD, particularly when there is coincident infection, or following surgery or other treatment manipulations [79]. Acute akinesia should be considered when there is sudden deterioration in parkinsonian symptoms that are refractory to dopaminergic therapy. Intensive treatment includes management of the underlying comorbidity, rehydration, reduction of hyperthermia and antithrombotic prophylaxis.

Life-threatening hypothermia is a very uncommon condition in PD. A few case reports available on literature have been summarized in Table 30.3, some associated with peculiar signs such as the electrocardiographic Osborn J wave, a positive deflection seen on the downsloping section of the QRS complex [81–83].

Dyshidrosis in PD

Sweating disturbances occur in 30 to 50% of patients with PD, and hyperhidrosis, manifested by excessive sweating affecting the axillae, palms, soles of the feet and face or even the entire body (so-called drenching sweats), is a common and distressing symptom of PD [45]. Although drenching sweats have been well recognized in PD, hypohidrosis may be

Table 30.3 Published cases of life-threatening hypothermia in Parkinson's disease

	Case 1	Case 2	Case 3	Case 4
Author(s)	Gubbay and Barwick [81]	Gubbay and Barwick [81]	Hama et al. [82]	Sehara [83]
Age (years)	73	61	58	80
Treatment for PD	Benzhexol and benztropine	Nortriptylene	Levodopa, cabergoline, quetiapine	Levodopa, pramipexole, selegiline
Neuropsychiatric comorbidities	Progressive dementia	Depression	Dementia	–
Onset	1 week	Weeks	Weeks	A few days
Level of consciousness	Stupor	Conscious, but mute	Stupor	Lethargy
T_c (°C)	32.8	35.9	33.1	29.7
Pulse rate (beats/minute)	100	70	45	38
Electrocardiography	Flat T waves, no J waves	Left ventricular hypertrophy	J waves	Sinus bradycardia, QT prolongation, J waves
Electroencephalography	Generalized repetitive and triphasic sharp complexes synchronous in all channels	Generalized repetitive and triphasic sharp complexes synchronous in all channels	–	–
Therapy	Gradual warming, hydrocortisone, penicillin	–	Warming and saline infusion	Warming
Recovery	Yes	Yes	Yes	Yes

a more common form of dyshidrosis [84]. The progressive involvement of sweat function in PD as the disease progresses may reflect the spread from the central nervous system or pre-ganglionic fibres to the peripheral post-ganglionic fibres [85]. Although there is growing evidence of progression of the neurodegenerative process mediated via seeding of misfolded proteins, including α-synuclein, from the periphery to the central nervous system, it is possible that the process may also occur in the reverse direction [86]. Dysfunction of the sympathetic post-ganglionic cholinergic system has been suggested by an abnormal sweat response, using SSR, to intradermal acetylcholine [87]. In contrast to MSA, which is characterized by more autonomic symptoms at baseline and progression to global anhidrosis, in PD patients anhidrosis, as measured by the TST, remains regional, often distal, which is typical of a length-dependent neuropathic pattern [88–90]. In a Mayo Clinic series of autopsy-confirmed MSA cases, the most common pattern was global anhidrosis on TST (45%), followed by regional (13.6%) and segmental (4.5%) anhidrosis [89]. While anhidrosis is often greater than 30% on TST in MSA patients, in PD subjects it is often less than 10% [88,90]. A cutoff of anhidrosis greater than 9% on TST derived from receiver operating characteristic analysis has shown high accuracy in differentiating MSA patients from PD patients, especially at later time points of the disease when autonomic dysfunction becomes more severe [90]. Anhidrosis detected by TST may represent a valid tool in differential diagnosis between PD and MSA, and it may be more specific than ^{123}I-metaiodobenzylguanidine myocardial scintigraphy [90]. Sympathetic post-ganglionic adrenergic and cholinergic systems may in fact be independently affected in PD with dysautonomia [91].

A defect in the neurovascular control of distal extremities has been highlighted in MSA patients, in whom the detection of the 'cold hand sign' represents a characteristic clinical feature [92]. However, the skin blood flow rate after local cooling may not be different in MSA versus PD [93]. The vasoconstrictive neural response may decrease with sympathetic sudomotor activity in PD subjects compared with controls [94].

Treatment of thermoregulatory dysfunction associated with PD

Treatment of thermoregulatory dysfunction in PD may require different approaches targeting central thermoregulatory systems and peripheral effectors (principally the cholinergic innervations of the eccrine sweat glands). T_c dysregulation in PD often requires an optimization of the dopaminergic pharmacological regimen once a secondary cause has been excluded. There is a paucity of evidence-based data to support a specific pharmacological intervention for primary dysfunction of the central thermoregulatory systems in PD. Dopaminergic drugs may counteract hyperthermia-induced fatigue, consequently allowing an improvement in thermal discomfort and exercise performance [95]. Bupropione has been shown to exert ergogenic and thermogenic central effects, acting on dopamine and noradrenaline central pathways [95]. Other possible therapeutic strategies may focus on therapeutic compounds that act as anorectic and thus thermogenic agents, including sibutramine (a selective serotonin and noradrenaline reuptake inhibitor), topiramate (a GABA-ergic agonist and glutamate antagonist) and rimonabant (an inverse agonist at the cannabinoid-1 receptor) [1]. Antagonists of the melanin-concentrating hormone, a hypothalamic neuropeptide, have also shown thermogenic effects [1].

Treatment of dyshidrosis is often quite challenging as there is no proven pharmacological therapy. Treatment efficacy for secretory disorders can be assessed quantitatively using techniques like gravimetric quantification of sweat production or Minor's iodine-starch test to detect colour changes at skin surfaces depending on sweat production, as well as subjectively by a health-related quality of life scale such as the Hyperhidrosis Disease Severity Scale (HDSS), a single-item four-point scale rating the tolerability of hyperhidrosis and its interference with daily activities [96,97]. Since dyshidrosis seems to be worse in PD patients with motor fluctuations, smoothing out the response to levodopa should be the first step in the management of this symptom. Conservative treatments for focal hyperhidrosis include topical application of aluminium chloride hexahydrate, anticholinergics (glycopyrrolate) and iontophoresis [45]. Botulinum neurotoxin (BoNT) has shown to be a safe and effective treatment for focal hyperhidrosis, including axillary, palmar and gustatory (facial) hyperhidrosis [97,98]. BoNT serotype A (BoNT-A) has been found to be effective for the treatment of axillary hyperhidrosis, with a Level A recommendation based on the American Academy of Neurology classification of evidence for therapeutic intervention [97]. It is usually well tolerated, with a mean duration of effect ranging between 3 and 9 months. Effective doses of BoNT-A are 50–100 U for onabotulinumtoxinA and incobotulinumtoxinA, 150–400 U for abobotulinumtoxinA and 2500–5000 U for rimabotulinumtoxinB. For palmar hyperhidrosis, there are three placebo-controlled and one comparative study available for BoNT-A and one comparative study for BoNT serotype B (BoNT-B). However, all these Class II studies are relative small with a short follow-up period. The evidence supports a Level B recommendation for BoNT-A and a Level C recommendation for BoNT-B [97].

Seborrhea, also frequently observed in patients with PD, seems to be more related to plasma androgen levels than abnormalities of the autonomic nervous system, although cholinergic innervation of the skin may play a role [45,99,100]. BoNT injections into the affected skin area may be useful, as it has been also found to be effective in acne [101].

Conclusion

Thermoregulation is critical for the normal homeostasis and survival of a living organism. The architecture of the thermoregulatory circuitry includes afferent pathways, central control nuclei and output systems with effectors. Dysregulation of thermal homeostasis can result from dysfunctions originating at each of these levels, leading to variations in central body temperature (hyperthermia or hypothermia), dysthermesthesia or dyshidrosis. Although there are many aetiological mechanisms for thermal dysregulation, in this chapter we have focused on neurological disorders, particularly PD, which is associated with autonomic dysfunction. Patients with PD are at risk for developing both hyperthermia and hypothermia. Dysthermesthesia can also be present, being ascribed to the documented altered sensory processing in PD. Sweating disturbances frequently occur in patients with PD, and are often manifested by focal or generalized excessive sweating. Comorbidities should be screened first in patients with PD to correctly identify and treat possible secondary causes of thermal dysfunction. While the mechanisms of thermoregulatory dysfunction in PD remain poorly understood, symptomatic treatments are available. BoNT represents a first demonstrated efficacious therapeutic option for dyshidrosis in PD.

References

1 **Clapham JC**. Central control of thermogenesis. Neuropharmacology 2012; **63**: 111–23.

2 **Romanovsky AA**. Thermoregulation: some concepts have changed. Functional architecture of the thermoregulatory system. Am J Physiol Regul Integr Comp Physiol 2007; **292**: R37–R46.

3 **Mekjavic IB, Eiken O**. Contribution of thermal and nonthermal factors to the regulation of body temperature in humans. J Appl Physiol 2006; **100**: 2065–72.

4 **Weinert D**. Circadian temperature variation and ageing. Ageing Res Rev 2010; **9**: 51–60.

5 **Jain S**. Multi-organ autonomic dysfunction in Parkinson disease. Parkinsonism Relat Disord 2011; **17**: 77–83.

6 **Bell DG, Tikuisis P, Jacobs I**. Relative intensity of muscular contraction during shivering. J Appl Physiol 1992; **72**: 2336–42.

7 **Meigal AY, Oksa J, Hohtola E, Lupandin YV, Rintamäki H**. Influence of cold shivering on fine motor control in the upper limb. Acta Physiol Scand 1998; **163**: 41–7.

8 **Haman F, Legault SR, Weber JM**. Fuel selection during intense shivering in humans: EMG pattern reflects carbohydrate oxidation. J Physiol 2004; **556**: 305–13.

9 **Nakamura K, Morrison SF**. Central efferent pathways for cold-defensive and febrile shivering. J Physiol 2011; **589**: 3641–58.

10 **McAllen RM, Tanaka M, Ootsuka Y, McKinley MJ**. Multiple thermoregulatory effectors with independent central controls. Eur J Appl Physiol 2010; **109**: 27–33.

11 **Silva JE**. Thermogenic mechanisms and their hormonal regulation. Physiol Rev 2006; **86**: 435–64.

12 **Flouris AD**. Functional architecture of behavioural thermoregulation. Eur J Appl Physiol 2011; **111**: 1–8.

13 **Schlader ZJ, Stannard SR, Mündel T**. Human thermoregulatory behavior during rest and exercise—a prospective review. Physiol Behav 2010; **99**: 269–75.

14 **Suttrup I, Oberdiek D, Suttrup J, Osada N, Evers S, Marziniak M**. Loss of sensory function in patients with idiopathic hand dystonia. Mov Disord 2011; **26**: 107–13.

15 **Shibasaki M, Wilson TE, Crandall CG**. Neural control and mechanisms of eccrine sweating during heat stress and exercise. J Appl Physiol 2006; **100**: 1692–701.

16 **Shibasaki M, Crandall CG**. Mechanisms and controllers of eccrine sweating in humans. Front Biosci (Schol Ed) 2011; **2**: 685–96.

17 **Illigens BM, Gibbons CH**. Sweat testing to evaluate autonomic function. Clin Auton Res 2009; **19**: 79–87.

18 **Kaufman MP, Hayes SG**. The exercise pressor reflex. Clin Auton Res 2002; **12**: 429–39.

19 **Vetrugno R, Liguori R, Cortelli P, Montagna P**. Sympathetic skin response. Basic mechanisms and clinical applications. Clin Auton Res 2003; **13**: 256–70.

20 **Gibbons CH, Illigens BM, Wang N, Freeman R**. Quantification of sweat gland innervation: a clinical-pathologic correlation. Neurology 2009; **72**: 1479–86.

21 **Gibbons CH, Illigens BM, Wang N, Freeman R**. Quantification of sudomotor innervation: a comparison of 3 methods. Muscle Nerve 2010; **42**: 112–19.

22 Gillman PK. Neuroleptic malignant syndrome: mechanisms, interactions, and causality. Mov Disord 2010; **25**: 1780–90.

23 Glazer JL. Management of heatstroke and heat exhaustion. Am Fam Physician 2005; **71**: 2133–42.

24 Waln O, Jankovic J. An update on tardive dyskinesia. From phenomenology to treatment. Tremor Other Hyperkinet Mov (NY) 2013; 3: http://tremorjournal.org/article/view/161

25 Perry PJ, Wilborn CA. Serotonin syndrome vs neuroleptic malignant syndrome: a contrast of causes, diagnoses and management. Ann Clin Psychiatry 2012; **24**: 155–62.

26 Burke S, Hanani M. The actions of hyperthermia on the autonomic nervous system: central and peripheral mechanisms and clinical implications. Auton Neurosci 2012; **168**: 4–13.

27 Romanovsky AA. Do fever and anapyrexia exist? Analysis of set point-based definitions. Am J Physiol Regul Integr Comp Physiol 2004; **287**: R992–R995.

28 Clemmer TP, Fisher CJ Jr, Bone RC, Slotman GJ, Metz CA, Thomas FO. Hypothermia in the sepsis syndrome and clinical outcome. The Methylprednisolone Severe Sepsis Study Group. Crit Care Med 1992; **20**: 1395–401.

29 Sessler DI. Defeating normal thermoregulatory defenses induction of therapeutic hypothermia. Stroke 2009; **40**: e614–21.

30 Wu TC, Grotta JC. Hypothermia for acute ischaemic stroke. Lancet Neurol 2013; **12**: 275–84.

31 Magnifico F, Pierangeli G, Barletta G, et al. Paroxysmal episodic central thermoregulatory failure. Neurology 2002; **58**: 1300–2.

32 White KD, Scoones DJ, Newman PK. Hypothermia in multiple sclerosis. J Neurol Neurosurg Psychiatry 1996; **61**: 369–75.

33 Davis SL, Wilson TE, White AT, Frohman EM. Thermoregulation in multiple sclerosis. J Appl Physiol 2010; **109**: 1531–7.

34 Sansing LH, Tuzun E, Ko MW, Baccon J, Lynch DR, Dalmau J. A patient with encephalitis associated with NMDA receptor antibodies. Nat Clin Pract Neurol 2007; **3**: 291–6.

35 Jacob S, Irani SR, Rajabally YA, et al. Hypothermia in VGKC antibody-associated limbic encephalitis. J Neurol Neurosurg Psychiatry 2008; **79**: 202–4.

36 Shenoy C. Shapiro syndrome. Q J Med 2008; **101**: 61–2.

37 Pazderska A, O'Connell M, Pender N, Gavin C, Murray B, O'Dowd S. Insights into thermoregulation: a clinico-radiological description of Shapiro syndrome. J Neurol Sci 2013; **329**: 66–8.

38 Danel T, Libersa C, Touitou Y. The effect of alcohol consumption on the circadian control of human core body temperature is time dependent. Am J Physiol Regul Integr Comp Physiol 2001; **281**: R52–R55.

39 Ellrich J, Ristic D, Yekta SS. Impaired thermal perception in cluster headache. J Neurol 2006; **253**: 1292–9.

40 Patel N, Jankovic J, Hallett M. Sensory aspects of movement disorders. Lancet Neurol 2014; **13**: 100–12.

41 Schattschneider J, Bode A, Wasner G, Binder A, Deuschl G, Baron R. Idiopathic restless legs syndrome: abnormalities in central somatosensory processing. J Neurol 2004; **251**: 977–82.

42 Jamal GA, Weir AI, Hansen S, Ballantyne JP. Sensory involvement in motor neuron disease: further evidence from automated thermal threshold determination. J Neurol Neurosurg Psychiatry 1985; **48**: 906–10.

43 Lair L, Gibbons C, Freeman R. Phantom sweating: a novel autonomic paresthesia. Clin Auton Res 2008; **18**: 352–4.

44 Wenzel FG, Horn TD. Nonneoplastic disorders of the eccrine glands. J Am Acad Dermatol 1998; **38**: 1–17.

45 Mostile G, Jankovic J. Treatment of dysautonomia associated with Parkinson's disease. Parkinsonism Relat Disord 2009; **15**(Suppl 3): S224–S232.

46 Low PA, Tomalia VA, Park KJ. Autonomic function tests: some clinical applications. J Clin Neurol 2013; **9**: 1–8.

47 Sage JI, Mark MH. Drenching sweats as an off phenomenon in Parkinson's disease: treatment and relation to plasma levodopa profile. Ann Neurol 1995; **37**: 120–2.

48 Swinn L, Schrag A, Viswanathan R, Bloem BR, Lees A, Quinn N. Sweating dysfunction in Parkinson's disease. Mov Disord 2003; **18**: 1459–63.

49 Pursiainen V, Haapaniemi TH, Korpelainen JT, Sotaniemi KA, Myllylä VV. Sweating in Parkinsonian patients with wearing-off. Mov Disord 2007; **22**: 828–32.

50 Cox B, Kerwin R, Lee TF. Dopamine receptors in the central thermoregulatory pathways of the rat. J Physiol 1978; **282**: 471–83.

51 Takubo H, Harada T, Hashimoto T, et al. A collaborative study on the malignant syndrome in Parkinson's disease and related disorders. Parkinsonism Relat Disord 2003; **9**(Suppl 1): S31–S41.

52 Schwartz PJ, Erk SD. Regulation of central dopamine-2 receptor sensitivity by a proportional control thermostat in humans. Psychiatry Res 2004; **127**: 19–26.

53 Collins GT, Newman AH, Grundt P, et al. Yawning and hypothermia in rats: effects of dopamine D3 and D2 agonists and antagonists. Psychopharmacology (Berl) 2007; **193**: 159–70.

54 Parada MA, de Parada MP, Rada P, Hernandez L. Sulpiride increases and dopamine decreases intracranial temperature in rats when injected in the lateral hypothalamus: an animal model for the neuroleptic malignant syndrome? Brain Res 1995; **674**: 117–21.

55 Nirenberg MJ. Dopamine agonist withdrawal syndrome: implications for patient care. Drugs Aging 2013; **30**: 587–92.

56 Cagnacci A, Bonuccelli U, Melis GB, et al. Effect of naloxone on body temperature in postmenopausal women with Parkinson's disease. Life Sci 1990; **46**: 1241–7.

57 Ben V, Bruguerolle B. Effects of bilateral striatal 6-OHDA lesions on circadian rhythms in the rat: a radiotelemetric study. Life Sci 2000; **67**: 1549–58.

58 Donadio V, Nolano M, Elam M, et al. Anhidrosis in multiple system atrophy: a preganglionic sudomotor dysfunction? Mov Disord 2008; **23**: 885–8.

59 Pierangeli G, Provini F, Maltoni P, et al. Nocturnal body core temperature falls in Parkinson's disease but not in multiple-system atrophy. Mov Disord 2001; **16**: 226–32.

60 Suzuki K, Miyamoto T, Miyamoto M, Hirata K. The core body temperature rhythm is altered in progressive supranuclear palsy. Clin Auton Res 2009; **19**: 65–8.

61 Carmel PW. Sympathetic deficits following thalamotomy. Arch Neurol 1968; **18**: 378–87.

62 Ludwig J, Remien P, Guballa C, et al. Effects of subthalamic nucleus stimulation and levodopa on the autonomic nervous system in Parkinson's disease. J Neurol Neurosurg Psychiatry 2007; **78**: 742–5.

63 Trachani E, Constantoyannis C, Sirrou V, Kefalopoulou Z, Markaki E, Chroni E. Effects of subthalamic nucleus deep brain stimulation on sweating function in Parkinson's disease. Clin Neurol Neurosurg 2010; **112**: 213–17.

64 Maruo T, Saitoh Y, Hosomi K, et al. Deep brain stimulation of the subthalamic nucleus improves temperature sensation in patients with Parkinson's disease. Pain 2011; **152**: 860–5.

65 Kim JH, Kwon TH, Koh SB, Park JY. Parkinsonism-hyperpyrexia syndrome after deep brain stimulation surgery: case report. Neurosurgery 2010; **66**: E1029.

66 Jankovic J. Parkinson's disease: clinical features and diagnosis. J Neurol Neurosurg Psychiatry 2008; **79**: 368–76.

67 Sanghera MK, Ward C, Stewart RM, Mewes K, Simpson RK, Lai EC. Alleviation of drenching sweats following subthalamic deep brain stimulation in a patient with Parkinson's disease—a case report. J Neurol Sci 2009; **285**: 246–9.

68 Storch A, Schneider CB, Wolz M, et al. Nonmotor fluctuations in Parkinson disease: severity and correlation with motor complications. Neurology 2013; **80**: 800–9.

69 Schestatsky P, Valls-Solé J, Ehlers JA, Rieder CR, Gomes I. Hyperhidrosis in Parkinson's disease. Mov Disord 2006; **21**: 1744–8.

70 Shishido T, Ikemura M, Obi T, et al. alpha-synuclein accumulation in skin nerve fibers revealed by skin biopsy in pure autonomic failure. Neurology 2010; **74**: 608–10.

71 Ha AD, Jankovic J. Pain in Parkinson's disease. Mov Disord 2012; **27**: 485–91.

72 Mylius V, Engau I, Teepker M, et al. Pain sensitivity and descending inhibition of pain in Parkinson's disease. J Neurol Neurosurg Psychiatry 2009; **80**: 24–8.

73 Lenz FA, Gracely RH, Baker FH, Richardson RT, Dougherty PM. Reorganization of sensory modalities evoked by microstimulation in region of the thalamic principal sensory nucleus in patients with pain due to nervous system injury. J Comp Neurol 1998; **399**: 125–38.

74 Borsook D, Upadhyay J, Chudler EH, Becerra L. A key role of the basal ganglia in pain and analgesia—insights gained through human functional imaging. Mol Pain 2010; **6**: 27.

75 Nandhagopal R, Troiano AR, Mak E, Schulzer M, Bushnell MC, Stoessl AJ. Response to heat pain stimulation in idiopathic Parkinson's disease. Pain Med 2010; **11**: 834–40.

76 Stamelou M, Dohmann H, Brebermann J, et al. Clinical pain and experimental pain sensitivity in progressive supranuclear palsy. Parkinsonism Relat Disord 2012; **18**: 606–8.

77 Yamashita S, Uchida Y, Kojima S, et al. Heatstroke in patients with Parkinson's disease. Neurol Sci 2012; **33**: 685–7.

78 Ikebe S, Harada T, Hashimoto T, et al. Prevention and treatment of malignant syndrome in Parkinson's disease: a consensus statement of the malignant syndrome research group. Parkinsonism Relat Disord 2003; **9**(Suppl 1): S47–S49.

79 Onofrj M, Thomas A. Acute akinesia in Parkinson disease. Neurology 2005; **64**: 1162–9.

80 Simonetto M, Ferigo L, Zanet L, et al. Acute akinesia, an unusual complication in Parkinson's disease: a case report. Neurol Sci 2008; **29**: 181–3.

81 Gubbay SS, Barwick DD. Two cases of accidental hypothermia in Parkinson's disease with unusual E.E.G. findings. J Neurol Neurosurg Psychiatry 1966; **29**: 459–66.

82 Hama K, Miwa H, Kondo T. Life-threatening hypothermia in Parkinson's disease. Mov Disord 2009; **24**: 945–6.

83 Sehara Y. Hypothermia with Osborn waves in Parkinson's disease. Intern Med 2009; **48**: 615–18.

84 Hirayama M. Sweating dysfunctions in Parkinson's disease. J Neurol 2006; 253(Suppl 7): VII42–VII47.

85 Mano Y, Nakamuro T, Takayanagi T, Mayer RF. Sweat function in Parkinson's disease. J Neurol 1994; **241**: 573–6.

86 Walker LC, Diamond MI, Duff KE, Hyman BT. Mechanisms of protein seeding in neurodegenerative diseases. Arch Neurol 2013; **70**: 304–10.

87 Hirashima F, Yokota T, Hayashi M. Sympathetic skin response in Parkinson's disease. Acta Neurol Scand. 1996;93:127–32.

88 Lipp A, Sandroni P, Ahlskog JE, et al. Prospective differentiation of multiple system atrophy from Parkinson disease, with and without autonomic failure. Arch Neurol 2009; **66**: 742–50.

89 Iodice V, Lipp A, Ahlskog JE, et al. Autopsy confirmed multiple system atrophy cases: Mayo experience and role of autonomic function tests. J Neurol Neurosurg Psychiatry.2012; **83**: 453–9.

90 Kimpinski K, Iodice V, Burton DD, et al. The role of autonomic testing in the differentiation of Parkinson's disease from multiple system atrophy. J Neurol Sci 2012; **317**: 92–6.

91 Sharabi Y, Li ST, Dendi R, Holmes C, Goldstein DS. Neurotransmitter specificity of sympathetic denervation in Parkinson's disease. Neurology 2003; **60**: 1036–9.

92 Klein C, Brown R, Wenning G, Quinn N. The 'cold hands sign' in multiple system atrophy. Mov Disord 1997; **12**: 514–18.

93 Pietzarka K, Reimann M, Schmidt C, et al. The cold hand sign in multiple system atrophy: skin perfusion revisited. J Neural Transm 2010; **117**: 475–9.

94 Shindo K, Iida H, Watanabe H, Ohta E, Nagasaka T, Shiozawa Z. Sympathetic sudomotor and vasoconstrictive neural function in patients with Parkinson's disease. Parkinsonism Relat Disord 2008; **14**: 548–52.

95 Meeusen R, Roelands B. Central fatigue and neurotransmitters, can thermoregulation be manipulated? Scand J Med Sci Sports 2010; **20**(Suppl 3): 19–28.

96 Bhidayasiri R, Truong DD. Evidence for effectiveness of botulinum toxin for hyperhidrosis. J Neural Transm 2008; **115**: 641–5.

97 Naumann M, Dressler D, Hallett M, et al. Evidence-based review and assessment of botulinum neurotoxin for the treatment of secretory disorders. Toxicon 2013; **67**: 141–52.

98 Jankovic J. Disease-oriented approach to botulinum toxin use. Toxicon 2009; **54**: 614–23.

99 Martignoni E, Godi L, Pacchetti C, et al. Is seborrhea a sign of autonomic impairment in Parkinson's disease? J Neural Transm 1997; **104**: 1295–304.

100 Fischer M, Gemende I, Marsch WC, Fischer PA. Skin function and skin disorders in Parkinson's disease. J Neural Transm 2001; **108**: 205–13.

101 Diamond A, Jankovic J. Botulinum toxin in dermatology—beyond wrinkles and sweat. J Cosmetic Dermatol 2006; **5**: 169.

102 Tascilar N, Tekin NS, Erdem Z, Alpay A, Emre U. Unnoticed dysautonomic syndrome of the face: Harlequin syndrome. Auton Neurosci 2007; **137**: 1–9.

103 Davis D, Jabbari B. Significant improvement of stiff-person syndrome after paraspinal injection of botulinum toxin A. Mov Disord 1993; **8**: 371–3.

104 Rotthier A, Baets J, De Vriendt E, et al. Genes for hereditary sensory and autonomic neuropathies: a genotype-phenotype correlation. Brain 2009; **132**; 2699–711.

105 Santos-Bento M, de Carvalho M, Evangelista T, Sales Luís ML. Sympathetic sudomotor function and amyotrophic lateral sclerosis. Amyotroph Lateral Scler Other Motor Neuron Disord 2001; **2**: 105–8.

106 Palm F, Löser C, Gronau W, Voigtländer V, Grau AJ. Successful treatment of acquired idiopathic generalized anhidrosis. Neurology 2007; **68**: 532.

Chapter 31

The role of continuous dopaminergic stimulation in the management of non-motor symptoms in Parkinson's disease

P. Reddy, A. Antonini and P. Odin

Introduction

Non-motor symptoms (NMS) in Parkinson's disease (PD) have a significant impact on the quality of life of patients and yet they are under-recognized and under-treated [1–5]. This is mainly due to poor awareness and an insufficient evidence base for treating them [6].

The motor features of PD largely arise from dopamine deficiency in the substantia nigra and related dysfunction in the striato-cortical loops. Other neurotransmitter systems are also involved in PD, with depletion of acetylcholine, norepinephrine and serotonin levels [7]. However, current treatment has largely focused on replacing endogenous dopamine via the administration of levodopa or other dopaminergic drugs [8–12]. Some, but not all, non-motor features (sleep disorders, autonomic dysfunction and fatigue) have a dopaminergic basis (Table 31.1) [13,14].

The term continuous dopaminergic stimulation (CDS) is used for treatments which can provide relatively steady plasma levels of dopaminergic drugs, and thereby continuous dopamine receptor stimulation. Options for such treatment are subcutaneous apomorphine (Apo) infusion, intrajejunal levodopa/carbidopa gel (LCIG) infusion, a rotigotine skin patch and deep brain stimulation (DBS) (note that this is not dopaminergic but provides continuous stimulation).

CDS is a very effective option for patients with severe motor fluctuations that are poorly controlled by oral therapy [15]. The giving of drugs via a non-oral approach has made it possible to achieve steady plasma levels of dopaminergic drugs, thereby achieving continuous drug delivery. These approaches have in turn reduced side effects and increased the efficacy of the drugs [16]. Motor fluctuations complicate levodopa-treated PD. A non-motor aspect of these fluctuations has also been described by several workers such as Witjas et al. [17], who classified them into three subtypes: dysautonomic, cognitive and psychiatric, and sensory or pain. NMS such as pain and excessive daytime sleepiness may

Table 31.1 The individual non-motor symptoms in Parkinson's disease and their responsiveness to dopaminergic therapy. (Courtesy Professor R. Chaudhuri)

	Responsive to dopaminergic treatment
Neuropsychiatric symptoms	
Depression, apathy, anxiety	Yes
Anhedonia	Yes
Cognitive dysfunction	"
Attention deficit	"
Hallucinations, illusions, delusions	"
Dementia	"
Confusion	"
Panic attacks	Yes (when related to "off" period)
Sleep disorders	
Restless legs and periodic limb movements	Yes
REM behaviour disorder	Yes?
REM loss of atonia	"
Non-REM sleep-related movement disorders	"
Excessive daytime somnolence	"
Vivid dreaming	"
Insomnia	"
Sleep-disordered breathing	"
Autonomic symptoms	
Bladder disturbances	"
Urgency	Yes (detrusor overactivity)
Nocturia	Yes
Frequency	"
Sweating	"
Orthostatic hypotension	"
Erectile impotence	Yes
Gastrointestinal symptoms	
Dribbling of saliva	Yes?
Ageusia	"
Dysphagia, choking	"
Reflux, vomiting	"
Nausea	"
Constipation	Yes
Unsatisfactory voiding of bowel	Yes
Faecal incontinence	
Sensory symptoms	
Pain	"
Primary pain related to Parkinsons's disease (central pain)	Yes
Secondary pain	"
Fluctuation-related pain (wearing off, dyskinesias)	Yes
Paraesthesia	"
Olfactory disturbance	"
Visual dysfunction (contrast sensitivity, colour vision)	"

Table 31.1 (continued) The individual non-motor symptoms in Parkinson's disease and their responsiveness to dopaminergic therapy. (Courtesy Professor R. Chaudhuri)

	Responsive to dopaminergic treatment
Other symptoms	
Non-motor fluctuations	Yes
Autonomic symptoms	"
Cognitive or psychiatric symptoms	"
Sensory symptoms including pain	"
Fatigue	Yes

Yes? some anecdotal reports of response to dopaminergic treatment. Some unmarked symptoms might also respond to treatment.

result from 'off' periods. Witjas and colleagues reported that anxiety (66%), drenching sweats (64%), slowness of thinking (58%), fatigue (56%) and akathisia (54%) were the most common non-motor fluctuations, and these correlated with motor disability and pulsatile levodopa treatment [18,19].

While there is significant evidence for the efficacy of long-acting dopamine agonists in reducing some of these NMS, there is still a paucity of controlled trials focusing on the effect of CDS on NMS. Currently no consensus exists as to whether there is a difference in the effect of the various CDS therapies on NMS. No randomized head to head trials exist comparing the effects of the various therapies offering CDS [20]. The mechanisms of the effects of CDS on NMS probably vary depending on the individual NMS, one of these certainly being that the patients spend more time in the 'on' state and have fewer NMS in the 'on' state compared to 'off'.

Intrajejunal levodopa/carbidopa infusion

LCIG (trade name Duodopa) represents a physiological option for dopamine replacement by providing a more stable levodopa plasma concentration than oral therapy. Striatal dopamine terminals normally store dopamine and buffer the plasma dopamine fluctuations seen with oral levodopa therapy. However, these terminals degenerate in advanced PD exposing dopamine receptors to the fluctuating dopamine concentrations resulting from per oral levodopa therapy [21]. By administering levodopa directly into the proximal part of the small intestine, the drug bypasses the erratic gastric emptying and can be quickly and continuously transported over the intestinal wall. This results in more stable plasma concentrations and most likely a more stable stimulation at the dopamine receptor level. Moving from per oral levodopa to LCIG therapy thus reduces 'off' periods and peak-dose dyskinesias and provides more predictable clinical benefits for patients [22]. There are also results indicating that the non-motor symptomatology does improve with LCIG. A recent 6-month open-label study of LCIG demonstrated improvement in six of the nine domains of the Non-motor Symptom Scale (NMSS) and for the total NMS burden score, in addition

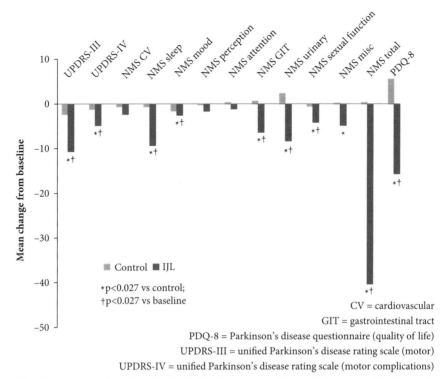

Fig. 31.1 Mean change from baseline in Unified Parkinson's Disease Rating Scale (UPDRS) and Non-motor Symptoms Scale (NMSS) scores in the intrajejunal levodopa/carbidopa gel (IJL in the figure) versus the control group [24]. The y-axis represents the mean change from baseline in the UPDRS scores, NMSS scores and the PDQ-8 scores.

to improvements in the Parkinson's Disease Sleep Scale (PDSS) and PDQ-8 quality of life scores [23] (Fig. 31.1).

Apo infusion

Apo is a dopamine agonist with effects on the D2 and D3 receptors. It is the only available dopamine agonist with an antiparkinsonian effect comparable to levodopa. Apo is normally administered as a subcutaneous injection on demand or as a continuous subcutaneous infusion with a portable pump. It has been shown to be effective in reducing time in 'off' compared with oral therapies, but reports suggest that it can reduce dyskinesias (both their severity and duration) if monotherapy is achieved [25–33]. Recently, Apo has also been shown to have an effect on NMS, particularly mood and urinary symptoms [34], similar to intrajejunal therapy [35]. However, it must be considered that unlike LCIG, Apo is commonly used in combination with oral levodopa.

Change in the items of the NMSS in patients treated with continuous Apo infusion are shown in Table 31.2.

Table 31.2 Effect of apomorphine infusion on individual non-motor symptoms. The symptoms which improve significantly as measured on the Non-motor Symptoms Scale on apomorphine therapy are given in bold type

	Items and domains	Baseline	Follow-up	$P*$
	CARDIOVASCULAR			
1	Light-headedness	3.53 ± 3.98	2.29 ± 3.06	0.03
2	Fainting	1.23 ± 2.63	0.47 ± 0.94	0.27
	SLEEP/FATIGUE			
3	Daytime sleeping	4.12 ± 4.44	2.88 ± 2.82	0.06
4	**Fatigue**	**7.29 ± 3.93**	**2.82 ± 2.86**	**0.0004†**
5	**Difficult falling asleep**	**5.12 ± 5.04**	**2.47 ± 3.22**	**0.008†**
6	**Restless legs**	**5.53 ± 4.02**	**2.53 ± 3.54**	**0.003†**
	MOOD/COGNITION			
7	**Lost interest surroundings**	**2.94 ± 4.25**	**0.82 ± 2.13**	**0.009†**
8	**Lack motivation**	**3.65 ± 4.26**	**1.18 ± 1.74**	**0.009†**
9	**Nervous**	**6.12 ± 5.43**	**3.23 ± 3.47**	**0.003†**
10	**Sad**	**5.53 ± 4.98**	**2.88 ± 3.71**	**0.001†**
11	Flat mood	2.23 ± 2.93	1.47 ± 2.87	0.09
12	**Difficult experiencing pleasure**	**2.76 ± 4.38**	**1.71 ± 3.22**	**0.015†**
	PERCEPTUAL PROBLEMS			
13	Hallucinations	1.41 ± 2.45	0.53 ± 1.12	0.09
14	Delusions	1.53 ± 2.72	1.00 ± 1.87	0.3
15	Double vision	1.65 ± 3.26	0.35 ± 1.06	0.08
	ATTENTION/MEMORY			
16	**Problems with concentration**	**5.47 ± 4.49**	**3.29 ± 3.69**	**0.002†**
17	Forget recent events	4.06 ± 3.53	2.88 ± 2.59	0.1
18	Forget doing things	3.29 ± 3.51	2.53 ± 2.65	0.2
	GASTROINTESTINAL			
19	**Dribbling saliva**	**2.23 ± 2.36**	**1.35 ± 1.97**	**0.015†**
20	Swallowing	2.00 ± 2.52	1.00 ± 1.58	0.026
21	Constipation	3.12 ± 4.03	2.06 ± 3.44	0.026
	URINARY			
22	**Urgency**	**3.71 ± 3.88**	**1.88 ± 2.87**	**0.005†**
23	**Frequency**	**2.59 ± 3.00**	**1.41 ± 3.32**	**0.015†**
24	**Nocturia**	**4.41 ± 3.78**	**2.41 ± 2.67**	**0.005†**
	SEXUAL FUNCTION			
25	Altered interest in sex	1.59 ± 3.41	0.82 ± 1.74	0.05

Table 31.2 (continued) Effect of apomorphine infusion on individual non-motor symptoms. The symptoms which improve significantly as measured on the Non-motor Symptoms Scale on apomorphine therapy are given in bold type

	Items and domains	Baseline	Follow-up	*P**
26	Problems having sex	0.94 ± 3.01	1.18 ± 2.65	0.5
	MISCELLANEOUS			
27	Unexplained pains	1.76 ± 3.99	2.59 ± 4.11	0.6
28	Lost taste/smell	4.41 ± 4.27	3.41 ± 4.18	0.05
29	Change in weight	3.00 ± 4.55	1.29 ± 2.23	0.05
30	**Excessive sweating**	**7.59 ± 4.43**	**3.23 ± 3.77**	**0.001†**

Reproduced from Martinez-Martin et al. [34].

*Wilcoxon test.

†Significant after Benjamini–Hochberg correction; $P < 0.025$.

Deep brain stimulation

While DBS is not really a form of continuous dopaminergic therapy, it does continuously modulate dopaminergic transmission. DBS is currently most commonly administered via bilateral subthalamic nucleus (STN) stimulation. STN DBS reduces 'off' time, dyskinesia time and intensity, as well as the amount of dopaminergic medication required. It may also reduce fluctuation-related anxiety [36], depression [37], 'off' period-associated pain and pain intensity [38]. A recent paper by Ashkan et al. [39] showed that STN DBS reduced the overall NMS load as measured by the NMSS, along with the motor improvements. Improvements have been seen concerning sleep, pain and urinary problems, with a few studies also demonstrating improved bladder control in PD patients on DBS [39–42].

The outcome for NMS after DBS in PD varies across studies. Some symptoms improve (sleep disorders, pain or sensory complaints, obsessive–compulsive disorder) but other aspects worsen (verbal fluency) or appear for the first time (apathy, weight gain). Isolated studies note mild improvements in working memory, visuomotor sequencing and conceptual reasoning and some gastrointestinal, urogenital, sweating and olfactory disturbances; whereas other studies have reported declines in verbal memory (long-delay recall), visuospatial memory, processing speed and executive function, with orthostatic hypotension (OH) remaining unchanged. The reasons for such a variability in effect on different NMS is probably due to the multifactorial aetiology of the NMS, including pre-operative vulnerability, changes in dopaminergic medications, surgical and stimulation effects, and underlying PD-related factors and psychosocial effects. Specific patient subgroups may be at greater risk of cognitive deficits, for example patients older than 69 years, or with cognitive impairment prior to surgery, or pre-operative psychiatric symptoms [43].

The suggestion of a differential effect of target (globus pallidus versus STN) on cognition and mood was seen in the COMPARE trial, particularly when more ventral stimulation was used in the STN [44].

Effects of CDS on individual NMS

Restless legs syndrome, periodic limb movements of sleep and early morning akinesia

Sleep disturbances are very common in patients with PD, and include restless legs syndrome (RLS), periodic limb movements of sleep (PLMS), insomnia, excessive daytime sleepiness (EDS) and rapid eye movement (REM) sleep behaviour disorder (RBD).

The prevalence/occurrence of RLS in PD is controversial, but observational uncontrolled studies suggest a two-fold increase compared with subjects without PD [45]. Neuroimaging has pointed to a pre-synaptic striatal pathology underlying idiopathic RLS and PLMS [46]. However, RLS has not been associated with cell loss in the substantia nigra or the presence of Lewy body pathology [47].

Sensory RLS symptoms can fluctuate along with motor status, being particularly bad during 'off' periods. A study by Tan et al. [48] showed that 0.8% of PD patients had RLS-like symptoms during 'wearing off', while Witjas et al. [18] observed that 22% of patients experienced symptoms consistent with RLS relating to 'off' periods, although 18% experienced them independent of treatment.

RLS in PD occurs in several forms. 'Typical' RLS is uncommon, while an RLS-like syndrome is common. The latter may either not respond to dopaminergic therapy or may result from nocturnal motor fluctuations which may benefit from extended/continuous release dopamine agonists.

Dopamine agonists are currently the first-line choice for the treatment of RLS and PLMS [49]. In comparative studies, cabergoline, a long-acting dopamine agonist (no longer used due to the risk of heart-valve fibrosis) [50] and a rotigotine transdermal patch have been shown to provide more effective relief from nocturnal painful dystonia, akinesia and early morning dystonia than controlled-release levodopa [51,52]. The recent RECOVER study [53] was the first large-scale, double-blind trial to investigate sleep as a primary outcome measure. It demonstrated that 24-hour transdermal rotigotine treatment significantly improved nocturnal disturbances and reduced nighttime disabilities including pain, immobility, cramps and limb restlessness.

Continuous dopaminergic stimulation can improve overall sleep quality [54] and sleep/fatigue symptoms as measured by the NMSS and PDSS [23]. These have been reported after the use of slow-release ropinirole, rotigotine patch, Apo infusion and intrajejunal levodopa, suggesting that nocturnal NMS may occur as a result of inadequate dopaminergic stimulation, which might be alleviated by CDS.

Pain

Pain is a major component of the NMS complex in PD [55], with one large study showing it to be reported by 29% of patients [56]. Although a number of neurotransmitters and tracts control and transmit the perception of pain, dopamine modulates pain at various levels including the spinal cord, thalamus, periaqueductal grey, basal ganglia and cingulate cortex [57,58]. This may explain why PD patients have a lower pain threshold compared with a healthy control population [59]. Further, Tinazzi et al. [60] have shown that nociceptive input processing is abnormal in pain-free PD patients independent of motor signs and is not affected by dopaminergic drugs.

The majority of pain in PD is caused by motor fluctuations and dyskinesias secondary to dopaminergic therapy [61]. 'Fluctuation-related pain' can be further categorized into dyskinetic pain, 'off' period dystonia-related pain, and 'off' period generalized pain [62,63]. RLS or akathisia can also be a cause of pain in PD.

There are no trials specifically investigating the effect of CDS on pain. However, in a small overnight study Apo infusion alleviated pain in six patients with RLS [64]. Studies have shown that the pain threshold in PD patients may increase with the administration of levodopa [59]. CDS, either by subcutaneous Apo infusion or duodenal levodopa infusion may be more effective. A 12-month prospective study of Duodopa infusion in seven patients with PD showed a significant improvement in bodily discomfort [22,65]. The RECOVER study reported improvement of pain with rotigotine compared with placebo, as measured on a Likert scale [53]. The RECOVER study is actually the first controlled trial to address pain as an independent secondary outcome variable [53].

Gastrointestinal disturbances and dysphagia

Gastrointestinal symptoms such as constipation, anorexia, nausea, dysphagia and reduced gastric motility are very common NMS and can also occur as a side effect of dopaminergic therapy.

Aspiration of saliva does not correlate with the severity of PD, indicating that autonomic phenomena in PD dysphagia are likely to be unrelated to motor progression [66]. There is not much evidence that the classical drugs used to treat PD can decrease or postpone silent laryngeal penetration/silent aspiration and there are controversies regarding the capacity of dopamine to decrease swallowing disturbances in PD patients [67,68].

Patients suffering from constipation during 'off' periods may relieve their symptoms with subcutaneous Apo injections, suggesting a role for dopaminergic treatment in improving gastric motility [69]. One non-controlled study has described the efficacy of CDS in reducing gastrointestinal symptoms in PD [23].

Orthostatic hypotension

OH is one of the most disabling NMS. Noradrenergic and neurocirculatory degeneration results in cardiac vagal reflex anomalies and altered sympathetic reflexes with decreased levels of serum norepinephrine. OH in PD has been observed independent of levodopa [70–72], while vasodilation with hypotension and bradycardia can also result from dopaminergic therapy [73]. This suggests that the autonomic dysfunction may be caused by the disease itself, by the effect of medication or by both. Furthermore, studies have shown varying supine and standing blood pressure measurements in 'on' versus 'off' states, suggesting that more stable, prolonged-release dopaminergic therapy may be beneficial in some patients. Anecdotal observations suggest that in some patients with advanced PD the use of levodopa infusion and concurrent withdrawal of oral therapies may lead to improvement of OH.

Peripheral oedema

Peripheral oedema may be seen in advanced PD, particularly as a side effect of dopamine agonist therapy. It most commonly presents as a unilateral painful swollen leg, mimicking thrombosis or a complex regional pain syndrome. Levodopa significantly reduces venous tone in the lower extremities and non-ergot dopamine agonists, including pramipexole and ropinirole, cause a dose-dependent oedema. However, 10% of patients may experience fluctuations in oedema as 'off'-period phenomena, suggesting that CDS may be beneficial [74].

Visual hallucinations

Visual hallucinations (VH) are common in patients with PD, affecting a third of patients with fluctuations. VH may result from a combination of reduced perceptual input and lowered attention [75]. Some studies have shown that subcutaneous infusion of Apo may not worsen VH [76,77], and may in fact improve contrast sensitivity [78] and VH in PD [34,79]. Some study results indicate that VH might also improve when moving from per oral therapy to LCIG infusion [22].

Insomnia

Sleep problems are present in 60–98% of patients with PD [80]. A study by Gjerstad et al. [81] reported a prevalence of insomnia in 54–60% of PD patients. Insomnia also fluctuates over time and the cause is often multifactorial. Coexisting depression is a common cause [82]. Garcia Ruiz [83] showed that overnight use of Apo infusion improved sleep architecture and Zibetti et al. [84] showed improvements in nocturnal sleep in patients started on intrajejunal levodopa infusion. All these studies show that there is a direct link between the dopaminergic pathways and sleep. Therefore improving dopaminergic stimulation at night can play a major role in improving insomnia and quality of sleep.

Depression and anxiety

The effect of dopaminergic therapy on mood disorders and apathy in PD can partly be explained by the knowledge that levodopa is taken up and decarboxylated in serotoninergic neurons, which also convert levodopa to dopamine [63]. Anxiety often coexists with depression and can respond to dopaminergic therapy [85]. In clinical practice anxiety is seen to occur as a dopamine-dependent event as part of 'wearing off' (presenting as panic attacks) and would therefore respond to dopaminergic strategies aimed to prevent wearing off, best achieved by the CDS strategies [63]. Similarly, depression-related anxiety might also respond to dopaminergic treatment, although in some patients anxiety can remain a constant underlying problem that is independent of dopaminergic state and that might not respond to dopaminergic therapy [86].

A randomized but unblinded study showed a significant improvement in anxiety after STN DBS compared with the best conventional medical treatment at 6 months of follow-up [37]. In an observational study by Witjas et al. [36], fluctuation-related anxiety was reported to be significantly lowered after STN DBS in advanced PD. These findings once again support that idea that CDS is useful in treating anxiety in PD.

Cognition and attention

The early cognitive changes of PD might involve the caudate and corticostriatal pathways [87]. Abnormalities of dopamine uptake and brain metabolism in cortical targets of striatal dopaminergic fibres have been reported [88,89]. A gradual increase in dopamine levels in the striatum improves motor function and memory when there is saturation of the dorsal striatum. Dopaminergic stimulation of the ventral striatum, however, has a detrimental effect on cognitive function, particularly impairment in learning new stimulus associations [90]. In view of these findings, a CDS strategy to optimize dopaminergic stimulation and prevent the peaks obtained with oral therapies, thus preventing excessive effects on the ventral striatum, would be most useful.

Urological symptoms

Dopaminergic stimulation has a varied effect on micturition. Striatal D1 receptor stimulation inhibits micturition and D2 stimulation activates it [91]. Hence urge incontinence and urgency can be worsened by dopaminergic therapy while voiding difficulties are improved [92]. Seif et al. [40] showed that STN DBS has a beneficial effect on bladder function in PD. These improvements were thought to be due to improvements in bladder capacity and reflex volume, possibly secondary to improved sensory motor integration and afferent activity. However, recent studies looking at the non-motor effects of LCIG and Apo infusion showed improvement in the urinary domain with both therapies [24,34].

Sustained-release dopaminergic therapy

The recently introduced dopamine agonists given by sustained drug delivery mechanisms, such as extended release ropinirole XL, pramipexole prolonged release and the rotigotine transdermal patch, may reduce the NMS burden in patients with PD. Although they do not provide a strictly 'continuous' form of dopaminergic stimulation they may be particularly effective in relieving sleep-related NMS including RLS, RBD and nocturia, and improving PDSS scores [8,93]. However, the benefits of these dopamine agonists have to be balanced against some sleep-related adverse events, including EDS, VH and the risk of impulse control disorders.

Conclusion

Treating NMS in PD remains a significant unmet challenge. Some NMS, especially those associated with 'off' periods, may be relieved using CDS. Both the pump-based therapies and DBS can achieve considerable improvements in many NMS, as well as improvements in motor symptomatology. While there are a few studies assessing the efficacy of CDS in treating NMS, there are none that directly compare them. The rotigotine transdermal patch may offer an alternative CDS strategy for those who are unsuitable for invasive therapies. Further research is needed to elucidate the specific benefits of each therapy and its role in treating NMS in PD.

References

1 Antonini A, Colosimo C, Marconi R, Morgante L, Barone P; PRIAMO Study Group. The PRIAMO study: background, methods and recruitment. Neurol Sci 2008; **29**: 61–5.

2 Barone P, Antonini A, Colosimo C, et al. The PRIAMO study: a multicenter assessment of nonmotor symptoms and their impact on quality of life in Parkinson's disease. Mov Disord 2009; **24**: 1641–9.

3 Chapuis S, Ouchchane L, Metz O, Gerbaud L, Durif F. Impact of the motor complications of Parkinson's disease on the quality of life. Mov Disord 2005; **20**: 224–30.

4 Chaudhuri KR, Healy DG, Schapira AH; National Institute for Clinical Excellence. Non-motor symptoms of Parkinson's disease: diagnosis and management. Lancet Neurol 2006; **5**: 235–45.

5 Chaudhuri KR, Odin P. The challenge of non-motor symptoms in Parkinson's disease. Prog Brain Res 2010; **184**: 325–41.

6 Antonini A, Barone P, Marconi R, et al. The progression of non-motor symptoms in Parkinson's disease and their contribution to motor disability and quality of life. J Neurol 2012; **259**: 2621–31.

7 Winogrodzka A, Booij J, Wolters E. Disease-related and drug-induced changes in dopamine transporter expression might undermine the reliability of imaging studies of disease progression in Parkinson's disease. Parkinsonism Relat Disord 2005; **11**: 475–84.

8 Poewe W. Non-motor symptoms in Parkinson's disease. Eur J Neurol 2008; **15**(Suppl 1): 14–20.

9 Agid Y, Ahlskog E, Albanese A, et al. Levodopa in the treatment of Parkinson's disease: a consensus meeting. Mov Disord 1999; **14**: 911–13.

10 Rascol O, Goetz C, Koller W, Poewe W, Sampaio C. Treatment interventions for Parkinson's disease: an evidence based assessment. Lancet 2002; **359**: 1589–98.

11 Nutt JG, Holford NH. The response to levodopa in Parkinson's disease: imposing pharmacological law and order. Ann Neurol 1996; **39**: 561–73.

12 Fabbrini G, Brotchie JM, Grandas F, Nomoto M, Goetz CG. Levodopa-induced dyskinesias. Mov Disord 2007; 22: 1379–89; quiz 1523.

13 Wolters E, Braak H. Parkinson's disease: premotor clinico-pathological correlations. J Neural Transm 2006; **70**(Suppl): 309–19.

14 Braak H, Del Tredici K, Rub U, de Vos RA, Jansen Steur EN, Braak E. Staging of brain pathology related to sporadic Parkinson's disease. Neurobiol Aging 2003; **24**: 197–211.

15 Antonini A, Chaudhuri KR, Martinez-Martin P, Odin P. Oral and infusion levodopa-based strategies for managing motor complications in patients with Parkinson's disease. CNS Drugs 2010; **24**: 119–29.

16 Gershanik O, Jenner P. Moving from continuous dopaminergic stimulation to continuous drug delivery in the treatment of Parkinson's disease. Eur J Neurol 2012; **19**: 1502–8.

17 Witjas T, Kaphan E, Azulay JP. Non-motor fluctuations in Parkinson's disease. Rev Neurol (Paris) 2007; **163**: 846–50.

18 Witjas T, Kaphan E, Azulay JP, et al. Nonmotor fluctuations in Parkinson's disease: frequent and disabling. Neurology 2002; **59**: 408–13.

19 Storch A, Schneider CB, Wolz M, et al. Nonmotor fluctuations in Parkinson disease: severity and correlation with motor complications. Neurology 2013; **80**: 800–9.

20 Volkmann J, Albanese A, Antonini A, et al. Selecting deep brain stimulation or infusion therapies in advanced Parkinson's disease: an evidence-based review. J Neurol 2013; **260**: 2701–14.

21 Antonini A, Odin P. Pros and cons of apomorphine and L-dopa continuous infusion in advanced Parkinson's disease. Parkinsonism Relat Disord 2009; **15**(Suppl 4): S97–S100.

22 Antonini A, Isaias IU, Canesi M, et al. Duodenal levodopa infusion for advanced Parkinson's disease: 12-month treatment outcome. Mov Disord 2007; **22**: 1145–9.

23 Honig H, Antonini A, Martinez-Martin P, et al. Intrajejunal levodopa infusion in Parkinson's disease: a pilot multicenter study of effects on nonmotor symptoms and quality of life. Mov Disord 2009; **24**: 1468–74.

24 Reddy P, Martinez-Martin P, Rizos A, et al. Intrajejunal levodopa versus conventional therapy in Parkinson disease: motor and nonmotor effects. Clin Neuropharmacol 2012; **35**: 205–7.

25 Katzenschlager R, Hughes A, Evans A, et al. Continuous subcutaneous apomorphine therapy improves dyskinesias in Parkinson's disease: a prospective study using single-dose challenges. Mov Disord 2005; **20**: 151–7.

26 Tyne HL, Parsons J, Sinnott A, Fox SH, Fletcher NA, Steiger MJ. A 10 year retrospective audit of long-term apomorphine use in Parkinson's disease. J Neurol 2004; **251**: 1370–4.

27 Manson AJ, Hanagasi H, Turner K, et al. Intravenous apomorphine therapy in Parkinson's disease: clinical and pharmacokinetic observations. Brain 2001; **124**: 331–40.

28 Nutt JG, Carter JH. Apomorphine can sustain the long-duration response to L-DOPA in fluctuating PD. Neurology 2000; **54**: 247–50.

29 van Laar T, van der Geest R, Danhof M, Bodde HE, Goossens PH, Roos RA. Stepwise intravenous infusion of apomorphine to determine the therapeutic window in patients with Parkinson's disease. Clin Neuropharmacol 1998; **21**: 152–8.

30 Pfeiffer RF, Gutmann L, Hull KL Jr, Bottini PB, Sherry JH. Continued efficacy and safety of subcutaneous apomorphine in patients with advanced Parkinson's disease. Parkinsonism Relat Disord 2007; **13**: 93–100.

31 Colosimo C, Merello M, Hughes AJ, Sieradzan K, Lees AJ. Apomorphine responses in Parkinson's disease and the pathogenesis of motor complications. Neurology 1998; **50**: 573–4.

32 Trosch RM, Silver D, Bottini PB. Intermittent subcutaneous apomorphine therapy for 'off' episodes in Parkinson's disease: a 6-month open-label study. CNS Drugs 2008; **22**: 519–27.

33 De Gaspari D, Siri C, Landi A, et al. Clinical and neuropsychological follow up at 12 months in patients with complicated Parkinson's disease treated with subcutaneous apomorphine infusion or deep brain stimulation of the subthalamic nucleus. J Neurol Neurosurg Psychiatry 2006; **77**: 450–3.

34 Martinez-Martin P, Reddy P., Antonini A, et al. Chronic subcutaneous infusion therapy with apomorphine in advanced Parkinson's disease compared to conventional therapy: a real life study of non motor effect. J Parkinson's Dis 2011; **1**: 197–203.

35 Reddy P, Martinez-Martin P, Antonini A. A multicentre European comparative survey of motor and non motor effects of subcutaneous apomorphine infusion and intrajejunal levodopa infusion in Parkinson's disease. Mov Disord 2012; **27**(Suppl 1): 160.

36 Witjas T, Kaphan E, Regis J, et al. Effects of chronic subthalamic stimulation on nonmotor fluctuations in Parkinson's disease. Mov Disord 2007; **22**: 1729–34.

37 Witt K, Daniels C, Reiff J, et al. Neuropsychological and psychiatric changes after deep brain stimulation for Parkinson's disease: a randomised, multicentre study. Lancet Neurol 2008; **7**: 605–14.

38 Gierthmuhlen J, Arning P, Binder A, et al. Influence of deep brain stimulation and levodopa on sensory signs in Parkinson's disease. Mov Disord 2011; **25**: 1195–202.

39 Ashkan K, Samuel M, Reddy P, Ray Chaudhuri K. The impact of deep brain stimulation on the nonmotor symptoms of Parkinson's disease. J Neural Transm 2013; **120**: 639–42.

40 Seif C, Herzog J, van der Horst C, et al. Effect of subthalamic deep brain stimulation on the function of the urinary bladder. Ann Neurol 2004; **55**: 118–20.

41 Winge K, Nielsen KK, Stimpel H, Lokkegaard A, Jensen SR, Werdelin L. Lower urinary tract symptoms and bladder control in advanced Parkinson's disease: effects of deep brain stimulation in the subthalamic nucleus. Mov Disord 2007; **22**: 220–5.

42 Borgohain R, Kandadai RM, Jabeen A, Kannikannan MA. Nonmotor outcomes in Parkinson's disease: is deep brain stimulation better than dopamine replacement therapy? Ther Adv Neurol Disord 2012; **5**: 23–41.

43 Sevillano-Garcia MD, Manso-Calderon R. Nonmotor symptoms in Parkinson's disease and deep brain stimulation. Rev Neurol 2010; **50**(Suppl 2): S95–S104.

44 Okun MS, Fernandez HH, Wu SS, et al. Cognition and mood in Parkinson's disease in subthalamic nucleus versus globus pallidus interna deep brain stimulation: the COMPARE trial. Ann Neurol 2009; **65**: 586–95.

45 Chaudhuri KR. Nocturnal symptom complex in PD and its management. Neurology 2003; **61**: S17–S23.

46 Ruottinen HM, Partinen M, Hublin C, et al. An FDOPA PET study in patients with periodic limb movement disorder and restless legs syndrome. Neurology 2000; **54**: 502–4.

47 Connor JR, Boyer PJ, Menzies SL, et al. Neuropathological examination suggests impaired brain iron acquisition in restless legs syndrome. Neurology 2003; **61**: 304–9.

48 Tan EK, Lum SY, Wong MC. Restless legs syndrome in Parkinson's disease. J Neurol Sci 2002; **196**: 33–6.

49 Hening W, Allen R, Earley C, Kushida C, Picchietti D, Silber M. The treatment of restless legs syndrome and periodic limb movement disorder. An American Academy of Sleep Medicine Review. Sleep 1999; **22**: 970–99.

50 Antonini A, Poewe W. Fibrotic heart-valve reactions to dopamine-agonist treatment in Parkinson's disease. Lancet Neurol 2007; **6**: 826–9.

51 Rinne UK, Bracco F, Chouza C, et al. Early treatment of Parkinson's disease with cabergoline delays the onset of motor complications. Results of a double-blind levodopa controlled trial. The PKDS009 Study Group. Drugs 1998; 55(Suppl **1**): 23–30.

52 Pal S, Bhattacharya KF, Agapito C, Chaudhuri KR. A study of excessive daytime sleepiness and its clinical significance in three groups of Parkinson's disease patients taking pramipexole, cabergoline and levodopa mono and combination therapy. J Neural Transm 2001; **108**: 71–7.

53 Trenkwalder C, Kies B, Rudzinska M, et al. Rotigotine effects on early morning motor function and sleep in Parkinson's disease: a double-blind, randomized, placebo-controlled study (RECOVER). Mov Disord 2011; **26**: 90–9.

54 Nyholm D, Jansson R, Willows T, Remahl IN. Long-term 24-hour duodenal infusion of levodopa: outcome and dose requirements. Neurology 2005; **65**: 1506–7.

55 Defazio G, Berardelli A, Fabbrini G, et al. Pain as a nonmotor symptom of Parkinson disease: evidence from a case-control study. Arch Neurol 2008; **65**: 1191–4.

56 Martinez-Martin P, Schapira AH, Stocchi F, et al. Prevalence of nonmotor symptoms in Parkinson's disease in an international setting; study using nonmotor symptoms questionnaire in 545 patients. Mov Disord 2007; **22**: 1623–9.

57 Chudler EH, Dong WK. The role of the basal ganglia in nociception and pain. Pain 1995; **60**: 3–38.

58 Shyu BC, Kiritsy-Roy JA, Morrow TJ, Casey KL. Neurophysiological, pharmacological and behavioral evidence for medial thalamic mediation of cocaine-induced dopaminergic analgesia. Brain Res 1992; **572**: 216–23.

59 Djaldetti R, Shifrin A, Rogowski Z, Sprecher E, Melamed E, Yarnitsky D. Quantitative measurement of pain sensation in patients with Parkinson disease. Neurology 2004; **62**: 2171–5.

60 Tinazzi M, Del Vesco C, Defazio G, et al. Abnormal processing of the nociceptive input in Parkinson's disease: a study with CO_2 laser evoked potentials. Pain 2008; **136**: 117–24.

61 Quinn NP, Koller WC, Lang AE, Marsden CD. Painful Parkinson's disease. Lancet 1986; **1**: 1366–9.

62 Chaudhuri KR, Healy DG, Schapira AH. Non-motor symptoms of Parkinson's disease: diagnosis and management. Lancet Neurol 2006; **5**: 235–45.

63 Chaudhuri KR, Schapira AH. Non-motor symptoms of Parkinson's disease: dopaminergic pathophysiology and treatment. Lancet Neurol 2009; **8**: 464–74.

64 Reuter I, Ellis CM, Ray Chaudhuri K. Nocturnal subcutaneous apomorphine infusion in Parkinson's disease and restless legs syndrome. Acta Neurol Scand 1999; **100**: 163–7.

65 Antonini A. Continuous dopaminergic stimulation—from theory to clinical practice. Parkinsonism Relat Disord 2007; 13(Suppl): S24–S28.

66 Ali GN, Wallace KL, Schwartz R, DeCarle DJ, Zagami AS, Cook IJ. Mechanisms of oral-pharyngeal dysphagia in patients with Parkinson's disease. Gastroenterology 1996; **110**: 383–92.

67 Monte FS, da Silva-Junior FP, Braga-Neto P, Nobre e Souza MA, de Bruin VM. Swallowing abnormalities and dyskinesia in Parkinson's disease. Mov Disord 2005; **20**: 457–62.

68 Hunter PC, Crameri J, Austin S, Woodward MC, Hughes AJ. Response of parkinsonian swallowing dysfunction to dopaminergic stimulation. J Neurol Neurosurg Psychiatry 1997; **63**: 579–83.

69 Merello M. Non-motor disorders in Parkinson's disease. Rev Neurol 2008; **47**: 261–70.

70 Goldstein DS. Orthostatic hypotension as an early finding in Parkinson's disease. Clin Auton Res 2006; **16**: 46–54.

71 Goldstein DS, Eldadah BA, Holmes C, et al. Neurocirculatory abnormalities in Parkinson disease with orthostatic hypotension: independence from levodopa treatment. Hypertension 2005; **46**: 1333–9.

72 Pursiainen V, Korpelainen JT, Haapaniemi TH, Sotaniemi KA, Myllyla VV. Blood pressure and heart rate in parkinsonian patients with and without wearing-off. Eur J Neurol 2007; **14**: 373–8.

73 Polakowski JS, Segreti JA, Cox BF, et al. Effects of selective dopamine receptor subtype agonists on cardiac contractility and regional haemodynamics in rats. Clin Exp Pharmacol Physiol 2004; **31**: 837–41.

74 Tan EK, Ondo W. Clinical characteristics of pramipexole-induced peripheral edema. Arch Neurol 2000; **57**: 729–32.

75 Collerton D, Perry E, McKeith I. Why people see things that are not there: a novel perception and attention deficit model for recurrent complex visual hallucinations. Behav Brain Sci 2005; 28: 737–57; discussion 757–94.

76 Di Rosa AE, Epifanio A, Antonini A, et al. Continuous apomorphine infusion and neuropsychiatric disorders: a controlled study in patients with advanced Parkinson's disease. Neurol Sci 2003; **24**: 174–5.

77 Morgante L, Basile G, Epifanio A, et al. Continuous apomorphine infusion (CAI) and neuropsychiatric disorders in patients with advanced Parkinson's disease: a follow-up of two years. Arch Gerontol Geriatr 2004; Suppl **9**: 291–6.

78 Geerligs L, Meppelink AM, Brouwer WH, van Laar T. The effects of apomorphine on visual perception in patients with Parkinson disease and visual hallucinations: a pilot study. Clin Neuropharmacol 2009; **32**: 266–8.

79 Ellis C, Lemmens G, Parkes JD, et al. Use of apomorphine in parkinsonian patients with neuropsychiatric complications to oral treatment. Parkinsonism Relat Disord 1997; **3**: 103–7.

80 Mondragon-Rezola E, Arratibel-Echarren I, Ruiz-Martinez J, Marti-Masso JF. [Sleep disorders in Parkinson's disease: insomnia and sleep fragmentation, daytime hypersomnia, alterations to the circadian rhythm and sleep apnea syndrome]. Rev Neurol 2010; **50**(Suppl 2): S21–S26.

81 Gjerstad MD, Wentzel-Larsen T, Aarsland D, Larsen JP. Insomnia in Parkinson's disease: frequency and progression over time. J Neurol Neurosurg Psychiatry 2007; **78**: 476–9.

82 Caap-Ahlgren M, Dehlin O. Insomnia and depressive symptoms in patients with Parkinson's disease. Relationship to health-related quality of life. An interview study of patients living at home. Arch Gerontol Geriatr 2001; **32**: 23–33.

83 Garcia Ruiz PJ. Nocturnal subcutaneous apomorphine infusion for severe insomnia in Parkinson's disease. Mov Disord 2006; **21**: 727–8.

84 Zibetti M, Rizzone M, Merola A, et al. Sleep improvement with levodopa/carbidopa intestinal gel infusion in Parkinson disease. Acta Neurol Scand 2013; **127**: e28–e32.

85 Lemke MR, Brecht HM, Koester J, Kraus PH, Reichmann H. Anhedonia, depression, and motor functioning in Parkinson's disease during treatment with pramipexole. J Neuropsychiatry Clin Neurosci 2005; **17**: 214–20.

86 Richard IH, Schiffer RB, Kurlan R. Anxiety and Parkinson's disease. J Neuropsychiatry Clin Neurosci 1996; **8**: 383–92.

87 Emre M. What causes mental dysfunction in Parkinson's disease? Mov Disord 2003; **18**(Suppl 6): S63–S71.

88 Lewis SJ, Dove A, Robbins TW, Barker RA, Owen AM. Cognitive impairments in early Parkinson's disease are accompanied by reductions in activity in frontostriatal neural circuitry. J Neurosci 2003; **23**: 6351–6.

89 Rinne JO, Portin R, Ruottinen H, et al. Cognitive impairment and the brain dopaminergic system in Parkinson disease: [18F]fluorodopa positron emission tomographic study. Arch Neurol 2000; **57**: 470–5.

90 MacDonald PA, MacDonald AA, Seergobin KN, et al. The effect of dopamine therapy on ventral and dorsal striatum-mediated cognition in Parkinson's disease: support from functional MRI. Brain 2011; **134**: 1447–63.

91 Seki S, Igawa Y, Kaidoh K, Ishizuka O, Nishizawa O, Andersson KE. Role of dopamine D1 and D2 receptors in the micturition reflex in conscious rats. Neurourol Urodyn 2001; **20**: 105–13.

92 Uchiyama T, Sakakibara R, Hattori T, Yamanishi T. Short-term effect of a single levodopa dose on micturition disturbance in Parkinson's disease patients with the wearing-off phenomenon. Mov Disord 2003; **18**: 573–8.

93 Pahwa R, Stacy MA, Factor SA, et al. Ropinirole 24-hour prolonged release: randomized, controlled study in advanced Parkinson disease. Neurology 2007; **68**: 1108–15.

Index

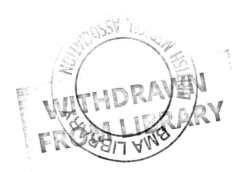
WITHDRAWN
FROM LIBRARY
BMA LIBRARY
BRITISH MEDICAL ASSOCIATION